JAPANESE CANCER ASSOCIATION

GANN Monograph on Cancer Research No.17

RECENT TOPICS IN CHEMICAL CARCINOGENESIS

IN MEMORY OF PROFESSOR TOMIZO YOSHIDA

Edited by
SHIGEYOSHI ODASHIMA
SHOZO TAKAYAMA
HARUO SATO

UNIVERSITY OF TOKYO PRESS

Published by
UNIVERSITY OF TOKYO PRESS
7-3-1 Hongo, Bunkyo-ku, Tokyo, Japan

August 30, 1975

RECENT TOPICS IN
CHEMICAL CARCINOGENESIS

GANN Monograph on Cancer Research

The series of GANN Monograph on Cancer Research was initiated in 1966 by the late Dr. Tomizo Yoshida (1903-73) for the purpose of publishing proceedings of international conferences and symposia on cancer and allied research fields, and papers on specific subjects of importance in cancer research.

The decision to publish a monograph is made by the Editorial Board of the Japanese Cancer Association, with the final approval of the Board of Directors. It is hoped that the series will serve as an important source of information in cancer research.

Japanese Cancer Association

Publication of this monograph is supported
by the Kazushige Higuchi Fund.

PREFACE

It is said that there are no boundries in science, however, it is also true that there exist some characteristic individualities in scientific research in each country and in individual scientists. The late Professor Tomizo Yoshida preferred held this concept and philosophy.

In the summer of 1973, just after we experienced the loss of Professor Yoshida, the decision on the publication of this memorial issue of GANN Monograph on Cancer Research was reached by the Editorial Board of the Japanese Cancer Association followed by the final approval of the Board of Directors.

Responding to the requests of the editors of this issue, a total of 29 papers were received; 14 from foreign countries, including 4 from the U.S.A., 3 from Germany, 2 each from Canada, England, and France, and 1 from the U.S.S.R., and 15 from Japanese scientists.

These contributions were subgrouped into the following 4 major topics:

I. Mutagenicity and *in vitro* carcinogenesis; 7 papers.
II. Chemistry and metabolism of N-nitroso compounds; 4 papers.
III. Environmental carcinogenesis; 5 papers.
IV. Experimental model of tumors in various organs such as digestive tract, liver, urinary tract, hematopoietic organs, and skin; 13 papers.

In addition memorial papers were submitted by old friends of Professor Yoshida, Professor Sir Alexander Haddow of England, Professor Herwig Hamperl of Germany, Dr. Harold L. Stewart of the United States, and Dr. Waro Nakahara of Japan.

The editors of this memorial issue would like to express their sincere thanks for cooperation and friendship of all contributors, and hope that this will be a milestone for future research in cancer in the world.

Professor Yoshida started his research in carcinogenesis, and extended his research fields to pathobiology and experimental chemotherapy. He was not only a man of the laboratory, but was also a man of deep thinking, suggesting, and exploiting ways of furthering cancer research. It should be recalled once more that there are so many approaches, nevertheless, the final aim of cancer research is the cure of cancer.

August 1975

Shigeyoshi Odashima
Shozo Takayama
Haruo Sato

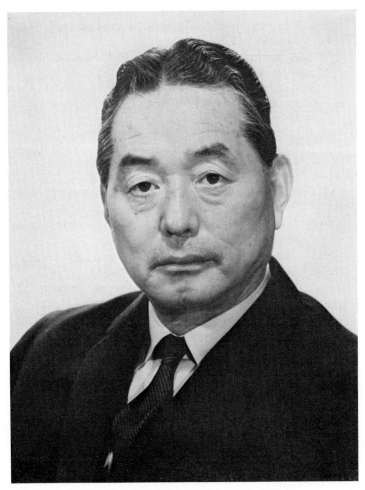

Tomizo Yoshida, M.D. (1903–1973)

February 10, 1903   Born in Asakawa-machi, Fukushima Prefecture

1927   Graduated from the Tokyo Imperial University, School of Medicine. Appointed assistant in the Medical School, Tokyo Imperial University (Department of Pathology).

1929   Became research member in the Sasaki Institute and started work on rat experimental hepatocarcinogenesis.

1935   Returned to the Tokyo Imperial University (Department of Pathology) as an assistant.
Appointed Assistant Professor of Nagasaki Medical College, chair of pathology.
Received the Yamagiwa Award of the Japanese Cancer Association, Hattori Hokokai Award, and Imperial Academy Award (1936) for his work on the production of liver carcinoma by oral administration of *o*-aminoazotoluene.
Went to Germany and studied under Prof. Rössle in Berlin.

1938   Returned to Japan and appointed Professor of Nagasaki Medical College. Started work on rat ascites tumor.

1944   Appointed Professor of Tohoku Imperial University, School of Medicine (Department of Pathology).

1952   Appointed Professor of The University of Tokyo, School of Medicine (Department of Pathology).

1952   Received the Asahi Newspaper Scientific Award.

1953   Received the Japan Academy Award.
These two awards for his work on pathological studies on Yoshida sarcoma.

1953   Became concurrently Director of Sasaki Institute, Tokyo.

1955   Elected an honorary member of the American Cancer Association.

1956   Received the Scheele Medal from the Swedish Chemical Society.

1959   Decorated with the Order of Cultural Merit.

1960   Appointed Dean of the Medical School, The University of Tokyo, and concurrently professor of the Institute for Infectious Diseases, The University of Tokyo.

1960   Elected a member of the Japan Science Council.

1961   Conferred the honorary degree from the University of Perugia, Italy.

1962   Received the Fujiwara Award for his work on ascites hepatoma.

1963   Elected Vice President of the Japan Science Council.
Retired from the professorship at The University of Tokyo and became the Director of Cancer Institute, Japanese Foundation for Cancer Research.
Received the Robert Koch Medal from Germany.
Served as a member of the Commission on Japanese Language Problems, Ministry of Education.

1965   Elected a member of the Japan Academy.

1966   Served as President of the Ninth International Cancer Congress held in Tokyo.

April 27, 1973   Died after six months of hospitalization.

Dedication to Tomizo Yoshida, M. D.

PROFESSOR TOMIZO YOSHIDA

All concerned with cancer research will have learned with sorrow of the death of Professor Tomizo Yoshida.

I regard it as a great honour to be invited to write this preface in a special number of GANN Monograph on Cancer Research devoted to the memory of an old friend and colleague.

Born at Fukushima in 1903, he was educated at the Tokyo Imperial University. He was Assistant Professor at Nagasaki Medical College from 1935–1938 and Professor from 1938–1944; became Professor at Tohoku Imperial University 1944–1952, Professor at the University of Tokyo from 1952 to his death. He was Director of the Sasaki Institute from 1953, Dean of the Faculty of Medicine at the University of Tokyo in the year 1958, Director of the Cancer Institute, Japanese Foundation for Cancer Research (1963) and Adviser, Minister of Education (1963) until his death. He gained the Order of Cultural Merit in 1959 and the Imperial Prize of the Japan Academy 1931, 1953, the Scheele Medal in 1956 and the Koch Medal (Germany) 1963. Perhaps the height of his career was reached in 1966, when he became President of the 9th International Cancer Congress in Tokyo, where he proved an outstanding success.

As an experimental pathologist and observer he was pre-eminent and his massive contributions included the description of the Yoshida sarcoma, the discovery of the azo-carcinogens, and his translation of Virchow's *Cellular Patologie*; naturally he was greatly influenced by the German schools.

I first of all met him at the Second International Cancer Congress (of the present series), held in Brussels in 1936. At once we became firm friends but inevitably were separated in our contacts by the Second World War, and I well recall his visit to London (to see Kennaway) on the advent of peace.

He was a devoted advocate of the Union Internationale contre le Cancer.

Apart from his scientific work, he had numerous other interests, especially in Japanese tradition, art, theatre and architecture. He showed special concern with reform of the Japanese language and its many thousands of ideograms.

In the conduct of Union affairs he travelled widely and, incidentally, attended the Congress held in Houston, Texas, in 1970.

On numerous visits to Japan one recollects his companionship not only in visits to Tokyo, Osaka, Nara and Kyoto, but also to see the indescribable beauty of the Japanese islands, with their mountains, forests, lakes, artificial gardens, and the shrines and temples of old Japan. Amusing stories could be told of travels together in many other parts, especially perhaps, in India.

On one occasion we travelled together by plane from Bombay to New Delhi, but had to land at Jaipur because of fog at Delhi Airport. We spent a full day or more together in Jaipur at one of the most miserable hotels (although with a splendid name) which I have ever encountered, with vultures and carrion crows near the front door. On the Airport being cleared at New Delhi we set forth again and eventually landed safely. Being rather disenchanted with the squalor of the preceding day, I asked Tomizo if I might take charge and arrange our accommodation at one of Delhi's splendid hotels. When we got there, I enquired which was the best, to which we made instant tracks. We were then told by the Clerk that the hotel was completely full. This was a disappointment, but before leaving at least we had a good shower. While this was going on the same Clerk came running down to say that after all they had a luxurious flat with separate bedrooms, dressing rooms, a dining room and a kitchen, with separate entry to one of the most beautiful gardens I have ever seen. He explained it was distinctly expensive, but I replied "this exactly what we want." Thus, it turned out that proceeding from our previous squalor we ascended to the heights of comfort, and spent several days there before the time came when we had to part company. Each time I met Tomizo we regaled ourselves on this experience.

Tomizo was a splendid and genial host, introducing one to all his friends, and in the presence of his charming wife and family inviting one on many occasions to the delights of the tea ceremony in his home. During one such occasion, I remember the glories of his red waistcost on his 60th birthday—a picture retained for us in a never-to-be-forgotten portrait.

Some 35 years ago, Tomizo reported the appearance of liver cancers in rats maintained on diets to which "Butter Yellow" and related azo dyes had been added. The news was popularised by Kinosita, who was on a lecture tour in the United States. Practically all the cancer research laboratories existent at that time attempted to repeat the work. In the United States, however, rats placed on diets to which azo dyes were added refused to develop liver tumours. Consultations and investigations soon showed that the key discrepancy between Japan and the United States was in the diet to which the azo dyes were added. In Japan, the rats were maintained on a Spartan diet based on polished rice. In the United States, the animals were pampered on carefully balanced diets designed for optimum growth. Further investigations pinpointed riboflavin as the main protector against the carcinogenic effects of azo dyes. Rats on riboflavin-deficient diets to which azo dyes were added promptly developed liver tumours as originally described and thereafter proved a powerful armamentarium for the study of carcinogenesis.

Liver is, of course, a popular organ for the biochemical study of cancerous change, being easily used as homogenates, slides, or extracts. Normal livers, embryonic livers, livers regenerating after partial hepatectomy, and livers obtained after timed exposure to carcinogenic chemicals, provided a rich spectrum of experimental material for identifying biochemical events related to carcinogenesis.

Our sympathies extend to his wife and family, and he will be deeply mourned. However, we pray they will derive great solace from the fact that when the history of cancer research comes to be written, the name of Tomizo Yoshida will occupy an ever-enduring place.

Alexander Haddow

TOMIZO YOSHIDA AND GERMAN SCIENCE
AND SCIENTISTS

In November, 1935, a stocky young Japanese doctor knocked at the door of my room in the Pathological Institute of the Charité-Hospital in Berlin in order to present himself. It was my first meeting with Tomizo Yoshida. Instead of a calling card, he handed me a little box made of ebony containing a set of histological slides from his just completed experiments (10). They represented in fact a great discovery and opened entirely new possibilities for the investigation on carcinogenesis.

Such great scientific achievements seem to illuminate in a flash a wide field, making visible new paths along which research may proceed. But just as lightning needs clouds for its generation, scientific discovery also is in some way dependent on the existing circumstances and the knowledge that has accumulated from the past for its propagation. Each discovery is a link, connected with the past on the one side and with the progressing knowledge on the other side, where it ultimately proves its usefulness. Such was true for many of the contributions Yoshida made to oncology, whereby he has secured for himself his share of fame. Without mentioning all of his discoveries, only one will be dwelt on here, which has a special connection with past and present oncology in Germany.

Yoshida originally followed a path opened years before (1906) by Fischer (3–5) and Schmidt (9), when they tried to produce tumors with Biebricher-Scharlach, a dye widely used at that time by clinicians to promote proliferation and regeneration of tissue and the healing of wounds. Since everybody's thinking then was influenced by Virchow's theory, that cancers were caused by chronic irritation, it seemed only logical to try to produce such a chronic irritation by using a substance known also to induce proliferation, with the hope that such proliferation would finally turn into malignant growth. Both German authors succeeded, it is true, in provoking the proliferation of cells, but they failed in initiating genuine tumorous growths—at least with the animals they used, with the way they applied the substance, and with the duration of their experiments. At first Yoshida (11) also could only provoke epithelial metaplasia in the thyroid by injecting the main component of Biebricher-Scharlach, o-aminoazotoluene, into guinea pigs. By varying the experiment with infinite patience, Sasaki and Yoshida (10) finally were able to succeed where others had failed; they fed o-aminoazotoluene in chemically pure form to rats and produced a high percentage of hepatomas. In fact the little box Yoshida handed me as an introductory gift contained slides of just such experimentally produced liver tumors.

Immediately after the Japanese authors published their results Fischer (6) and his group (1, 7) tried to repeat their previous experiments, substituting the purer substance used by Yoshida and Sasaki for the Biebricher-Scharlach. The result was at first negative and became positive only after the procedure of the Japanese experiments of feeding the animals unpolished rice was meticulously followed.

Stimulated by the success of the experiments with o-aminoazotoluene, chemically related substances were tried. One of them, dimethylaminoazobenzene, proved especially potent (8). These experiments were immediately repeated by German researchers who were stimulated by the fact that the substance was widely used in the German dairly industry under the name "Butter Yellow."

The prevailing tendency in German cancer research to study the different aspects of chemical cancerogenesis dates back to that time. I was fortunate enough to partake in those endeavours from the beginning (2) and also to have personally gotten to know one of the initiators of that kind of experiment, Dr. Tomizo Yoshida.

Yoshida had come to the German Pathological Institute of the Charité to complete his knowledge in pathology by working with Rössle, thus following a Japanese tradition dating back to the close cooperation of Aschoff with many of the most outstanding Japanese pathologists of his time. Yoshida stayed with us almost three fateful years—fateful particularly for the further development of cancer research in Germany. Both of us were younger then and more open to contacts and friendships than in later years. As usual, personal relations established at that time in life have the advantage of persisting life-long.

Yoshida proved to be a very sociable fellow and was quickly accepted in the family of assistants at Rössle's Institute. His success in making friends was greatly helped by his keen sense of humor, which induced him to laugh heartily, not only at all the jokes we told him, but also at his own hilarious mistakes. He himself retained a happy and grateful memory of that time and of his young colleagues. When we met 30 and 40 years later somewhere in the scientific circuit he never failed to inquire about the destiny of all the persons, whom he remembered by family and Christian name, and the incidents, both cheerful and serious, he experienced with them.   His main concern, of course, was for Professor Rössle, whom he referred to as his teacher in an article written on the occasion of Rössle's birthday (12).

In Germany, Yoshida and his accomplishments were never forgotten; in 1963, he was invited to give the Ludwing Aschoff Lecture (13) and was awarded the Robert Koch Medal (14). More meaningful than all the honors conferred on him all over the world, however, are his discoveries, his ideas, and the impulse he gave to the emerging science of oncology. In that sense he is remembered in Germany as a loving and stimulating friend.

Herwig Hamperl

1. Brass, K. A. Zellwucherungen in Leber und Schilddrüse durch enterale oder parenterale Zufuhr von Scharlachrot. *Frankf. Z. Pathol.*, **50**, 63–85 (1936).
2. Brock, N., Druckrey, H., and Hamperl, H. Die Erzeugung von Leberkrebs durch den Farbstoff 4-Dimethylamino-azobenzol. *Z. Krebsforsch.*, **50**, 431–456 (1940).
3. Fischer, B. Experimentelle Erzeugung atypischer Epithelwucherungen und die Entstehung bösartiger Geschwülste. *Münch. Med. Wochschr.*, **53**, 2041 (1906).
4. Fischer, B. Experimentelle Erzeugung von Epithelwucherung und Epithelmetaplasie. *Dtsch. Pathol. Ges.*, **10**, 20–22 (1920).
5. Fischer, B. Über experimentelle Erzeugung großer Flimmerepithelblasen der Lunge. *Frankf. Z. Pathol.*, **27**, 98–184 (1922).
6. Fischer-Wasels, B. Die experimentelle Erzeugung maligner Leberzelladenome durch o-Aminoazotoluol. *Verh. Dtsch. Pathol. Ges.*, **29**, 182–187 (1936).
7. Heep, W. Zellwucherungen in Leber und Schilddrüse durch enterale oder parenterale Zufuhr von o-Aminoazotoluol. *Frankf. Z. Pathol.*, **50**, 48–62 (1936).
8. Kinosita, R. Studies on cancerogenic chemical substances. *Nippon Byōri Gakkai Kaishi* (*Trans. Japan. Pathol. Soc.*), **27**, 665–727 (1937) (in Japanese).
9. Schmidt, M. B. Über vitale Fettfärbung in Geweben und Sekreten und geschwulstartige Wucherungen der ausscheidenden Drüsen. *Virchows Arch.*, **253**, 432–445 (1924).
10. Sasaki, T. and Yoshida, T. Experimentelle Erzeugung des Lebercarcinoms durch Fütterung mit o-Aminoazotoluol. *Virchows Arch.*, **295**, 175–200 (1935).
11. Yoshida, T. Experimenteller Beitrag zur Frage der Epithelmetaplasie. *Virchows Arch.*, **283**, 29–40 (1932).
12. Yoshida, T. Studien über das Ascites-Hepatom. *Virchows Arch.*, **295**, 175–200 (1935).
13. Yoshida, T. Zelluläre Multizentrizität der Krebsentstehung. *Dtsch. Med. Wochschr.*, **88**, 2229–2238 (1963).
14. Yoshida, T. Transformation of malignant growth. *Klin. Wochschr.*, **49**, 621–628 (1971).

TOMIZO YOSHIDA, A GIFTED " GLÜCKSKIND "

In discussing the forms that human destiny may take, Arthur Schopenhauer referred to the saying of "an ancient writer" that there are three great powers in the world: Sagacity, Strength, and Luck, the last being the most efficacious.

"A man's life is like a voyage of a ship, where luck—*secunda aut adversa fortuna*—acts the part of the wind, speeds the vessel on its way or drives it far out of its course. All that the man can do for himself is of little avail; like the rudder, which, if worked hard and continuously may help in the navigation of the ship; and yet all may be lost again by a sudden squall. But if the wind is only in the right quarter, the ship will sail on so as not to need any steering. The power of luck is nowhere better expressed than in a certain Spanish proverb: *Da ventura a tu hijo, y echa lo en el mar*—give your son luck and throw him into the sea."

The life of Tomizo Yoshida was a remarkable example for the substantiation of this Schopenhauerian opinion.

It is not only far beyond the scope of this brief commentary but also quite unnecessary to go into Yoshida's activities within and without the field of cancer research, since these are too wide and varied as well as too well known. At least the high reputation and numerous honors he won for himself in his lifetime need no mention for the readers of this Yoshida memorial volume of GANN Monographs. Yoshida did have in himself Sagacity and Strength, two of the three great powers which Schopenhauer named as important in determining human destiny. Now let us see how the third power, Luck, played its role in the life of Yoshida.

I have before me a booklet compiled and published in commemoration of Yoshida's retirement from Professorship of the University of Tokyo. In it is the record of what he said at the dinner given in honor of the occasion (February 10, 1963), in which he gave, among other things, his own account of many things that happened in his life. I can now borrow from it without fear of misrepresenting the actual facts.

When he graduated from the University of Tokyo (1927), Yoshida and five other classmates wanted to be admitted to the Pathology Department to do postgraduate work. Professor Mataro Nagayo, who was Chairman of the Department, asked if they meant to take up pathology as their speciality. Yoshida said honestly that he would like to study pathology for two years or so before going into internal medicine. He was told that the Pathology Department was full, and there was no room for such a dubious student. In the end, however, through the mediation of Professor Tomosaburo Ogata, second in command of the Department, Yoshida did obtain an appointment as assistant without pay. Trivial as it was, this was the first of the series of lucks for Yoshida, for had he been turned down in pathology and had to go into internal medicine there would not have been the Yoshida we now know.

About a year after his admission to the Pathology Department, Yoshida's father, who had been suffering from hypertension, suddenly died. This unfortunate event induced him to seek a position with some stipend; apparently he had depended on his father for financial support so far. Professor Ogata obtained for him an assistantship with stipend of 100 Yen a month in the laboratory of Professor Sasaki. Little did anybody dream that this was to prove to be the most important, great good fortune for Yoshida in forming the starting point of his successful career as a leading cancerologist. Here Luck played its most decisive role.

Professor Takaoki Sasaki was a wealthy clinician, private owner of the great Kyoundo Hospital, but was a biochemist of high reputation at the same time. His work on the use of bacteria for decomposition of amino acids and separation and identification of some of the intermediate metabolites is a classic. Earlier he had spent several years in Germany, where he worked in the laboratory of Emil Fischer. In later years his interest turned to what he called " Chemical Morphopathology," by which he intended to combine biochemistry with experimental pharmacology and pathology. He conducted his researches in his private laboratory built within the compound of his residence, which was the forerunner of the present Sasaki Institute for Medical Research. It was during this chemical morphopathology period of scientific activity that Yoshida joined Sasaki's private laboratory. One day, Sasaki handed to Yoshida a bottle containing some yellowish powder and asked that its morphopathologic effects be tested. The content of the bottle was o-aminoazotoluene!

We all know the rest of the story. In 1932, only three years after Yoshida came under the instruction of Sasaki, a short preliminary note on the azo dye hepatocarcinogenesis appeared: "Über experimentelle Erzeugung von Hepatom durch die Fütterung mit o-Amidoazotoluol" (Proc. Imperial Academy, Vol. 8, pp. 464–467 (1932)). This paper was published under Yoshida's sole authorship. The full paper on the subject later appeared as a joint work of Sasaki and Yoshida: "Experimentelle Erzeugung des Lebercarzinoms durch Fütterung mit o-Amidoazotoluol," *Virchows Archiv.*, **295**, 175–200 (1935). Sasaki, talking of those days, said that although the original idea of using o-aminoazotoluene as a tool in morphopathological study was his own, it was actually through the extraordinary industry and endurance on the part of Yoshida that the work progressed to the experimental production of hepatoma. Yoshida made full use of azo dye hepatocarcinoma throughout his later scientific activities, as may be seen in his long sustained studies on ascites hepatomas.

I should not fail to mention another incidence in Yoshida's life which shows how Luck plays its part in determining the fate of a man. I preface this story by recalling the historical facts. Yoshida left the Sasaki laboratory in 1935, when he received appointment as Assistant Professor at the Nagasaki Medical College; from Nagasaki he was sent to Germany for study in Pathology for two years, and upon return was raised to full Professorship. In June, 1944, he was called to Tohoku Imperial University, Sendai, as Professor of Pathology. This transfer from Nagasaki to Sendai at that time was a most fateful event, for although Yoshida's Sendai appointment was officially dated June, 1944, actually he had not left Nagasaki until less than a year before the Nagasaki bombing. Japan's unconditional surrender was announced on August 15, 1945. The Nagasaki bombing killed many of Yoshida's former colleagues.

To quote from Yoshida's talk in the booklet afore mentioned (translated from the original Japanese): "I visited Nagasaki in December of that year (1945). There were about five men in the Sendai faculty who had been transferred from Nagasaki, but I, as the youngest among them, was chosen as probably capable of standing the hardship of travelling to Nagasaki. (Travelling by railway in those immediate post-war days was no easy task!) Upon reaching Nagasaki I saw that the non-clinical section of the Medical College, being of wooden structure, was completely reduced to ashes. Everything was leaning or falling down, even very large trees, in the direction of the path of explosion blast. . . ."

"The successor to my post at Nagasaki, Professor Umeda, died there. Umeda and I were of the same age and of the same school. We were together in Berlin, where we worked in the same laboratory for a year and a half. When I moved to Sendai, Umeda came to Nagasaki to take my place. He was giving lecture at 11 in the morning of that fatal day and was blown off along with students and the whole buildings. His favorite Dunhill pipe was found where the lecture hall was, still holding its shape, I was told."

"I walked over to the place a short distance from the Medical College where my family and I used to live. The house was no longer there, but bones of perhaps three people laid unrecovered in what was probably the living room. . . ."

Some children, they say, are born under a lucky star. But only when such children are endowed with Sagacity and Strength can they accomplish something of real value to the world. Our esteemed friend Tomizo Yoshida was one such gifted "Glückskind."

Waro Nakahara

AN APPRECIATION

To understand a great man one needs to know something about the circumstances that surrounded his life, those who influenced his career, and those whose career he influenced. In the late 20's and early 30's of this century, at the time that Tomizo Yoshida embarked on cancer research, the environment of Japan was highly conductive to the encouragement of this endeavor. The medical science then taught and practiced had been imported from Germany by scholars who had gone abroad to study following the Meiji Restoration in 1868. Upon their return they began to test the theories that they had listened to while abroad and they enlarged their knowledge by the perusal of current medical and scientific publications. This combination of sound learning and avid reading, coupled with a natural bent for scientific investigation, a special mode of approach to the study of problems, and a natural patience and perseverance contributed pioneer discoveries of great significance. Among the medical disciplines followed, pathology had an especial appeal and of the numerous lines of investigation pursued cancer research became preeminent. Three areas intensely explored were tumor transplantation, and viral and chemical carcinogenesis. The early studies of tumor transplantation bore fruit in 1910 when Fujinami and his collaborators independently found a transplantable chicken sarcoma that by 1913 they proved to be transmissible by cell-free filtrates. Two years later, Yamagiwa and Ichikawa reported the induction of cutaneous carcinoma in rabbits painted with coal tar and three years later, Tsutsui introduced the mouse as a suitable animal for carcinogenicity testing. Earlier, in 1907, the intense interest in cancer research had led to the establishment of the journal "Gann" and in the following year to the organization of what is presently named the "Japanese Cancer Association." Then in 1924, under the patronage of H.I.H. Prince Hiroyasu Fushimi and Prince Fumimaro Konoe the "Japanese Foundation for Cancer Research" was established. The first president was Mataro Nagayo, an influential cancer investigator of that day. Cancer research had thus become a way of life, patronized by the Imperial family and successfully pursued by many scientists who were producing new observations, discoveries, and practical innovations unsurpassed in any country of the world. This was the environment into which Tomizo Yoshida made his debut in 1929, an environment well suited to nurture his intellectual creativity, for research ability, like talent in art, requires a touch of genius that must be nurtured. History teaches that great achievements have often followed group efforts applied to a single purpose as has proven true in many fields of endeavor including painting, poetry, the theater, architecture, sculpture, and navigation. Apart from opportunity and physical facilities, the

investigator needs the motivation that can be supplied by understanding colleagues who can offer encouragement, appreciation, criticism, and competition.
These are some of the circumstances that influenced Yoshida's successful career
in cancer research.

Tomizo Yoshida was born on February 10, 1903, into a well-to-do family
living in the small village of Asakawa situated in a mountainous agricultural
area in Fukushima Prefecture which lies between Tokyo and Sendai. His parents
early recognized his potential for learning and following his graduation from
the village elementary school they enrolled him first at the Kinjoo Middle School
and later at the First High School in Tokyo. During these 5 years he lived at the
home of his uncle, his mother's brother, who was a teacher in a private woman's
medical college. Hence young Tomizo not only received his education at the
best middle school and high school of prewar Japan but where he was residing
he came under the influence of a teacher of medicine from whom he must have
absorbed ideas that influenced his later career. With the intelligence that he
inherited from his parents combined with his natural industry he did well in
his studies. He received his medical education at the Tokyo Imperial University,
and there too his subsequent training in pathology under Professor Tomosaburo
Ogata. Professor Ogata thought highly enough of Yoshida to recommend him
in 1952 as his successor to the chair of pathology of Tokyo Imperial University.

Beyond doubt, the greatest single influence on Yoshida's scientific career
was his early mentor, Professor Takaoki Sasaki, who later founded the Sasaki
Institute. Attesting to his research ability, Professor Sasaki had, in 1924, received
the Imperial Prize from the Japanese Imperial Academy for his studies of the
end products formed by the action of bacteria on amino acids. He was the
third generation of the brilliant family of Sasaki who themselves pursued and
where in addition the public spirited benefactors of scholarship and research in
the fields of medicine and basic science. Beginning in 1876, the grandfather,
Tōyō Sasaki, initiated and later his son, Masakichi Sasaki, supported and enlarged
the medical investigation facilities at Kyoundo Hospital out of which grew the
present Sasaki Institute. The third in line, Professor T. Sasaki, Yoshida's
mentor, had trained in biochemistry in Strassburg and Berlin, and upon his
return to Japan he took up research at Kyoundo Hospital in 1916, after a brief
period as professor of medicine at Kyoto Imperial University School of Medicine.
It was at the Kyoundo Hospital that Yoshida, among other young physicians,
came under the influence of Professor Sasaki's wide scientific knowledge, stimulating research ideas, and humanistic personality. Here Yoshida made his first great
discovery in cancer research and here later in 1952 he returned as director when
he was appointed to the chair of pathology at the University of Tokyo.

Yoshida did not have long to wait for the reward of this association with his
mentor T. Sasaki. Together in 1929 they embarked on studies of the pathologic
effects of the ingestion of *o*-aminoazotoluene on the epithelial cells of the organs
of a number of species of animals. In the course of these studies Yoshida detected
hepatic cancers in rats. He published this epoch-making discovery in 1932.
Probably no animal model in cancer research has been so thoroughly investigated
from so many points of view by so many scientists, in so many lands as this

model discovered by Yoshida. The influence of Professor Sasaki on young Yoshida exemplifies what Anne Roe discovered from her studies of the lives of many top scientists. She learned that most of them somehow or other while young, often as students, found a teacher or an associate along the way who induced them or permitted them to find out things on their own. After that beginning they learned to rely upon themselves. The opportunity to engage in experimentation provides an outlet for the potential scientist's undeveloped energies of mind. This experience enables him to find out for himself whether he possesses the imagination, needed initiative, motivation, and enthusiasm for intellectual success. Research therefore is largely self learning but at its beginnings it often requires a primer in the form of a capable mentor, a role that Sasaki played in Yoshida's career. Thereafter Yoshida pursued his ideas with assurance and vigor.

It is to the everlasting credit of those in control of support for promising talent in Japan, that they recognized the genius of young Yoshida and arranged for him to go abroad for postgraduate study. At the Charité in Berlin (1935–1938) he came under the tutelage of Robert Rössle who introduced him to the deep speculations of the great minds in pathology. More than 30 years later in 1972, in his last published paper, Yoshida was still reflecting on these philosophies and attempting to correlate them with the most modern views about the processes of cancer. In this paper he speculated about the integration of the virus genome into the host chromosome or the host genome in relation to the earlier views about the "Seat of Disease" held by Morgani (1682–1771), the pursuit of this idea down to the microscopic cell level by Virchow (1821–1902), and the "New Cell Race" by Hauser (1903). These speculations personify Yoshida; whatever he put his mind to was bound to be important, and he pursued ideas in depth and for as long as he lived.

One cannot overemphasize the importance of these two periods in his scientific life, the one spent with T. Sasaki and the other with R. Rössle. From them he learned much. Ever afterward in the design and conduct of his experiments, he continued to ask questions in order that he might obtain answers. He learned that research must be undertaken in the faith that ultimately the fragmentary knowledge being revealed today will somehow combine with other knowledge to provide an innovation of practical value. He was to realize the truth of this in 1943 at Nagasaki when he successfully transplanted to other rats the scrotal neoplasm and tumor cell-containing milky ascites fluid that he had induced in one of his experimental rats. By that act he provided a tool of such value for fundamental research and practicality for cancer chemotherapy, that after 1945 when the Yoshida sarcoma was first presented to the scientific community, approximately 30% of the investigations reported for several years at the annual meetings of the Japanese Cancer Association dealt with studies of ascites tumors. In 1971, in a publication of 60 pages dealing with the comparative studies of the Yoshida sarcoma and ascites hepatomas, he concluded that cancer can be "regarded as a rapidly changing, very unstable, and perhaps fragile creation." Thus the discovery of the Yoshida sarcoma ranks with the discovery of those transplantable neoplasms bearing the names of others such as Erlich, Krebs, Jensen, and Walker that over the years have achieved immortality.

Yoshida spent the years 1944–1952 as Professor of Pathology at the School of Medicine at Tohoku University in Sendai. Here fate seems to have intervened in his behalf. For had he remained as professor at Nagasaki he would in all likelihood have shared the fate of many of his former colleagues there who perished in the bomb attack of 1945. The period spent at Sendai was a happy one and most productive for him and his new found associates. It was here that he attracted to his department associates who are now among the top scientific and educational leaders in Japan: Dr. Isaka of the Sasaki Institute, Professor Nakamura of Fukushima Medical College, Dr. Odashima of the National Institute of Hygienic Sciences, Professor Sato of Tohoku University, and Dr. Satoh of the Sasaki Institute. It was this small band of original, eager, and industrious young investigators who learned from the master and in collaboration with him succeeded in establishing lines of ascites hepatoma in rats which have been widely used in the pursuit of investigations of cancer chemotherapy screening. This marks the period of Yoshida's greatest influence in the development of young investigators excepting for Dr. Sugano and Dr. Takayama who joined him later in Tokyo. Both of the latter are at the Cancer Institute of Tokyo where Dr. Sugano succeeded to the directorship, a position Yoshida had occupied in 1963 when he retired as Professor of Pathology and Dean of the Medical College of the University of Tokyo.

H. A. Krebs has written that scientists are not so much born as made by those who teach them and that there is such a thing as a scientific genealogy. This is exemplified by the career of Yoshida. One line of his genealogy begins in 1876 with the first of three important members of the Sasaki family, followed in turn by the son and the grandson, each of whom influenced his successor, the combined influence being transmitted to Yoshida. The other genealogical line is that of Professor Rössle and his scientific antecedents. Then follows the generation of scientists whose careers Yoshida influenced while at Sendai and Tokyo. And now there are indications that the scientific descendants of this later generation of cancer investigators are demonstrating their worth in present day Japan. These then are those who influenced Yoshida and those in turn who were influenced by him. The importance of scientific genealogy was clearly recognized by Yoshida when he said, "A person who was able to meet with a good teacher has (himself) to try to be a good teacher for younger generations."

In the small space allotted to me in this publication I cannot possibly go into details about the many facets of my close friend Tomizo, this great man, the type of genius who appears once in a century; the numerous and important awards, prizes; and honors that he received both inside Japan and from foreign countries in recognition of his work; the high regard in which he was held by his fellow countrymen and his many friends abroad; his later career as science statesman of Japan; his wide circle of friends from fields outside of medicine, including economics, journalism, politics, entertainment, and sports; his superb style in writing English; his warm friendship; his ability for deep concentration; his fertile and lively imagination; and his flair for the unusual. To illustrate Yoshida's flair for the unusual I repeat an anecdote told me by a young research fellow working in an American laboratory. He was eagerly looking forward to the advice he would receive during a promised visit from the great professor. They spent the entire day together. Finally just before his departure Yoshida imparted this unusual piece of advice: "Read American History."

I close this brief "Appreciation" with verses from an "Epitaph on a Friend" by my favorite poet Robert Burns:

An honest man here lies at rest
As e'er God with his image blest!
The friend of man, the friend of truth;
The friend of age, and guide of youth;

Few hearts like his, with virtue warmed,
Few heads with knowledge so informed:
If there's another world, he lives in bliss;
If there is none, he made the best of this.

Harold L. Stewart

CONTENTS

ENVIRONMENTAL CARCINOGENESIS

EXPERIMENTAL MODEL OF TUMORS IN VARIOUS ORGANS

MUTAGENICITY AND
IN VITRO CARCINOGENESIS

GANN Monograph on Cancer Research 17, 3–15 (1975)

DNA REPAIR OF HUMAN CELLS AS A RELEVANT, RAPID, AND ECONOMIC ASSAY FOR ENVIRONMENTAL CARCINOGENS

H. F. Stich, D. Kieser, B. A. Laishes, R. H. C. San, and P. Warren

*Cancer Research Center, University of British Columbia**

The possibility of using DNA repair synthesis (unscheduled uptake of ^{3}HTdR into arrested cultured cells) as a rapid and economic assay for chemical carcinogens was explored. This procedure appears highly relevant in assessing a potential carcinogenic or mutagenic hazard to man because the response of cultured cells of normal and sensitive persons can be examined. Precarcinogens can be readily detected when the compounds are incubated with activation mixtures prior to their addition to cultured human cells. A new combined *in vivo* and *in vitro* system for the detection of organotropic carcinogens and their target tissues is described. A protocol for testing the capacity of a compound to interact with DNA is proposed.

It is generally assumed that chemical and physical mutagens interact with DNA and thereby initiate processes resulting in mutations. Similarly, many, if not all, properly examined chemical carcinogens seem to bind to DNA, cause DNA breakage, and elicit DNA repair synthesis. Although at present the involvement of these early cell responses in carcinogenesis is unknown this interaction of chemical carcinogens with the nuclear DNA of treated cells may be utilized in a rapid prescreening test.

In this paper we would like to discuss the pros and cons of using DNA repair in a large scale monitoring program for chemical carcinogens. This procedure may have several advantages: DNA repair can be readily estimated, it would lend itself to a semi-mechanized treatment, and the required technical facilities and manpower are minimal. Furthermore mammalian cells respond with a DNA repair synthesis to many different DNA lesions which were induced by a great variety of chemical compounds. This uniform response appears to be a good indicator for the DNA damaging effect of carcinogens. Its estimation does not require a detailed knowledge of the type of carcinogen-DNA interaction.

Methodologic Considerations

From the many techniques available to measure DNA repair only a few fullfil the criteria required for a bioassay to be applicable to a large-scale test

---

* Vancouver 8, British Columbia, Canada.

program. The most promising procedures are (1) the adaptation of the alkaline or neutral sucrose gradient techniques for examining shifts in molecular weight profiles of DNA and (2) the detection of an unscheduled incorporation of nucleotides (*e.g.*, ³HTdR) by autoradiography.

The first technique which reveals changes in the molecular weight of DNA can be applied to cells *in vitro* and tissues *in vivo* (Fig. 1(a) and 1(b)). Since one of the prerequisites is the ability to label DNA with a radioactive precursor the technique can be only used on proliferating tissue. This restriction can be overcome by injecting radioactive DNA precursors into young animals in which many tissues are in a state of rapid proliferation. Thus their DNA can be readily labelled.

As a rule, intact cells are placed into an overlay of lysing solution on top of a preformed sucrose gradient (*3, 10, 11, 14, 21*). Thus a gentle lysis of cells and concomitant release of DNA, with a minimum of mechanical shearing, is facilitated. The profiles illustrated in Fig. 1(a) and 1(b) were derived from the same alkaline sucrose gradient technique employing a 5–20% sucrose gradient layered on top of a 1-ml cushion of 2.3 M sucrose. This particular technique requires only 30 min of centrifugation at 20,000 rpm (20°) and, with further development of rotors and accessories, could lend itself to a large-scale screening program. Analysis of the distribution of ³H-DNA within the gradients could be easily adapted to automation.

The second procedure which meets many of the prerequisites of a screening

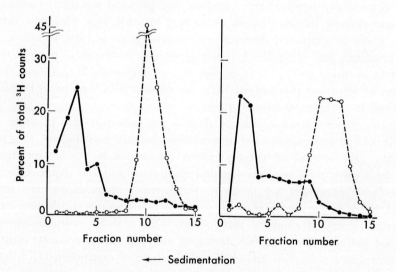

FIG. 1a (left). Shift in alkaline sucrose gradient sedimentation profiles of ³H-DNA released from cultured human fibroblasts

Exposure to 5×10^{-6} M 4NQO for 30 min. ○ control; ● non-exposed fibroblasts.

FIG. 1b (right). Shift in alkaline sucrose gradient sedimentation profiles of ³H-DNA of mouse livers

Sample was taken 4 hr after one intraperitoneal injection of 10 μg/g DMN. ○ control; ● non-exposed fibroblasts.

test is the unscheduled incorporation of [3]HTdR with subsequent detection by autoradiography (20, 22): it is simple and can be easily handled by low-skilled technicians; it requires only few cells (about 200 cells per sample) which can be readily obtained from human beings (e.g., lymphocytes, fibroblasts from skin biopsies, cells from amniocenteses samples), it can be applied to *in vitro* and *in vivo* systems, it can reveal variations within a cell population, it is highly economic, and it can be completed within a 10-day period (or within 2 days if a rapid autoradiographic method is employed).

DNA Repair Synthesis in the Identification of Active Carcinogens

The use of DNA repair synthesis as a rapid and economic monitoring system is based on the observations that many, if not all, chemical carcinogens and mutagens interact with DNA and that the ensuing DNA changes will initiate a DNA repair synthesis (32, 33). There is evidence to suggest that a great variety of DNA alterations will lead to one type of DNA repair synthesis which can be detected by an unscheduled uptake of labelled DNA precursors. Thus, by measuring DNA repair synthesis one obtains quantitative data about a DNA damage without going through the difficult and time-consuming task of analysing the type of carcinogen-DNA bondage and the type of DNA alterations.

A correlation between the oncogenicity of a compound and its capacity to induce DNA repair synthesis was examined on about 65 different compounds. Cultured diploid mammalian fibroblasts including human ones, which were obtained from skin biopsies, were employed as test subjects.

A positive correlation between degree of oncogenicity and extent of DNA repair capacity becomes particularly evident when chemicals which belong to one category are compared with each other. One of the most thoroughly examined compounds are 4-nitroquinoline 1-oxide (4NQO) and its highly, weakly, and non-oncogenic derivatives (19, 23, 29, 31). The parental compound 4NQO and its strongly oncogenic derivatives elicited a high level of unscheduled [3]HTdR uptake in cultured mammalian fibroblasts. Following application of weakly carcinogenic 4NQO derivatives the unscheduled DNA synthesis occurred to a smaller extent. The non-oncogenic 4NQO derivatives and 4NQO isomers failed to evoke any detectable response in this respect.

A good correlation was also obtained with several precarcinogens of aromatic polycyclic hydrocarbons, their epoxides which seem to represent the reactive metabolites (5, 7, 13), and their non-oncogenic diol forms (27) (Table I).

Similarly the proximate N-hydroxy metabolites and the ultimate N-acetoxy metabolites of 2-acetylaminofluorene (15, 16) induced DNA alterations which resulted in a measurable level of DNA repair synthesis, whereas the parental compounds lack this capacity, when applied at equimolar concentrations (25). Two more examples are given in Table I.

These results suggest that DNA repair synthesis of cultured mammalian fibroblasts including human ones will detect chemical carcinogens which are directly active and reactive metabolites of precarcinogens.

Thus a successful application of DNA repair in a prescreening test would

TABLE I. DNA Repair Synthesis in Cultured Human Cells (Controls and
Xeroderma Pigmentosum) Following Exposure to Precarcinogens
and Proximate Carcinogens

Compound	Concentration (3 hr)	DNA repair (grains/nucleus)	
		Control	XP-E
AAP	1×10^{-4} M	0	0
N-OH-AAP	,,	20	3.5
N-Ac-AAP	,,	39	6.9
AS	5×10^{-5} M	0	0
AAS	,,	0	0
N-OH-AAS	,,	13	2.7
N-Ac-AAS	,,	35	6.3
MCA	1×10^{-3} M	0	0
MCA-diol	,,	0	0
MCA-epoxide	,,	41	7.2

AAP: 2-acetylaminophenanthrene. AS: 4-aminostilbene. AAS: 4-acetylaminostilbene.
MCA: 20-methylcholanthrene. XP-E: Xeroderma pigmentosum (Edmonton).

require the availability of carcinogens in their reactive form. Unfortunately the reactive metabolites of most carcinogens are neither known nor can they be readily synthesized. This situation restricts the simple use of cultured fibroblast and DNA repair synthesis as a generally applicable prescreening test. To cope with the problem of active forms of carcinogens a more complex assay system was designed. Its advantages are discussed in the following section.

DNA Repair in the Identification of Chemicals Which Require Metabolic Activation to Proximate Carcinogens

Most foreign compounds ingested by mammals are metabolized along a multiformity of chemical pathways. The liver appears to be the major site for the metabolic transformation of foreign compounds including carcinogens. To a lesser extent foreign compound metabolism occurs in other tissues and is also accomplished by the bacterial populations of the gastrointestinal tract. The enzyme systems in the hepatocytes transform seemingly harmless compounds into potent, reactive metabolites as exemplified by various polycyclic aromatic hydrocarbons, nitrosamines, and several naturally occurring fungal toxins (e.g., aflatoxins, sterigmatocystin). The application of in vitro assays that use fibroblasts as indicator cells must, therefore, include a means of producing and detecting various reactive metabolites of precarcinogens.

A successful approach to this problem is to mix the chemical which is being tested with a fresh isolate of mammalian liver microsomes, fortified with any necessary co-factors and to expose the indicator cells to this mixture (10, 12). A mouse liver microsomal fraction, fortified with NADPH, was used to activate dimethylnitrosamine (DMN), aflatoxin-B_1, and sterigmatocystin. A moderate level of DNA repair synthesis, reduced cell survival, and an increase in chromosome

TABLE II. DNA Repair Synthesis in Cultured Human Fibroblasts Following a 30-Min Exposure to Carcinogens Plus Complete and Incomplete Activation Mixtures

Treatment	Grains/nucleus		Chromosome aberration[a]
	DMN $(5 \times 10^{-2}$ M$)$	Sterigmatocystin $(5 \times 10^{-4}$ M$)$	Aflatoxin $(6 \times 10^{-5}$ M$)$
Chemicals alone	0.5	0.0	1.5
Activation system alone	0.3	0.0	1.7
Chemicals plus activation system	23.2	27.4	22.2
Chemicals plus activation system but without NADPH	1.0	—	1.7

[a] Percentage of metaphase plates with at least one chromatid break or one chromatid exchange.

aberrations was evoked in human skin fibroblasts following short (30 min) exposure to the chemical " precarcinogens " combined with the complete activation system. Exposure to the precarcinogens alone produced virtually no detectable effects. Table II illustrates typical examples.

An extensive body of work remains before the general validity of this procedure can be fully assessed. Activation preparations derived from different tissues must be compared because the possibility cannot be neglected that some of the organotropic carcinogens may require enzyme systems that occur in organs other than the liver. A second improvement of this method can be achieved by increasing the metabolic activity of the liver through the administration of drug-metabolizing enzymes (1). It is also likely that exposure of the animal to particular inducers of drug-metabolizing enzymes *in vivo* may alter the level of sensitivity of the technique. In this manner the effect of various environmental chemicals which function as either inducers (halogenated hydrocarbon insecticides, polycyclic aromatic hydrocarbons, dyes, food preservatives) or repressors (organophosphorus insecticides, carbon monoxide, carbon tetrachloride) of the metabolism of carcinogens, can be studied in order to clarify the role of such environmental chemicals in carcinogenesis.

Importance of the Employed Endpoint

A reliable and relevant assessment of the carcinogenic or mutagenic hazard should be based on bioassays that employ different endpoints. The irrelevance of conclusions that rely only on one test system is best illustrated by the combined effects of the carcinogen, 4NQO, and human or simian adenovirus type-12 (AD12) (26).

Three different endpoints were employed: the level of DNA repair synthesis, the frequency of chromatid aberrations, and the incidence of neoplastic transformation of embryonal hamster cells. These criteria are relatively well defined, lend themselves to a quantitative evaluation, and reflect different types of genetic anomalies. A DNA repair synthesis indicates physically or chemically induced DNA changes. In the process of correction, copying errors of the excised nu-

TABLE III. Response of Cultured Syrian Hamster Cells to Adenovirus (AD12 or SA7), 4NQO, and the Combination of AD12 and 4NQO

	DNA repair (grains/nucleus)	Chromosome aberrations (%)	Transformation frequency[a]
Virus[b]	0	37	13
4NQO	61	20	0
Virus[b]+4NQO	57	55	300

[a] Number of colonies per 2×10^6 surviving cells. [b] AD12 was used for DNA repair and chromosome studies; SA7 was employed for the transformation experiments.

cleotide segments or strand interruptions, which may occur if DNA with unrepaired alterations enters into replication, can result in mutations. Chromatid breakage and exchanges will lead to deletion and duplication of larger gene sequences or to translocations which may affect gene function by the so-called position effect. Finally, the virus-transformed cells exemplify a genetic change resulting from the addition of new partially transcribed DNA.

The three endpoints were differently affected by the combined application of 4NQO and adenovirus (Table III).

1) As previously described, DNA repair synthesis followed the application of 4NQO. The oncogenic virus had no detectable stimulating or supressing effect on this 4NQO-initiated DNA repair synthesis. Thus DNA repair synthesis as an endpoint would reveal the effect of the chemical carcinogen but would not detect the presence of viral oncogens.

2) The enumeration of chromosome aberrations detected the action of 4NQO and that of AD12. There was an additive effect of chromatid breaks and exchanges when a cell was exposed to the chemical and viral carcinogens.

3) Neoplastic transformation as an endpoint revealed an enhancing effect of 4NQO on the transforming capacity of simian adenovirus (SA7).

Combined in Vivo and in Vitro System for the Detection of Organotropic Carcinogens or Precarcinogens

It is likely that compounds with a highly specific organotropic action may be activated in various target tissues. If this is truly the case then activation preparation obtained from livers may not be able to change all precarcinogens into active metabolites. Such compounds may give "false negatives" when incubated with a liver post-mitochondrial fraction and tested on cultured fibroblasts.

To detect organotropic carcinogens or organotropic precarcinogens an *in vivo*/*in vitro* combination system was designed (*31, 33*). The test procedure consists of (a) administering (injecting, force-feeding, *etc.*) the compound to mice, hamsters, or rats for a short period (2 to 5 hr), (b) taking biopsies of various organs, (c) tearing these tissue samples into tiny pieces, (d) incubating these pieces in a standard tissue culture medium which contains 10 μCi/ml ³HTdR for 3 to 5 hr at 37°, (e) fixing the tissue pieces with ethanol: acetic acid (3:1), (f) preparing sections or squashes on microscopic slides, and (g) coating with an autoradio-

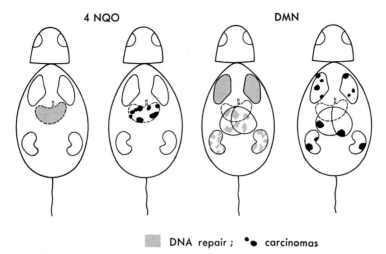

DNA repair ; • carcinomas

FIG. 2. Schematic drawings showing the occurrence of DNA repair synthesis in only those organs from which tumors arise
Mice were force-fed 4NQO (200 mg/kg body weight) or DMN (1,500 mg/kg body weight). The DNA repair synthesis was estimated 4 hr after the application of the carcinogens with the new *in vivo/in vitro* combination assay (*33*).

graphic emulsion. As a rule cells in DNA repair (lightly labelled) can be readily distinguished from cells in DNA-replication during S-phase (heavily labelled). The incorporation of ³HTdR into nuclear DNA was checked by treating the tissue preparation with deoxyribonuclease prior to autoradiography. The general validity of this new *in vivo/in vitro* combination system is being currently examined by using several carcinogens of known organotropic action.

Comparing the occurrence of DNA repair in various tissues and the location of tumors a positive correlation emerged: a few examples may illustrate this point (Fig. 2).

1) After subcutaneous (s.c.) administration of a single dose of 4NQO the only site of DNA repair as detected by the *in vivo/in vitro* test system is the lung. Tumors reported after s.c. injection of 4NQO arise mainly, if not exclusively, in the lung (*17*). If on the other hand, 4NQO is force-fed, cells of the stomach show an unscheduled ³HTdR uptake and only stomach tumors arise (*18*).

2) Subcutaneous injection of DMN into mice (C3H) leads to DNA repair in the lung, and to a lesser extent in the liver and kidney. Lung and kidney tumors are reported by Terracini (*35*). Vesselinovitch (*37*) found liver tumors after injection of DMN. No stomach tumors appeared after single or repeated DMN injections and also no DNA repair synthesis was observed in the stomach epithelium. Unscheduled DNA repair synthesis was found in most cells of the lung after force-feeding of DMN and was present to a much lesser extent in kidney and liver. After applying DMN in drinking water a great number of lung tumors developed followed in frequency by liver and kidney tumors (*34–36*).

3) 4-Aminoquinoline 1-oxide which has been tested and found to be a non-carcinogenic metabolite of 4NQO (*8*) gave no DNA repair response in our system.

The simplest interpretation of these results is to assume that precarcinogens are submitted to an organ-specific activation into ultimate carcinogens in those tissues in which they cause DNA alterations and that these DNA changes in turn initiate a DNA repair which is finally measured by the unscheduled uptake of ^{3}HTdR. On the other hand the possibility cannot be discarded that the precarcinogen becomes activated in the liver but accumulates (9) and induces DNA alterations in another receptor organ. If a causal relationship between the measured DNA alterations and the site of the tumor origin exists, our *in vivo/in vitro* combination system would yield a quick, reliable system for the detection of organ-specific carcinogens which could be easily missed by tests that rely on cultured fibroblasts.

Importance of the Sensitivity of Indicator Cell

Results of bioassays can be strongly influenced by the sensitivity of the employed indicator cells. Up to 100-fold differences in response to chemical carcinogens are quite common among different bacterial or yeast mutants. Thus, one of the crucial points in the introduction of a prescreening or screening program will be the choice of cells with a sensitivity that is comparable to that found in "average cells" of the "average human being." A too sensitive test system as well as a too insensitive one may easily lead to erroneous conclusions about the actual carcinogenic or mutagenic hazard of a compound.

The sensitivity of indicator cells can be affected by genetic factors as well as external ones. A profound understanding of these modifying factors is a prerequisite of any successful application of cultured cells in a screening or prescreening program.

A genetic influence on the response of cells to chemical carcinogens is exemplified by Xeroderma pigmentosum (XP) which is a genetic disease (recessive) linked to a defect in the DNA repair mechanism (2). The level of DNA repair synthesis following UV irradiation varies among different patients; from close to 0% to about 80% as compared to that of control persons (review in

TABLE IV.   Unscheduled Uptake of ^{3}HTdR and Frequency of Chromosome Aberrations of Cultured Cells from Various Xeroderma Pigmentosum Patients after Exposure to 4NQO

	DNA repair (%) of controls[a]	Metaphase plates with chromosome aberrations (%)[b]
Control	100	0.7
Heterozygote (XP-Edmonton)	102	1.1
XP-Kamloops	56	12.8
XP-Calgary	33	20.3
XP-Edmonton	21	57.1
XP-Hamilton	12	68.5

[a] Unscheduled incorporation of ^{3}HTdR was measured after 90-min exposure to 2×10^{-6} M 4NQO.   [b] Chromosome aberrations (breaks and exchanges) were counted on cell cultures exposed to 5×10^{-7} M 4NQO.

Ref. *31*). The DNA repair capacity also varies when cultured cells of various patients are exposed to chemical carcinogens (*28*) (Table IV).

Thus a low level of DNA repair can either indicate a small extent of DNA damage or it may reveal an impaired response to the carcinogen-induced DNA damage. If it is unknown which of these two phenomena is involved in the response of a cell then a wrong interpretation of the results can easily occur.

Recently, several examples showing a non-genetic influence on the cell response to physical or chemical carcinogens have become known. Elkind (*4*) has reported that the repair of X irradiation in Chinese hamster cells can be affected by shifting the temperature during and after irradiation. Lethality of cells exposed at 0° or 42° increases after ionizing irradiation, whereas temperatures between 34° and 41° show only a slight effect on lethality as compared to 37°. This is taken to indicate that at extremes in temperature the repair system is not capable of fully repairing the DNA damage.

The way of applying carcinogens to the indicator cells may also strongly affect their response (*6*). An example will show the response to one and two consecutive doses of the carcinogen, 4NQO. Cultured human fibroblasts were exposed to one low dose of 4NQO and were then given a second identical dose, with the time interval between doses varying from 0 to 12 hr. The lethal effect of the carcinogens was measured by the clone-forming capacity of the treated cells. After the first dose a highly sensitive period occurred whereby the cells were unable to cope normally with a second dose of 4NQO.

This sensitive period following the application of 4NQO is characterized by a reduced DNA repair synthesis (Fig. 3). The peak of unscheduled incor-

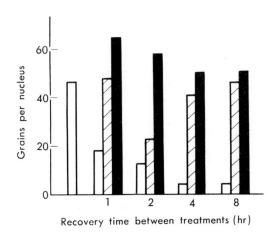

Fig. 3.   Level of DNA repair synthesis in cultured human fibroblasts following one dose of 4NQO (60 min) and two doses of 4NQO given at different time intervals

DNA repair synthesis was measured as unscheduled incorporation of ^{3}HTdR (grains/nucleus in autoradiographs) □ average number of grains per nucleus following one 4NQO dose and sampled 0, 1, 2, 4, or 8 hr after treatment; ▨ average grain number per nucleus after two consecutive 4NQO treatments which were 1, 2, 4, or 8 hr apart of each other; ■ expected grain number per nucleus if the two 4NQO doses were additive.

poration of ³HTdR has been shown to occur in the first few hours after treatment with a chemical carcinogen. If a second dose of 4NQO is given during *e.g.*, a 2-hr period, the cells do not respond at a normal level. It would seem that when a cell has initiated the process of DNA repair it is incapable for a certain time period of repairing at a normal level a further damage, yet when repair of the first dose is completed further DNA damage can be repaired effectively.

We have further noted that the "nutritional" status of a cell can significantly affect its response to a second dose of a chemical carcinogen. Cells that are exposed to two doses of 4NQO in an arginine-deficient medium do not repair the second dose effectively during the sensitive period. Yet cells exposed to two doses of 4NQO in a complete culture medium containing 5% fetal calf serum are able to repair the second dose to a greater extent.

The results show that the experimental conditions must be well defined prior to the application of cultured fibroblasts and DNA repair synthesis in a large-scale monitoring program. No response to a carcinogen or a reduced one could reflect the genetic or physiological state of the cell rather than the oncogenic capacity of the examined compound.

Proposed Schedule of Using DNA Repair Synthesis as an Economic and Rapid Bioassay for Carcinogens and Mutagens

Based on the presented and published results (*22–33*), we propose the following protocol for testing the capacity of a compound to interact with DNA and to initiate a DNA repair synthesis. Since these two phenomena appear to be linked to neoplastic transformation and mutagenesis, they actually seem to reveal the carcinogenic and/or mutagenic property of a compound.

Step 1: Add different concentrations of the test chemical to monolayer cultures of non-dividing mammalian cells for 1 to 3 hr and estimate the unscheduled incorporation of ³HTdR (10 μCi/ml for 90 min). If no DNA repair synthesis can be detected proceed with Step 2.

Step 2: Mix test chemical with an activation preparation (*e.g.*, fortified post-mitochondrial liver fraction), add this mixture to monolayer cultures of non-dividing mammalian cells and estimate the unscheduled incorporation of ³HTdR. If no DNA repair synthesis can be detected proceed with Step 3a.

Step 3a: The test chemical is added to tiny pieces of various mammalian organs for 1 to 5 hr and thereafter these organ pieces are placed for 90 min into culture medium containing ³HTdR. If no DNA repair can be detected proceed with Step 4.

Step 3b: Instead of organ pieces, cultured cells of different tissue could be used. However, the scarcity of differentiated cells which can be maintained *in vitro* severely restricts this approach.

Step 4: Apply the afore-mentioned combined *in vivo/in vitro* system.

Undoubtedly there remain many unanswered questions which cannot be simply ignored. For example the assumption that all chemical carcinogens produce DNA alterations which are followed by a DNA repair synthesis must be proved or disproved on a larger number of carcinogens. Although a good correlation has been observed with about 65 different compounds the final answer is still outstanding. Furthermore, it is unknown whether there are compounds which elicit DNA repair but lack a carcinogenic effect.

The sensitivity of the test system is another unresolved problem. If cultured cells of "normal" persons are employed in a screening program one could extrapolate to the sensitivity of an "average person" to chemical carcinogens. However, one may miss the population segment which has an increased sensitivity. But this is precisely the population group that shows a higher cancer risk and needs protection. On the other hand the use of the most sensitive indicator cells (*e.g.*, cells of patients with XP) may lead to an overestimation of a carcinogenic hazard.

This report would appear to be more incomplete without mentioning the recent design of a new method to estimate DNA repair in mammalian cells. This procedure is based on the repair of UV-irradiated viruses that depends on the repair capacity of the host cell. This method is highly sensitive, it lends itself to an easy quantitative evaluation, and it may reveal defects at various steps of the entire repair process. Thus chemicals that interfere with later steps of the repair process could be possibly detected with this method. Although this procedure was successfully used by us to estimate the repair capacity of XP cells its possible role in a bioassay of chemical carcinogens remains to be examined.

In spite of the many open questions the use of DNA repair synthesis in a prescreening test for chemical carcinogens appears to be a highly promising approach and worthy of a careful consideration. Since this test can be performed on human cells the results can be more readily used in assessing a carcinogenic hazard to man. The economy and speed of this assay fulfill two other prerequisites of a prescreening assay. Furthermore the possibility of automation would facilitate the application of the assay in a large-scale screening program.

REFERENCES

1. Ames, B. N., Durston, W. E., Yamasaki, E., and Lee, F. D. Carcinogens are mutagens: A simple test system combining liver homogenates for activation and bacteria for detection. *Proc. Natl. Acad. Sci. U.S.*, **70**, 2281–2285 (1973).

2. Cleaver, J. E. Defective repair replication of DNA in Xeroderma pigmentosum. *Nature*, **218**, 652–656 (1968).

3. Cox, R., Damjanov, I., Abanobi, S. E., and Sarma, D. S. R. A method for measuring DNA damage and repair in the liver *in vivo*. *Cancer Res.*, **33**, 2114–2121 (1973).

4. Elkind, M. M., Bronk, B. V., and Ben-Hur, E. Thermally enhanced radiosensitivity of cultured Chinese hamster cells. *Nature New Biol.*, **238**, 209 (1972).

5. Heidelberger, C. *In vitro* studies on the role of epoxides in carcinogenic hydrocarbon activation. *In* "Topics in Chemical Carcinogenesis," ed. by W. Nakahara, S. Takayama, T. Sugimura, and S. Odashima, University Park Press, Baltimore, pp. 371–386 (1972).

6. Heidelberger, C. and Thilly, W. G. Cytotoxicity and mutagenicity of ultraviolet

irradiation as a function of the interval between split doses in cultured Chinese hamster cells. *Mutat. Res.*, **17**, 287–290 (1973).

7. Huberman, E., Aspiras, L., Heidelberger, C., Grover, P. L., and Sims, P. Mutagenicity to mammalian cells of epoxides and other derivatives of polycyclic hydrocarbons. *Proc. Natl. Acad. Sci. U.S.*, **68**, 3195–3199 (1971).

8. Kawazoe, Y., Tachibana, M., Aoki, K., and Nakahara, W. The structure-carcinogenicity relationship among derivatives of 4-nitro- and 4-hydroxyamino-quinoline 1-oxides. *Biochem. Pharmacol.*, **16**, 631–636 (1967).

9. Kawazoe, Y., Uehara, N., and Araki, M. Studies on chemical carcinogens. XI. Metabolism of tritiated carcinogenic 4-nitroquinoline 1-oxide and distribution of its metabolites in mouse. *Gann*, **60**, 617–629 (1969).

10. Laishes, B. and Stich, H. F. Repair synthesis and sedimentation analysis of DNA of human cells exposed to dimethylnitrosamine and activated dimethylnitrosamine. *Biochem. Biophys. Res. Commun.*, **52**, 827–833 (1973).

11. Laishes, B. A. and Stich, H. F. Relative DNA damage induced in cultured human skin fibroblasts by exposure to the precarcinogen, 2-acetylaminofluorene, the proximate carcinogen, N-hydroxy-2-acetylaminofluorene and the ultimate carcinogen, N-acetoxy-2-acetylaminofluorene. *Can. J. Biochem.*, **51**, 990–994 (1973).

12. Malling, H. V. Dimethylnitrosamine: Formation of mutagenic compounds by interaction with mouse liver microsomes. *Mutat. Res.*, **13**, 425–429 (1971).

13. Marquardt, H., Kuroki, T., Huberman, E., Selkirk, J. K., Heidelberger, C., Grover, P. L., and Sims, P. Malignant transformation of cells derived from mouse prostate by epoxides and other derivatives of polycyclic hydrocarbons. *Cancer Res.*, **32**, 716–720 (1972).

14 McGrath, R. A. and Williams, R. W. Reconstruction *in vivo* of irradiated *Escherichia coli* deoxyribonucleic acid; the rejoining of broken pieces. *Nature*, **212**, 534–535 (1966).

15. Miller, J. A. Carcinogenesis by chemicals: An overview. *Cancer Res.*, **30**, 559–576 (1970).

16. Miller, J. A. and Miller, E. C. Metabolic activation of carcinogenic amines and amides *via* N-hydroxylation and N-hydroxyesterification and its relationship of ultimate carcinogens as electrophilic reactants. *In* "The Jerusalem Symposia on Quantum Chemistry and Biochemistry. Physico-chemical Mechanisms of Carcinogenesis," ed. by E. D. Bergmann and B. Pullman, Israel Academy of Sciences and Humanities, Jerusalem, Vol. 1, p. 237 (1969).

17. Mori, K. and Kondo, M. Induction of pulmonary tumors by a single dose of 4-nitroquinoline 1-oxide injected in newborn mice. A consideration on renewal of tissue cells in carcinogenesis. *Gann*, **57**, 543–548 (1966).

18. Mori, K. Carcinoma of the glandular stomach of mice by instillation of 4-nitro-quinoline 1-oxide. *Gann*, **58**, 389–393 (1967).

19. Nakahara, W., Fukuoka, F., and Sakai, S. The relation between carcinogenicity and chemical structure of certain quinoline derivatives. *Gann*, **49**, 33–41 (1958).

20. Rasmussen, R. E. and Painter, R. B. Radiation-stimulated DNA synthesis in cultured mammalian cells. *J. Cell Biol.*, **29**, 11–19 (1966).

21. Stewart, B. W. and Farber, E. Induction by a hepatic carcinogen, 1-nitroso-5,6-dihydrouracil, of single- and double-strand breaks of liver DNA with rapid repair. *Biochem. Biophys. Res. Commun.*, **53**, 773–779 (1973).

22. Stich, H. F. and San, R. H. C. DNA repair and chromatid anomalies in mammalian cells exposed to 4-nitroquinoline 1-oxide. *Mutat. Res.*, **10**, 389–404 (1970).

23. Stich, H. F., San, R. H. C., and Kawazoe, Y. DNA repair synthesis in mammalian

cells exposed to a series of oncogenic and non-oncogenic derivatives of 4-nitro-quinoline 1-oxide. *Nature*, **229**, 416–419 (1971).

24. Stich, H. F. and San, R. H. C. DNA repair synthesis in Xeroderma pigmentosum cells exposed to the oncogenic 4-nitroquinoline 1-oxide. *Mutat. Res.*, **13**, 279–282 (1971).

25. Stich, H. F., San, R. H. C., Miller, J. A., and Miller, E. C. Various levels of DNA repair synthesis in Xeroderma pigmentosum cells exposed to the carcinogenic N-hydroxy- and N-acetoxy-2-acetylaminofluorene. *Nature New Biol.*, **238**, 9–10 (1972).

26. Stich, H. F., Hammerberg, O., and Casto, B. The combined effect of chemical mutagen and virus on DNA repair, chromosome aberration and neoplastic trans-formation. *Can. J. Genet. Cytol.*, **14**, 911–917 (1972).

27. Stich, H. F. and San, R. H. C. DNA repair synthesis and cell survival of repair deficient human cells exposed to the K-region epoxide of benz(a)anthracene. *Proc. Soc. Exp. Biol. Med.*, **142**, 155–158 (1973).

28. Stich, H. F., San, R. H. C., and Kawazoe, Y. Increased sensitivity of Xeroderma pigmentosum cells to some chemical carcinogens and mutagens. *Mutat. Res.*, **17**, 127–137 (1973).

29. Stich, H. F. The link between oncogenicity of 4NQO and 4NPO derivatives, induction of DNA lesion and enhancement of viral transformation. *In* "Topics in Chemical Carcinogenesis," ed. by W. Nakahara, S. Takayama, T. Sugimura, and S. Odashima, University Park Press, Baltimore, pp. 17–28 (1972).

30. Stich, H. F., Stich, W., and San, R. H. C. Chromosome aberrations in Xeroderma pigmentosum cells exposed to the carcinogens 4-nitroquinoline 1-oxide and N-methyl-N'-nitro-nitrosoguanidine. *Proc. Soc. Exp. Biol. Med.*, **142**, 1141–1144 (1973).

31. Stich, H. F., Kieser, D., Laishes, B. A., and San, R. H. C. The use of DNA repair in the identification of carcinogens, precarcinogens and target tissue. *In* "Proc. 10th Cancer Conference," ed. by P. S. Scholefield, Univ. of Toronto Press, Toronto, Vol. 10, pp. 83–110 (1973).

32. Stich, H. F. and Laishes, B. A. DNA repair and chemical carcinogens. *In* "Patho-biology Annual," ed. by H. L. Ioachim, Appleton-Century-Crofts, New York, pp. 341–376 (1973).

33. Stich, H. F. and Kieser, D. Use of DNA repair synthesis in detecting organotropic actions of chemical carcinogens. *Proc. Soc. Exp. Biol. Med.*, in press (1974).

34. Takayama, S. and Oota, K. Induction of malignant tumors in various strains of mice by oral administration of dimethylnitrosamine and diethylnitrosamine. *Gann*, **56**, 189–199 (1965).

35. Terracini, B., Palestro, G., Gigliardi, M. R., and Montesano, R. Carcinogenicity of dimethylnitrosamine in Swiss mice. *Brit. J. Cancer*, **20**, 871–876 (1966).

36. Toth, B., Magee, P. N., and Shubik, P. Carcinogenesis study with dimethylnitro-samine administered orally to adult and subcutaneously to newborn BALB/c mice. *Cancer Res.*, **24**, 1712–1721 (1964).

37. Vesselinovitch, S. D. The sex-dependent difference in the development of liver tumors in mice administered dimethylnitrosamine. *Cancer Res.*, **29**, 1024–1027 (1969).

GANN Monograph on Cancer Research 17, 17–29 (1975)

AN APPROACH TO THE DETECTION OF POSSIBLE ETIOLOGIC FACTORS IN HUMAN GASTRIC CANCER[*1]

Hideya ENDO, Koichi TAKAHASHI, Norihiko KINOSHITA, Tadami UTSUNOMIYA, and Tsuneo BABA

Cancer Research Institute, Faculty of Medicine, Kyushu University[*2]

In view of the potent gastric carcinogenicity of the well-known mutagen, N-methyl-N′-nitro-N-nitrosoguanidine (MNNG) which is formed by nitrosation of N-methyl-N′-nitroguanidine (MNG) under acidic conditions, MNNG-like compounds were surveyed by examining the mutagenicity of some food components structurally similar to MNG after nitrosation in actual and simulated human gastric juice. Among 15 food components having a guanido group in their molecules, methylguanidine showed a potent mutagenicity after nitrosation for a strain of *Salmonella typhimurium*, at neutral pH, and the mutagenic principle was identified to be methylnitrosocyanamide (MNC). The mutagenic activity of MNC was about 10 times higher for the strain than that of MNNG. MNC was shown to be similar to MNNG in its mutagenic quality. MNC obtained by organic synthesis in analytically pure form was given orally to rats by dissolving it in drinking water (6.9 mg/day/kg body weight). In all cases of 14 rats that survived more than 11 months, tumors were seen in the forestomach. They were diagnosed as squamous cell carcinoma except for one case that was still in a papillomatous stage. In the glandular stomach, a bean-sized tumor was seen in one and small nodules in 5 cases among the 14. The former was of malignant nature and the latter were polyploid hyperplasia of mucosa. Minute esophageal cancers were also seen in 3 out of 7 cases so far examined.

Regarding the cause for the high incidence of gastric cancer in Japan, peculiar food custom of the Japanese has been discussed on the basis of epidemiological studies but we are still quite ignorant not only of the etiologic factors for human gastric cancer but also of rational means to detect them.

Working Hypothesis and Experimental Design

In order to approach the solution of the problem, the present study was undertaken following two series of works that suggested an essential clue. One

---

[*1] A part of work outlined in this paper was published in *Nature*, **245**, 325 (1973), *Biochem. Biophys. Res. Commun.*, **54**, 1384 (1973), and *Proc. Japan Acad.*, **50**, 497 (1974).

[*2] Maidashi 3-1-1, Higashi-ku, Fukuoka 812, Japan (遠藤英也, 高橋耕一, 木下徳彦, 宇都宮忠実, 馬場恒男).

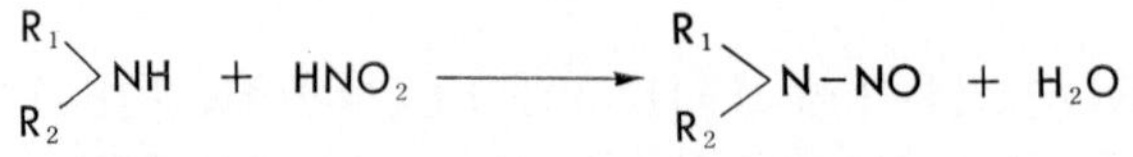

$$\begin{array}{c} R_1 \\ R_2 \end{array}\!\!>\!\!NH \ + \ HNO_2 \longrightarrow \begin{array}{c} R_1 \\ R_2 \end{array}\!\!>\!\!N-NO \ + \ H_2O$$

FIG. 1. Intragastric formation of N-nitroso compounds from nitrite and secondary amine

$$NO_2\,NH-C\!\!\begin{array}{c} \\ \\ \| \\ NH \end{array}\!\!\begin{array}{c} CH_3 \\ >N-NO \\ \\ \end{array}$$

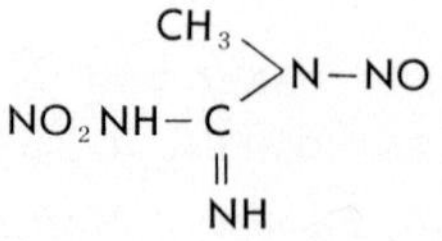

FIG. 2.   N-Methyl-N′-nitro-N-nitrosoguanidine (MNNG)

$$NO_2\,NH-C\!\!\begin{array}{c} CH_3 \\ >NH \\ \| \\ NH \end{array} + \ HNO_2 \longrightarrow NO_2\,NH-C\!\!\begin{array}{c} CH_3 \\ >N-NO \\ \| \\ NH \end{array} + \ H_2O$$

MNG   MNNG

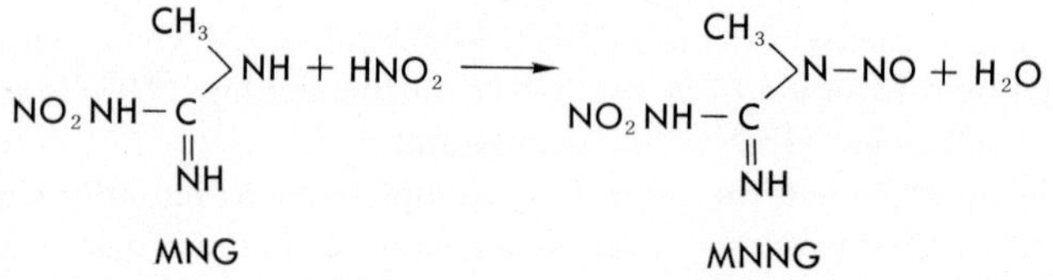

FIG. 3.   Nitrosation of MNG with sodium nitrite under acidic conditions

is the intragastric formation of N-nitroso compounds from nitrite and secondary amine or amides (Fig. 1) which have been extensively studied since the pioneering works of Druckrey et al. (4) and Sander (16). The other is the study of Sugimura et al. (19–21) on an animal model of gastric cancer. They succeeded in demonstrating a high frequency of cancer in the glandular stomach of rodents and the stomach of dogs by oral application of the well-known mutagen, N-methyl-N′-nitro-N-nitrosoguanidine (MNNG) (1, 11) (Fig. 2). This compound, MNNG, is a typical N-nitroso compound and was reported by McKay et al. (12) to be synthesized easily and in a good yield by nitrosation of N-methyl-N′-nitro-guanidine (MNG) under acidic conditions (Fig. 3).

Based on these facts, we assumed that human gastric cancer may at least partly be caused by MNNG-like compounds which could be formed by intragastric nitrosation of certain food components structurally similar to MNG (Fig. 4). It seems reasonable to expect that such MNNG-like compound would be mutagenic. From this point of view, we designed our experiments as follows: (1) to list food components structurally similar to MNG, (2) to select such compounds that show mutagenicity after nitrosation in human gastric juice out of food components listed above, (3) to identify the active principle responsible for mutagenicity, (4) to synthesize the identified compounds, and (5) to subject them to carcinogenesis experiment in animals by oral administration.

$$\begin{array}{ccc} \text{MNG-like} & & \text{MNNG-like} \\ & + \ HNO_2 \longrightarrow & \\ \text{food component} & & \text{compound} \end{array}$$

FIG. 4.   Proposed mechanism for the formation of possible etiologic factors in human gastric cancer

Mutagenic Assay of MNG-like Food Components Nitrosated in Gastric Juice

First, 15 naturally occurring guanidine derivatives (Table I) were selected, since they were considered to be more or less similar to MNG in structure in such a sense as to contain guanido group in their molecules. Each guanidine derivative was incubated for 2 hr at 37° with sodium nitrite in simulated gastric juice (VII Japanese Pharmacopoeia) in a molar ratio of 1: 1: 1.3 (as hydrochloric acid in simulated gastric juice). The reaction mixture was then neutralized with

TABLE I.   Naturally Occurring Guanidines

1. L-Arginine
2. Acetyl-L-arginine
3. Agmatine
4. Canavanine
5. D-Octopine
6. Creatine
7. Creatine phosphate
8. Creatinine
9. γ-Guanidinobutyric acid
10. γ-Guanidino-β-hydroxybutyric acid
11. Glycocyamine
12. Methylguanidine
13. Phosphoarginine
14. Arginosuccinate
15. Taurocyamine

sodium carbonate, sterilized by Millipore filtration, serially diluted, and spotted on the lawns of test bacteria which had been plated on semi-enriched minimal agar (2), 1 hr in advance. After incubation of the bacterial plate at 37° for about 2 days, the appearance of revertants was examined and the maximum dilution showing the mutagenicity was determined. The test bacteria used for the mutagenicity assay were deep rough derivatives of histidine-requiring strains of *Salmonella typhimurium* carrying gal-bio-uvrB deletion (3). Strain TA1535 is to identify mutagens causing base-pair substitutions and TA1536, TA1537, and TA1538 are to identify mutagens causing various types of frameshift mutations. As shown in Photo 1(a), a large number of colonies of strain TA1535 appeared after spotting with undiluted reaction mixture containing nitrite and methyl-guanidine (MG). Ten colonies randomly picked from the plate were all his[+] and as sensitive to ultraviolet radiation as TA1535. Controls lacking MG (Photo 1(b)) or nitrite (Photo 1(c)) produced an average of only 6 or 7 colonies. There-fore, the colonies shown in Photo 1(a) are almost certainly his[+] revertants of TA1535 which appear because a mutagen causing base-pair substitutions is pro-duced in the reaction mixture. Nitrosated MG was found to be mutagenic up to 16-fold dilution of the original reaction mixture. All the other guanidines tested failed to show mutagenicity detectable by this spot test. Mutagenicity of MG nitrosated in human gastric juice was also studied by the spot test for TA1535.

H. ENDO ET AL.

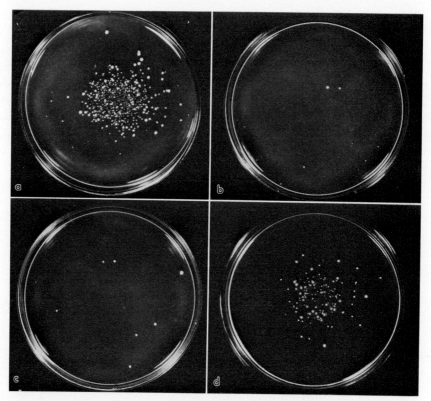

PHOTO 1. Spot tests demonstrating mutagenicity of nitrosated MG

(a) Reaction mixture, containing 4 ml of simulated gastric juice, 0.2 mmole of MG, and 0.22 mmole of $NaNO_2$ in a total volume of 5 ml, was spotted on TA1535 after treating it as described. (b) Control mixture lacking MG was spotted in the same manner with (a). (c) Control mixture lacking $NaNO_2$ was spotted in the same manner with (a). (d) The same reaction mixture with (a) except that human gastric juice, pH 1.2, was used instead of simulated gastric juice was spotted in the same manner with (a).

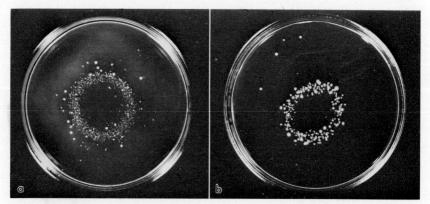

PHOTO 2. Spot test demonstrating mutagenicity of nitrosated MNG

(a) The same reaction mixture with Photo 1 (a) except that 0.2 mmole of MNG was used instead of MG and spotted in the same manner as in Photo 1. (b) The same reaction mixture with Photo 1 (d) except that 0.2 mmole of MNG was used instead of MG and spotted in the same manner as in Photo 1.

Fresh samples of gastric juice with pH 1.2, 1.3, 1.4, and 3.4 were obtained from 4 patients with gastric ulcer and used in the reaction mixture instead of simulated gastric juice. The reaction mixture containing human gastric juice of pH 1.2 again showed the appearance of many revertant colonies (Photo 1(d)). Those with pH 1.3 and 1.4 showed the same results whereas that with pH 3.4 failed to show the revertant colony formation. MG nitrosated in human gastric juice of pH 1.2 was mutagenic up to 16-fold dilution of the reaction mixture, like MG nitrosated in simulated gastric juice.

Next, in order to compare the mutagenic potency of nitrosated MG with that of nitrosated MNG, MNG was treated with nitrite in both gastric juice with pH 1.2 in the same conditions as described above. As shown in Photo 2(a) and Photo 2(b), a ring of revertant colonies was formed on TA1535 plate by spotting MNG nitrosated in simulated gastric juice and human gastric juice undiluted. MNG nitrosated in human gastric juice was mutagenic up to 32-fold dilution. This means that the mutagenic activity of nitrosated MG is about one-half of that of nitrosated MNG.

Identification of the Mutagenic Principle of Nitrosated MG

Now, the question is, what is the active principle responsible for the mutagenicity of MG nitrosated in both kinds of gastric juice. In previous papers (*5, 6*) we reported that two arginine derivatives, benzoylarginineamide (BAA) and acetylarginineamide (AAA), when nitrosated under weakly acidic conditions, showed a powerful mutagenicity for TA1535 and their mutagenic principles were 4-benzoylamido-4-carboxamido-N-nitrosobutylcyanamide and 4-acetamido-4-carboxamido-N-nitrosobutylcyanamide, respectively. These results led us immediately to assume that the mutagenic principle of nitrosated MG may be methylnitrosocyanamide (MNC).

Regarding MNG, Mirvish (*13*) first observed its transient formation spectrophotometrically during nitrosation of MG in weakly acidic conditions. He also demonstrated that the final product of nitrosation reaction of MG to be methylnitrosourea (MNU). Mirvish suggested, however, that *in vivo* nitrosation of MG may be not significant for the etiology of human gastric cancer, since the kinetics for *in vitro* nitrosation of MG to give MNU is too slow. Our data on the nitrosated BAA rather suggest that it is the MNC that is the biologically important compound. Bearing this in mind, we attempted to identify the mutagenic principle of MG nitrosated, first, in weakly acidic conditions on a large scale (Table II). From the results of the spot test of the aliquot, the total mutagenic activity of the reaction mixture was 5.12×10^6 units when the critical

TABLE II.   Reaction Mixture (0° for 2 hr)

Methylguanidine hydrochloride	22 g	(200 mmoles)
Sodium nitrite	45.5 g	(660 mmoles)
Conc. HCl	80 ml	(810 mmoles)
Distilled water	500 ml	

Total mutagenic activity: 5.12×10^6 units.

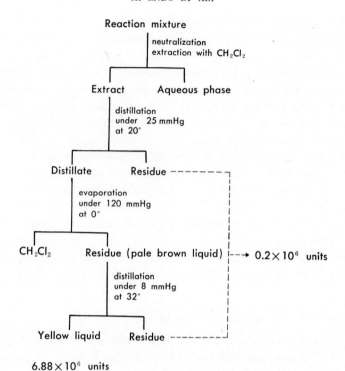

Reaction mixture
│ neutralization
│ extraction with CH_2Cl_2

Extract   Aqueous phase

│ distillation
│ under 25 mmHg
│ at 20°

Distillate   Residue - - - - - - -

│ evaporation
│ under 120 mmHg
│ at 0°

CH_2Cl_2 Residue (pale brown liquid) ⊢→ 0.2×10^6 units

│ distillation
│ under 8 mmHg
│ at 32°

Yellow liquid   Residue - - - - - - - -

6.88×10^6 units

FIG. 5.   Fractional distillation of the mutagenic principle of nitrosated MG

TABLE III.   Physical Properties of Active Principle Responsible for
Mutagenicity of Nitrosated Methylguanidine

Yellow liquid, distilled at 32° under 8 mm Hg
UV, λ_{max} (ε), 402 (106.0), 385 (133.9), and 373 (80.6) nm in ethanol
IR spectrum, typical CN band at 2240 cm^{-1}
Elementary analysis, calcd. for $C_2H_3ON_3$:
              C, 28.24;   H, 3.55;   N, 49.40%
      Found: C, 28.51;   H, 3.54;   N, 48.80%

TABLE IV.   Comparison of the Mutagenicity of MNC with

Tester strain	2.5 μmoles/ml	$\times 1$	$\times 2$	$\times 4$	$\times 8$
TA1535	MNC	K	+	+	+
	MNNG	+	+	+	+
TA1536	MNC	K	−		
	MNNG	−			
TA1537	MNC	K	+	+	+
	MNNG	+	+	+	+
TA1538	MNC	K	−		
	MNNG	−			

Plus and minus signs mean positive and negative revertant formations, respectively, and K means concentration to show mutagenicity for TA1535 is defined as 1 unit/ml. Meanwhile, the reaction mixture was extracted with methylene chloride and the extract was subjected to fractional distillation as shown in Fig. 5. It was found that the mutagenic activity of the final yellowish distillate was 6.88×10^6 units. This means that the total mutagenic activity of the original reaction mixture was almost completely recovered in this fraction. The physical properties of this yellowish distillate was analyzed and it was identified to be MNC (Table III). The same identification experiments were also carried out using simulated gastric juice on a large scale, and we reached the same conclusion as above although, in this case, the yield of MNC in the reaction mixture was calculated by comparing UV absorption at 385 nm with that of authentic MNC.

Comparison of the Properties of MNC with Those of MNNG

The mutagenic activity of MNC was surprisingly high. Namely, 2.5 μmoles/ml of MNC showed mutagenicity for TA1535 at up to 2,560-fold dilution, while the same concentration of MNNG was mutagenic up to 256-fold dilution. This means that the mutagenic activity of MNC is about 10 times higher than that of MNNG at neutral pH. MNC and MNNG also showed mutagenic effect for TA1537 up to 256- and 16-fold dilutions, respectively, but no activity for TA1536 and TA1538 strains. These results are summarized in Table IV. Especially noteworthy is the fact that the ratio of mutagenic potency of MNC and MNNG for TA1535 is about the same as that for TA1537. This implies the qualitative similarity of the two compounds in their mutagenicity.

MNC is stable in water under interception of light, but considerably labile in gastric juice compared with MNNG. Chemical half-life of MNC in simulated gastric juice was spectrophotometrically found to be 5.5 min, while that of MNNG was 110 min.

Organic Synthesis of MNC

Regarding the organic synthesis of MNC, we followed the method of Mirvish et al. (14). Crude methylcyanamide was synthesized from methylamine and cyano-

That of MNNG for *S. typhimurium* Strains

	Dilution								
×16	×32	×64	×128	×256	×512	×1,024	×2,048	×2,560	×4,096
+	+	+	+	+	+	+	+	+	−
+	+	+	+	+	−				
+	+	+	+	+	−				
+	−								

no colony was formed by killing action of the drug.

TABLE V. Physical Properties of the Compound Used for
the Carcinogenesis Experiment

IR spectrum, typical CN band at 2240 cm^{-1}
Elementary analysis, calcd. for $C_2H_3ON_3$:
        C, 28.24; H, 3.55; N, 49.40
   Found: C, 27.99; H, 3.64; N, 48.83
GC-MS[a]

Retention time (min)	m/e of M$^+$
0.7	28
1.4	57
9.2	85 main peak

MS[b] of peak 9.2 min, m/e (relative intensity):
  85 (4), 57 (2), 56 (7), 55 (12), 54 (18), 53 (64),
  43 (4), 41 (2), 40 (2), 32 (3), 30 (100), 29 (9)

   [a] Conditions: instrument, JEOL, JOC-2O-K; OV-17 10% on Chromosorb W AWDMCS; column temp. 50°. [b] Instrument: JEOL, JMS-D100; ionizing voltage 25 eV.

gen bromide, and then nitrosated. The MNC thus obtained was further subjected to differential distillation since they reported that MNC could not be prepared in analytically pure state. The fraction distilled under 8 mm Hg, at 32° was identified to be analytically pure as shown in Table V and was used for the carcinogenesis experiment.

Induction of Gastric and Esophageal Cancer in Rats by the Administration of MNC

The following carcinogenesis experiments were carried out; twenty Sprague-Dawley female rats initially weighing an average of 200 g were fed commercial CE-2 animal diet freely and given 25 ml/rat/day of drinking water in which MNC

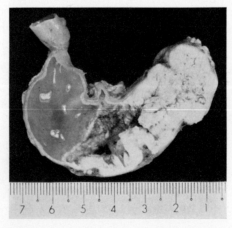

PHOTO 3. Stomach of a rat killed after administration of MNC solution (6.9 mg/rat/day) for 358 days
Note a huge tumor formation in the forestomach.

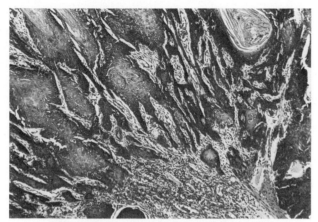

PHOTO 4. Histological appearance of the tumor shown in Photo 3; typical squamous cell carcinoma
Extensive invasion to the underlying connective tissues is evident.

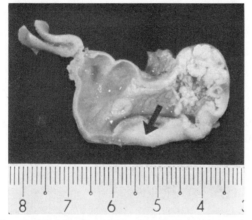

PHOTO 5. Three independent tumors seen in the stomach; one in the forestomach (right), other two in the glandular stomach
The larger tumor (arrow) of the glandular stomach corresponds to Photo 6.

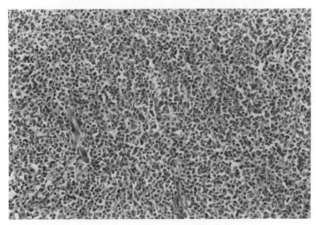

PHOTO 6. A malignant reticulum cell sarcoma-like lesion
Uniform distribution of irregularily shaped tumor cells which invade normal structures.

was dissolved so as to contain 1/10 of its oral LD_{50} (69 mg/kg) for mice (initial concentration, 56 mg/liter). Experimental rats grew at the same rate as controls. The effective 14 animals surviving more than 11 months on continuous MNC had large tumors in their forestomach (Photo 3), some of which reached the size of a hen's egg and were histologically diagnosed as squamous cell carcinoma (Photo 4), except one which was a squamous cell papilloma. In the glandular region of the stomach, a bean-sized tumor with a shallow ulcer was seen in one case (Photo 5) and small nodules in five cases among the 14, one of which is

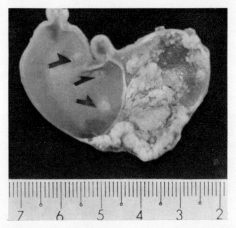

PHOTO 7. Three different mucosal lesion (arrows) in the glandular stomach, associated with forestomach carcinoma

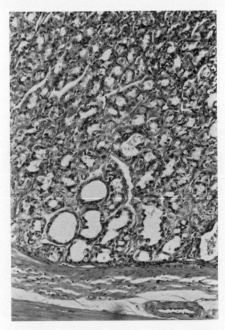

PHOTO 8. A basal portion of the mucosa of a hyperplastic nodular lesion of the glandular stomach indicated in Photo 7

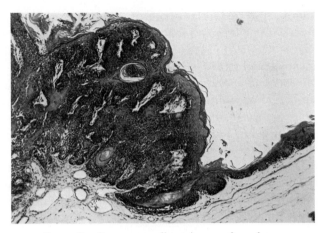

PHOTO 9.   Squamous cell carcinoma of esophagus

shown in Photo 7. The former was of malignant nature, but its histological diagnosis was difficult to make in spite of the use of various staining methods as to whether it was a reticulum cell sarcoma or an anaplastic carcinoma (Photo 6). The latter was polypoid hyperplasia with small foci of cystic dilatation and atypical arrangements in the mucosa (Photo 8). In the esophagus of 7 rats so far examined, 3 to 4 millet-like tiny nodules were seen in each case. In 3 cases, they were diagnosed as squamous cell carcinoma (Photo 9). Organs other than the stomach and the esophagus were unaffected. Among the other animals which died by the 200th day, papillomas were found in the forestomach in two cases. These results clearly indicate that MNC is strongly carcinogenic, especially to the forestomach of rats. The production of esophageal cancer by MNC seems to be reasonable, since the epithelium of esophagus and forestomach is histologically of the same origin. From the environmental point of view, rather noteworthy is the fact that in the glandular region of the stomach, precancerous change does occur by MNC in several cases besides malignant tumor formation in one case. This implies that the carcinogenic actions of MNC and MNNG to the stomach may be essentially the same and their apparent difference in the frequency for cancer induction in the forestomach or in the glandular stomach may be merely due to the difference in the reactivity and stability of the two compounds.

Source of MG and Nitrite

MG has been reported to be contained in fresh beef (*7, 9*), ray (*8*), cod (*7*), sardine (*17*), and especially in shark (*8*) in high concentrations (1,900 mg/kg wet weight), but contrary to these old positive results, there have also been negative reports on its natural occurrence (*10, 18*). So, the careful reinvestigation should be made on the quantitative estimation of MG in various foodstuffs. Regarding the origin of nitrite capable of reacting with MG in stomach, the first to consider is nitrite added to food as a preservative. This does not seem, however, to be important because the amount of nitrite as food additive is strictly limited legally.

Attention should be directed to the fact that instead of nitrite, nitrate and halophilic bacteria with high nitrate reductase activity are added to certain food-stuff. The second is nitrite converted by bacterial reduction from nitrate in food (15). This seems to be more important in connection with a peculiar food habit of the Japanese who eat *tsukemono* (vegetables pickled in salt or in salted rice bran). In fact, Tanimura *et al.* demonstrated the great increase in the amount of nitrite in cucumbers and cabbages 20 hr after salting them (personal communication). The third is nitrite which is formed by *in vivo* reduction from nitrate in ingested vegetables, circulated in blood, and secreted from salivary gland. Recently, Tanimura and Harada (22) also showed a transient but great increase of nitrate with concomitant rise of nitrite in saliva after ingesting vegetables. Considering that the daily amount of saliva swallowed in our stomach reaches about 1.5 liters, this route may eventually be the most important for the source of nitrite.

Further Studies

The present study provided evidence that gastric cancer, though not adeno-carcinoma, was produced in animals by MNC, which is formed from a possible food component, MG, after nitrosation in human gastric juice. It is quite interesting but we do not yet know whether MNC is really involved in the incidence of human gastric cancer. We are performing now following experiments.
1) Quantitative estimation of MG in various foodstuffs.
2) Quantitative estimation of MNC intragastrically formed by concurrent administration of MG and sodium nitrite.
3) Oral administration of MNC to rabbits and guinea pigs both with only a glandular stomach, in expectation of occurrence of adenocarcinoma with metastasis.
4) Concurrent administration of MG and sodium nitrite to rats and rabbits in expectation of gastric cancer formation.

Acknowledgments

This work was supported by grants from the Ministry of Education and the Ministry of Health and Welfare of Japan, from the Society for the Promotion of Cancer Research, and from the Princess Takamatsu Cancer Research Fund. We are indebted to Dr. B. N. Ames, Biochemistry Department, University of California, for his gift of tester bacteria. Grateful acknowledgment is also made to Dr. M. Hamana and Dr. K. Aoki in Kyushu University for their invaluable suggestions on this work.

REFERENCES

1. Adelberg, E. A., Mandel, M., and Ching Chen, G. C. Optimal conditions for mutagenicity by N-methyl-N'-nitro-N-nitrosoguanidine in *Escherichia coli* K12. *Biochem. Biophys. Res. Commun.*, **18**, 788–795 (1965).
2. Ames, B. N. The detection of chemical mutagens with enteric bacteria. *In* "Chemical Mutagen; Principles and Methods for their Detection," ed. by A. Hollaender, Plenum Press, New York, Vol. 1, pp. 267–282 (1971).
3. Ames, B. N., Lee, G. D., and Durston, W. E. An improved bacterial test system

for the detection and classification of mutagens and carcinogens. *Proc. Natl. Acad. Sci. U.S.*, **70**, 782–786 (1973).

4. Druckrey, H., Steinhoff, D., Beuthner, H., Schneider, H., and Klärner, P. Prüfung von Nitrit auf chronisch-toxische Wirkung an Ratten. *Arzneimittel-forschung*, **13**, 320–323 (1963).

5. Endo, H. and Takahashi, K. A nitrosated arginine derivative, a powerful mutagen. *Biochem. Biophys. Res. Commun.*, **52**, 254–262 (1973).

6. Endo, H., Takahashi, K., and Aoyagi, H. Screening of compounds structurally and functionally related to N-methyl-N'-nitro-N-nitrosoguanidine, a gastric carcinogen. *Gann*, **65**, 45–54 (1974).

7. Kapeller-Adler, R. and Krael, J. Untersuchungen über die Stickstoffverteilung in den Muskeln verschiedener Tierklassen. I. *Biochem. Z.*, **221**, 437–460 (1930).

8. Kapeller-Adler, R. and Krael, J. Untersuchungen über die Stickstoffverteilung in den Muskeln verschiedener Tierklassen. II. Über die Stickstoffverteilung im Rochen- und Haifisch-muskel. *Biochem. Z.*, **224**, 364–377 (1930).

9. Komarrow, S. A. Über das Vorkommen des präformierten Methylguanidins im Muskelgewebe. *Biochem. Z.*, **211**, 326–351 (1929).

10. Makizumi, S. Paper chromatography of guanidine compounds. *Nippon Kagaku Zasshi*, **73**, 737–739 (1952) (in Japanese).

11. Mandell, J. D. and Greenberg, J. A. A new chemical mutagen for bacteria, 1-methyl-3-nitro-1-nitrosoguanidine. *Biochem. Biophys. Res. Commun.*, **3**, 575–577 (1960).

12. McKay, A. F. and Wright, G. F. Preparation and properties of N-methyl-N-nitroso-N'-nitroguanidine. *J. Am. Chem. Soc.*, **69**, 3028–3030 (1947).

13. Mirvish, S. S. Kinetics of nitrosamide formation from alkylureas, N-alkylurethans and alkylguanidines: Possible implications for the etiology of human gastric cancer. *J. Natl. Cancer Inst.*, **46**, 1183–1193 (1971).

14. Mirvish, S. S., Nagel, D. L., and Sams, J. Methyl- and ethylnitrosocyanamide, some properties and reactions. *J. Org. Chem.*, **38**, 1325–1329 (1973).

15. Raineri, R. and Weisburger, J. H. Role of the reduction of dietary nitrate to nitrite in the etiology of gastric cancer. *Proc. Am. Assoc. Cancer Res.*, **15**, 39 (1974).

16. Sander, J. Kann Nitrit in der menschlichen Nahrung Ursache einer Krebsentstehung durch Nitrosaminbildung sein? *Arch. Hyg. Bakteriol.*, **151**, 22–28 (1967).

17. Sasaki, A. Über die Extraktivstoffe des Sardinenfleisches (Maiwashi, *Sardinia melanosticta*). *Tohoku J. Exp. Med.*, **34**, 561–570 (1938).

18. Shibuya, S. and Makizumi, S. Biochemical studies on guanidine compounds (VIII). *Seikagaku (Japan. J. Biochem. Soc.)*, **25**, 210–213 (1953) (in Japanese).

19. Sugimura, T. and Fujimura, S. Tumour production in glandular stomach of rat by N-methyl-N'-nitro-N-nitrosoguanidine. *Nature*, **216**, 943–944 (1967).

20. Sugimura, T., Fujimura, S., and Baba, T. Tumor production in the glandular stomach and alimentary tract of the rat by N-methyl-N'-nitro-N-nitrosoguanidine. *Cancer Res.*, **30**, 455–465 (1970).

21. Sugimura, T., Fujimura, S., Kosuge, K., Baba, T., Saito, T., Nagao, M., Hosoi, H., Shimosato, Y., and Yokoshima, T. Production of adenocarcinomas in glandular stomach of experimental animals by N-methyl-N'-nitro-N-nitrosoguanidine. *GANN Monograph*, **8**, 157–196 (1969).

22. Tanimura, A. and Harada, M. Studies on *in vivo* formation of nitroso compounds. Nitrite and nitrate contained in human saliva. *Shokuhin Eiseigaku Zasshi (J. Food Hyg. Soc. Japan)*, **15**, 206–207 (1974) (in Japanese).

GANN Monograph on Cancer Research 17, 31–38 (1975)

CHROMOSOME ABERRATIONS OF CULTURED YOSHIDA SARCOMA CELLS INDUCED BY 4-NITROQUINOLINE 1-OXIDE AND RELATED CHEMICALS[*1]

Hidehiko Isaka[*2]

*Sasaki Institute[*3]*

Chromosome aberrations of cultured Yoshida sarcoma cells induced by 4-nitroquinoline 1-oxide (4NQO) derivatives were mainly chromatid gaps, chromatid breaks, and chromatid exchanges. Frequencies of chromatid breaks and exchanges induced by most carcinogenic 4NQO derivatives were greater than those by non-carcinogenic 4NQO derivative, as far as examined.

Carcinogenicity of chemical substances can be ascertained only by animal experiments, although the organ and incidence of tumors induced by chemical carcinogens can vary greatly according to the method of administration and animal species used. It is a problem whether a chemical substance capable of inducing malignant tumors in experimental animals may show any carcinogenicity in man. However, the chemical should be considered as a potential carcinogen.

In order to select potential carcinogens from numerous chemical substances, it is hoped that suspicious substances could be screened adequately before performing animal experiments. A simple and reliable method for screening is strongly required, but none of the methods available at present is sufficient by its single criterion alone.

Many agents including X rays, alkylating agents, and viruses are cytotoxic and capable of inducing chromosome aberrations such as chromatid breaks and exchanges, which suggest mutagenic action of the agents on mammalian cells *in vitro*. It is likely that chromosomally aberrant cells induced by certain carcinogens may no longer proliferate, but some of the slightly damaged cells, even though invisibly injured, may have proliferating potency and develop to cancer cells with visible chromosome rearrangement during their subsequent growth. When chromosome aberrations are induced in cultured cells by a chemical carcinogen, it is probable that similar types of aberrations can also be induced on the same cells by related and derivative carcinogens. If so, a capacity to induce chromosome aberrations may provide an indicator for screening carcinogens from

[*1] This work was supported by the Subsidy for Cancer Research from the Ministry of Health and Welfare and a Grant-in-Aid for Cancer Research from the Ministry of Education, Japan.

[*2] Present address: Department of Pathology, Kagoshima University School of Medicine, Kagoshima 890, Japan.

[*3] Surugadai 2-chome, Kanda, Chiyoda-ku, Tokyo 101, Japan (井坂英彦).

suspicious related compounds, although different series of carcinogens may show discrepancies in relationship between their mutagenicity and carcinogenicity.

In the present experiment, chromosome aberrations in Yoshida sarcoma cells induced *in vitro* by 4-nitroquinoline 1-oxide (4NQO) and its related compounds were studied. 4NQO has a wide variety of carcinogenic and non-carcinogenic relatives and is capable of inducing chromosome aberrations on various kinds of cells (*3, 5, 9, 17*).

Chromosome Aberrations of 4NQO-treated Cells

Chromosome aberrations of cultured Yoshida sarcoma cells induced by 4NQO, a strong carcinogen, were studied (*5*). Yoshida sarcoma cells with 40

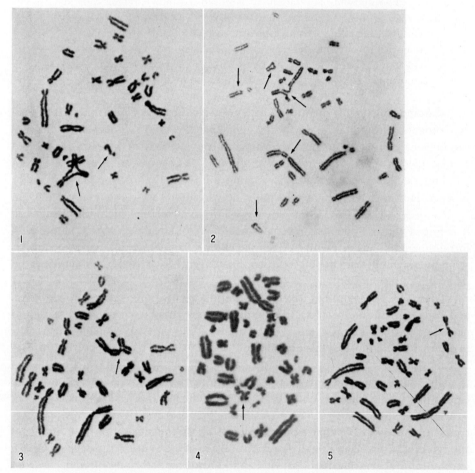

Chromatid break and chromatid exchange in cultured Yoshida sarcoma cells (indicated by arrows)
PHOTO 1.   Control, 48 hr
PHOTO 2.   4NQO-treated, 48 hr
PHOTO 3.   6 Cl·4NQO-treated, 8 hr
PHOTO 4.   3 Me·4NQO-treated, 8 hr
PHOTO 5.   3 F·4NQO-treated, 8 hr. Satellite association

chromosomes in the modal region were used because these rapidly growing tumor cells are easily cultured. Methods for this experiment were as follows: tumor cells were harvested from Donryu rats bearing the Yoshida ascites sarcoma 4 days after intraperitoneal transplantation. The cells were cultured in a petri dish of 50 mm diameter at 37° in a static culture with a gas phase of 5% CO_2 and 95% air. Culture medium was Eagle's minimum essential medium (Nissui Seiyaku Co., Tokyo), supplemented with 10% calf serum and 0.1% Bactopeptone (Difco, U.S.A.). Inoculum size was 5×10^4 cells/ml. They grew floating as individually isolated cells. An almost exponential growth was seen for 48 hr after 24 culture hour (Fig. 1). 4NQO was added to the medium 10 min before the cultivation of cells in a final concentration of 10^{-4}, 10^{-5}, 10^{-6}, $10^{-6.5}$, 10^{-7}, 10^{-8}, $10^{-8.5}$, or 10^{-9} M. 4NQO was dissolved in a drop of ethanol and diluted with the fresh medium. The final concentration of ethanol in the culture medium was less than 0.1%. The number of cells was counted every 24 hr by the aid of a hemocytometer, in order to examine the minimum concentration of 4NQO which caused the slightest inhibition of growth of cultured cells compared to the control. Thus the minimum growth-inhibitory concentration was determined as 10^{-8} M for 4NQO (Fig. 1).

Chromosome examinations were made on cells treated with 10^{-8} M, the minimum growth-inhibitory concentration, of 4NQO for various periods such as 4, 13, 15, 24, 30, 48, 72, and 90 hr. Specimens were made by the air-drying method. A final concentration of colchicine, 10^{-6} M, was added to the medium 2 hr before collecting the cells. They were agitated in 0.05 M NaCl solution for 10 min at 37°. After staining with Giemsa solution, well-spread metaphase plates were studied as many as possible, and photomicrographic records were made with a 35-mm film camera.

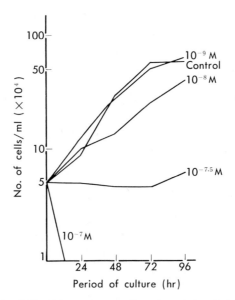

Fig. 1. Growth of Yoshida sarcoma cells cultured *in vitro* in a medium containing various concentrations of 4NQO

H. ISAKA

TABLE I. Chromosome Aberrations in Yoshida Sarcoma Cells
Induced *in Vitro* by 10^{-8} M 4NQO

Period (hr)	4NQO				Control			
	Chromatid break		Chromatid exchange		Chromatid break		Chromatid exchange	
	No.	%	No.	%	No.	%	No.	%
4	13/104	12.5	0/104					
13	3/15	20.0	4/15	26.7				
15	13/69	18.8	24/69	34.8	5/74	6.8	1/74	1.4
24	10/75	13.3	35/75	46.7	3/40	7.5	5/40	12.5
30	0/7		4/7	57.1				
48	3/43	7.0	4/43	9.3	15/163	9.2	20/163	12.3
72	7/98	7.1	7/98	7.1	18/137	13.1	4/137	2.9
90	1/60	1.7	0/60					
96					5/73	6.8	0/73	
Total	50/471	10.6	78/471	16.6	46/487	9.4	30/487	6.2

No. of cells with aberrant chromosomes/total No. of cells examined.

In this examination 471 4NQO-treated cells and 487 control cells were examined for their chromosomes. The predominant chromosome aberrations caused by this chemical were increased chromatid gaps, chromatid breaks, and chromatid exchanges. The abnormalities were found at random in chromosomes of treated cells, as far as examined. Similar aberrant chromosomes occurred spontaneously in the control (Photos 1 and 2), but their frequency was significantly lower compared to the 4NQO-treated group. It was considered that chromatid breaks and chromatid exchanges were the most conspicuous and important chromosome aberrations induced by 4NQO. In the 4NQO-treated group chromatid breaks reached the highest level at 13 culture hour of 20% (Table I), and then chromatid exchanges followed to increase up to 30 culture hour. However, the occurrence of chromatid breaks and exchanges was lower as 13.1% or less in the control. After 72 hr, any differences in frequencies of these chromatid aberrations were not found between the 4NQO-treated and control groups, both groups showing the same karyotype specific to the Yoshida sarcoma. This may imply that Yoshida sarcoma cells with aberrant chromosomes can no longer proliferate and/or those with unchanged chromosomes have the growth advantage.

Chromosome Aberrations Induced by 4NQO and Related Chemicals

Chromosome abnormalities of cultured Yoshida sarcoma cells induced by 4NQO and related substances were studied for comparative purpose. A total of 8 chemicals were tested, including 4NQO, 4-hydroxyaminoquinoline 1-oxide (4HAQO), 6-chloro-4-nitroquinoline 1-oxide (6Cl·4NQO), 6-methyl-4-nitro-quinoline 1-oxide (6Me·4NQO), 3-fluoro-4-nitroquinoline 1-oxide (3F·4NQO), 3-methyl-4-nitroquinoline 1-oxide (3Me·4NQO), 4-nitroquinoline (4NQ), and 4-nitropyridine 1-oxide (4NPO), as indicated in Table II. According to Nakahara

TABLE II.   Carcinogenicity 4NQO and Its
Related Compounds

Compound	Carcinogenicity
4NQO	+
4HAQO	+
6Cl·4NQO	+
6Me·4NQO	+
3F·4NQO	±
3Me·4NQO	±
4NQ	±
4NPO	−

TABLE III.   Chromatid Aberration of Yoshida Sarcoma Cells Induced *in Vitro*
by 4NQO and Its Related Compounds

Substance	Concn. (M)	Nuclei examined	Gap[a]	%	Break and exchange[a]	%	Break and exchange per chromatid (%)[b]
4NQO	10^{-8}	37	2		4		
	$10^{-7.5}$	32	11		2		
		69	13	19.4	6	9.0	0.0023
4HAQO	10^{-7}	51	7		1		
	10^{-6}	11	3		3		
		62	10	16.9	4	6.5	0.0026
6Cl·4NQO	10^{-8}	35	8		0		
	10^{-7}	44	12		7		
		79	20	25.3	7	8.9	0.0062
6Me·4NQO	10^{-7}	36	9	25.0	5	13.5	0.0075
3F·4NQO	10^{-7}	30	5		4		
	10^{-6}	22	4		1		
		52	9	17.3	5	9.6	0.0086
3Me·4NQO	10^{-6}	34	4		0		
	10^{-5}	32	8		4		
		66	12	18.2	4	6.1	0.0033
4NQ	$10^{-6.5}$	17	2	11.8	0		
4NPO	10^{-6}	49	1		0		
	10^{-5}	9	6		0		
		58	7	12.1	0		
Control		48	4	8.3	1	2.1	0.0010

[a] No. of cells with gaps, or, with breaks and/or exchanges.   [b] No. of breaks and/or exchanges × 1/2 × total No. of chromosomes.

and his coworkers (*2, 4, 7, 10–12, 15*), the former four substances are carcinogenic while the last one is non-carcinogenic. The remaining three are weak carcinogens.

The method for chromosome examination was the same as mentioned before, but the examination was made at 8 culture hour exclusively, without paying attention to any prolongation of S and/or G_2 phase of the treated cells. The minimum growth-inhibitory concentration and another slightly higher concentration of the chemicals were used as a rule. The solvent for the chemicals was ethanol or dimethyl sulfoxide and the final concentration of the solvents in the medium never exceeded 0.1%.

Increased chromatid gaps, chromatid breaks, and chromatid exchanges were also found and they were the predominant chromosome aberrations of cells treated with 4NQO and 7 related substances, as shown in Table III. It is interesting that any carcinogenic chemicals, either strong or weak, are capable of frequent chromatid aberrations when compared to the control. 4NQ, a weak carcinogen, and 4NPO, a non-carcinogen, induced no chromatid breaks and/or exchanges. The ratio of chromatid breaks and exchanges to all chromatids of examined cells exceeded 0.002% in 6 carcinogens such as 4NQO, 4HAQO, 6Cl·4NQO, 6Me·4NQO, 3F·4NQO, and 3Me·4NQO, while it was less than 0.001% in 4NQ, 4NPO, and the control. The abnormal features in cells treated with 6Cl·4NQO, 3Me·4NQO, and 3F·4NQO are shown in Photos 3–5.

COMMENTS

The present study was only a preliminary work, comparing chromosome aberrations induced by carcinogenic and non-carcinogenic 4NQO derivatives. These results indicated that 4NQO and its related carcinogens induced frequent chromosome aberrations such as chromatid breaks and exchanges on cultured Yoshida tumor cells, compared to a non-carcinogenic substance, 4NPO. 4NQ was the only exception. The capacity of inducing chromatid aberrations varied in carcinogenic 4NQO derivatives.

Yosida *et al.* (*17*), among Japanese workers who have examined early chromosome aberrations of various cells by 4NQO, stated that the major chromosome abnormalities of Yoshida sarcoma *in vivo* were abnormal elongation of chromosomes, and breakage and translocation of chromatid. In the present study, however, increased gaps, chromatid breaks, and chromatid exchanges were the main features of 4NQO-induced chromosome aberrations. This was also the case in cells treated with 4NQO derivatives. Breaks at chromosome level were not observed in the present study, though reported in human lymphocytes *in vitro* by 4NQO treatment. It is not possible that the solvents for 4NQO derivatives used in this study were responsible for the chromatid aberrations observed (*1*).

Stich *et al.* (*16*) studied DNA synthesis in hamster cells *in vitro* exposed to a variety of oncogenic and non-oncogenic derivatives of 4NQO. They showed a link between the oncogenicity of 4NQO derivatives and their capacity to provoke DNA repair synthesis, and also indicated a positive relationship between their oncogenicity and colony-forming capacity of cells treated with 4NQO derivatives. To compare the present results with those of Stich *et al.*, however, further studies are needed. The present examination of chromatid aberrations was carried out exclusively at 8 culture hour without paying attention to any prolongation of G_2 phase of cells treated with 4NQO derivatives, so that a true feature of chromatid aberrations induced might be not shown. According to Yosida *et al.* (*17*), 4NQO prolongs the duration of G_2 phase because of the delayed mitosis of cells due to 4NQO treatment. It should be noted here that both hamster and rat cells are sensitive to the treatment with 4NQO and they show malignant transformation *in vitro* by the treatment (*6, 13, 14*), although rat tumor cells were used in the present study.

The mechanism of chemically induced chromosome break and rejoining have been well reviewed by Kihlman (*8*) and by Cohen *et al.* (*1*), though the exact mechanism for the formation of aberrant chromosomes by 4NQO derivatives is not known (*3, 5, 9, 17*).

Further structurally related mutagenic chemicals should be studied for their capacity to induce chromosome aberrations and their carcinogenicity comparatively.

Acknowledgment

The author wishes to thank Dr. Yutaka Kawazoe, National Cancer Center Research Institute, for the gift of 4NQO derivatives.

REFERENCES

1. Cohen, M. M., Hirschhorn, R., and Freeman, A. I. Mechanisms of chemically induced chromosome abnormalities. *In* "Genetic Concepts and Neoplasia" (23rd Annu. Symp. on Fundamental Cancer Res., 1969), Williams & Wilkins Co., Baltimore, pp. 238–252 (1970).
2. Endo, H. and Kume, F. Comparative studies on the biological actions of 4-nitroquinoline 1-oxide and its reduced compound, 4-hydroxyaminoquinoline 1-oxide. *Gann*, **54**, 443–453 (1963).
3. Hiragun, A. and Nishimoto, Y. Induction of chromosome aberrations in cultured human lymphocytes by 4-nitroquinoline 1-oxide. *Gann*, **64**, 183–187 (1973).
4. Hoshino, H., Kawazoe, Y., and Fukuoka, F. Detection of potential weak carcinogens and precarcinogens. I. Effect of the derivatives of 4-nitroquinoline 1-oxide on submanifestational dose of 4-nitroquinoline 1-oxide. *Gann*, **60**, 523–527 (1969).
5. Isaka, H. Chromosome aberrations and persistent nucleoli of Yoshida sarcoma cells induced by 4-nitroquinoline 1-oxide *in vitro*. *Gann*, **61**, 193–196 (1970).
6. Kamahora, J. and Kakunaga, T. *In vitro* carcinogenesis of 4-nitroquinoline 1-oxide with golden hamster cells. *Proc. Japan Acad.*, **42**, 1079–1081 (1966).
7. Kawazoe, Y. and Araki, M. Chemical problems in 4NQO carcinogenesis. *In* "Chemical Tumor Problems," ed. by W. Nakahara, Japan Society for Promotion of Science, Tokyo, pp. 43–104 (1970).
8. Kihlman, B. A. Molecular mechanisms of chromosome breakage and rejoining. *In* "Advances in Cell and Molecular Biology," ed. by E. J. DuPraw, Academic Press, New York/London, Vol. 1, pp. 59–107 (1971).
9. Kurita, Y., Shisa, H., Matsuyama, M., Nishizuka, Y., Tsuruta, R., and Yosida,

T. H. Carcinogen-induced chromosome aberrations in hematopoietic cells of mice. *Gann*, **60**, 91–95 (1969).

10. Mori, K., Kondo, M., Tamura, M., Ichimura, H., and Ohta, A. Induction of sarcoma in mice by a new carcinogen, 4-nitroquinoline. *Gann*, **60**, 663–664 (1969).

11. Nakahara, W., Fukuoka, F., and Sakai, S. The relation between carcinogenicity and chemical structure of certain quinoline derivatives. *Gann*, **49**, 33–41 (1958).

12. Nakahara, W., Fukuoka, F., and Sugimura, T. Carcinogenic action of 4-nitro-quinoline N-oxide. *Gann*, **48**, 129–137 (1957).

13. Namba, M., Masuji, H., and Sato, J. Carcinogenesis in tissue culture. IX. Malignant transformation of cultured rat cells treated with 4-nitroquinoline 1-oxide. *Japan. J. Exp. Med.*, **39**, 253–265 (1969).

14. Sato, H. and Kuroki, T. Malignization *in vitro* of hamster embryonic cells by chemical carcinogens. *Proc. Japan Acad.*, **42**, 1211–1216 (1966).

15. Shirasu, Y. Further studies on carcinogenic action of 4-hydroxyaminoquinoline 1-oxide. *Gann*, **54**, 487–495 (1963).

16. Stich, H. F., San, R. H. C., and Kawazoe, Y. DNA repair synthesis in mammalian cells exposed to a series of oncogenic and non-oncogenic derivatives of 4-nitro-quinoline 1-oxide. *Nature*, **229**, 416–419 (1971).

17. Yosida, T. H., Kurita, Y., and Moriwaki, K. Chromosomal aberrations in Yoshida sarcoma cells treated with 4-nitroquinoline 1-oxide. *Gann*, **56**, 523–528 (1965).

GANN Monograph on Cancer Research 17, 39–58 (1975)

CHEMICAL ONCOGENESIS IN CULTURES[*1]

Charles HEIDELBERGER[*2] and Patricia F. BOSHELL

*McArdle Laboratory for Cancer Research and Wisconsin Clinical Cancer Center,
University of Wisconsin[*3]*

This review of oncogenesis in culture traces the early stages in the history of chemical carcinogenesis, with particular emphasis on the major research of Professor Yoshida and other Japanese workers in this field. The need to elucidate the cellular and molecular mechanisms whereby chemical agents such as the polycyclic aromatic hydrocarbons exert their oncogenic activity in mammalian tissues has led to the development of a number of cell culture systems which permit quantitative measurements of malignant transformation under rigidly controlled conditions. Several critical questions concerning the cellular mechanisms of malignant transformation have been asked and answered. The review emphasizes the work carried out in the authors' laboratory.

The use of cell cultures as experimental models to probe the cellular and molecular mechanisms underlying the transformation of a normal cell to malignancy represents a relatively new approach to the study of chemical oncogenesis. It was only in 1963 that the first unequivocal demonstration was made by Berwald and Sachs (*4*) of the malignant transformation of cells in culture by means of chemical oncogens. It may at first sight seem inappropriate to have selected this topic as a contribution to the memorial volume in honor of Professor Tomizo Yoshida, whose brilliant scientific career spanned the years from 1929 until his untimely death earlier this year (1973), and whose first contribution to the field of chemical carcinogenesis was his epic discovery in 1932 that cancers of the liver could be induced in laboratory animals by administration of *o*-aminoazotoluene (*79*). Yet Professor Yoshida himself clearly pointed out the link between this newer cell culture approach and the more traditional methods making use of intact animals when, in 1964, he offered us his reflections on the problem of malignancy, and predicted that the era of cell populations as material for cancer research was at hand (*82*). Even so, as he indicated, the only certain means available at that time to characterize individual cells as cancer cells was to transplant them into animals and see whether or not proliferation to form a tumor took place, a procedure he defined as a "retrospective" determination of carcinogenicity. Today, refined cell culture techniques have made such identification

[*1] The work described in this review has been supported in part by Grants CA-07175 and CRTY-5002 from the National Cancer Institute, N.I.H., U.S.A., by Contract NCI-72-2022 from the National Cancer Institute, and by Grant BC-2C from the American Cancer Society.
[*2] American Cancer Society, Professor of Oncology.
[*3] Madison, Wisconsin 53706, U.S.A.

possible in cell cultures, yet we have frequently stressed (*32*) that it is still necessary to verify the findings made in cultures by transplantation of the cells into
suitable animals. At present, good correlations have emerged between the data
collected on the activity of chemicals in producing malignant transformation of
cells in culture, and their ability to induce tumors in experimental animals.

It is particularly appropriate that the editors of this memorial monograph
have chosen the subject of chemical carcinogenesis, a field to which Professor
Yoshida and other Japanese scientists have, throughout its history, made pre-
eminent contributions.

Japanese Contributions to Chemical Carcinogenesis

The beginning of the field of experimental chemical carcinogenesis dates
from 1915, when two Japanese researchers, Yamagiwa and Ichikawa, painted
the skin of a rabbit's ear with coal tar and thus induced, for the first time, a
squamous cell carcinoma at a site where no spontaneous tumor had ever been
observed (*78*). It was Yoshida who first induced hepatomas in rats by feeding
them *o*-aminoazotoluene (*79*), an important landmark in cancer research. Yoshida
considered the "fortuitous" occurrence, in 1943, of the first Yoshida sarcoma in
one of 20 rats fed an aminoazo dye followed by painting with arsenite, to be
the outcome of a long search by himself and his coworkers for what he termed
the "ultimate or essential feature of malignant growth in a pure cell colony of
malignant cells without resulting in any tissue formation" (*80*). This was the
ascites tumor, proliferating in the rat peritoneum as single cell suspensions,
and of which the Yoshida sarcoma was his first example. Nine years later,
stimulated by the dearth of experimental tumors available to Japanese investigators in the post-war period, Yoshida and his group (*83*) also developed the
ascites hepatomas, formed through ascitic conversion of an azo dye-induced
hepatoma in the Japanese albino rat. This led to a series of studies of ascites
hepatomas, mainly at the Sasaki Institute in Tokyo, and the establishment
of some 60 different lines (*61*). Strains of ascites hepatomas, which are both
transmissible and easily reproducible and hence are probably the most valuable
transplantable ascitic tumors available for cancer research, have been distributed
to investigators all over the world. Studies on these many transplanted strains
made it clear that each strain has its own individual biological and morphological characteristics (ascitic properties (*61*), metastatic capability (*72*), chromosome pattern (*41*), drug sensitivity (*40*)) differentiating it from other strains.
This brought confirmation to Yoshida's "individuality of cancer" concept which
he had first introduced in 1957 (*81*); in other words, the individuality of the
tumor strains as a variant within the overall framework of the malignant tumor.

Japanese Contributions to Oncogenesis in Culture

Japanese scientists have also made important contributions to the development of the field of chemical oncogenesis in culture, the major researchers here
being Katsuta, Takaoka, Kuroki, Sato, and Kakunaga.

Three years following Berwald and Sachs' demonstration of the direct malignant transformation of hamster embryo cells in culture by polycyclic hydrocarbons (4), Kamahora and Kakunaga (44), and Sato and Kuroki (73) independently reported similar transformations of the same cell species by means of 4-nitroquinoline 1-oxide (4NQO). These investigations were extended to a series of derivatives of 4NQO and here again morphological transformation and neoplastic development were achieved; all the transformed cultures gave rise to fibrosarcomas upon inoculation into newborn and/or adult hamsters, although the time periods differed from culture to culture and in some instances the morphological transformation occurred prior to the ability of the cells to induce tumors (51). Kuroki *et al.* also described certain chromosomal alterations in cells transformed by 4NQO and derivatives (84).

4NQO was also the agent responsible for the eventual successful malignant transformation (47) in 1972 by Katsuta and Takaoka of rat liver cells, such as those that they had succeeded in growing in culture as early as 1963 (45). Their previous attempts to transform liver cells using 4-dimethylaminoazobenzene (DAB) had given rise to a proliferation of parenchymal-like cells, but no tumor on subsequent inoculation into animals (46). Katsuta and Takaoka ascribed the discrepancies observed in the behavior of cultured liver parenchymal cells as compared to fibroblasts in the oncogenic process to the fact that such cells show different characteristics (*e.g.*, adhesiveness) from the more widely investigated fibroblasts, and they advocated the adoption of new and more reliable criteria for the identification of malignancy in epithelial cell systems (47).

A third cell culture system for quantitative assays of chemical oncogenesis is that of the 3T3 cells, introduced by Todaro and Green (76), and other permanent mouse cell lines. Recently, Kakunaga (43) reported the establishment of a quantitative system using a subclone derived from the A31 clone of BALB/3T3 (1). Four chemical oncogens produced transformation to malignancy: 4NQO, 3-methylcholanthrene (MCA), benzo[a]pyrene (BP), and N-methyl-N'-nitro-N-nitrosoguanidine (MNNG). The dose-response curves he established for determining the transformation frequency and cloning efficiency showed no direct correlation between the two phenomena as had been observed by many others. However, all the transformed cell lines exhibited characteristics (criss-crossing and piling up of cells, increase in saturation density, and ability to grow in soft agar) that are recognized indices of malignantly transformed cells, and all produced fibrosarcomas on injection into newborn or adult mice, within 3 to 6 weeks (43). In this system, therefore, there was a close relation between morphological transformation and malignant transformation. DiPaolo has described somewhat similar results with another clone of BALB/3T3 cells (18).

Turning now to an appreciation of the contribution of non-Japanese workers to this field, only a few highlights can be listed. Following the pioneering publication of Berwald and Sachs (4), in which malignant transformation by polycyclic hydrocarbons was first reported, they presented a much more detailed description (5) of their quantitative cloning assay, which has been the basis for all subsequent quantitative work with fibroblastic cells. When small numbers of control hamster embryo secondary cultures were plated and allowed to form colonies, the colonial morphology showed that the individual cells remained flat on the plastic surface. However, some of the colonies obtained after treatment with MCA or BP were piled up, with an irregular criss-cross pattern. This characteristic picture has been the classically accepted criterion of transformation, which, however, probably only pertains to fibroblasts. Mass cultures of such transformed cells gave rise to fibrosarcomas on inoculation into hamsters. A high incidence of spontaneous transformation of mouse embryo cells was observed (5), which did not occur with hamster embryo cells, which were adopted by Sachs et al. for all subsequent work. In the case of BP, Berwald and Sachs observed that up to 10% of the surviving cells could be transformed. Huberman and Sachs (38) carried out quantitative dose-response studies on the toxicity and transformation produced by BP and concluded, since the shapes of the curves were different, that toxicity and transformation were separate phenomena and that transformation followed "one-hit" kinetics.

Gelboin et al. (23) showed that the hamster embryo cells contained arylhydrocarbon hydroxylase (AHH) activity, and concluded that 3-hydroxy-BP was responsible for the cytotoxicity observed. Borek and Sachs also produced transformation by means of X rays (6). Much of the rest of Sachs' research has been reviewed (8, 32).

Although Berwald and Sachs did not report that they had picked transformed clones and produced tumors with them, this was demonstrated by DiPaolo et al. (16), who have made major contributions to this field, which have also been reviewed (8, 32). Quantitative studies in this system with a variety of polycyclic hydrocarbons were reported by DiPaolo et al. (14), who found a good correlation between the numbers of transformed colonies produced by the hydrocarbons and their oncogenic activities in vivo. The same authors also described the oncogenic and karyological characteristics of the transformed clones (17), and have made numerous other contributions to the field. A widely used, but thus far non-quantitative system for studying chemical transformation that involves the use of lines of rat embryo fibroblasts infected with the Rauscher leukemia virus has been used by Freeman et al. (21).

Diverse other mammalian cell systems have been used over the years for the study of chemical oncogenesis; indeed, their very variety, coupled with the lack of uniformity in experimental methods and materials, have made comparisons of results and assessments of the efficacy of the various oncogenic agents a difficult task. These different systems have been extensively reviewed by Heidelberger (32) and recently Casto and DiPaolo published a comprehensive survey of the relationships among virus, chemicals, and cancer (8). The evident need for the setting up of well-defined parameters for the identification and evaluation of conversion to malignancy of cells treated with chemical oncogens in culture prompted Sanders (71) to propose a novel series of criteria, based on mathematical analyses of specific dose-response curves. At present, considerable efforts are being expended in many laboratories to try to develop quantitative systems for the malignant transformation by chemical oncogens of various types of epithelial cells. Success in this endeavor will be of great importance.

Studies Carried Out in Authors' Laboratory

1. Systems

The remainder of this paper will be devoted to studies carried out in the authors' laboratory. The stimulus to the initiation of this research came from a conviction of the inherent limitations to posing and answering critical questions about the cellular and molecular mechanisms of hydrocarbon carcinogenesis imposed by working with intact animals (*29, 30, 32*). At that time the major clue came from the pioneering studies of Lasnitzki (*52*) who found that organ cultures of mouse prostates underwent histological changes of hyperplasia and squamous metaplasia after treatment with MCA. After studying in her laboratory, the senior author returned to Wisconsin and set up the organ culture system using the anterior prostates from inbred C3H mice. Although we obtained very striking histological changes suggestive of malignancy, these specimens failed to give tumors on implantation into isologous mice under a variety of conditions (*70*). However, when such pieces of prostate that had been treated in organ culture with MCA were dispersed and put into cell culture, permanent lines were obtained that did give rise to sarcomas when inoculated into C3H mice (*34*). Thus, oncogenesis in culture had been obtained, but it was impossible to quantitate this system. Accordingly, we succeeded in obtaining permanent aneuploid lines of mouse prostate fibroblasts that were highly susceptible to density-dependent inhibition of cell division, did not pile up when confluent, and did not give rise to tumors on inoculation into irradiated C3H mice. These cells underwent spontaneous transformation very rarely and only after cultivation for more than a year (*10*). When these cells were treated with MCA and other polycyclic hydrocarbons they piled up in cultures and produced highly malignant fibrosarcomas on injection into non-irradiated C3H mice (*11*). These prostate cells could be studied by quantitative cloning techniques and were scored for transformation by the production of distinct piled-up colonies after the culture dishes had been allowed to become confluent (*9*). The appearance of fixed and stained control and treated dishes is shown in Photo 1, and the edge of a transformed colony at higher magnification is shown in Photo 2 (*9*). A good correlation between the

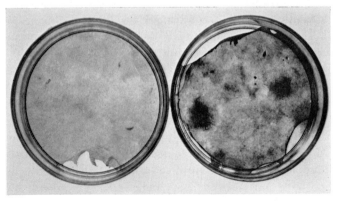

Photo 1. Photograph of confluent stained dishes of C3H mouse prostate fibroblasts: left, acetone control; right, treated with MCA (*9*)

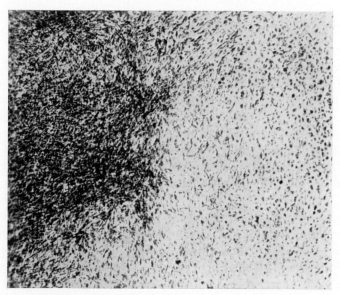

PHOTO 2.   Photomicrograph of the edge of a transformed colony in the dish
shown in Photo 1 (9). ×45

number of transformed colonies produced by a series of polycyclic aromatic
hydrocarbons (PAH) and their tumor-inducing activity was found, and individual
transformed colonies gave rise to fibrosarcomas on injection into C3H mice (9).
In agreement with the observations of Huberman and Sachs (38) in the hamster
embryo cells, the dose-response curves of cytotoxicity and transformation did
not correspond (9), again indicating that those two processes are different.

Much more recently we have described in detail (35, 69) the establishment
and characterization of clones of cell lines with high cloning efficiency that we
prepared from the embryos of C3H mice, and which exhibit unusually high
stability of properties in culture, including excellent density-dependent inhibition
of cell division; spontaneous transformation has never been observed in these
cells, which we have termed C3H/10Tl/2, and which do not give rise to tumors
on inoculation into irradiated C3H mice. These cells are hypotetraploid. Their
growth characteristics and saturation density are shown in Fig. 1 (69). On treatment with PAH, distinct piled up colonies are observed which are similar in
gross appearance to those obtained from the prostate fibroblasts (Photo 1), and
these isolated colonies give rise to fibrosarcomas in C3H mice. A detailed description of factors influencing malignant transformation has been given (68).

In the prostate, hamster embryo, and mouse embryo fibroblasts it was possible to study the conversion of various PAH into water-soluble metabolites,
doubtless mediated by AHH, followed by conjugation with glutathione and other
substances. In all cases, the PAH were metabolized to a greater or lesser extent,
which varied among the species. However, all the transformed cells carried out
this conversion to a considerably lesser extent than did their nontransformed
counterparts (39). The covalent binding of several PAH to DNA, RNA, and
proteins of the various cultures was also measured. The embryo cells gave rise

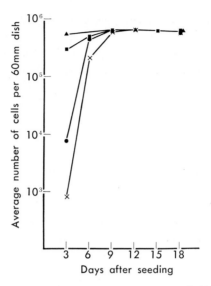

FIG. 1. Effect of seeding different numbers of C3H/10T1/2 CL8 cells on the growth rate and final saturation density

The cells were seeded in 60-mm petri dishes. A medium change was made every 3rd day. × 500 cells seeded; ● 5,000 cells seeded; ■ 50,000 cells seeded; ▲ 500,000 cells seeded (69).

to more binding than the prostate cells, and there was much greater binding to these macromolecules in the nontransformed than in the transformed cells. There was also a rough correspondence between the activity of the PAH and the extent to which they were bound (48). We also showed that the nontransformed cells bound MCA covalently to the "h-protein"; there was no such binding detectable in the transformed cells (49). The possible role of this h-protein in hydrocarbon oncogenesis is currently under intensive investigation in our laboratory.

In the type of research discussed here, it is always important to validate the model system by comparing it with various corresponding properties of *in vivo* oncogenesis. One of the most complicated and sophisticated properties of hydrocarbon-induced sarcomas is their cell-surface tumor-specific transplantation antigens (TSTA), described systematically by Prehn (65). The remarkable property of these TSTA's is that they are all individual and non-crossreacting. We investigated whether our transformed clones exhibited TSTA's, and found by transplantation techniques that most of the transformed clones were antigenic, and in a series of paired clones derived from the same culture dishes that the antigens were non-crossreacting (58). Less malignant revertant clones lost their TSTA's (56). We could now ask a question that had not been asked in whole animals. Are TSTA's produced during the process of transformation or does the transformation select clones of cells with preexisting antigens? The former was found to be true when we demonstrated by lymphocyte-mediated cytotoxicity and indirect immunofluorescence methods that 17 clones transformed independently from a single clone of prostate fibroblasts had individual antigens (20). Furthermore, spontaneously transformed clones were not detectably antigenic.

However, since they were malignant, we can conclude that in our system the TSTA's are not essential for malignancy (20). We have recently found that the TSTA's are also non-crossreacting in C3H/10Tl/2 cells (Embleton and Heidelberger, in preparation), which also express common cell-surface embryonic antigens.

2. *Mechanisms*

One of the simplest and most fundamental questions concerning the cellular mechanisms of chemical carcinogenesis could not be approached in whole animals, but is admirably suited for examination in cell culture: does a chemical oncogen transform normal cells to malignant cells or, as proposed by Prehn (64), does the chemical select for preexisting malignant cells? Although most workers in the field would intuitively support the former alternative, no evidence one way or the other was available. We succeeded in growing with high cloning efficiency individual prostate fibroblasts all by themselves in separate dishes. When they were treated with MCA for one day at the single cell stage, 100% of the clones were transformed to malignancy without toxicity. Furthermore, recloning experiments showed that all the progeny of the single cell were potentially transformed (57). This demonstrates conclusively that in this system the MCA carried out direct transformation to malignancy and did not select for preexisting malignant cells. DiPaolo has come to the same conclusion from his experiments with hamster embryo cells (15).

A second fundamental question is: does the chemical accomplish the transformation by itself, or does it act by "switching on" a "latent" oncogenic virus? In collaboration with Dr. R. Nowinski of this laboratory we have examined a large number of nontransformed clones of mouse prostate, 10Tl/2 cells derived from C3H mice, and transformed clones derived therefrom by a variety of chemical oncogens. None of these clones expressed group-specific (gs1) antigens or infectious C-type RNA oncogenic viruses. By contrast, AKR clones derived from the strain that naturally carries the Gross leukemia virus all expressed infectious virus, whether or not they were transformed (Ref. 33 and Heidelberger et al., unpublished). From these experiments we can conclude that the genome of the cells determines the expression of intact virus particles, and that the transformed phenotype does not. Since the chemical oncogen does not "switch on" intact viruses during the process of malignant transformation in C3H cells it is next necessary to determine whether the chemical "switches on" viral information. This is currently being studied by appropriate nucleic acid hybridization experiments.

If it turns out that the chemical can produce malignant transformation without the intervention of an oncogenic virus or its informational precursors, then the question can be asked: is the mechanism a mutational one, strictly defined as an alteration in the primary sequence of DNA, or does it act by altering gene expression, *i.e.*, by producing a perpetuated derepression (64) or by producing abnormal differentiation? This question will be discussed below.

It is also of considerable interest to determine whether there are phases of the cell cycle that are sensitive or resistant to transformation. Using 10Tl/2 cells

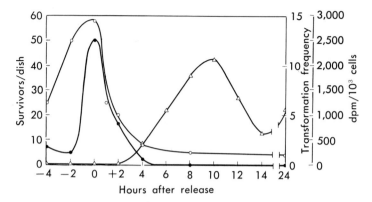

FIG. 2.   Transformation frequency (●) and number of survivors/dish (○) obtained in replicate cultures treated with 4 μg/ml of MNNG at various times prior to, at, and after release from the cell cycle block induced by 48-hr arginine deprivation

Progression of cells through the cell cycle was monitored in blocked but otherwise untreated cells by measuring the uptake of tritiated thymidine into acid-insoluble material (△) at 2-hr intervals after release.

synchronized by a variety of procedures and a short-acting oncogen, MNNG, it has been found (3) that the most sensitive phase occurs quite sharply when the MNNG is added 4 hr prior to the onset of DNA synthesis. A typical experiment is shown in Fig. 2. Synchrony was achieved by maintaining cells for 48 hr in a medium devoid of arginine; when arginine is added at zero time, DNA synthesis, as determined by tritiated thymidine labeling, started 4 hr after release from the block and the cells divided synchronously at about 12 hr after release. When MNNG was added 4 hr before or 4 hr after release of the block, no transformation was observed. However, when MNNG was added at the time of release of the block, a sharp peak of transformation was obtained (3). Thus, transformation is highly phase-specific. Three other methods of synchronization gave comparable results.

Using this highly specific system, we are now critically examining the role of DNA repair in the process of malignant transformation (62, 63).

3.   Metabolic activation of hydrocarbons

We now turn to a consideration of the concept of metabolic activation, which arose from the research of my colleagues, the Millers (53). According to this concept, all chemical oncogens that are not themselves chemically reactive must be converted metabolically to a form that reacts as an electrophile directly with cellular macromolecules. The Millers have elucidated the mechanisms of metabolic activation of several types of chemical oncogens (cf. Ref. 53), and we were interested to identify the metabolically activated form of PAH. Our initial contributions to this field have been reviewed (31).

That metabolic activation of PAH is carried out by the microsomal mixed-function oxidases was demonstrated simultaneously and independently by Grover and Sims (26) and by Gelboin (22), who incubated labeled PAH with microsomes

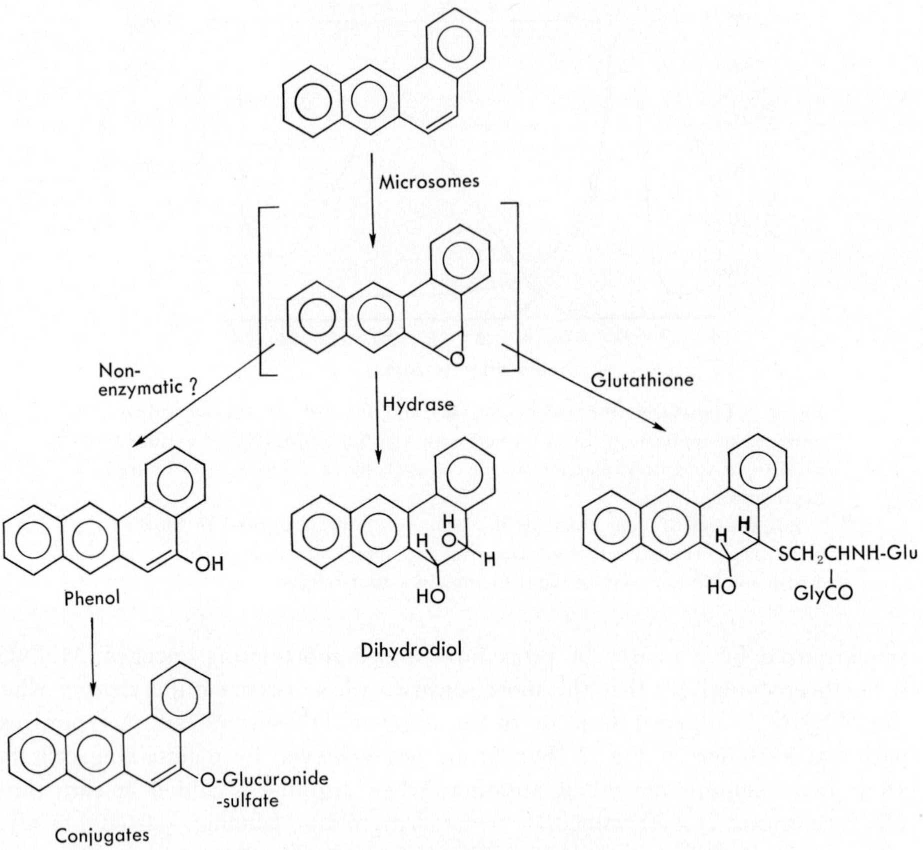

FIG. 3. Scheme of metabolism of benz[a]anthracene (BA) (31)

and observed covalent binding to exogenously added DNA, which did not occur in the absence of the microsomal system.

As a result of extensive studies on the metabolism of K-region (67) derivatives of PAH, which he and his colleagues had shown were converted to *trans*-dihydrodiols, phenols, and glutathione conjugates (illustrated for BA in Fig. 3), Boyland postulated in 1950 (7) that an epoxide (arene oxide) could be a metabolic intermediate. Because of their chemical reactivity, epoxides could also be metabolically activated metabolites of PAH, and indeed, our group (74) and Grover *et al.* (25) have isolated them as intermediates in microsomal metabolism. Moreover, Jerina *et al.* (42) had shown that an epoxide is an obligatory intermediate in the microsomal hydroxylation of naphthalene. Grover and Sims (27) then demonstrated that the epoxides of phenanthrene and dibenz[a,h]anthracene (DBA) reacted in the test tube to bind covalently with DNA and histones, and bound covalently with DNA, RNA, and proteins of cultured BHK-21 cells (24).

It was then necessary, in order to establish the role of epoxides as metabolically activated compounds, to show that they have the requisite biological activity. This was established in a fruitful international collaboration between our group

TABLE I.   Transformation and Toxicity to Mouse Prostate Fibroblasts
Produced by Chemicals (55)

Compound	Dose (μg/ml)	% plating efficiency	No. transformed colonies/ No. dishes
Control	DMSO[a] 0.5%	25	0/30
MNNG	0.2	11	25/17
BA	5.0	15	0/18
BA-5,6-epoxide	1.0	3.0	23/25
BA-8,9-epoxide	1.0	13	0/14
BA-trans-5,6-dihydrodiol	5.0	27	0/10
5-Hydroxy-BA	3.0	3.0	0/18
MCA	10.0	17	10/33
MCA-11,12-epoxide	0.75	17	38/27
Phenanthrene	5.0	20	0/12
Phenanthrene-9,10-epoxide	5.0	1.5	0/15

[a] DMSO: dimethylsulfoxide.

and P. L. Grover and P. Sims of the Chester Beatty Institute in London. We tested for the ability to produce malignant transformation of hamster embryo and mouse prostate fibroblast cells, several series of compounds that included the parent hydrocarbon, the K-region epoxide, the corresponding cis- and trans-dihydrodiols, and phenols. In all cases, particularly in a clone of prostate cells that metabolized PAH very poorly, the epoxides of unsubstituted PAH were much more active at producing malignant transformation than any of the other compounds tested (28). Table I documents this for the mouse prostate fibroblasts; it was found that the epoxide of phenanthrene, a non-oncogenic hydrocarbon, did not produce transformation, whereas K-region epoxides of BA and MCA did (55). MNNG was added as a positive control, because it does not require metabolic activation. Very similar results were obtained with hamster embryo fibroblasts (37).

As mentioned above, the metabolic activation is carried out by the mixed-function oxidases, which are known to be inducible in liver and in cultured cells (60). Accordingly, we studied the effect of inducing the cells with BA and with diphenyloxazole (PPO), as demonstrated by an increase in the production of water-soluble metabolites of MCA, on the toxicity and malignant transformation produced by MCA in the mouse prostate cells. As shown in Table II (54), MCA produced considerably more toxicity and transformation in the induced, than in the non-induced cells. It had been previously shown by Wiebel et al. (77) that α-naphthoflavone (ANF) inhibits AHH activity immediately after addition to cells, and we found (Table II) that it abolished the toxicity and transformation produced by MCA (54). Thus, we can conclude with considerable assurance that metabolism of MCA by the microsomal mixed-function oxidases is required in order for it to produce toxicity and transformation in these mouse prostate fibroblasts. These experiments show that epoxides are a major metabolically activated form of PAH. Nevertheless, other types of metabolic activation

TABLE II.   Effect of Induction and Inhibition of AHH on Toxicity and Transformation Produced by MCA in Mouse Prostate Fibroblasts (54)

Compounds	Dose (µg/ml)	% plating efficiency	No. transformed colonies/ No. dishes	Water-soluble metabolites[a]
No induction				
DMSO	0.5%	23.5	0/29	36
MCA	10.0	20.0	7/18	
Induction with BA, 0.25 µg/ml				
DMSO	0.5	26.5	0/19	61
MCA	10.0	14.0	15/8	
Induction with PPO, 2.5 µg/ml				
DMSO	0.5	23.5	0/17	60
MCA	10.0	15.0	37/19	
Inhibition with ANF, 1.5 µg/ml				
DMSO	0.5	20.0	0/10	5
MCA	10.0	23.0	0/10	

[a] pmoles formed in 24 hr by 10^6 cells from 260 pmoles of ^{3}H-MCA.

have been considered, but have not yet been established to play a role in hydrocarbon oncogenesis, since Dipple *et al.* (*19*) have proposed that PAH containing *meso*-methyl groups (such as 7,12-dimethylbenz[a]anthracene) may be activated on the methyl groups, and Nagata *et al.* (*59*) have shown that the free radical from 6-hydroxy-BP is formed during microsomal oxidation.

The rather complicated situation of activation of PAH by microsomal mixed-function oxidases through epoxides is shown in Fig. 4. The parent hydrocarbon, which is biologically innocuous *per se*, is converted to the epoxide by a microsomal P448 or P450 oxygenase. The epoxide can then react chemically with a critical cellular macromolecule to initiate cancer (the exact target has not yet been identified with certainty), it can be converted nonenzymatically by an acid-catalyzed reaction to the phenol (which is highly toxic and does not transform), it can be converted by a microsomal-bound epoxide hydrase to the dihydrodiol (which is nontoxic), or it can be converted by a soluble enzyme to the glutathione

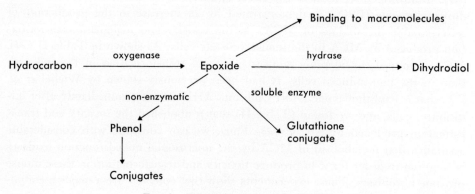

FIG. 4.   Metabolic activation of PAH

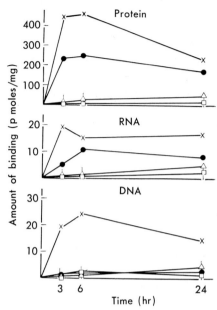

FIG. 5.   Binding of BA and K-region derivatives to DNA, RNA, and proteins of mouse prostate cells (*50*)

× epoxide ;   ● phenol ;   △ BA ;   □ diol.

conjugate (which is also nontoxic and represents the first step of metabolism towards the mixture of water-soluble metabolites). Whether a given hydrocarbon produces oncogenic transformation in a given cell or tissue is probably the resultant of this complicated network of competing enzymatic and chemical reactions; thus, a simple correlation between the activity or inducibility of AHH and the production of transformed cells or tumors is not to be expected. Nevertheless, if the original oxygenase were completely inhibited, or the activity of epoxide hydrase were significantly and specifically induced, oncogenesis by chemicals that require metabolic activation might be prevented.

We have also found, as shown in Fig. 5, that epoxides are bound to DNA, RNA, and proteins of transformable cells to a greater extent than the other compounds in the series, as expected (*50*). The binding of the phenol might be explained by free radical formation. The epoxides are also more rapidly metabolized in these cells than PAH (*75*).

4.   *Mutagenic or nonmutagenic mechanism?*

Finally, returning to the question of whether the molecular mechanism of chemical oncogenesis involves a somatic mutation or a perpetuated effect on gene expression (*66*), we can seek a correlation between the mutagenic and oncogenic activities of compounds. Since mutagenesis is commonly tested in bacteria and bacteriophages, which obviously do not have microsomes, little correlation between these processes was found prior to the concept of metabolic activation. Now, however, a much better correlation is emerging. In all cases where metabolically activated products have been identified they have been found to have mutagenic activity. However, not all mutagens are carcinogens, as illustrated by the base analogues and the acridine dyes. The mutagenic activity of epoxides of PAH has been demonstrated in bacteriophage by Cookson *et al.* (*13*) and in *Salmonella* by Ames *et al.* (*2*).

In our laboratory we have studied the mutagenic activity of hydrocarbons and their derivatives in mammalian cells—the Chinese hamster V79 cell system

A. Cytotoxicity

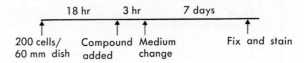

B. Mutagenesis

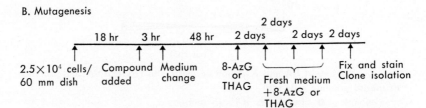

Fig. 6.   Scheme for assay of cytotoxicity and mutagenicity in Chinese hamster V-79 cells (*36*)

8-AzG: 8-azaguanine.   THAG: thymidine, hypoxanthine, aminopterine, glycine.

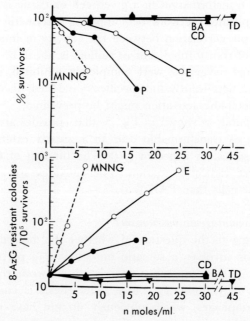

Fig. 7.   Cytotoxicity and mutagenicity to V-79 cells by MNNG and by BA and its K-region derivatives (*36*)

developed by Chu and Malling (*12*). The experimental setup is shown in Fig. 6. Cytotoxicity and forward mutagenesis to 8-AzG resistance are measured. The data we obtained (*36*) are shown in Fig. 7. BA and its K-region *cis*- and *trans*-dihydrodiols were not toxic or mutagenic to these cells. However, the epoxide was highly mutagenic and the phenol was highly toxic but weakly mutagenic. MNNG was included as a positive control, and similar results were obtained with the epoxides of other PAH. However, correlations do not constitute proof, and if a mutagenic mechanism of chemical oncogenesis is to be established it is necessary to carry out critical experiments.

We hope that this brief review has succeeded in conveying some of the present sense of excitement in the field of chemical oncogenesis and the important role that cell culture studies are playing at the current time. This importance will undoubtedly increase in the future for studies of fundamental mechanisms, and also as a potentially rapid method of screening environmental chemicals for oncogenic activity. Thus, the foresight of Professor Yoshida (*82*) in visualizing that research on cancer should emphasize work on cells has been realized, and his Japanese colleagues and students will certainly continue to be at the forefront of important research on chemical oncogenesis.

REFERENCES

1. Aaronson, S. A. and Todaro, G. J. Basis for the acquisition of malignant potential by mouse cells cultured *in vitro*. *Science*, **162**, 1024–1026 (1968).
2. Ames, B. N., Sims, P., and Grover, P. L. Epoxides of carcinogenic polycyclic hydrocarbons are frameshift mutagens. *Science*, **176**, 47–49 (1972).
3. Bertram, J. S. and Heidelberger, C. Cell cycle dependency of oncogenic transformation reduced by N-methyl-N'-nitro-N-nitrosoguanidine in culture. *Cancer Res.*, **34**, 526–537 (1974).
4. Berwald, Y. and Sachs, L. *In vitro* transformation with chemical carcinogens. *Nature*, **200**, 1182–1184 (1963).
5. Berwald, Y. and Sachs, L. *In vitro* transformation of normal cells to tumor cells by carcinogenic hydrocarbons. *J. Natl. Cancer Inst.*, **35**, 641–661 (1965).
6. Borek, C. and Sachs, L. *In vitro* cell transformation by X-irradiation. *Nature*, **210**, 276–278 (1966).
7. Boyland, E. The biological significance of metabolism of polycyclic compounds. *Symp. Biochem. Soc.*, **5**, 40–54 (1950).
8. Casto, B. C. and DiPaolo, J. A. Virus, chemicals and cancer. *Prog. Med. Virol.*, **16**, 1–47 (1973).
9. Chen, T. T. and Heidelberger, C. Quantitative studies on the malignant transformation of mouse prostate cells by carcinogenic hydrocarbons *in vitro*. *Int. J. Cancer*, **4**, 166–168 (1969).
10. Chen, T. T. and Heidelberger, C. Cultivation *in vitro* of cells derived from adult C3H mouse ventral prostate. *J. Natl. Cancer Inst.*, **42**, 903–914 (1969).
11. Chen, T. T. and Heidelberger, C. *In vitro* malignant transformation of cells derived from mouse prostate in the presence of 3-methylcholanthrene. *J. Natl. Cancer Inst.*, **42**, 915–925 (1969).
12. Chu, E. H. Y. and Malling, H. V. Mammalian cell genetics. II. Chemical induc-

tion of specific locus mutations in Chinese hamster cells *in vitro*. *Proc. Natl. Acad. Sci. U.S.*, **61**, 1306–1312 (1968).

13. Cookson, M. J., Sims, P., and Grover, P. L. Mutagenicity of epoxides of polycyclic hydrocarbons correlates with carcinogenicity of parent hydrocarbons. *Nature New Biol.*, **234**, 186–187 (1971).

14. DiPaolo, J. A., Donovan, P., and Nelson, R. Quantitative studies of *in vitro* transformation by chemical carcinogens. *J. Natl. Cancer Inst.*, **42**, 867–874 (1969).

15. DiPaolo, J. A., Donovan, P. J., and Nelson, R. L. *In vitro* transformation of hamster cells by polycyclic hydrocarbons: Factors influencing the number of cells transformed. *Nature New Biol.*, **230**, 240–242 (1971).

16. DiPaolo, J. A., Nelson, R. L., and Donovan, P. J. Sarcoma producing cell clones derived from clones transformed *in vitro* by benzo[a]pyrene. *Science*, **165**, 917–918 (1969).

17. DiPaolo, J. A., Nelson, R. L., and Donovan, P. J. Morphological, oncogenic, and karyological characteristics of Syrian hamster embryo cells transformed *in vitro* by carcinogenic polycyclic hydrocarbons. *Cancer Res.*, **31**, 1118–1127 (1971).

18. DiPaolo, J. A., Takano, K., and Popescu, N. C. Quantitation of chemically induced neoplastic transformation of BALB/3T3 cloned cell lines. *Cancer Res.*, **32**, 2686–2695 (1972).

19. Dipple, A., Lawley, P. D., and Brookes, P. Theory of tumor initiation by chemical carcinogens: dependence of activity on structure of ultimate carcinogen. *Eur. J. Cancer*, **4**, 493–506 (1968).

20. Embleton, M. J. and Heidelberger, C. Antigenicity of clones of mouse prostate cells transformed *in vitro*. *Int. J. Cancer*, **9**, 8–18 (1972).

21. Freeman, A. E., Price, P. J., Igel, H. J., Young, T. C., Maryak, J. M., and Huebner, R. J. Morphological transformation of rat embryo cells induced by diethylnitrosamine and murine leukemia viruses. *J. Natl. Cancer Inst.*, **44**, 65–78 (1970).

22. Gelboin, H. V. Microsome-dependent binding of benzo[a]pyrene to DNA. *Cancer Res.*, **29**, 1272–1276 (1969).

23. Gelboin, H. V., Huberman, E., and Sachs, L. Enzymatic hydroxylation of benzopyrene and its relationship to toxicity. *Proc. Natl. Acad. Sci. U.S.*, **64**, 1188–1194 (1969).

24. Grover, P. L., Forrester, J. A., and Sims, P. Reactivity of the K-region epoxides of some polycyclic hydrocarbons towards the nucleic acids and proteins of BHK 21 cells. *Biochem. Pharmacol.*, **20**, 1297–1302 (1971).

25. Grover, P. L., Hewer, A., and Sims, P. Epoxides as microsomal metabolites of polycyclic hydrocarbons. *FEBS Letters*, **48**, 76–80 (1971).

26. Grover, P. L. and Sims, P. Enzyme-catalyzed reactions of polycyclic hydrocarbons with deoxyribonucleic acid and proteins *in vitro*. *Biochem. J.*, **110**, 159–160 (1968).

27. Grover, P. L. and Sims, P. Interaction of the K-region epoxides of phenanthrene and dibenz[a,h]anthracene with nucleic acids and histone. *Biochem. Pharmacol.*, **19**, 2251–2259 (1970).

28. Grover, P. L., Sims, P., Huberman, E., Marquardt, H., Kuroki, T., and Heidelberger, C. *In vitro* transformation of rodent cells by K-region derivatives of polycyclic hydrocarbons. *Proc. Natl. Acad. Sci. U.S.*, **68**, 1098–1101 (1971).

29. Heidelberger, C. Chemical carcinogenesis, chemotherapy: Cancer's continuing core challenges—G. H. A. Clowes Memorial Lecture. *Cancer Res.*, **30**, 1549–1569 (1970).

30. Heidelberger, C. Studies on the cellular and molecular mechanisms of hydrocarbon carcinogenesis. *Eur. J. Cancer*, **6**, 161–172 (1970).

31. Heidelberger, C. *In vitro* studies on the role of epoxides in carcinogenic hydrocarbon activation. *In* "Topics in Chemical Carcinogenesis," ed. by W. Nakahara, S. Takayama, T. Sugimura, and S. Odashima, University of Tokyo Press, Tokyo, pp. 371–386 (1972); discussion, pp. 387–388.

32. Heidelberger, C. Chemical oncogenesis in culture. *Adv. Cancer Res.*, **18**, 317–366 (1973).

33. Heidelberger, C. Current trends in chemical carcinogenesis. *Fed. Proc.*, **32**, 2154–2161 (1973).

34. Heidelberger, C. and Iype, P. T. Malignant transformation *in vitro* by carcinogenic hydrocarbons. *Science*, **155**, 214–217 (1967).

35. Heidelberger, C., Reznikoff, C. A., and Krahn, D. F. Malignant transformation of cells in culture using oncogenic chemicals. *In* "Tissue Culture Methods and Applications," ed. by P. F. Kruse, Jr. and M. K. Patterson, Jr., Academic Press, New York, pp. 644–653 (1973).

36. Huberman, E., Aspiras, L., Heidelberger, C., Grover, P. L., and Sims, P. Mutagenicity to mammalian cells of epoxides and other derivatives of polycyclic hydrocarbons. *Proc. Natl. Acad. Sci. U.S.*, **68**, 3195–3199 (1971).

37. Huberman, E., Kuroki, T., Marquardt, H., Selkirk, J. K., Heidelberger, C., Grover, P. L., and Sims, P. Transformation of hamster embryo cells by epoxides and other derivatives of polycyclic hydrocarbons. *Cancer Res.*, **32**, 1391–1396 (1972).

38. Huberman, E. and Sachs, L. Cell susceptibility to transformation and cytotoxicity by the carcinogenic hydrocarbon benzo[a]pyrene. *Proc. Natl. Acad. Sci. U.S.*, **56**, 1123–1129 (1966).

39. Huberman, E., Selkirk, J. K., and Heidelberger, C. Metabolism of polycyclic aromatic hydrocarbons in cell cultures. *Cancer Res.*, **31**, 2161–2167 (1971).

40. Isaka, H. " Natural" drug resistance of the ascites hepatoma in the rat. *Natl. Cancer Inst. Monogr.*, **16**, 131–148 (1964).

41. Isaka, H. Deviation in chromosomal pattern of ascites tumors. *GANN Monograph*, **1**, 89–99 (1966).

42. Jerina, D. M., Daly, J. W., Witkop, B., Zaltzman-Nirenberg, P., and Udenfriend, S. 1,2-Naphthalene oxide as an intermediate in the microsomal hydroxylation of naphthalene. *Biochemistry*, **9**, 147–155 (1970).

43. Kakunaga, T. A quantitative system for assay of malignant transformation by chemical carcinogens using a clone derived from BALB/3T3. *Int. J. Cancer*, **12**, 463–473 (1973).

44. Kamahora, J. and Kakunaga, T. *In vitro* carcinogenesis of 4-nitroquinoline-1-oxide with golden hamster whole embryonic cells. *Proc. Japan Acad.*, **42**, 1079–1087 (1966).

45. Katsuta, H. and Takaoka, T. Carcinogenesis in tissue culture. I. Cultivation of normal rat liver cells. *Japan. J. Exp. Med.*, **33**, 265–275 (1963).

46. Katsuta, H. and Takaoka, T. Carcinogenesis in tissue culture. II. Proliferation-inducing effect of 4-dimethylaminoazobenzene on normal rat liver cells in culture. *Japan. J. Exp. Med.*, **35**, 209–230 (1965); III. Effects of the second treatments on DAB-induced proliferating liver cells of normal rats in culture. *Japan. J. Exp. Med.*, **35**, 231-248 (1965).

47. Katsuta, H. and Takaoka, T. Carcinogenesis in culture. XIV. Malignant trans-

formation of rat liver parenchymal cells treated with 4-nitroquinoline-1-oxide in tissue culture. *J. Natl. Cancer Inst.*, **49**, 1563–1576 (1972).

48. Kuroki, T. and Heidelberger, C. The binding of polycyclic aromatic hydrocarbons to the DNA, RNA, and proteins of transformable cells in culture. *Cancer Res.*, **31**, 2168–2176 (1971).

49. Kuroki, T. and Heidelberger, C. Determination of the h-protein in transformable and transformed cells in culture. *Biochemistry*, **11**, 2116–2124 (1972).

50. Kuroki, T., Huberman, E., Marquardt, H., Selkirk, J. K., Heidelberger, C., Grover, P. L., and Sims, P. Binding of K-region epoxides and other derivatives of benz[a]anthracene and dibenz[a,h]anthracene to DNA, RNA, and proteins of transformable cells. *Chem.-Biol. Interact.*, **4**, 389–397 (1971/72).

51. Kuroki, T. and Sato, H. Transformation and neoplastic development *in vitro* of hamster embryonic cells by 4-nitroquinoline-1-oxide and its derivatives. *J. Natl. Cancer Inst.*, **41**, 53–71 (1968).

52. Lasnitzki, I. Growth pattern of the mouse prostate gland in organ culture and its response to sex hormones, vitamin A, and 3-methylcholanthrene. *Natl. Cancer Inst. Monogr.*, **12**, 318–403 (1963).

53. Miller, J. A. Carcinogenesis by chemicals: an overview—G. H. A. Clowes Memorial Lecture. *Cancer Res.*, **30**, 599–676 (1970).

54. Marquardt, H. and Heidelberger, C. Influence of "feeder cells" and inducers and inhibitors of microsomal mixed-function oxidases on hydrocarbon-induced malignant transformation of cells derived from C3H mouse prostate. *Cancer Res.*, **32**, 721–725 (1972).

55. Marquardt, H., Kuroki, T., Huberman, E., Selkirk, J. K., Heidelberger, C., Grover, P. L., and Sims, P. Malignant transformation of cells derived from mouse prostate by epoxides and other derivatives of polycyclic hydrocarbons. *Cancer Res.*, **32**, 716–720 (1972).

56. Mondal, S., Embleton, M. J., Marquardt, H., and Heidelberger, C. Production of variants of decreased malignancy and antigenicity from clones transformed *in vitro* by methylcholanthrene. *Int. J. Cancer*, **8**, 410–420 (1971).

57. Mondal, S. and Heidelberger, C. *In vitro* malignant transformation by methylcholanthrene of the progeny of single cells derived from C3H mouse prostate. *Proc. Natl. Acad. Sci. U.S.*, **65**, 219–225 (1970).

58. Mondal, S., Iype, P. T., Griesbach, L. M., and Heidelberger, C. Antigenicity of cells derived from mouse prostate cells after malignant transformation *in vitro* by carcinogenic hydrocarbons. *Cancer Res.*, **30**, 1593–1597 (1970).

59. Nagata, C., Inomata, M., Kodama, M., and Tagashira, Y. Electron spin resonance study on the interaction between chemical carcinogens and tissue components. III. Determination of the structure of the free radical produced either by stirring 3,4-benzopyrene with albumin or incubating it with liver homogenates. *Gann*, **59**, 289–298 (1968).

60. Nebert, D. W. and Gelboin, H. V. Substrate-inducible microsomal aryl hydroxylase in mammalian cell culture. *J. Biol. Chem.*, **243**, 6242–6249, 6250–6261 (1968).

61. Odashima, S. Establishment of ascites hepatomas in the rat, 1951–1962. *Natl. Cancer Inst. Monogr.*, **16**, 51–94 (1964).

62. Peterson, A. R., Bertram, Y. S., and Heidelberger, C. DNA damage and its repair in transformable mouse fibroblasts treated with N-methyl-N′-nitro-N-nitrosoguanidine. *Cancer Res.*, **34**, 1592–1599 (1974).

63. Peterson, A. R., Bertram, Y. S., and Heidelberger, C. Cell cycle dependency of

DNA damage and repair in transformable mouse fibroblasts treated with N-methyl-N′-nitro-N-nitrosoguanidine. *Cancer Res.*, **34**, 1600–1607 (1974).

64. Prehn, R. T. A clonal selection theory of chemical carcinogenesis. *J. Natl. Cancer Inst.*, **32**, 1–17 (1964).

65. Prehn, R. T. Tumor-specific antigens of putatively nonviral tumors. *Cancer Res.*, **28**, 1326–1330 (1968).

66. Pitot, H. C. and Heidelberger, C. Metabolic regulatory circuits and carcinogenesis. *Cancer Res.*, **23**, 1694–1700 (1963).

67. Pullman, H. and Pullman, B. A quantum chemist's approach to the mechanism of chemical carcinogenesis. Proc. Int. Symp. on Physico-chemical Mechanisms of Carcinogenesis, Jerusalem, 1968, Academic Press, New York, pp. 9–24 (1969).

68. Reznikoff, C. A., Bertram, J. S., Brankow, D. W., and Heidelberger, C. Quantitative and qualitative studies of chemical transformation of cloned C3H mouse embryo cells sensitive to postconfluence inhibition of cell division. *Cancer Res.*, **33**, 3239–3249 (1973).

69. Reznikoff, C. A., Brankow, D. W., and Heidelberger, C. Establishment and characterization of a cloned line of C3H mouse embryo cells sensitive to postconfluence inhibition of division. *Cancer Res.*, **33**, 3231–3238 (1973).

70. Röller, M. R. and Heidelberger, C. Attempts to produce carcinogenesis in organ cultures of mouse prostate with polycyclic hydrocarbons. *Int. J. Cancer*, **2**, 509–520 (1967).

71. Sanders, F. K. The effect of some nonviral oncogenic agents on mammalian cells *in vivo*. *In* "Topics in Chemical Carcinogenesis," ed. by W. Nakahara, S. Takayama, T. Sugimura, and S. Odashima, University of Tokyo Press, Tokyo, pp. 429–444 (1972).

72. Sato, H. Cancer metastasis and ascitic tumors. *Natl. Cancer Inst. Monogr.*, **16**, 241–262 (1964).

73. Sato, H. and Kuroki, T. Malignization *in vitro* of hamster embryonic cells by chemical carcinogens. *Proc. Japan Acad.*, **42**, 1211–1216 (1966).

74. Selkirk, J. K., Huberman, E., and Heidelberger, C. An epoxide is an intermediate in the microsomal metabolism of the chemical carcinogen, dibenz[a,h]anthracene. *Biochem. Biophys. Res. Commun.*, **43**, 1010–1016 (1971).

75. Sims, P., Grover, P. L., Kuroki, T., Huberman, E., Marquardt, H., Selkirk, J. K., and Heidelberger, C. The metabolism of benz[a]anthracene and dibenz[a,h]-anthracene and their related "K-region" epoxides, *cis*-dihydrodiols and phenols by hamster embryo cells. *Biochem. Pharmacol.*, **22**, 1–8 (1973).

76. Todaro, G. J. and Green, H. Quantitative studies of the growth of mouse embryo cells in culture and their development into established lines. *J. Cell. Biol.*, **17**, 299–313 (1963).

77. Wiebel, F. J., Leutz, J. C., Diamond, L., and Gelboin, H. V. Aryl hydrocarbon (benzo[a]pyrene) hydroxylase in microsomes from rat tissue: Differential inhibition and stimulation by benzoflavones and organic solvents. *Arch. Biochem. Biophys.*, **144**, 78–86 (1971).

78. Yamagiwa, K. and Ichikawa, K. Experimentelle Studien über die Pathogenese der Epithelialgeschwürste (II Mitteilung). *Mitteil. Med. Fakultät Kaiserl. Univ. Tokyo*, **17** (I), 19 (1917).

79. Yoshida, T. Über die experimentelle Erzeugung von Hepatom durch die Fütterung mit *o*-Aminoazotoluol. *Proc. Imp. Acad. (Tokyo)*, **8**, 464 (1932).

80. Yoshida, T. Studies on an ascites (reticuloendothelial cell?) sarcoma of the rat. *J. Natl. Cancer Inst.*, **12**, 947–961 (1952).

81. Yoshida, T. Studien über das Ascites Hepatom. Zugleich ein Beitrag zum Begriff der cellulären Autonomie und der Individualität der einzelnen Geschwulst anderseits. *Arch. Pathol. Anat. Physiol.*, **330**, 85–105 (1957).

82. Yoshida, T. Some thoughts on malignant growth. *Natl. Cancer Inst. Monogr.*, **16**, 1–6 (1964).

83. Yoshida, T., Sato, H., and Aruji, T. On the origin of Yoshida sarcoma. I. Experimental production of ascites hepatoma in the rat. *Proc. Japan Acad.*, **27**, 485–492 (1951).

84. Yosida, T. H., Kuroki, T., Masuji, H., and Sato, H. Chromosomal alteration and the development of tumors. XX. Chromosome change in the course of malignant transformation *in vitro* of hamster embryonic cells by 4-nitroquinoline-1-oxide and its derivative, 4-hydroxyaminoquinoline-1-oxide. *Gann*, **61**, 131–163 (1970).

GANN Monograph on Cancer Research 17, 59–65 (1975)

CHEMICAL CARCINOGENESIS OF MAMMALIAN EPITHELIAL CELLS IN TISSUE CULTURE[*1]

Hajim KATSUTA and Toshiko TAKAOKA

Department of Cancer Cell Research, Institute of Medical Science, University of Tokyo[*2]

The cultivation in tissue culture of normal rat liver cells and the effect of chemical carcinogens on these cells are described. Proliferation was induced when resting liver cells were treated with 4-dimethylaminoazobenzene (DAB). Mutant cells were produced in some of the cultures by the cultivation of liver cells with no subculturing, for 1 or 2 months. The treatment of cells with DAB, after prolonged culture, resulted in the production of mutant cells in each culture tube. These cells, however, did not produce tumors on back-transplantation into animals. The treatment of liver cells in culture with 4-nitroquinoline 1-oxide resulted in transformation of the cells into malignant cells. A single treatment of 30 min also produced this same effect.

Tissue culture is a valuable method for investigating the mechanism of chemical carcinogenesis at the cellular level. Many works have been carried out along these lines to transform normal cells into malignant cells in culture. In most of them, however, cultures of fibroblasts have been employed. Thus they were not studies on "carcinogenesis" but "sarcomagenesis." The results of our work will be described, together with those of other workers, to transform rat liver cells into malignant cells in tissue culture.

Induction of the Proliferation of Rat Liver Cells by 4-Dimethylaminoazobenzene (DAB)

We found that, when small fragments of rat liver tissue were cultivated by the roller tube culture method and treated with 1 μg/ml of DAB for the initial 4 days of primary culture, the proliferation of liver cells was abruptly initiated about 7 to 10 days after the treatment (*3*). This proliferation continued indefinitely and many cell strains were established by this method (Photo 1).

These proliferating cells, however, did not produce tumors on back-transplantation into rats. Various second treatments of the cells, including no renewal of culture fluid, addition of hormones, DAB, or thalidomide into culture medium, also did not transform them into malignant cells (*4*). Inbred rats of JAR-1 line were employed in these studies (*13*). Sato confirmed these findings by the use of

---

[*1] This work was supported in part by a grant from the Japanese Ministry of Education.
[*2] Shirokanedai 4-6-1, Minato-ku, Tokyo 108, Japan (勝田　甫, 高岡聰子).

Donryu rats and with 3′-methyl-DAB (12). We later developed a method to grow normal rat liver cells and established many cell strains from inbred rats (Photo 2). These strains have been used in various experiments on chemical carcinogenesis.

Transformation of Rat Liver Cells by Nagisa Culture

We found that normal rat liver cells were morphologically transformed without use of chemical carcinogens or viruses (7). When liver cells were cultivated in glass tubes with flattened surfaces without subculturing for a long time, i.e., 1 or 2 months, and kept slanted at an angle of 5° in stationary culture, marked changes appeared in the morphology of the cells scattering near the air-liquid interphase; abnormal and multipolar mitosis, endomitosis, endoreduplication, unequal division of nuclei, and others. We eventually found the production of mutant cells which were piling up on the cell sheet of untransformed liver cells. We call this method of cultivation a Nagisa culture. These transformed cells proliferated very rapidly and became predominant in the cultures. Many mutant cell strains have been established by this method (Photo 3). The transformed cells closely resembled hepatoma cells in morphology, but did not give rise to tumors on back-transplantation. This suggests that not all the instances of morphological transformation of cells are malignant transformation.

We also treated the cultures of liver cells, after Nagisa culture, with high concentrations of DAB (5). In all of these culture tubes, mutant cell strains were produced after 1 week of DAB treatment. They exhibited tremendous differences in cell properties from each other; in cell morphology, in shift of the modal number of chromosomes, and especially in the activity of metabolizing DAB added to the medium. Some mutant cell strains grew rapidly receiving no effect of the presence of 4 μg/ml of DAB, whereas others also grew metabolizing DAB completely into non-azo compounds within 4 days. These cell strains closely resembled hepatoma cells morphologically. However, all of them did not produce tumors on back-transplantation.

Malignant Transformation of Rat Liver Cells by 4-Nitroquinoline 1-Oxide (4NQO)

Namba et al. treated cell strains of rat liver cells repeatedly with 4NQO for a long period and obtained malignant transformation of the cells (11). The cells produced tumors in animals about 6 months after back-transplantation. We employed one of the cell strains, RLC-10, derived from normal rat liver cells preserving a diploid number of chromosomes as a mode. These cultures were given 3.3×10^{-6} M 4NQO, each time for 30 min. Five lines of experiments were carried out and, in all of them, liver cells were found to have been transformed into malignant cells about 3 or 4 months after the treatment with 4NQO, as confirmed by intraperitoneal back-transplantation into rats and by tumor death of the animals (2, 6). We tried to decrease the number of treatment as little as possible. It was striking that one of them was transformed by single treatment with 4NQO for 30 min.

In cell morphology, no marked change was induced by the transformation (Photo 4). By cinemicrography, however, decrease in adhesiveness between cells was noticed. The cells exhibited active locomotion, as if they were swimming among the cells in the crowded cell sheet. This suggested a distinct change in cell membrane.

In the modal number of chromosomes, the transformed cells showed a little shift; reduction of a few number of chromosomes. The control cultures had maintained diploid number of chromosomes with high frequency.

Changes in cytoelectrophoretic mobility of liver cells were examined by our co-worker, T. Yamada, at certain intervals after the treatment with 4NQO (2, 8, 9, 15, 16): 4NQO-treated cells gradually became to simulate ascites hepatoma cells in their electric mobility with time of culture.

DISCUSSION

A system for cultivating rat liver cells has been established in our laboratory and we have also been engaged in developing new techniques. The culture strains of rat liver cells obtained have greatly contributed to the investigation of chemical carcinogenesis in tissue culture.

The experiments utilizing DAB suggested a certain stepwise increase in tumorigenicity of cells by their treatment with chemical carcinogens. The transformation of liver cells by *Nagisa* culture also gave us an unknown clue to open the field of "spontaneous transformation" of cells, not only in culture but also *in vivo*. The finding obtained with 4NQO that the cells were transformed into malignant cells by a single treatment for 30 min was striking. This suggests that human beings may be exposed to such dangers.

Iype (1) described another method for culturing liver cells from normal adult rats. Weisburger and his collaboraters (14) also obtained carcinoma-conversion of rat liver cells by the treatment with Aflatoxin B_1, dimethylnitrosamine, N-nitrosomethylurea, N-hydroxy-N-2-fluorenylacetamide, or 7, 12-dimethylbenz(a)anthracene. Montesano *et al.* reported the malignant transformation in culture of epithelial-like cells derived from rat liver tissues by the addition of dimethylnitrosamine or N-methyl-N'-nitrosoguanidine (10).

These observations will contribute to the understanding of carcinogenesis and the identification of cell properties between cancers and sarcomas.

Acknowledgment

The authors sincerely thank the late Professor Tomizo Yoshida for his kind and warm advices in carrying out these works.

REFERENCES

1. Iype, P. T. Cultures from adult rat liver cells. I. Establishment of monolayer cell-cultures from normal liver. *J. Cell. Physiol.*, **78**, 281–288 (1971).
2. Katsuta, H. Liver carcinogenesis in vitro. *In* "Oncology 1970," ed. by R. L. Clark, R. W. Cumley, J. E. McCay, and M. M. Copeland, Year Book Medical Publishers, Inc., Chicago, Vol. 1, pp. 103–109 (1971).

3. Katsuta, H. and Takaoka, T. Carcinogenesis in tissue culture. II. Proliferation-inducing effect of 4-dimethylaminoazobenzene on normal rat liver cells in culture. *Japan. J. Exp. Med.*, **35**, 209–230 (1965).

4. Katsuta, H. and Takaoka, T. Carcinogenesis in tissue culture. III. Effects of the second treatments on DAB-induced proliferating liver cells of normal rats in culture. *Japan. J. Exp. Med.*, **35**, 231–248 (1965).

5. Katsuta, H. and Takaoka, T. Cytobiological transformation of normal rat liver cells by treatment with 4-dimethylaminoazobenzene after Nagisa culture. *In* "Cancer Cells in Culture," ed. by H. Katsuta, University of Tokyo Press, Tokyo, pp. 321–334 (1968).

6. Katsuta, H. and Takaoka, T. Carcinogenesis in tissue culture. XIV. Malignant transformation of rat liver parenchymal cells treated with 4-nitroquinoline 1-oxide in tissue culture. *J. Natl. Cancer Inst.*, **49**, 1563–1576 (1972).

7. Katsuta, H., Takaoka, T., Doida, Y., and Kuroki, T. Carcinogenesis in tissue culture. VII. Morphological transformation of rat liver cells in Nagisa culture. *Japan. J. Exp. Med.*, **35**, 513–544 (1965).

8. Katsuta, H., Takaoka, T., and Yamada, T. Malignant transformation of rat liver parenchymal cells by chemical carcinogens in tissue culture. *In* "Chemical Carcinogenesis," ed. by P. O. P. Ts'o and J. A. DiPaolo, Marcel Dekker, Inc., New York, Part B, pp. 473–481 (1974).

9. Katsuta, H., Takaoka, T., and Yasumoto, S. Toxic metabolites released from rat hepatoma cells in culture. I. Effects of metabolites of hepatomas on various cells. *J. Natl. Cancer Inst.*, **51**, 1841–1844 (1973).

10. Montesano, R., Vincent, L. S., and Tomatis, L. Malignant transformation *in vitro* of rat liver cells by dimethylnitrosamine and N-methyl-N′-nitro-N-nitroso-guanidine. *Brit. J. Cancer*, **28**, 215–220 (1973).

11. Namba, M., Masuji, H., and Sato, J. Carcinogenesis in tissue culture. IX. Malignant transformation of cultured rat cells treated with 4-nitroquinoline 1-oxide. *Japan. J. Exp. Med.*, **39**, 253–265 (1969).

12. Sato, J. Carcinogenesis in tissue culture. IV. Proliferation-inducing effect of 4-dimethylaminoazobenzene and 3′-methyl-4-dimethylaminoazobenzene on liver cells from normal Donryu rats in culture. *Japan. J. Exp. Med.*, **35**, 433–444 (1965).

13. Takaoka, T. and Katsuta, H. Establishment of two inbred strains of the rat for cancer research in tissue culture. *Japan. J. Exp. Med.*, **43**, 403–411 (1973).

14. Williams, G. M., Elliott, J. M., and Weisburger, J. H. Carcinoma after malignant conversion *in vitro* of epithelial-like cells from rat liver following exposure to chemical carcinogens. *Cancer Res.*, **33**, 606–612 (1973).

15. Yamada, T., Takaoka, T., and Katsuta, H. Carcinogenesis in tissue culture. 23. Population analysis in the cultures of transformed rat liver cells by cell electrophoresis. *Japan. J. Exp. Med.*, **44**, 199–210 (1974).

16. Yamada, T., Takaoka, T., Katsuta, H., Namba, M., and Sato, J. Carcinogenesis in tissue culture. 20. Electrokinetic changes in cultured rat liver cells associated with malignant transformation *in vitro*. *Japan. J. Exp. Med.*, **42**, 377–388 (1972).

EXPLANATION OF PHOTOS

PHOTO 1.   Rat liver cells which initiated their proliferation after DAB treatment.

PHOTO 2.   The strain RLC-2 cells derived from a normal rat liver tissue.

PHOTO 3.   The strain JTC-22 cells derived from a normal rat liver but transformed by *Nagisa* culture.

PHOTO 4.   The strain RLC-10 cells derived from a normal rat liver but transformed into malignant cells by treatment with a chemical carcinogen (Exp. CQ-39), 4NQO in culture.

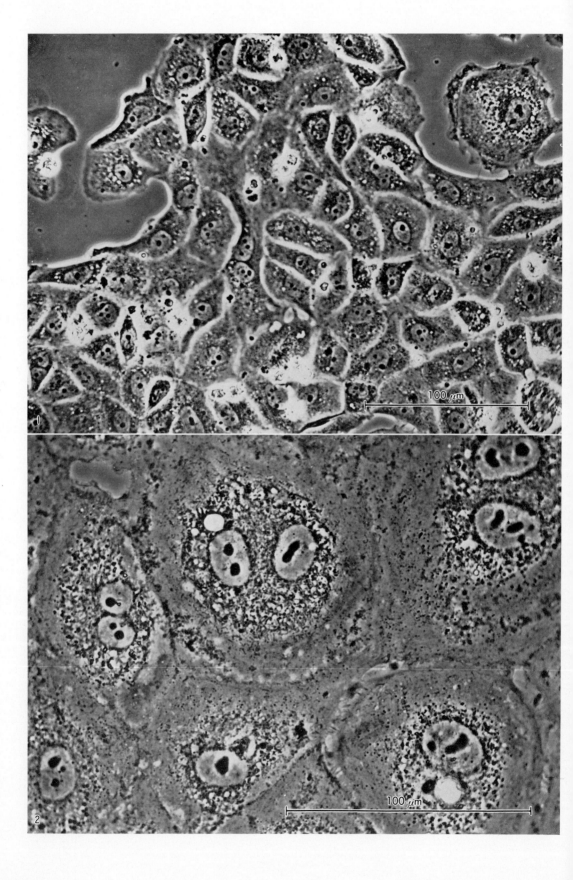

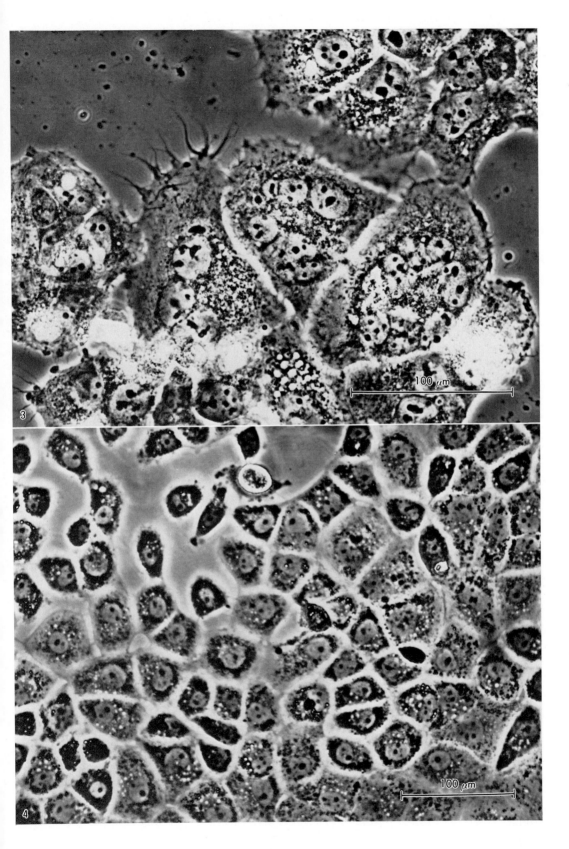

100 μm

100 μm

CHEMISTRY AND METABOLISM OF N-NITROSO COMPOUNDS

GANN Monograph on Cancer Research 17, 69–85 (1975)

CONTRIBUTIONS OF TISSUE CULTURE TO THE STUDY OF CHEMICAL CARCINOGENESIS: A REVIEW

Toshio KUROKI

*Department of Cancer Cell Research, Institute of Medical Science, University of Tokyo**

In this paper, contributions of tissue culture in the field of chemical carcinogenesis are reviewed. The most important contributions that tissue culture have made is the achievement of "chemical carcinogenesis in tissue culture"; that is, the conversion of normal cells or cells having normal characteristics to malignant cells or cells having malignant characteristics by treatment with chemicals. Experimental systems can be classified as follows:

1. Qualitative transformation using diploid fibroblastic cells.
2. Quantitative transformation using diploid fibroblastic cells.
3. Quantitative transformation using aneuploid fibroblastic cells.
4. Qualitative transformation using diploid epithelial cells.
5. Qualitative transformation using organ culture.

Future problems in this field are also discussed.

Almost four decades have passed since the great discovery of o-aminoazotoluol by Dr. T. Yoshida (*98*). However, we are still far from understanding the mechanisms by which cells undergo neoplastic transformation. We know that some chemicals and viruses cause cancer in humans and experimental animals, and it is significant that these chemicals and viruses are found in our environment. An understanding of the mechanisms of carcinogenesis would help us to prevent the occurrence of cancer and to eliminate these carcinogenic compounds and viruses from our environment. In this decade, marked progress has been made in the study of chemical carcinogenesis, using a variety of experimental systems for organic synthesis of possible metabolites of carcinogens, microbial assay systems of chemical mutagens and carcinogens, and tissue culture techniques. The most important contribution that tissue culture studies have made in this field is the achievement of "chemical carcinogenesis in tissue culture," that is, the conversion of normal cells or cells having normal characteristics to malignant cells or cells having malignant characteristics by treatment with chemicals. This seems to provide a reliable model of chemical carcinogenesis at a cellular level under controlled *in vitro* conditions. From the viewpoint of transformation experimental systems can be classified as either qualitative or quantitative, the cells used are either diploid or aneuploid and either fibroblastic or epithelial, and either in cell culture or in organ culture. In this paper I will

---

* Shirokanedai 4-6-1, Minato-ku, Tokyo 108, Japan (黒木登志夫).

briefly review the experimental systems by classifying into following five systems and will attempt to single out their advantages and, when appropriate, their disadvantages. Heidelberger (*32*) has recently reviewed the subject of chemical oncogenesis in culture.

Qualitative Systems for Chemical Transformation Using Diploid Fibroblastic Cells (*Table I*)

In 1965, Berwald and Sachs (*3*) reported the first successful malignant transformation of hamster embryo cells by treatment with carcinogenic hydrocarbons. The following year, Kamahora and Kakunaga (*47*), and we (*87*) reported independently that hamster embryo cells could be transformed by treatment with 4-nitroquinoline 1-oxide (4NQO) or its derivatives. Although malignant transformation has also been achieved with cells from rats (*5, 75, 81, 89, 92, 93*) and mice (*3, 29, 30, 33*), hamster cells have proved preferable because of their relatively low incidence of spontaneous transformation.

Morphological transformation usually appears within several weeks after treatment. The duration of effective treatment was successfully shortened to 15 min in the case of 4-hydroxyaminoquinoline 1-oxide (4HAQO), a proximate

TABLE I. Qualitative Systems for Chemical Transformation of Diploid Fibroblastic Cells

Cells	Chemicals	References
Hamster embryo	HC	Berwald and Sachs (*3*)
,,	4NQO, 4HAQO	Sato and Kuroki (*87*), Kuroki et al. (*54, 56, 57*)
,,	4NQO	Kamahora and Kakunaga (*47, 48*)
,,	HC	DiPaolo and Donovan (*18*)
,,	HC	Sivak and Van Duuren (*91*)
,,	DMN	Huberman et al. (*39*)
,,	NaNO$_2$	Tsuda et al. (*94*)
,,	Inhibitors of DNA synthesis[a]	Jones et al. (*43*)
Hamster lung	Cigarette tar	Inui and Takayama (*41*)
,,	MNNG	Inui et al. (*42*)
Mouse embryo	HC	Berwald and Sachs (*3*)
,,	NMU	Frei and Oliver (*29*)
,,	4NQO	Fujimoto (*30*)
Mouse prostate cells	HC	Heidelberger and Iype (*33*)
Rat embryo	4NQO	Namba et al. (*75*)
,,	HC	Rhim and Huebner (*81*)
,,	FAA	Sekely et al. (*89*)
Rat thymus, lung	MNNG	Takii et al. (*92*)
Rat kidney	DMN[b]	Borland and Hard (*5*)
Rat liver	AFB	Toyoshima et al. (*93*)

HC: carcinogenic polycyclic hydrocarbons. DMN: dimethylnitrosamine. MNNG: N-methyl-N'-nitro-N-nitrosoguanidine. NMU: nitrosomethylurea. FAA: fluorenylacetamide. AFB: aflatoxin B$_1$. [a] Inhibitors of DNA synthesis: 1-β-D-arabinofuranosylcytosine, 5-fluorodeoxyuridine, and hydroxyurea. [b] Host-mediated application.

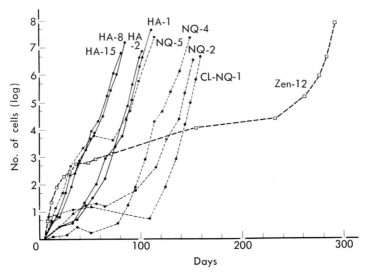

FIG. 1.   Cumulative growth curves of the carcinogen-treated and -untreated control cultures of hamster embryo cells

The ordinate shows cumulative increase in cell number with the cell number at the first subculture referred to one. NQ- and HA- indicate the cells treated with 4NQO and 4HAQO, respectively. Zen-12 shows the control cells which, during the first three or four weeks, grew rapidly, then gradually lost their ability to proliferate and finally transformed spontaneously. In our system, the spontaneous transformation of hamster cells was observed in 2 out of 12 cultures, after 260 days in culture.

carcinogen of 4NQO (*56*). In general, the transformed cells are characterized by the following characteristics: loss of contact inhibition in terms of a criss-crossed arrangement of cells and piling up growth, ability to grow *in vitro* beyond the normal life span (Fig. 1), cell agglutination with plant agglutinin, formation of colonies in soft agar medium, and production of fibrosarcomas on inoculation into suitable animals. Among these characters, piling up growth of cells seems to be a reliable parameter *in vitro* for assessing malignant transformation of fibroblastic cells. A criss-crossed arrangement of cells, another expression of loss of contact inhibition, usually appears in the early stage of transformation, but sometimes it becomes obscure after transfer of cells. In a later stage of transformation, however, the cells tended to pile up with a parallel rather than a random orientation.

Chromosomal analysis has indicated that cells at an early stage of transformation have a diploid or near-diploid distribution, but later their karyotypes shift more or less from those of normal cells (*100*). DiPaolo *et al.* (*23*) reported that chemically transformed cells were generally near-diploid and had 10 marker chromosomes that were recognizable by the banding technique.

In studies on the kinetics of glucose and amino acid uptake, we found that the maximum velocity of 2-deoxy-D-glucose uptake in chemically transformed cells was 1.5- to 2.8-fold that of control cells, though the apparent K_m was unchanged (*58*). This increase in uptake of glucose after chemical transformation seems to result from increased uptake, rather than increased phosphorylation after transport, since the isozymes and activity of hexokinase before and after chemical transformation were similar. We also found that the chemically transformed cells showed increased aerobic glycolysis compared to normal cells and a Crabtree effect (88).

The process through which the cells acquire a neoplastic potential is a progressive change. We found that malignancy is enhanced with time of cultivation or through cell divisions (56, 57). From the clonal analysis, it seems likely that at least two mechanisms may operate in the progressive development of malignancy; (1) progressive change in malignancy within a clone and (2) selective overgrowth of the cells from highly malignant clones. Kakunaga and Kamahora (46) reported progression from small to large colonies in soft agar. It is not known whether these changes in chromosomal constitutions and glucose utilization, mentioned above, are results of transformation or further progression of the transformed cells.

Thus, these systems have the advantage that the whole course of transformation from normal to malignant cells can be investigated at a cellular level, but the disadvantage that quantitative measurements are not possible.

Quantitative Systems for Chemical Transformation Using Diploid Fibroblastic Cells (Table II)

A technique for quantitative transformation by chemical carcinogens was established by Berwald and Sachs using Syrian hamster embryo cells (2, 3). This system has since been used extensively by DiPaolo et al. (19–22). In this system, 8–10 days after treatment with a carcinogen, the transformation of colonies is judged as a random pattern of cell orientation, particularly at the edge of colonies. In this case, piling up of cells is not considered as a good indicator of transformation. DiPaolo et al. (20) showed that the isolated transformed colonies subsequently developed into cell lines that, unlike control cultures, produced fibrosarcomas on injection into hamsters.

TABLE II. Quantitative Systems for Chemical Transformation of Diploid Fibroblasts

Cells	Chemicals	References
Hamster embryo	HC	Berwald and Sachs (2, 3)
,,	HC	Huberman and Sachs (36)
,,	HC, AFB, N-acetoxy-FAA, MNNG, (urethan, DEN)[a]	DiPaolo et al. (19–21)
,,	N-acetoxy-FAA	Huberman et al. (34)
,,	HC	Umeda and Iype (95)
,,	Epoxides of HC	Huberman et al. (35)
,,	Epoxides of HC	Grover et al. (31)
,,	(HC, DEN, ENU, AFB, FAA, DAB, 4NQO, BPL, PPS)[a]	DiPaolo et al. (22)
Mouse embryo	HC	Berwald and Sachs (3)

DEN: diethylnitrosamine. ENU: ethylnitrosourea. DAB: dimethylaminoazobenzene. BPL: β-propionolactone. PPS: propane sultone. [a] Transplacental application.

Transformation was achieved by diverse chemical carcinogens, such as AFB, a proximate form of FAA, 11-methylcyclopenta[a]phenanthrene, and MNNG. Although urethan, N-hydroxyurethan, DEN, and DAB failed to transform cells when added to tissue cultures, transplacental administration of these chemicals produced transformation of cells derived from the embryos, suggesting that these chemicals require *in vivo* activation (21, 22).

Huberman and Sachs (36) demonstrated that the slope of the linear dose-response curve of transformation with benzo[a]pyrene (BP) concentrations of up to 10 μg/ml differed significantly from that of cytotoxicity. This suggests that transformation and cytotoxicity caused by this carcinogen are two different events. Similar results were obtained on quantitative transformation of aneuploid fibroblasts (11, 79).

This system also has advantages and disadvantages. An advantage is that using diploid cells transformation can be estimated within 10 days after treatment. However, the system involves heterogeneous secondary cultures of cells derived from the noninbred hamster, and in practice it may be difficult to distinguish transformed colonies from normal ones. For the latter reason, this system has not been widely used.

Quantitative Systems for Chemical Transformation Using Aneuploid Fibroblastic Cells (Table III)

In these systems, transformation is estimated quantitatively by scoring piled up, multilayered foci, which are easily distinguished from the surrounding monolayer of control cells (Photo 1). The cells used in these systems were C3H mouse prostate cells, BALB 3T3 cells, and C3H mouse embryo 10T1/2 cells.

TABLE III.   Quantitative Systems for Chemical Transformation of Aneuploid Fibroblastic Cells

Cells	Chemicals	References
C3H mouse prostate cells	HC	Chen and Heidelberger (11)
,,	HC	Mondal and Heidelberger (73)
,,	Epoxides of HC	Grover et al. (31)
,,	Epoxides of HC	Marquardt et al. (68, 69)
M2 clone of C3H mouse prostate	HC	Marquardt (66, 67)
,,	Epoxides of HC	Marquardt et al. (70)
BALB 3T3	HC, MNNG, N-acetoxy-FAA, AFB	DiPaolo et al. (24)
,,	4NQO, MNNG, HC	Kakunaga (45)
10T1/2	HC	Reznikoff et al. (79)
,,	MNNG	Bertram and Heidelberger (1)
Chinese hamster cell line	HC	Borenfreund et al. (4)
,,	NMU	Sanders and Burford (84, 85)
,,	UV, NMU, HC, nitroso compounds	Sanders (83)

UV : ultraviolet.

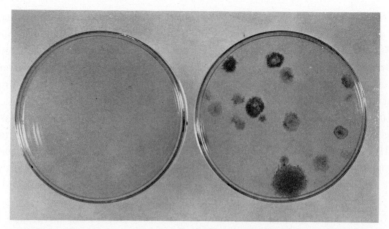

PHOTO 1.   The control (left) and BP (1 μg/ml) treated culture of 10T1/2 cells
   The distinct transformed foci that formed a dense layer are seen in the
treated dish, which makes striking contrast to the flat, lightly stained control
dish, cultured for 5 weeks.

These cells are aneuploid fibroblast cell lines with high sensitivity to contact inhibition.

A quantitative system for transformation of C3H mouse prostate cells was developed by Chen and Heidelberger (9–11). These cells underwent transformation within 8 weeks after treatment with various kinds of carcinogenic hydrocarbons. Morphologically transformed clones produced fibrosarcomas on injection into isologous mice, while control cells did not. No transformation was observed when the carcinogen was applied after confluent monolayers had been formed, suggesting that cell division is required to "fix" the transformation. It was demonstrated from Heidelberger's laboratory (26, 72, 73) that the chemically transformed clones of mouse prostate cells are highly antigenic and their tumor-specific transplantation antigens are non-crossreacting. Thus, the concept of "individuality of cancer cells" proposed by Yoshida (99) was also confirmed using tissue culture technique.

This system has since been extensively used for the studies on metabolic activation of carcinogenic hydrocarbons. It was demonstrated from Heidelberger's laboratory (31, 35, 69) that the K-region epoxides of benz[a]anthracene, dibenz[a,h]anthracene (DBA), and 3-methylcholanthrene (MCA) may be the activated metabolites. The enzyme system involved in this metabolic activation is known as arylhydrocarbon hydroxylase or BP hydroxylase. Marquardt and Heidelberger (68) demonstrated that MCA-induced transformation was enhanced when the prostate cells had been pretreated with inducers of this enzyme or plated on an irradiated "feeder layer" of rodent fibroblasts that metabolize the carcinogen, while transformation produced by the K-region epoxide of MCA was decreased. This and other experiments suggest that in the system of arylhydrocarbon hydroxylase, there are at least two enzymes, an epoxide-forming enzyme and epoxide hydrase which are involved, respectively, in metabolic activation and detoxication of polycyclic hydrocarbons.

Recently, Marquardt (66) established a transformable cell line of mouse fibroblasts from C3H mouse prostate using the procedures described by Chen and Heidelberger (9). With a clone of this cell line, Marquardt (67) demonstrated cell cycle dependence of chemical transformation; i.e., when the cells were synchronized by double thymidine block and then treated with a short-lasting chemical such as 7,12-dimethylbenz[a]anthracene-5,6-epoxide or MNNG at various times after release of the block, malignant transformation was observed only in the G_1 and S phases of the cell cycle.

A quantitative system using BALB 3T3 cells was developed independently by DiPaolo et al. (24) and by Kakunaga (45). Transformation of cells in this system was observed with the carcinogenic hydrocarbons, AFB, N-acetoxy-FAA, MNNG, and 4NQO. Fibrosarcomas were produced at the site of injection of the transformed cells, while no tumor was obtained with control cells. DiPaolo et al. (24) found a Poisson frequency of distribution in transformed colonies per dish, suggesting that transformation is due to induction.

A third quantitative transformation system was recently developed by Reznikoff et al. (79, 80) using C3H mouse embryo 10T1/2 cells, which were established by transferring cells at 10-day intervals at a cell density of 5×10^4 cells/60-mm dish. In this system transformation can be scored within 6 weeks after treatment with carcinogenic hydrocarbons (Photo 1). Transformed clones produced fibrosarcomas while control cells did not. 10T1/2 cells were negative with respect to spontaneous expression of C-type RNA murine viruses and viral antigens. Bertram et al. (1) recently demonstrated, by 4 synchrony-producing methods, that 10T1/2 cells are most sensitive to transformation by MNNG at the period of the G_1-S boundary. It was concluded by Peterson et al. (78) that there is no direct relationship in cell cycle between DNA repair, as measured by alkaline sucrose sedimentation, and susceptibility to transformation or lethality produced by MNNG.

In addition to these cells derived from mice, a Chinese hamster cell line has also been used by Borenfreund et al. (4) and Sanders (83–85) for studies on chemical transformation. This particular cell line can be induced to form morphologically abnormal colonies by treatment with polycyclic hydrocarbons, nitroso compounds, and a variety of other water-soluble substances, as well as by irradiation with X rays or UV ray. Sanders (83) proposed a value of efficacy of cell conversion that can be calculated from the dose-response curves for cytotoxicity and conversion.

These systems have the advantages that transformation, in most cases accompanied with malignancy, can be scored quantitatively within several weeks after treatment and that various fine techniques of cell culture, such as cloning and synchronous culture, are applicable in studies on chemical transformation. However, a disadvantage is the use of aneuploid cells, even though these cells are sensitive to contact inhibition. Another problem in practice is the difficulty of maintaining control cells with sensitivity to contact inhibition, since if the sera or transfer schedule is not adequate, these cells are readily replaced by cells which are not contact inhibited.

Quantitative Systems for Chemical Transformation Using Diploid Epithelial Cells (Table IV)

A limited variety of epithelial cells have been cultured and proved to be useful in studies on chemical carcinogenesis. As summarized in Table IV, most experiments have been carried out with epithelial cells derived from rat liver, and these are reviewed by Katsuta and Takaoka in another chapter of this Monograph. Transformation of liver cells usually took longer time than that of fibroblastic cells; in Katsuta and Takaoka's experiments (*49*), malignant transformation was obtained about 3.5 months after treatment with 4NQO and tumors developed after a latent period of 3.6 months. The tumors obtained were mainly diagnosed as hepatomas, though in some instances the histology of the tumors showed the co-existence of carcinomatous and sarcomatous features (*49, 74, 75, 97*). Such mixtures of histological types may result either from transformation of mesenchymal cells, co-existing with a cell line which has an epithelial-like morphology, or from further transformation of epithelial cells into sarcomatous cells. An example of the latter change is the conversion of a pure clone of mouse mammary carcinoma to a sarcomatous tumor (*86*). In some cases, adenocarcinomas were obtained on inoculation of epithelial cells derived from rat liver (*74, 97*). Although adenomatous type hepatocellular carcinomas are formed on transplantation of rat hepatomas (*71*), the possibility that the tumors were derived from bile duct cells cannot be disregarded.

TABLE IV. Quantitative Systems for Chemical Transformation of Diploid Epithelial Cells

Cells	Chemicals	References
Rat liver cells	4NQO	Namba *et al.* (*75*)
,,	4NQO	Katsuta and Takaoka (*49*)
,,	AFB, DMN, NMU, FAA, HC	Williams *et al.* (*97*)
,,	MNNG, DMN	Montesano *et al.* (*74*)
Submandibular gland of rat	HC	Brown (*7*)

One difficulty in studies on chemical transformation of epithelial cells is the lack of suitable *in vitro* parameters of malignant transformation. The concept of contact inhibition was deduced from studies on fibroblastic cells and is hardly applicable to epithelial cells. The discrepancy between *in vitro* parameters and *in vivo* malignancy was discussed by Katsuta and Takaoka (*50*). The lack of a suitable parameter makes it difficult to establish a quantitative transformation system with epithelial cells.

Qualitative Systems for Chemical Transformation Using Organ Culture (Table V)

The above-mentioned experiments were carried out in cell cultures or monolayer cultures in which cells usually lose many of their morphological and structural characteristics and specific functions. Studies on chemical carcinogenesis using organ culture may approximate more closely to conditions *in vivo* than

TABLE V. Qualitative Systems for Chemical Transformation Using Organ Culture

Cells	Chemicals	References
Mouse prostate	HC	Lasnitzki (*59, 63*)
,,	HC	Röller and Heidelberger (*82*)
,,	HC	Heidelberger and Iype (*33*)
Mouse lung	HC	Flaks *et al.* (*27, 28*), Laws and Flaks (*64*)
,,	HC	Davies *et al.* (*15*)
Mouse lung bud	HC	Chan *et al.* (*8*)
Mouse ovary	HC	Jull *et al.* (*44*)
Mouse kidney	HC	Shabad *et al.* (*90*)
Rat trachea	HC	Crocker and Sanders (*12*), Dirksen and Crocker (*25*), Palekar *et al.* (*77*)
Rat mammary gland	HC	Dao (*13*), Dao and Sinha (*14*), Koyama *et al.* (*52*)
Human lung	HC	Lasnitzki (*60*)
,,	Cigarette smoke	Lasnitzki (*61, 62*)

those using cell cultures. There have been a number of studies on organ cultures, as summarized in Table V. Lasnitzki (*59, 63*) made extensive studies on the morphological effects of carcinogenic hydrocarbons on mouse and rat prostate glands in organ cultures. She observed that MCA-induced hyperplasia and metaplasia of the alveolar epithelium of prostate glands, which closely resembled preneoplastic changes. Similar observations of hyperplasia and metaplasia of epithelium produced by carcinogens were obtained in organ cultures of lung, trachea, kidney, and mammary glands of mouse, rat, hamster, and man (*12, 25, 52, 60–62, 77, 90*). Lasnitzki (*59, 63*) and Crocker and Sanders (*12*) found that vitamin A compounds counteract the hyperplastic and metaplastic changes induced by carcinogens and the cells maintain normal differentiation. The mechanisms involved in the antagonistic effect of vitamin A remain to be determined.

In spite of these histological changes, after treatment with carcinogens, these fragments did not usually produce tumors on implantation. Röller and Heidelberger (*82*) reported that no tumors were obtained on implantation of 872 carcinogen-treated specimens from organ cultures into isologous hosts. Later, Heidelberger and Iype (*33*) prepared monolayer cultures from organ-cultured fragments by dispersing the cells with pronase. Cell lines obtained from the carcinogen-treated organ cultures showed loss of contact inhibition and formed sarcomas on inoculation into isologous mice, while the control failed to grow continuously in cell culture.

Formation of tumors by tissues from organ cultures, without subsequent cell culture as mentioned above, were reported by Jull *et al.* (*44*), Flaks group (*27, 28, 64*), Davies *et al.* (*15*), and Dao group (*13, 14*). In these experiments, tissue fragments were maintained in organ culture for relatively short periods (usually less than 4 days), and treated with a relatively high dose of carcinogen and then implanted into isologous mice. Tumors usually appeared after 1 year or more.

Thus, systems using organ cultures have the advantage that the morphological effects of carcinogens on epithelium can be observed while keeping the *in vivo* structural correlation between epithelium and mesenchyme. But they have the disadvantage that, in spite of morphological changes analogous to precancerous changes, malignancy is only observed either by transferring organ cultures to cell cultures or after a prolonged latent period on implantation.

Future Problems

The primary object of studies on chemical carcinogenesis in tissue cultures is to obtain a model system for studies on mechanisms of chemical carcinogenesis. A number of tissue culture systems have been established for this purpose, as described above. However, the variety of cell systems available is still limited; the cell lines used are mainly fibroblasts, and less often rat liver cells. Thus it seems important to establish new experimental systems using a variety of cells from various organs; for example, epithelial cells from the gastro-intestinal tract, cells of nervous tissues, functioning cells from endocrine glands, and blood cells. An adequate transformation system using epithelial cells would be valuable, since carcinomas represent almost 90% of naturally occurring human tumors and may involve many interesting problems, such as cellular differentiation and metabolic activation of chemicals.

Tissue culture systems have the advantage over experimental animals that they permit elucidation of mechanisms which are obscure in the whole animal. In the near future we should consider "reconstitution" of these model *in vitro* systems, by adding *in vivo* factors, such as immunity. In this way it should be possible to evaluate the roles of various *in vivo* factors in development of cancer.

Chemical transformation systems will provide convenient assay systems for screening large numbers of environmental chemicals. In the systems described above, good correlations were found between carcinogenic potency *in vivo* and transforming activity *in vitro*. However, no transformation was observed when some carcinogens, including azo dyes, nitrosamine, and urethan, were tested in tissue culture. Recently DiPaolo *et al.* (*22*) and Borland and Hard (*5*) demonstrated that assay of transformation of cells after host-mediated application of chemicals reduced false-negative results such as these, which may be metabolic activation *in vivo*.

It should be possible to assess the risk of chemicals and environmental hazards to man using tissue culture of human cells. It will also be possible to examine problems such as drug metabolism, and chemical carcinogenesis and mutagenesis of human cells. There are already some studies along these lines: Dietz and Flaxman (*17*) attempted to transform human epidermis cells with carcinogenic hydrocarbons, but they did not observe any evidence of malignant transformation. In organ culture, as described above (Table V), Lasnitzki (*60–62*) observed that BP and cigarette smoke cause hyperplasia and metaplasia of the bronchial epithelium of human fetal lung. Several papers have shown that arylhydrocarbon hydroxylase is found in human cells (*6, 16, 37, 51, 65, 76, 96*), although the enzyme activity varied according to individuals (*37, 51, 65*), type of cells (epithelial or fibroblastic) (*37*), cigarette smoking (*76, 96*), and patients with bronchogenic carcinoma (*51*). Diamond *et al.* (*16*) found that human fibro-blasts are resistant to the cytotoxic action of carcinogenic hydrocarbons, and their metabolism and bindings are much less in human cells than in rodent cells. Similarly, we found the lack of binding of DBA and its K-region epoxide to basic soluble protein of human cells, whose profile on gel electrophoresis differed from that of rodent cells (*55*). Marquardt and Heidelberger (*68*), and Huberman and Sachs (*38*) used X-irradiated human fibroblasts as mediators of drug metabolism in chemical transformation and mutation, but, unlike rodent cells, human cells failed to mediate drug metabolism. It is evident that much more work is needed on human cells. For this, stock cultures of a wide variety of human cells would be useful.

Literature accumulated in recent years has indicated that most, and perhaps all, chemical carcinogens are mutagens and that DNA lesions caused by these chemicals can be recognized and repaired by a similar mechanism to that involved in the repair of UV-irradiated damage. Thus, there seems to be a close, but complicated relationship among carcinogenesis, mutagenesis, and DNA repair. To elucidate this relationship, an experimental system must be established in which both mutagenesis and carcinogenesis can be investigated in the same cell line. Cell lines lacking a DNA-repair system would be useful for studies on the possible involvement of DNA repair in chemical carcinogenesis. Accordingly, we have recently established a Lederberg-style replica plating method for mammalian cells to isolate UV-sensitive clones (*53*).

Huebner and Todaro (*40*) suggested that genetic information of cancer might be integrated into all mammalian cells as "oncogenes" or "virogenes" and expressed as C-type RNA tumor viruses, and that chemical carcinogens and many other carcinogenic agents may merely activate or "switch-on" this integrated virus genome. It is very difficult to find evidence to prove or disprove Huebner and Todaro's suggestion, but the relation between viral and chemical carcinogeneses should be investigated carefully in the near future.

Acknowledgment

The author is deeply grateful to the late Dr. T. Yoshida for his continued interest and encouragement during studies on chemical transformation of hamster embryo cells.

REFERENCES

1. Bertram, J. S. and Heidelberger, C. Cell cycle dependency of oncogenic transformation induced by N-methyl-N'-nitro-N-nitrosoguanidine in culture. *Cancer Res.*, **34**, 526–537 (1974).
2. Berwald, Y. and Sachs, L. *In vitro* transformation with chemical carcinogens. *Nature*, **200**, 1182–1184 (1963).
3. Berwald, Y. and Sachs, L. *In vitro* transformation of normal cells to tumor cells by carcinogenic hydrocarbons. *J. Natl. Cancer Inst.*, **35**, 641–661 (1965).
4. Borenfreund, E., Krim, M., Sanders, F. K., Sternberg, S. S., and Bendich, A. Malignant conversion of cells *in vitro* by carcinogens and viruses. *Proc. Natl. Acad. Sci. U.S.*, **56**, 672–679 (1969).
5. Borland, R. and Hard, G. C. Early appearance of "transformed" cells from the

kidneys of rats treated with a "single" carcinogenic dose of dimethylnitrosamine (DMN) detected by culture *in vitro. Eur. J. Cancer*, **10**, 177–184 (1974).

6. Brookes, P. and Duncan, M. E. Carcinogenic hydrocarbons and human cells in culture. *Nature*, **234**, 40–43 (1971).

7. Brown, A. M. *In vitro* transformation of submandibular gland epithelial cells and fibroblasts of adult rats by methylcholanthrene. *Cancer Res.*, **33**, 2779–2789 (1973).

8. Chan, P. C., Sanders, F. K., and Wynder, E. L. Effect of 3,4-benzo[a]pyrene on mouse lung primordia *in vitro. Nature*, **223**, 847–848 (1969).

9. Chen, T. T. and Heidelberger, C. Cultivation *in vitro* of cells derived from adult C3H mouse ventral prostate. *J. Natl. Cancer Inst.*, **42**, 903–914 (1969).

10. Chen, T. T. and Heidelberger, C. *In vitro* malignant transformation of cells derived from mouse prostate in the presence of 3-methylcholanthrene. *J. Natl. Cancer Inst.*, **42**, 915–925 (1969).

11. Chen, T. T. and Heidelberger, C. Quantitative studies on the malignant transformation of mouse prostate cells by carcinogenic hydrocarbons *in vitro. Int. J. Cancer*, **4**, 166–178 (1969).

12. Crocker, T. T. and Sanders, L. L. Influence of vitamin A and 3,7-dimethyl-2,6-octadienal (citral) on the effect of benzo[a]pyrene on hamster trachea in organ culture. *Cancer Res.*, **30**, 1312-1318 (1970).

13. Dao, T. L. Induction of mammary cancer after *in vitro* exposure to 7,12-dimethylbenz[a]anthracene. *Proc. Soc. Exp. Biol. Med.*, **133**, 416–418 (1970).

14. Dao, T. L. and Sinha, D. Mammary adenocarcinoma induced in organ culture by 7,12-dimethylbenz[a]anthracene. *J. Natl. Cancer Inst.*, **49**, 591–593 (1972).

15. Davies, R. F., Major, I. R., and Aberdeen, E. R. Pulmonary adenomata induced by carcinogen treatment in organ culture. Influence of increasing amount of carcinogen. *Brit. J. Cancer*, **24**, 785–787 (1970).

16. Diamond, L., Defendi, V., and Brookes, P. The interaction of 7,12-dimethylbenz[a]anthracene with cells sensitive and resistant to toxicity induced by this carcinogen. *Cancer Res.*, **27**, 890–897 (1967).

17. Dietz, M. H. and Flaxman, B. A. Toxicity of aromatic hydrocarbons on normal human epidermal cells *in vitro. Cancer Res.*, **31**, 1206–1209 (1971).

18. DiPaolo, J. A. and Donovan, P. J. Properties of Syrian hamster cells transformed in the presence of carcinogenic hydrocarbons. *Exp. Cell Res.*, **48**, 361–377 (1967).

19. DiPaolo, J. A., Donovan, P. J., and Nelson, R. L. Quantitative studies of *in vitro* transformation by chemical carcinogens. *J. Natl. Cancer Inst.*, **42**, 867–874 (1969).

20. DiPaolo, J. A., Nelson, R. L., and Donovan, P. J. Sarcoma-producing cell lines derived from clones transformed *in vitro* by benzo[a]pyrene. *Science*, **165**, 917–918 (1969).

21. DiPaolo, J. A., Nelson, R. L., and Donovan, P. J. *In vitro* transformation of Syrian hamster embryo cells by diverse chemical carcinogens. *Nature New Biol.*, **235**, 278–280 (1972).

22. DiPaolo, J. A., Nelson, R. L., Donovan, P. J., and Evans, C. H. Host-mediated *in vivo-in vitro* assay for chemical carcinogenesis. *Arch. Pathol.*, **95**, 380–385 (1973).

23. DiPaolo, J. A., Popescu, N. C., and Nelson, R. L. Chromosomal banding patterns and *in vitro* transformation of Syrian hamster cells. *Cancer Res.*, **33**, 3250–3258 (1973).

24. DiPaolo, J. A., Takano, K., and Popescu, N. C. Quantitation of chemically induced neoplastic transformation of BALB/3T3 cloned cell lines. *Cancer Res.*, **32**, 2686–2695 (1972).

25. Dirksen, E. R. and Crocker, T. T. Ultrastructural alterations produced by poly-cyclic aromatic hydrocarbons on rat tracheal epithelium in organ culture. *Cancer Res.*, **28**, 906–923 (1968).

26. Embleton, M. J. and Heidelberger, C. Antigenicity of clones of mouse prostate cells transformed *in vitro*. *Int. J. Cancer*, **9**, 8–18 (1972).

27. Flaks, A. and Hamilton, J. M. *In vitro* effects of chemical carcinogens. *Eur. J. Cancer*, **6**, 151–153 (1970).

28. Flaks, A. and Laws, J. P. Pulmonary adenomata induced by carcinogen treatment in organ culture. Influence of duration of treatment. *Brit. J. Cancer*, **22**, 839–842 (1968).

29. Frei, J. V. and Oliver, J. Influence of methylnitrosourea on malignant transforma-tion of mouse embryo cells in tissue culture. *J. Natl. Cancer Inst.*, **47**, 857–863 (1971).

30. Fujimoto, J. Malignant transformations of C3H mouse cells *in vitro*. Development of transplantable ascites tumors from mouse embryo cells treated with 4-nitro-quinoline 1-oxide. *J. Natl. Cancer Inst.*, **50**, 79–85 (1973).

31. Grover, P. L., Sims, P., Huberman, E., Marquardt, H., Kuroki, T., and Hei-delberger, C. *In vitro* transformation of rodent cells by K-region derivatives of polycyclic hydrocarbons. *Proc. Natl. Acad. Sci. U.S.*, **68**, 1098–1101 (1971).

32. Heidelberger, C. Chemical oncogenesis in culture. *Adv. Cancer Res.*, **18**, 317–366 (1973).

33. Heidelberger, C. and Iype, P. T. Malignant transformation *in vitro* by car-cinogenic hydrocarbons. *Science*, **155**, 214–217 (1967).

34. Huberman, E., Donovan, P. J., and DiPaolo, J. A. Mutation and transformation of cultured mammalian cells by N-acetoxy-N-2-fluorenylacetamide. *J. Natl. Cancer Inst.*, **48**, 837–840 (1972).

35. Huberman, E., Kuroki, T., Marquardt, H., Selkirk, J. K., Heidelberger, C., Grover, P. L., and Sims, P. Transformation of hamster embryo cells by epoxides and other derivatives of polycyclic hydrocarbons. *Cancer Res.*, **32**, 1391–1396 (1972).

36. Huberman, E. and Sachs, L. Cell susceptibility to transformation and cytotoxicity by the carcinogenic hydrocarbon benzo[a]pyrene. *Proc. Natl. Acad. Sci. U.S.*, **56**, 1123–1129 (1966).

37. Huberman, E. and Sachs, L. Metabolism of the carcinogenic hydrocarbon benzo-[a]pyrene in human fibroblast and epithelial cells. *Int. J. Cancer*, **11**, 412–418 (1973).

38. Huberman, E. and Sachs, L. Cell-mediated mutagenesis of mammalian cells with chemical carcinogens. *Int. J. Cancer*, **13**, 326–333 (1974).

39. Huberman, E., Salzberg, S., and Sachs, L. The *in vitro* induction of an increase in cell multiplication and cellular life span by the water-soluble carcinogen dimethylnitrosamine. *Proc. Natl. Acad. Sci. U.S.*, **59**, 77–82 (1968).

40. Huebner, R. J. and Todaro, G. J. Oncogens of RNA tumor viruses as determinants of cancer. *Proc. Natl. Acad. Sci. U.S.*, **64**, 1087–1094 (1969).

41. Inui, N. and Takayama, S. Effect of cigarette tar upon tissue culture cells. Neo-plastic transformation of hamster lung cells by tobacco tar in tissue culture. *Brit. J. Cancer*, **25**, 574–583 (1971).

42. Inui, N., Takayama, S., and Sugimura, T. Neoplastic transformation and chro-mosomal aberrations induced by N-methyl-N'-nitro-N-nitrosoguanidine. *J. Natl. Cancer Inst.*, **48**, 1409–1417 (1972).

43. Jones, P. A., Taderera, J. V., and Hawtrey, A. O. Transformation of hamster

cells *in vitro* by 1-β-D-arabinofuranosylcytosine, 5-fluorodeoxyuridine and hydroxyurea. *Eur. J. Cancer*, **8**, 595–599 (1972).

44.   Jull, J. W., Hawryluk, A., and Russell, A. Mechanism of induction of ovarian tumors in the mouse by 7,12-dimethylbenz[a]anthracene. III. Tumor induction in organ culture. *J. Natl. Cancer Inst.*, **40**, 687–706 (1968).

45.   Kakunaga, T. A quantitative system for assay of malignant transformation by chemical carcinogens using a clone derived from BALB/3T3. *Int. J. Cancer*, **12**, 463–473 (1973).

46.   Kakunaga, T. and Kamahora, J. Properties of hamster embryonic cells transformed by 4-nitroquinoline 1-oxide *in vitro* and their correlations with the malignant properties of the cells. *Biken J.*, **11**, 313–332 (1968).

47.   Kamahora, J. and Kakunaga, T. *In vitro* carcinogenesis of 4-nitroquinoline 1-oxide with hamster embryonic cells. *Proc. Japan Acad.*, **42**, 1079–1081 (1966).

48.   Kamahora, J. and Kakunaga, T. Malignant transformation of hamster embryonic cells *in vitro* by 4-nitroquinoline 1-oxide. *Biken J.*, **10**, 219–242 (1967).

49.   Katsuta, H. and Takaoka, T. Carcinogenesis in tissue culture. XIV. Malignant transformation of rat liver parenchymal cells treated with 4-nitroquinoline 1-oxide in tissue culture. *J. Natl. Cancer Inst.*, **49**, 1563–1576 (1972).

50.   Katsuta, H. and Takaoka, T. Parameters for malignant transformation of mammalian cells treated with chemical carcinogenesis in tissue culture. *In* "Topics in Chemical Carcinogenesis," ed. by W. Nakahara, S. Takayama, T. Sugimura, and S. Odashima, University of Tokyo Press, Tokyo, pp. 389–400 (1972).

51.   Kellermann, G., Shaw, C. R., and Luyten-Kellermann, M. Aryl hydrocarbon hydroxylase inducibility and bronchogenic carcinoma. *New Engl. J. Med.*, **289**, 934–937 (1973).

52.   Koyama, H., Sinha, D., and Dao, T. L. Effect of hormone and 7,12-dimethylbenz-[a]anthracene on rat mammary tissue grown in organ culture. *J. Natl. Cancer Inst.*, **48**, 1671–1680 (1972).

53.   Kuroki, T. Colony formation of mammalian cells on agar plates and its application to Lederberg's replica plating. *Exp. Cell Res.*, **80**, 55–62 (1973).

54.   Kuroki, T., Goto, M., and Sato, H. Malignant transformation of hamster embryonic cells by 4-hydroxyaminoquinoline N-oxide in tissue culture. *Tohoku J. Exp. Med.*, **91**, 109–118 (1967).

55.   Kuroki, T. and Heidelberger, C. Determination of the h-protein in transformable cells and transformed cells in culture. *Biochemistry*, **11**, 2116–2124 (1972).

56.   Kuroki, T. and Sato, H. Transformation and neoplastic development *in vitro* of hamster embryonic cells by 4-nitroquinoline 1-oxide and its derivatives. *J. Natl. Cancer Inst.*, **41**, 53–71 (1968).

57.   Kuroki, T. and Sato, H. Carcinogenesis *in vitro* with nitroquinoline 1-oxide derivatives. *In* "Oncology 1970" (Proc. 10th Int. Cancer Congr.), ed. by R. L. Clark, R. W. Cumley, J. E. McCay, and M. M. Copeland, Year Book Medical Publishers Inc., Chicago, Vol. 1, pp. 91–103 (1971).

58.   Kuroki, T. and Yamakawa, S. Kinetics of uptake of 2-deoxy-D-glucose and 2-aminoisobutyric acid in chemically transformed cells. *Int. J. Cancer*, **13**, 240–245 (1974).

59.   Lasnitzki, I. The influence of a hypervitaminosis on the effect of 20-methylcholanthrene on mouse prostate glands grown *in vitro*. *Brit. J. Cancer*, **9**, 434–441 (1955).

60.   Lasnitzki, I. The effect of 3,4-benzpyrene on human foetal lung grown *in vitro*. *Brit. J. Cancer*, **10**, 510–516 (1956).

61. Lasnitzki, I. Observations on the effects of condensates from cigarette smoke on human foetal lung *in vitro*. *Brit. J. Cancer*, **12**, 547–552 (1958).

62. Lasnitzki, I. The effect of a hydrocarbon-enriched fraction of cigarette smoke condensate on human fetal lung grown *in vitro*. *Cancer Res.*, **28**, 510–516 (1968).

63. Lasnitzki, I. and Goodman, D. S. Inhibition of the effects of methylcholanthrene on mouse prostate in organ culture by vitamin A and its analogs. *Cancer Res.*, **34**, 1564–1571 (1974).

64. Laws, J. O. and Flaks, A. Pulmonary adenomata induced by carcinogen treatment in organ culture. *Brit. J. Cancer*, **20**, 550–554 (1966).

65. Levin, W., Conney, A. M., Alvares, A. P., Merkatz, L., and Kappas, A. Induction of benzo[a]pyrene hydroxylase in human skin. *Science*, **176**, 419–420 (1972).

66. Marquardt, H. The effect of X-irradiation on hydrocarbon metabolism and on hydrocarbon-induced lethality and transformation in cells derived from mouse prostate. *Z. Krebsforsch.*, **80**, 223–228 (1973).

67. Marquardt, H. Cell cycle dependence of chemically induced malignant transformation *in vitro*. *Cancer Res.*, **34**, 1612–1615 (1974).

68. Marquardt, H. and Heidelberger, C. Influence of "feeder cells" and inducers and inhibitors of microsomal mixed function oxidases on hydrocarbon-induced malignant transformation of cells derived from C3H mouse prostate. *Cancer Res.*, **32**, 721–725 (1972).

69. Marquardt, H., Kuroki, T., Huberman, E., Selkirk, J. K., Heidelberger, C., Grover, P. L., and Sims, P. Malignant transformation of cells derived from mouse prostate by epoxides and other derivatives of polycyclic hydrocarbons. *Cancer Res.*, **32**, 716–720 (1972).

70. Marquardt, H., Sodergren, J.E., Sims, P., and Grover, P. L. Malignant transformation *in vitro* of mouse fibroblasts by 7,12-dimethylbenz[a]anthracene and 7-hydroxymethylbenz[a]anthracene and by their K-region derivatives. *Int. J. Cancer*, **13**, 304–310 (1974).

71. Miyaji, H., Morris, H. P., and Wagner, B. P. Histological study of some primary and transplantable hepatic tumors in rats. *Methods Cancer Res.*, **4**, 153–178 (1968).

72. Mondal, S., Embleton, M. J., Marquardt, H., and Heidelberger, C. Production of variants of decreased malignancy and antigenicity from clones transformed *in vitro* by methylcholanthrene. *Int. J. Cancer*, **8**, 410–420 (1971).

73. Mondal, S. and Heidelberger, C. *In vitro* malignant transformation by methylcholanthrene of the progeny of single cells derived from C3H mouse prostate. *Proc. Natl. Acad. Sci. U.S.*, **65**, 219–225 (1970).

74. Montesano, R., Saint Vincent, L., and Tomatis, L. Malignant transformation *in vitro* of rat liver cells by dimethylnitrosamine and N-methyl-N'-nitro-N-nitroso-guanidine. *Brit. J. Cancer*, **28**, 215–220 (1973).

75. Namba, M., Masuji, H., and Sato, J. Carcinogenesis in tissue culture. IX. Malignant transformation of cultured rat cells treated with 4-nitroquinoline 1-oxide. *Japan. J. Exp. Med.*, **39**, 253–265 (1969).

76. Nebert, D. W., Winker, J., and Gelboin, H. V. Aryl hydrocarbon hydroxylase activity in human placenta from cigarette smoking and non-smoking woman. *Cancer Res.*, **29**, 1763–1769 (1969).

77. Palekar, L., Kuschner, M., and Laskin, S. The effect of 3-methylcholanthrene on rat trachea in organ culture. *Cancer Res.*, **28**, 2098–2104 (1968).

78. Peterson, A. R., Bertram, J. S., and Heidelberger, C. Cell cycle dependency of DNA damage and repair in transformable mouse fibroblasts treated with N-methyl-N'-nitro-N-nitrosoguanidine. *Cancer Res.*, **34**, 1600–1607 (1974).

79. Reznikoff, C. A., Bertram, J. S., Brankow, D. W., and Heidelberger, C. Quantitative and qualitative studies of chemical transformation of cloned C3H mouse embryo cells sensitive to post confluence inhibition of cell division. *Cancer Res.*, **33**, 3239–3249 (1973).

80. Reznikoff, C. A., Brankow, D. W., and Heidelberger, C. Establishment and characterization of a clone line of C3H mouse embryo cells sensitive to post-confluence inhibition of division. *Cancer Res.*, **33**, 3231–3238 (1973).

81. Rhim, J. S. and Huebner, R. J. Transformation of rat embryo cells *in vitro* by chemical carcinogens. *Cancer Res.*, **33**, 695–700 (1973).

82. Röller, M. R. and Heidelberger, C. Attempts to produce carcinogenesis in organ cultures of mouse prostate with polycyclic hydrocarbons. *Int. J. Cancer*, **2**, 509–520 (1967).

83. Sanders, F. K. The effect of some nonviral oncogenic agents on mammalian cells *in vitro*. *In* "Topics in Chemical Carcinogenesis," ed. by W. Nakahara, S. Takayama, T. Sugimura, and S. Odashima, University of Tokyo Press, Tokyo, pp. 429–444 (1972).

84. Sanders, F. K. and Burford, B. O. Morphological conversions of cells *in vitro* by N-nitrosomethylurea. *Nature*, **213**, 1171–1173 (1967).

85. Sanders, F. K. and Burford, B. O. Morphological conversion, hyperconversion and reversion of mammalian cells treated *in vitro* with N-nitrosomethylurea. *Nature*, **220**, 448–453 (1968).

86. Sanford, K. K., Dunn, T. B., Westfall, B. B., Covalesky, A. B., Dupree, L. T., and Earle, W. R. Sarcomatous change and maintenance of differentiation in long-term cultures of mouse mammary carcinoma. *J. Natl. Cancer Inst.*, **26**, 1139–1184 (1961).

87. Sato, H. and Kuroki, T. Malignization *in vitro* of hamster embryonic cells by chemical carcinogens. *Proc. Japan Acad.*, **42**, 1211–1216 (1966).

88. Sato, K., Kuroki, T., and Sato, H. Respiration and glycolysis of cells transformed with 4-nitroquinoline 1-oxide and its derivatives. *Proc. Soc. Exp. Biol. Med.*, **134**, 281–283 (1970).

89. Sekely, L. I., Malejka-Giganti, D., Gutmann, H. R., and Rydell, R. E. Malignant transformation of rat embryo fibroblasts by carcinogenic fluorenylhydroxamic acids *in vitro*. *J. Natl. Cancer Inst.*, **50**, 1337–1345 (1973).

90. Shabad, L. M., Sorokina, J. D., Golub, N. I., and Bogovski, S. P. Transplacental effect of some chemical compounds on organ cultures of embryonic kidney tissue. *Cancer Res.*, **32**, 617–627 (1972).

91. Sivak, A. and Van Duuren, B. L. Studies with carcinogens and tumor-promoting agents in cell culture. *Exp. Cell Res.*, **49**, 572–583 (1968).

92. Takii, M., Takaki, R., and Okada, N. Carcinogenesis in tissue culture. XVI. Malignant transformation of rat cells with N-methyl-N'-nitro-N-nitrosoguanidine. *Japan. J. Exp. Med.*, **41**, 563–579 (1971).

93. Toyoshima, K., Hiasa, Y., Ito, N., and Tsubura, Y. *In vitro* malignant transformation of cells derived from rat liver by means of aflatoxin B_1. *Gann*, **61**, 557–561 (1970).

94. Tsuda, H., Inui, N., and Takayama, S. *In vitro* transformation of newborn hamster cells by sodium nitrite. *Biochem. Biophys. Res. Commun.*, **55**, 1117–1124 (1973).

95. Umeda, M. and Iype, P. T. An improved expression of *in vitro* transformation rate based on cytotoxicity produced by chemical carcinogens. *Brit. J. Cancer*, **28**, 71–74 (1973).

96. Welch, R. M., Harrison, Y. E., Conney, A. H., Poppers, P. J., and Finster, M.

Cigarette smoking: stimulatory effect on metabolism of 3,4-benzopyrene by enzymes in human placenta. *Science*, **160**, 541–542 (1968).

97. Williams, G. M., Elliott, J., and Weisburger, J. H. Carcinoma after malignant conversion *in vitro* of epithelial-like cells from rat liver following exposure to chemical carcinogens. *Cancer Res.*, **33**, 606–612 (1973).

98. Yoshida, T. Über die experimentelle Erzeugung von Hepatoma durch die Fütterung mit *o*-Amido-azotoluol. *Proc. Imp. Acad. (Tokyo)*, **8**, 464–467 (1932).

99. Yoshida, T. Some thoughts on malignant growths. *Natl. Cancer Inst. Monogr.*, **16**, 1–6 (1964).

100. Yosida, T. H., Kuroki, T., Masuji, H., and Sato, H. Chromosomal alteration and development of tumor. XX. Chromosome change in the course of malignant transformation *in vitro* of hamster embryonic cells by 4-nitroquinoline 1-oxide and its derivative, 4-hydroxyaminoquinoline 1-oxide. *Gann*, **61**, 131–143 (1970).

GANN Monograph on Cancer Research 17, 87–106 (1975)

PRIMARY CULTURE AND CARCINOGENESIS *IN VITRO* BY N-METHYL-N′-NITRO-N-NITROSO-GUANIDINE OF GLANDULAR STOMACH CELLS OF *PRAOMYS* (*MASTOMYS*) *NATALENSIS*

Yuji KUROKAWA, Sachiko SAITO, and Haruo SATO

*Department of Oncology, Research Institute for Tuberculosis, Leprosy and Cancer, Tohoku University**

Glandular stomach cells of *Praomys* (*Mastomys*) *natalensis* were cultured and treated with N-methyl-N′-nitro-N-nitrosoguanidine (MNNG) (0.25–8.00 μg/ml) *in vitro*. From 4 control cell lines, 11 MNNG-treated lines were successfully established. Cultured cells exhibited almost similar morphology in both the control and treated cell lines. The majority of cells were oval in shape, others were spindle-shaped cells and multinucleated giant cells. Growth of treated cells was three times faster than control cells. Chromosomes distributed in a much wider range in treated cells than in control cells.

Subcutaneous, intramuscular, and intraperitoneal transplantation of cells into young mastomys was tried with cortisone-conditioning and X irradiation. Tumor take occurred in 2/4 of control cell lines and 6/11 of treated cell lines. Histological examinations showed that the tumors were mixed in type. They seemed to be of mesenchymal origin, the main component of which showed leiomyomatous appearance. By Bodian's Protargol technique, argyrophilic cells scattered in small number were found in the tumors. They were mostly oval cells with a large nucleus. Similar cells also existed in cultured cells. Biochemical examination revealed negligible histamine and histidine-decarboxylase in cultured cells, culture media, and tumor tissues. The incidence of argyrophilic cells greatly increased when maintained in histidine-rich medium.

The necessity of modifying culture medium and dissociation of mucosal epithelium of the stomach in future studies are discussed.

In 1955, Oettlé first reported the high incidence of spontaneous tumors of the glandular stomach in *Praomys* (*Mastomys*) *natalensis* (*25, 26*). Because of the rarity of spontaneous development of gastric tumors in experimental animals, this finding interested many workers in carcinogenesis. Several papers subsequently appeared concerning histological findings on stomach tumors (*27, 28, 36*) and, in 1969, these tumors were proved to be non-argentaffin argyrophilic cell carcinoids from both histochemical and ultrastructural studies (*34, 35, 37*).

---

* Hirose-machi 4-12, Sendai 980, Japan (黒川雄二, 斎藤祥子, 佐藤春郎).

Moreover, it was found that transplantable tumors derived from the carcinoids showed high activity of histidine-decarboxylase and stored large amounts of histamine (*14, 15*). Capella (*2*) and Hakånson (*11*) recently reported on the histogenesis of the carcinoids, concluding that probably enterochromaffin-like cells (argyrophilic cells) of the gastric oxyntic mucosa were the cells of origin.

Mastomys were first brought by Sato to our laboratory in 1963 from Dr. McPherson at the National Cancer Institute, U.S.A. They were probably from the stock of Family B (*32, 33*). They have been maintained by random-breeding in conventional circumstances. The incidence of stomach tumors in our stock was about 60% around 1957 (*27*), and gradually decreased to about 10% in 1973, accompanied with a shorter life span (*29*).

The recent advances in the field of *in vitro* carcinogenesis led us to undertake these experiments to ascertain the following: what will happen in tissue culture of mastomys' glandular stomach cells? Will the carcinoid tumor cells also arise *in vitro* as they spontaneously develop *in vivo*? We could not find any answers to these questions, *i.e.*, no work on *in vitro* carcinogenesis have been done dealing with cells derived from organs with high capacity for spontaneous development of tumors.

Reviewing the established cell lines in tissue culture, it is curious that only a few cell lines originated from the organs of the digestive tract; they were intestine 407 derived from human fetal intestine (*13*) and MC line derived from human stomach cancer (*24*). The culture techniques employed were explant and mincing-trypsinization methods.

Primary Culture of Glandular Stomach Cells

The culture of glandular stomach of mastomys was started as follows (*20*): 3- to 6-week-old animals of both sexes were sacrificed under chloroform anesthesia after 24-hr food restriction. The glandular portion of the stomach was separated from the forestomach and duodenum, and washed thoroughly in several changes of phosphate-buffered saline solution (PBS) with penicillin and chloramphenicol, and then minced into small pieces with a sharp razor. The cover slips coated with reconstituted rat tail collagen, according to the method of Ehrmann and Gey (*7*), were used as a substrate for primary culture of such minced fragments.

The medium used in this experiment was Eagle's minimal essential medium (MEM) (Nissui) supplemented with 20% calf serum (Kyokuto) and antibiotics (penicillin 100 U/ml, Kanamycin 60 μg/ml, chloramphenicol 0.025 μg/ml, Fungizone 2.5 μg/ml). Falcon plastic dishes and TD-40 bottles were ordinarily used for propagation of cells under constant flow of CO_2 and air with humidity at 37°. The medium was changed twice weekly, when confluent cells were subcultured with 0.025% pronase dissolved in Ca- and Mg-free PBS.

Untreated control cultures were prepared from 20 glandular stomachs, and 8 cases became contaminated within a week, probably due to minute food residues in the stomach. Within 30 days, or 3–4 generations, 8 more cases resulted in poor growth and were discarded. Four out of 20 cell lines showed rapid proliferation, were transferred twice weekly, and have been cultured up to 900 days *in vitro.* These cell lines consisted mostly of oval or polygonal cells with a large round nucleus, 3–5 prominent nucleoli, and clear cytoplasm (Photo 1). In later stages, when they showed malignancy in transplantation assay, the morphology of cells changed little with no criss-crossed arrangement and piling up of cells.

Treatment of Cells with N-Methyl-N'-nitro-N-nitrosoguanidine (MNNG)

In contrast to the *in vitro* carcinogenesis using cultured embryonic cells, it required 60–70 days in this experiment to collect several millions of cells at the same time. Actively growing cells of the control cell lines (designated as SS lines) were seeded at 30×10^4 per 60-mm plastic dish 24 hr before treatment.

MNNG was chosen as the carcinogen, because of the recent successful reports dealing with the specific carcinogenicity on the glandular stomach of various animals (*39*) and on the cultured cells *in vitro* (*17, 40*). The experiment on the carcinogenic action of MNNG given orally to mastomys has been presented briefly and will be published elsewhere (*19*).

MNNG (Aldrich Chemical Co., U.S.A.) was dissolved at a concentration of 1 mg/ml in pH 6.6 PBS as a stock solution and kept in a freezer. Then the solution was diluted with PBS and filtered through a Millipore filter, 0.5 ml of which was added to 4.5 ml of the medium to make the desired concentration by 10-fold dilution in dishes. The final concentration of MNNG ranged from 0.25 to 8.00 μg/ml in the medium. After 2 hr of incubation, the MNNG medium was discarded, and the cells were washed several times with PBS and refed with a fresh medium.

The time interval between carcinogen treatment and secondary subculture varied from 51 to 8 days. When treated cells seemed to revive from the initial attack, however, longer maintenance with sufficient medium changes resulted in better growth thereafter.

Morphology of MNNG-treated Cells

Cultured cells on cover glasses were routinely stained with May-Grünwald Giemsa after fixation with methanol. MNNG-treated cells (designated as PN lines) revealed some early changes depending on the concentration of the carcinogen. When treated with a higher concentration (8.0–4.0 μg/ml), pronounced cell necrosis occurred. There was a marked tendency of cells to change into fusiform or elongated form with fibrillar cytoplasmic processes, among which large oval cells with granulated cytoplasm intermingled. The cells affected with lower concentration (2.0–0.25 μg/ml) showed little cytopathic effects. They had, in general, quite similar appearance in shape compared with SS lines, but became smaller in size (Photo 2).

PN lines exhibited monotonous appearance of cells up to about 200 days after treatment; *i.e.*, oval or polygonal cells prevailed with round nuclei, prominent nucleoli, and clear cytoplasm (Photo 3). Mitotic figures were frequently observed. The criss-crossed arrangement and piling up of cells, usually explained as the

loss of contact inhibition, occurred as early as 30–40 days after MNNG treatment, while longer culture of the cells resulted in the change of cell types. After
300 days *in vitro*, two types of cells were distinguished; *e.g.*, polygonal cells with
clear cytoplasm and spindle-shaped cells with elongated nuclei and basophilic
fibrillar cytoplasm (Photo 4). The morphology of cells and changes in continuous
culture were almost similar in all PN lines independent of the concentration of
the carcinogen.

Growth of SS and PN Lines in Vitro

As shown in Fig. 1, cell growth of SS11 line was compared with PN265B
line which was derived from SS11 line and treated with 1 μg/ml of MNNG.
PN265B line was about three times higher than SS11 line in saturated cell
density. The doubling time of SS11 and PN265B line was approximately 48.0
and 28.8 hr, respectively. At that time, PN265B cells had the ability to produce
tumors when injected into mastomys, while SS11 cells did not, but, after 635
days *in vitro*, SS11 cells transformed spontaneously.

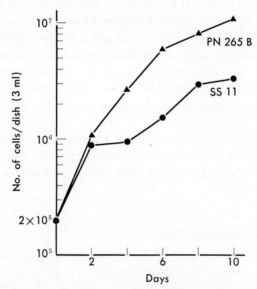

FIG. 1.   Growth curve of SS11 and PN265B cells
SS11: 64th gen., 427 days. PN265B: 65th gen., 357 days.

Chromosome Analysis of SS and PN Lines

For karyological studies, four cell lines were examined, *i.e.*, PN265B and
PN267A lines derived from SS11 and SS14 lines, respectively. The former two
lines were readily transplantable, but the latter two were not when chromosome
was examined. Chromosome preparations were made from cell cultures treated
with 10^{-6} M colchicine for 5 hr and with hypotonic solution for 20 min. They
were then stained with Aceto-orcein.

Results are summarized in Fig. 2. It is clear that chromosome number in

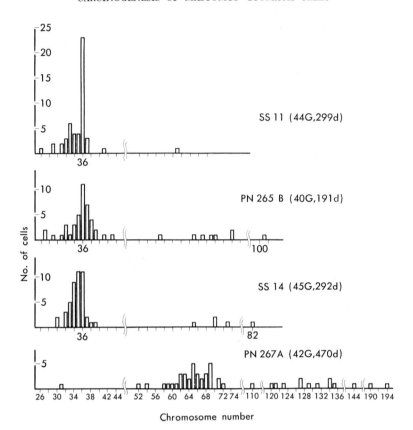

Fɪɢ. 2.   Chromosome distribution of SS and PN cell lines
50 metaphases counted.

the majority of non-transformed cells (SS11 and SS14) was 35 or 36. From the karyological points, these cells also seemed to be normal, as Huang *et al.* reported that diploid number of mastomys was 36 (*16*). The chromosomes of transformed cells (PN265B and PN267A) distributed in a much wider range than non-transformed cells. This phenomenon was more marked in PN267A cells than in PN265B cells. It might have resulted from the difference in distribution of chromosomes in the original cell lines, *i.e.*, chromosome distribution was wider in SS14 cells than in SS11 cells.

Transplantation Assay

The purpose of transplantation of cultured cells in this experiment was different from that of others in the following ways: it was concerned predominately with the time interval between treatment with carcinogen and appearance of neoplastic development *in vivo* and/or *in vitro*, correlation of transformation rate with the concentration of the carcinogen, and duration of the treatment. As Franks *et al.* (*9*) pointed out, reviewing the recent works of *in vitro* carcinogenesis, little attention has been called either to the true origin of cells transformed *in vitro* or the exact nature of the tumors formed by transplantation. Because the ultimate purpose of this experiment, as described previously, is the identification of transformed cells *in vitro*, either spontaneously or chemically, as carcinoid tumor cells or not, our interest was focused mainly on the histopathological examination of the transplanted tumors. The cells to be tested for tumorigenicity had been passed long enough in culture and the animals were conditioned in almost all cases.

The harvested cells were suspended in 0.2 to 0.4 ml of the medium. The inoculum ranged from $1-9 \times 10^6$ per animal. Intraperitoneal (i.p.), intramuscular (i.m.), and subcutaneous (s.c.) injections were given to 20- to 40-day-old young mastomys of both sexes, which were usually conditioned with daily administration of 5 mg of cortisone acetate (Upjohn) for 3 days before and after transplantation, and in some cases 500–240 R irradiation was given. Observation was continued for at least 1 year but, when animals were found moribund, they were sacrificed for morphological and biochemical examination.

Tables I and II summarize the results of transplantation of untreated and MNNG-treated cells. In SS cells, tumor formation occurred in 2 out of 4 cell lines. As long as about 300 days *in vitro*, however, were required to prove malignancy *in vivo*. It is probable that spontaneous transformation will develop in all, after 600 days *in vitro*. In PN cells, successful tumor take occurred in 6 out of 11 cell lines. In contrast to SS cells, PN265B cells produced tumors as early as 45 days after MNNG treatment. But in general, tumor formation by PN line was not related to the cultured days, concentration of MNNG, number of inoculated cells, or sites of transplantation.

TABLE I.   Transplantation Results of SS Line (Non-treated Cells)

Cell line	Generation (cult. days)	No. of cells ($\times 10^4$)	Site	Radiation (R)	Tumor take	Survival days
SS4	22 (296)	300	i.m.	—	0/3	
SS7	17 (154)	100	i.m.	—	0/3	
	,,	,,	i.p.	—	0/3	
SS11	36 (271)	200	i.m.	—	0/4	
	,,	,,	i.p.	—	0/3	
	46 (314)	540	s.c.	500	1/1	44[a]
	,,	,,	,,	240	0/1	
	,,	,,	,,	—	0/2	
	60 (398)	500	s.c.	—	0/4	
	,,	250	,,	—	0/4	
	85 (635)	300	s.c.	—	1/2	98[a]
	,,	250	,,	—	0/1	
SS14	38 (264)	200	i.m.	—	0/4	
	,,	,,	i.p.	—	0/4	
	47 (307)	300	s.c.	500	0/1	
	,,	,,	,,	240	0/2	
	,,	,,	,,	—	0/2	
	87 (609)	300	s.c.	—	3/3	106[a], 130, 148

[a] Sacrificed.

TABLE II. Transplantation Results of PN Line (MNNG-treated Cells)

Cell line	MNNG (μg/ml)	Generation (cult. days)	No. of cells (×10⁴)	Site	Tumor take	Survival days
PN265A[a]	0.5	9 (45)	250	i.m.	0/2	
		34 (213)	300	i.m.	1/2	378
		,,	600	,,	1/1	459
		56 (371)	500	s.c.	0/4	
PN265B	1.0	9 (45)	200	i.m.	1/2	56
		38 (189)	250	i.m.	2/2	47
		,,	,,	i.p.	1/1	34
		42 (208)	900	i.m.	2/2	27
		,,	,,	i.p.	2/2	29, 32
		54 (271)	400	i.m.	3/4	25, 32, 36
PN265C	2.0	9 (45)	250	i.m.	0/2	
PN267A[b]	2.0	24 (299)	800	s.c.	2/3	80, 99
PN267B	1.0	20 (210)	200	s.c.	0/3	
		39 (389)	600	s.c.	0/3	
PN267C	0.5	46 (364)	600	s.c.	1/3	19
PN267D	0.25	16 (231)	350	s.c.	0/1	
PN268A[c]	1.0	14 (131)	200	s.c.	0/2	
PN268C	4.0	31 (373)	500	s.c.	2/2	161, 161
PN268D	0.25	34 (250)	200	i.m.	0/2	
		,,	400	,,	0/2	
		56 (411)	500	s.c.	0/3	
PN269B[d]	1.0	13 (180)	300	i.m.	0/2	
		37 (407)	600	s.c.	2/2	47, 48

Origin: [a] PN265 from SS11 ; [b] PN267 from SS14 ; [c] PN268 from SS4 ; [d] PN269 from SS7.

Considering the fact that mastomys used were under continuous random-breeding, not by the brother-sister mating, the above phenomena could be reasonably explained. Moreover it is suspected from the same reason that if MNNG-treated cells were all similarly transformed *in vitro*, some cell lines were rejected by immunological resistance of the recipient.

The growth pattern of tumors also varied. PN265B cells showed the most progressive growth and animals were dead around 40 days, while the animals injected with PN265A cells survived more than a year bearing a tumor of 5×5 cm. In most cases, the tumors were found to be readily transplantable. The tumors were elastic soft in nature and the cut surface was whitish with slight hemorrhage.

Histological Findings of Transplanted Tumors

Tissues from all the tumors were fixed in 4% neutral formaldehyde solution or Bouin's fixative, embedded in paraffin, and sectioned. Staining methods used were Hematoxylin and Eosin (H-E), periodic acid-Schiff (PAS), Alcian Blue

PAS, Mucicarmine, Azan-Mallory, Masson's trichrome, Van-Gieson, Gomori's reticulin stain, and Masson-Fontana for argentaffin reaction. For the demonstration of argyrophilic granules, which are proved to be the most specific histochemical findings in mastomys' carcinoids, Bodian Protargol technique modified by Azzopardi (1) and Grimerius staining (10) were extensively employed to both sectioned materials and fixed cultured cells on cover glasses.

The tumors derived from SS cells and PN cells were almost similar in morphology. In the latter, also, concentration of MNNG did not influence the histological features. The histology exhibited marked resemblance to those described by Franks et al. (9). He noted the similarity of tumors, whatever the organ of origin.

The histological type of tumors in our series could be classified into predominantly leiomyomatous and anaplastic types, which were frequently found to be coexistent in the same tumor (Photos 5 and 6). In the leiomyomatous areas, spindle or oval cells formed structures with large strap-like cells arranged in interlacing bands and whorls. Appearance of giant cells was common in both tumor types. They were elongated or rosette-like in shape with usually a number of nuclei. The cytoplasm was eosinophilic (Photos 7 and 8). PAS staining was all negative. In tumors thick and short collagenous fibers were moderately distributed. No ulcers were detected in the stomach or duodenum. In several cases metastasis occurred in the lung, liver, kidney, and lymph nodes from tumors transplanted subcutaneously.

By the argyrophilic staining, cells with distinct dark grey or black granules in the cytoplasm were found in several areas of tumor. They were mostly oval cells with large nucleus, while some of the spindle cells and giant cells were also argyrophilic. They had, however, no tendency to accumulate in foci to form any carcinoid-like structures (Photo 9). They seemed to resemble the argyrophilic cells scattered in the hyperplastic zone of primary carcinoid of glandular stomach of mastomys (37). Similar argyrophilic cells were observed in cultured cells, which were also almost oval in shape (Photo 10). The incidence of such cells was higher in PN cells than in SS cells. Argentaffin staining was negative both in tumors and cultured cells.

For ultrastructural study, cultured cells and tumor tissues were fixed with 1.0% OsO_4 in Millonig's buffer (pH 7.4) for 2 hr at 4°. They were embedded in Epon epoxide resin after dehydration with ethanol.

At the ultrastructural level, secretory granules were found in only a few cells. They had densely stained central cores, some of which were surrounded by wavy limiting membranes. The diameter of granules ranged from 240 to 400 nm. In general, the number of granules in the cytoplasm was less than in the primary carcinoid of mastomys (Photo 11).

Histamine Assay

Table III shows the results of histamine assay in the medium, cultured cells, and transplanted tumors. It was evident that the content of histamine in the medium was less than in Eagle's minimum essential medium (MEM) and

TABLE III. Results of Histamine Assay

Medium	
PN265B	0.62 nmole/ml[a]
SS11	0.65 ,,
Eagle's MEM, CS20	0.86 ,,
Cultured cells	
PN265B	0 nmole/hr/mg protein[b]
SS11	0 ,,
Tumor tissue	
PN265B	0 ,,
Rat stomach	2.16 ,,

[a] Fluorometric assay by the method of Shore (31). [b] ^{14}C-Histidine uptake by the method of Kahlson (18).

histamine formation was negligible in either cultured cells or transplanted tumors. It may seem that negative demonstration of histamine resulted from the fact that the number of argyrophilic cells was too small to be detected biochemically, even if they actually produced histamine.

Culture in Histidine-rich Medium

As Laissue *et al.* showed in their experiments, histidine, the precurser of histamine, had effects on formation of histamine *in vitro* (6, 21, 30). They used mast cell tumors which produced histamine as well as serotonin and heparin. Thus the influence of histidine concentration in the culture medium to the incidence of argyrophilic cells was studied.

PN265B cells, which had been maintained in Eagle's MEM for 320 days, were used for this experiment. They were cultured for 5 days in the medium containing 2-, 5-, and 10-fold concentration of L-histidine compared to Eagle's MEM. Then argyrophilic cells were counted on fixed cover glasses after Bodian staining. It is noteworthy that the cells maintained in histidine-rich medium showed a marked increase of argyrophilic cells (Table IV). From these data, the dependence of histamine formation of the cells on the concentration of histidine was also evident.

PN287C cells, which were cultured for 112 days in the medium containing

TABLE IV. Comparison of Argyrophilic Cells in Different Levels of
L-Histidine in Medium

Medium	Cells	No. of cells/ ×400 field	Ratio
Eagle's MEM[a]	(PN265B)[e]	0.5	100
×2 Histidine[b]	(PN287A)	0.1	20
×5 ,, [c]	(PN287B)	9.8	1,960
×10 ,, [d]	PN287C	17.5	3,500

Concentration of L-histidine: [a] 42 mg/ml; [b] 84 mg/ml; [c] 210 mg/ml; [d] 420 mg/ml; [e] 62nd gen., 320 days.

10-fold concentration of L-histidine, were transplanted and formed tumors. In contrast to the cultured cells, the number of argyrophilic cells found in the tumor did not increase. The histological feature was similar to PN265B tumors, from which the cells were derived.

DISCUSSION AND CONCLUSIONS

Carcinogenesis experiment *in vitro* of glandular stomach cells did not result in the formation of similar carcinoid tumors as *in vivo*. Tumors were "mixed in type" as Franks mentioned for his tumors (*9*). Histological examination revealed that probably the main component of tumor tissue was of myogenic origin.

Argyrophilic cells were found scattered in small numbers, not forming any foci. Although carcinoid-like structures were not observed, the fact that argyrophilic cells did exist in tumors would suggest the possibility that they were also transformed cells. In this experiment cultured cells were routinely transplanted into subcutis or muscle. The fact that argyrophilic cells never pre-existed in transplanted sites would further support the view that they were neoplastic cells. The attempt to clone an argyrophilic cell line, however, has not been yet successful. This problem is also discussed by Azzopardi and Pollock (*1*), concluding that micro-focus of argyrophilic cells is neoplastic, but cell colonization is non-neoplastic.

Assuming that argyrophilic cells in the tumor were malignant, a question arises as to why their population was so small in mixed cells *in vitro* and *in vivo*.

In the search of the literature on tissue culture of carcinoid tumors, we could find only one paper written by Foley and Davis (*8*). They used ordinary fetal calf serum plus human serum with no specific nutritional supplements. Their results revealed the difficulty of maintaining the function to secrete 5-hydroxytryptamine and histamine *in vitro*. Establishment of cell line was probably unsuccessful.

Before beginning the present experiments, we expected the ability of mastomys' argyrophilic cells to proliferate and transform selectively *in vitro*. Thus, Eagle's MEM with 20% calf serum without any modification was used for all cultures. Later, it became evident that the incidence of argyrophilic cells *in vitro* was increased when cultured in histidine-rich medium, as already described. The effect of histidine-rich medium on selective growth of argyrophilic cells cultured primarily remains obscure. Similar carcinogenesis experiments *in vitro* using glandular stomach cells of mastomys maintained in such a medium are under study.

For the primary culture of glandular stomach cells, minced tissues were explanted on collagen-coated surface. Explant methods were employed by Monesi (*22, 23*) and Henle *et al.* (*13*). They used chicken plasma clot as a substrate. Although Henle *et al.* succeeded in separation of intestinal epithelium, there was always the difficulty to eliminate overgrowth of mesenchymal cells, such as fibroblasts, myoblasts, *etc.* The fact that one must inevitably encounter such problems in the process of establishing epithelial cell lines has been reported by many workers.

The method of Harrer *et al.* (*12*) and that modified by Stern (*38*) seem to be an excellent technique to collect mucosal epithelial cells of the stomach. However, it was impossible to maintain these cells *in vitro* for a long time and they ceased growing within a month.

For the purpose of epithelial cell culture, such concepts as "epithelio-mesenchymal relationships" proposed by Dawe *et al.* (*3–5*) are of great importance. He clearly demonstrated evidence that epithelial cell growth must be supported by mesenchymal elements, either cellular or humoral, based on a number of experiments dealing with carcinogenesis of salivary gland epithelium.

In conclusion, further studies to modify cultural conditions including dissociation of mucosal epithelium and culture media with some factors for the selective growth of argyrophilic cells *in vitro* will be necessary.

Acknowledgments

Grateful acknowledgment is made to Dr. Aizu, Department of Anatomy, Tohoku University Medical School, for his ultrastructural studies of cultured cells and tumor tissues, and also to Dr. Fukushima and Dr. Kawachi, Department of Biochemistry, National Cancer Center Research Institute, for their biochemical analysis of our materials for histamine.

REFERENCES

1. Azzopardi, J. G. and Pollock, D. J. Argentaffin and argyrophil cells in gastric carcinoma. *J. Pathol. Bacteriol.*, **86**, 443–451 (1963).
2. Capella, C., Solcia, E., and Snell, K. C. Ultrastructure of endocrine cells and argyrophil carcinoids of the stomach of *Praomys* (*Mastomys*) *natalensis. J. Natl. Cancer Inst.*, **50**, 1471–1485 (1973).
3. Dawe, C. J., Morgan, W. D., and Slatick, M. S. Influence of epitheliomesenchymal interactions on tumor induction by polyoma virus. *Int. J. Cancer*, **1**, 419–450 (1966).
4. Dawe, C. J., Morgan, W. D., and Slatick, M. S. Salivary gland neoplasms in the role of normal mesenchyme during salivary gland morphogenesis. *In* "Epithelial-Mesenchymal Interactions," ed. by R. Fleischmajer, Williams and Wilkins Co., Baltimore, pp. 295–312 (1968).
5. Dawe, C. J. Changes in cell interrelationships during epithelial carcinogenesis. *In* "Topics in Chemical Carcinogenesis," ed. by W. Nakahara, S. Takayama, T. Sugimura, and S. Odashima, University of Tokyo Press, Tokyo, pp. 401–427 (1972).
6. Day, M. and Green, J. P. The uptake of amino acids and the synthesis of amines by neoplastic mast cells in culture. *J. Physiol.*, **164**, 210–226 (1962).
7. Ehrmann, R. L. and Gey, G. O. The growth of cells on a transparent gel of reconstituted rat-tail collagen. *J. Natl. Cancer Inst.*, **16**, 1375–1403 (1956).
8. Foley, J. F. and Davis, R. B. Growth of carcinoid tumours in tissue culture. *Nature*, **205**, 785–786 (1965).
9. Franks, L. M., Chesterman, F. C., and Rowlatt, C. The structure of tumors derived from mouse cells after "spontaneous" transformation *in vitro. Brit. J. Cancer*, **24**, 843–847 (1970).
10. Grimerius, L. A silver nitrate stain for α_2 cells in human pancreatic islets. *Acta Soc. Med. Ups.*, **73**, 243–270 (1969).

11. Hakånson, R., Larsson, L. I., Owman, Ch., Snell, K. C., and Sundler, F. Fluo-
     rescence and electron microscopic histochemistry of endocrine-like cells in gastric
     mucosa and argyrophil tumor of *Praomys (Mastomys) natalensis*. Analysis of 5-
     hydroxytryptamine, histamine, histidine decarboxylase, and aromatic amino acid
     decarboxylase. *Histochemie*, **37**, 23–38 (1973).

12. Harrer, K. S., Stern, B. K., and Reilly, R. W. Removal and dissociation of epi-
     thelial cells from the rodent gastrointestinal tract. *Nature*, **203**, 319–320 (1964).

13. Henle, G. and Deinhardt, F. The establishment of strains of human cells in tissue
     culture. *J. Immunol.*, **79**, 54–59 (1957).

14. Hosoda, S., Nakamura, W., Snell, K. C., and Stewart, H. L. Histamine produc-
     tion by transplantable argyrophilic gastric carcinoid of *Praomys (Mastomys) na-
     talensis*. *Science*, **170**, 454–455 (1970).

15. Hosoda, S., Nakamura, W., Snell, K. C., and Stewart, H. L. Histidine decar-
     boxylase in the transplantable argyrophilic gastric carcinoid of *Praomys (Mastomys)
     natalensis*. *Pharmacology*, **20**, 2671–2676 (1971).

16. Huang, C. C. and Strong, L. C. Chromosomes of the African mouse. *J. Hered.*,
     53, 95–99 (1962).

17. Inui, N., Takayama, S., and Sugimura, T. Malignant transformation and cel-
     lular effects of hamster lung fibroblastic cells by N-methyl-N′-nitro-N-nitroso-
     guanidine and its derivatives. *Proc. Japan. Cancer Assoc., 29th Annu. Meet.*, 82
     (1972) (in Japanese).

18. Kahlson, G. and Rosengren, E. New approaches to the physiology of histamine.
     Physiol. Rev., **48**, 155–196 (1968).

19. Kurokawa, Y., Saito, S., and Sato, H. Induction of forestomach, duodenal and
     liver tumors in *Praomys (Mastomys) natalensis* by oral or intragastric administra-
     tion of N-methyl-N′-nitro-N-nitrosoguanidine. *Sci. Rep. Res. Inst. Tohoku Univ.
     -C*, **22**, 1–8 (1975).

20. Kurokawa, Y., Saito, S., Kimura, T., Sato, T., and Sato, H. *In vitro* carcino-
     genesis of cultured cells from glandular stomach of *Mastomys* by N-methyl-N′-
     nitro-N-nitrosoguanidine. *Proc. Japan. Cancer Assoc., 32nd Annu. Meet.*, 177
     (1973) (in Japanese).

21. Laissue, J., Marx, W., Grieder, A., and Schindler, R. Proliferation and specific
     functions of neoplastic mast cells in culture. *Exp. Cell Res.*, **69**, 57–64 (1971).

22. Monesi, V. The appearance of enterochromaffin cells in the intestine of the chick
     embryo. *Acta Anat.*, **41**, 97–114 (1960).

23. Monesi, V. Differentiation of argyrophil and argentaffin cells in organotypic cul-
     tures of embryonic chick intestine. *J. Embryol.*, **8**, 302–313 (1960).

24. Oboshi, S., Seido, T., and Shibata, H. *In vitro* culture of human cancer cells for
     cancer chemotherapy. I. A long-term cultured suspended cell line established from
     lymph node with metastasis from gastric cancer. *Gann*, **60**, 205–210 (1969).

25. Oettlé, A. G. Spontaneous carcinoma of the glandular stomach in a laboratory
     stock of *Rattus (Mastomys) natalensis*. *South Afr. J. Med. Sci.*, **20**, 36 (1955).

26. Oettlé, A. G. Spontaneous carcinoma of the glandular stomach in *Rattus (Mas-
     tomys) natalensis*, an African rodent. *Brit. J. Cancer*, **11**, 415–433 (1957).

27. Sato, H. and Fujii, K. Spontaneous development of stomach cancer in *Mastomys
     (Rattus) natalensis*. *GANN Monograph*, **3**, 37–44 (1967).

28. Sato, H., Fujii, K., Yamaura, H., and Kurokawa, Y. Malignant tumors of the
     stomach in *Praomys (Mastomys) natalensis*. *GANN Monograph*, **8**, 9–13 (1969).

29. Sato, H., Kurokawa, Y., and Saito, S. Life span of *Mastomys* and development
     of spontaneous tumors. *Exp. Animals*, **23**, 102 (1974) (in Japanese).

30. Schindler, R., Day, M., and Fischer, G. A. Culture of neoplastic mast cells and their synthesis of 5-hydroxytryptamine and histamine *in vitro*. *Cancer Res.*, **19**, 47–51 (1959).

31. Shore, P. A., Burkhalter, A., and Cohn, V. H. A method for the fluorometric assay of histamine in tissues. *J. Pharm. Exp. Ther.*, **127**, 182–186 (1959).

32. Simmers, M. H., Ibsen, K. H., and Berk, J. E. Concerning the incidence of "spontaneous" stomach cancer in *Praomys (Mastomys) natalensis*. *Cancer Res.*, **28**, 1573–1576 (1968).

33. Snell, K. C. Adenocarcinoma of the glandular stomach in *Mastomys*. *In* "Carcinoma of the alimentary tract, etiology and pathogenesis," ed. by W. J. Burdette, University of Utah Press, Salt Lake City, Utah, pp. 55–62 (1965).

34. Snell, K. C. and Stewart, H. L. Malignant gastric carcinoids of *Praomys (Mastomys) natalensis*. *Science*, **163**, 470 (1969).

35. Snell, K. C. and Stewart, H. L. Histology of primary and transplanted argyrophilic carcinoids of the glandular stomach of *Praomys (Mastomys) natalensis* and their physiologic effects on the host. *GANN Monograph*, **8**, 39–55 (1969).

36. Soga, J. Pathological analysis of spontaneous carcinogenesis in glandular stomach of *Praomys (Mastomys) natalensis*. *Acta Med. Biol.*, **15**, 181–206 (1968).

37. Soga, J., Tazawa, K., Kanahara, H., and Hiraide, K. Some characteristic features of spontaneous argyrophil cell carcinoids in glandular stomach of *Praomys (Mastomys) natalensis*. *GANN Monograph*, **8**, 15–38 (1969).

38. Stern, B. K. Some biochemical properties of suspension of intestinal epithelial cells. *Gastroenterology*, **51**, 855–867 (1966).

39. Sugimura, T., Fujimura, S., Kogure, K., Baba, T., Saito, T., Nagao, M., Hosoi, H., Simosato, Y., and Yokoshima, T. Production of adenocarcinomas in glandular stomach of experimental animals by N-methyl-N'-nitro-N-nitrosoguanidine. *GANN Monograph*, **8**, 157–196 (1969).

40. Takaki, R., Takii, M., and Ikegami, T. Preliminary studies on the *in vitro* carcinogenesis of rat thymus cells by N-methyl-N'-nitro-N-nitrosoguanidine. *Gann*, **60**, 661–662 (1969).

EXPLANATION OF PHOTOS

PHOTO 1.   Untreated cell line is composed mostly of oval or polygonal cells with round nuclei. SS11, 30th gen., 233 days *in vitro*. May-Grünwald Giemsa stain. ×200.

PHOTO 2.   Early changes 10 days after treatment with 1 μg/ml of MNNG. Most cells are oval with granulated cytoplasm. Spindle-shaped cells gradually decreased thereafter. PN265B derived from SS11. Phase contrast. ×100.

PHOTO 3.   Same cell line (PN265B), 194 days after treatment with MNNG. Monotonous appearance of cells similar to untreated cell line continued up to about 200 days. Piling up of cells is evident. May-Grünwald Giemsa stain. ×200.

PHOTO 4.   Two types of cells are intermingled in later stages. Cells with large oval nucleus are overlapped by spindle-shaped cells. PN267A, 21st gen., 454 days *in vitro*. May-Grünwald Giemsa stain. ×200.

PHOTO 5.   Leiomyomatous area with interlacing bands and whorls in tumor of SS14 cell line. Hematoxylin-Eosin stain (H-E). ×100.

PHOTO 6.   Anaplastic area in tumor of PN269B cell line. H-E. ×100.

PHOTO 7.   Area of multiple huge giant cells with a number of nuclei. PN267A tumor. H-E. ×100.

PHOTO 8.   Showing two types of giant cells in detail, rossete-like and elongated form. PN267A tumor. H-E. ×400.

PHOTO 9.   Oval argyrophilic cells, with dark grey granules in the cytoplasm, without any carcinoid-like structures. PN265B tumor. Bodian stain. ×400.

PHOTO 10.   Oval argyrophilic cells found in cultured cells fixed on cover glass. PN265B, 42nd gen., 248 days *in vitro*. Bodian stain. ×200.

PHOTO 11.   Secretory granules in the cytoplasm. Some are clearly surrounded by wavy limiting membranes. Diameter, 240–400 nm. PN265B tumor. ×35,000, original ×12,500.

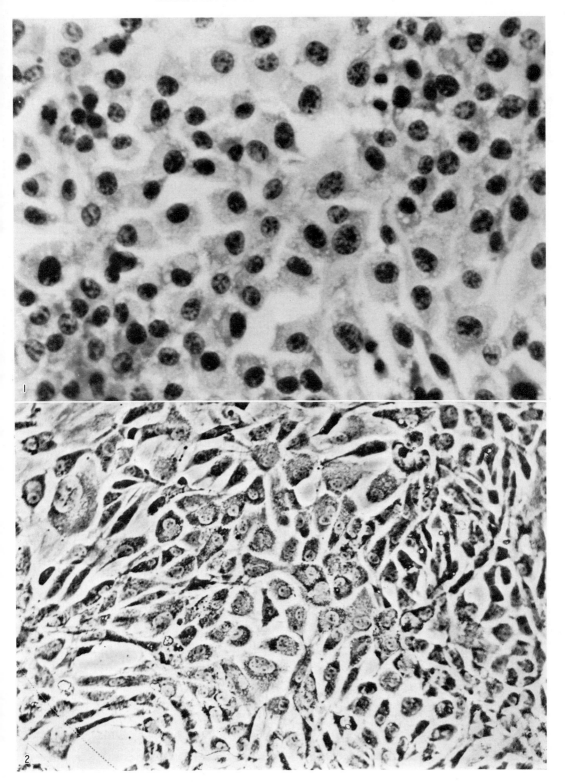

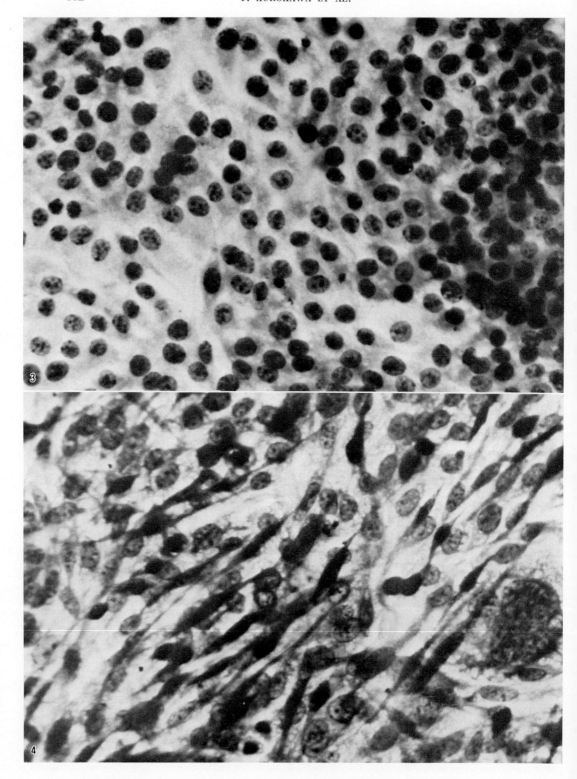

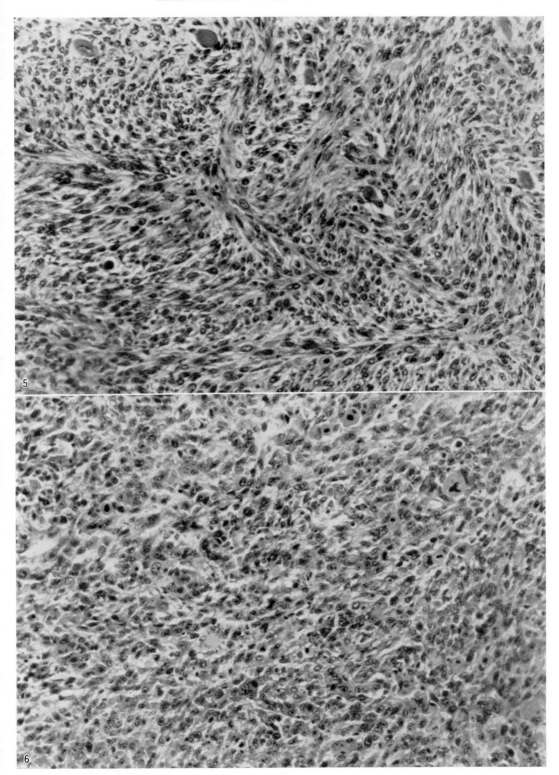

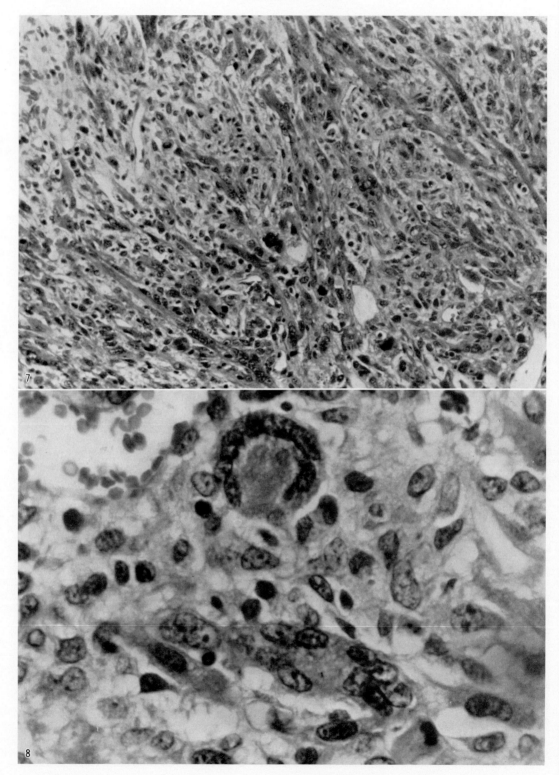

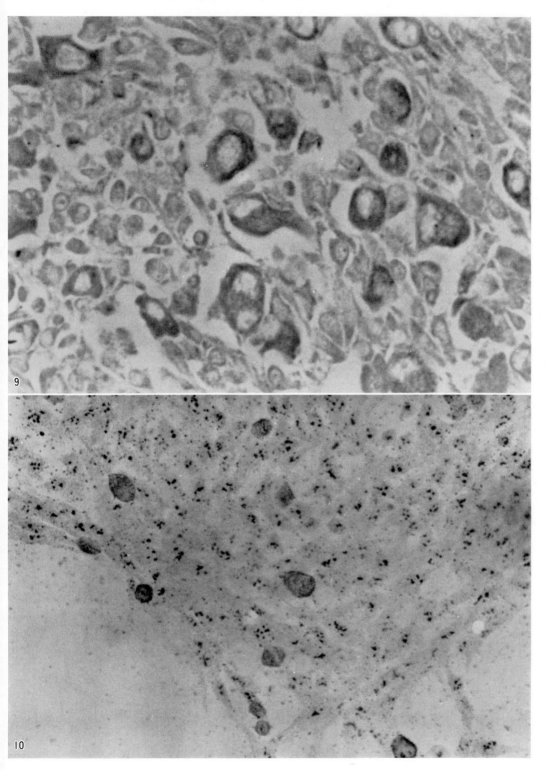

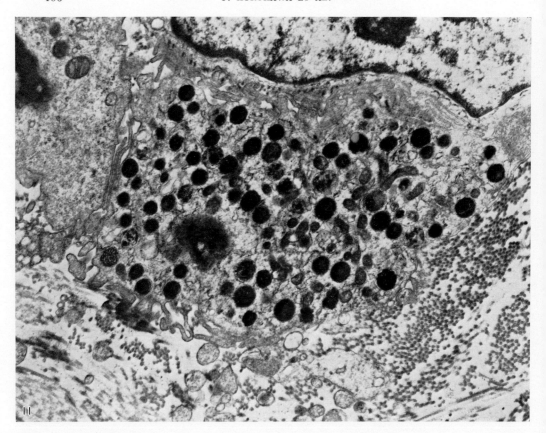

GANN Monograph on Cancer Research 17, 107–132 (1975)

CHEMICAL CARCINOGENESIS ON N-NITROSO DERIVATIVES

H. Druckrey

Forschergruppe Präventivmedizin, Max-Planck Institut für Immunologie*

" Die Präzise Formulierung eines Problems enthält meist schon seine Lösung.
Immer ist sie die Voraussetzung dafür."

Max Planck

In systematic studies with numerous dialkylnitrosamines striking organospecific carcinogenesis, dependent on chemical structure, has been observed. The results indicate that metabolic dealkylation, yielding the corresponding alkyldiazonium as "proximate" carcinogens, is initiated by enzymic α-hydroxylation, and that the hydroxylases involved probably are specific. In transplacental experiments, dialkylnitrosamines were not carcinogenic to rat fetus, except at the last day of gestation.

Acylalkylnitrosamides, which decompose by heterolysis without enzymic activation, proved to be potent topical carcinogens. Nevertheless, organospecific effects were observed, dependent on both the acyl and alkyl groups. For example, methylnitrosourea selectively produced malignant tumors of the brain. Ethylnitrosourea has been tested for transplacental and neonatal carcinogenicity in comprehensive studies on rats. One single low dose, when administered at one after the 12th day of gestation, exclusively produced neurogenic tumors in all offspring. The same susceptibility of the nervous system, surpassing that of adults about 60-fold, was observed in newborn rats.

Quantitative evaluations of the relations between dose (d) and medium induction time (t) corresponded regularly to the simple formula $dt^n =$ const. with $n > 2$, independent of whether chronic exposure to constant dosage or one single dose was used. Accordingly, carcinogenesis is to be considered an "accelerated process." The results provide strong support for the "genetic theory" of cancer.

The discovery made by Tomizo Yoshida in 1932 and 1935 (*93, 123, 124*) that *o*-aminoazotoluene after oral administration to rats regularly and specifically induced liver cancer opened a new epoch in experimental carcinogenesis research. At that time, when I had the pleasure of his visit in Berlin, even famous pathologists like R. Rössle refused to accept his discovery, objecting "cancer is a human disease, and what you have comes from rats." Nevertheless, it was the

---

* D-7802 Freiburg-Merzhausen, West Germany.

first example demonstrating the absorptive carcinogenicity of a well-known and defined aromatic amine to one specific internal organ. The exclusive observation of liver cancer should have suggested the assumption that the compound is metabolically activated in the liver and that the resulting "ultimate" carcinogen is too short-lived to exert its effects on other organs. Having this in mind, it is an honor for me to dedicate my contribution on organotropic carcinogenesis to the memory of the great pioneer in experimental cancer research, Tomizo Yoshida.

The specific and regular induction of cancer in certain organs undoubtedly is a fundamental problem. In general, such "organotropic" effects can be expected from substances that *per se* are inactive "transport forms" but become metabolically converted into an "active form" (*32*). An interesting example of this principle of action is dimethylnitrosamine (N-nitrosodimethylamine) (DMN), discovered as a specific liver carcinogen by Magee and Barnes (*73*). As demonstrated by Dutton and Heath (*42*), the simple molecule $O=N-N(CH_3)_2$ is enzymically demethylated predominantly in the liver, which explains its organotropic effect. The resulting monomethylnitrosamine is known to be extremely unstable and decomposes spontaneously to yield an alkylating intermediate, which was originally assumed to be diazomethane. Using ^{14}C-labeled DMN, methylation of nucleic acids of rat liver, predominantly on N(7) of guanine, was then demonstrated by Magee and Farber (*76*). Thus, the irreversible change of the "genetic code" in the affected cells was regarded as the carcinogenic primary process, which for the first time became experimentally accessible at the molecular level. This "alkylation theory" or, in a general term, "genetic theory," was later supported by many experimental results and proved to be one of the greatest achievements in carcinogenesis research.

Demethylation yielding formaldehyde, as is well known from many examples, was originally attributed to special demethylases. They are mainly found in the microsomal fraction of liver cells and belong to the group of "drug-metabolizing enzymes" described by Brodie *et al.* (*9*). However, the observation that diethylnitrosamine (DEN) and even N-nitrosopiperidine are also potent carcinogens (*35*) demonstrated that the enzymic process is not restricted to demethylation but is generally effective in dealkylation.

For biochemical reasons, an initial hydroxylation at one αC atom was assumed by Druckrey *et al.* (*35*). The resulting hydroxylated compounds are extremely unstable, and dealkylation by formation of the corresponding aldehyde occurs spontaneously. Accordingly, the enzymes involved probably are hydroxylases. This view then found strong support in the work of Gilette (*45*), Keberle *et al.* (*62*), McMahon (*77*), and Parke and Williams (*87*) on the oxidative dealkylation of various other alkylamino and alkoxy compounds, which in many respects parallels that of dialkylnitrosamines. Their oxidative degradation by the enzyme-free hydroxylase model of Udenfriend *et al.* (*116*) has been demonstrated in our institute, as reported by Preussmann (*90*).

Studies on relationships between chemical structure, reaction mechanisms, and biological actions are fundamental in pharmacology, and particularly in carcinogenesis research. For this purpose, comparative tests with a great number of systematically selected derivatives of one chemical group are required. The N-nitroso compounds were considered to be ideal models for the following reasons. (1) The molecular structure and the synthesis are generally simple. (2) The two valences of the central N atom offer innumerable possibilities for chemical variations in any direction. (3) The reaction mechanisms are controllable by well-known chemical and biochemical methods. (4) Hydroxylases, required for the activation of dialkylnitrosamines, are not restricted to the liver but exist in many specialized organs and tissues, as reviewed by Hayaishi and Nozaki (50). (5) There are many indications for substrate specificity of hydroxylases. Hence, specific carcinogenic effects on organs other than the liver, dependent on the chemical structure of the tested compound, were expected and have been observed in several animal species (32).

Chemistry and Biochemistry

The name "nitrosamines," though commonly used, is not correct. In fact they are dialkylamides of nitrous acid and have practically no basic properties. This deserves attention, because the metabolic hydroxylation and dealkylation, despite some similarities, is not identical to that of basic dialkylamino compounds. Nitrosamines have a high dipole moment, and the nitroso-oxygen reveals pronounced nucleophilic (55) and hydrogen-bonding properties. The molecular structure is coplanar and, accordingly, *cis* and *trans* isomers are possible. Furthermore, the grade of binding between N–N is considerably higher than that of a single bond, which indicates a $\overset{\oplus}{>}N=N-\overset{\ominus}{O}$ structure, comparable to that of azoxyalkanes. The two boundary structures, explained by Druckrey (16, 18), are formulated in Fig. 1.

As demonstrated by Keefer and Fodor (63) and by Seebach and Enders (100), one proton at an αC atom is unstable, and its fission leads to an α-carbanion, susceptible to various electrophilic substitutions and even to metalation, for example by lithium (100). These recent results provide strong support for

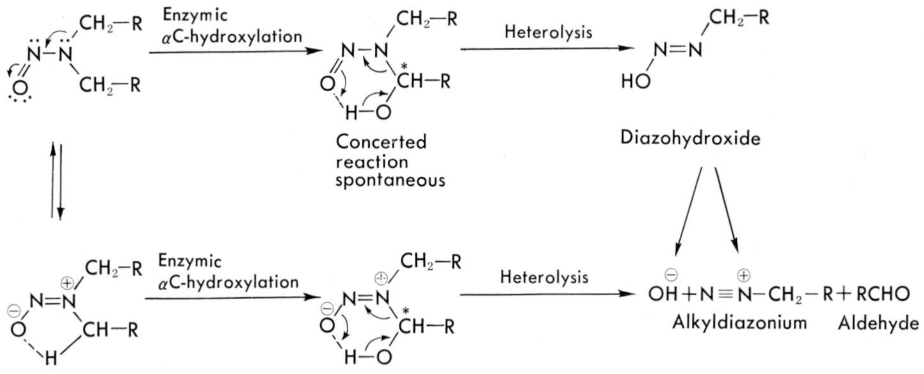

FIG. 1. Dialkylnitrosamines
Molecular structure and probable mechanism of action, yielding alkyldiazohydroxide and -diazonium as "proximate" alkylating carcinogen.

the assumption of α-hydroxylation, probably by an oxene mechanism, first proved by Ullrich *et al.* (*117*) using the example of phenacetin. Calculations of the electronic charges of several nitrosamines and their α-hydroxylated derivatives have been performed by Nagata and Imamura (*80*). α-Hydroxylation of an N–CH$_2$–R group necessarily leads to an asymmetric C atom (*18*). Hydroxy group is possible in the *cis* or *trans* position to the nitroso-oxygen. In the first case, the formation of a hydrogen bridge can be assumed, which probably leads to spontaneous degradation by concerted reaction, directly yielding the diazohydroxide or alkyldiazonium, as formulated in Fig. 1 (*16*, *18*). This view is in agreement with the findings of Lijinsky *et al.* (*69*), who conclusively demonstrated that the alkylating intermediate of DMN cannot be diazomethane.

In higher dialkylnitrosamines, hydroxylation in the β-position (*67*) or at one of the terminal C atoms is also possible (*6*, *86*). The resulting CH$_2$OH group may be either coupled, for example, by glucuronic acid, or oxidized to carboxyl (*49*). In the latter case, degradation by β-oxidation (similar to that of fatty acids) has been demonstrated by Okada and Suzuki (*86*) leading to different carboxylic products depending on whether the number of C atoms of the original alkyl group was even or odd. This can be important to some organotropic properties of the respective compounds, but cannot lead to an alkylating intermediate, with the exception of degradation to the highly reactive alkylnitrosocarbamic acid, which is possible only with an odd-numbered alkyl group.

Recently, direct reactions between hydroxylated nitrosamines and nucleic acids have been discussed by Schoental (*96*). Of special interest are former studies of Fahr *et al.* (*43*) on the specific reaction of intact dialkylnitrosamines with cytidylic acid *in vitro*, the mechanism of which is still unknown. Translocation of the nitroso group to an αC atom yielding an amidoxime was proposed by Neunhöffer *et al.* (*81*). Theoretically, there are many possibilities, but whatever mechanism is considered, it must be in accordance with the well-established fact that all dialkylnitrosamines produce cancer exclusively in certain remote organs and never at the site of application (*16*). Accordingly, they are "indirect" carcinogens, requiring metabolic activation.

The assumption of an initial α-hydroxylation as the only enzymic step of activation is well founded. It presumes the presence of at least one proton at one αC atom and depends on its accessibility. As will be shown, this is in perfect agreement with the results of the carcinogenicity tests. Beyond that, it explains the striking organotropic effects of certain nitrosamines, because there are many examples for the existence of organospecific hydroxylases with substrate-specific properties.

The alkylation of nucleic acids will be discussed by Farber and by Magee in this Monograph from the biochemical viewpoint (*72*). The apparent differences between the degree of alkylation of N-7 guanine and the localization of tumors, reported by Schoental (*95*) and by Swann and Magee (*107*), cannot refute the alkylation theory, since other alkylations are possible. That at 0–6 of deoxyguanosine probably is more relevant to carcinogenesis, as reported by Loveless (*71*) and by O'Connor *et al.* (*82*). Furthermore, alkylation of mitochondrial DNA, demonstrated by Wunderlich *et al.* (*122*), may also play an important role, which would be in accordance with the fundamental work of Warburg (*118*) on the impairment of respiration and the high aerobic glycolysis, the only common biochemical feature of all tumors. In any case, according to general pharmacological experience, it must be assumed that only a very few of the numerous alkylations can be relevant to the malignant transformation of the affected cells and that the vast majority of them are responsible for cytotoxic or lethal effects, generally observed with all carcinogens, dependent on concentration.

Acylalkylnitrosamides, in contrast to dialkylnitrosamines, are unstable in alkaline solution, and no enzymic activation is required. They become deacylated by heterolysis and have been widely used in chemistry as alkylating substances. Accordingly, they act as "direct" carcinogens. Five types of alkylnitrosamides have been tested, namely, carboxylamides (N–COR), urethans (N–COOR), ureas (N–CO–NH$_2$) (*8*), biurets (N–CO–NH–CO–NH$_2$), and N'-nitroguanidines (N–CNH–NH–NO$_2$). The breakdown of the urethans is considerably enhanced by thiol compounds, and the formation of the thio-half-acetal as an intermediate was demonstrated by Schoental and Rive (*98*). In contrast, we found the heterolysis of the urea compounds is not affected by cysteine, probably because the carbonyl groups is much less reactive (*16*).

Furthermore, whereas all other nitrosamides are liquid, the urea and biuret derivatives are crystalline. This indicates the existence of a hydrogen bridge to the nitroso-oxygen, which may also occur in the other compounds after reaction with thiols. With this assumption the probable structures and biochemical mechanisms of action are formulated for two examples in Fig. 2, in which a breakdown by concerted reaction is proposed, directly yielding alkyldiazohydroxide as the "proximate" alkylating carcinogen (*16*). The formation of isocyanate and an alkyl cation from alkylnitrosoureas was demonstrated by Montgomery *et al.* (*79*), and that of nitrocyanamide from N-methyl-N'-nitro-N'-nitrosoguanidine (MNNG) by Lawley and Thatcher (*68*) and by Wheeler and Bowdon (*120*), as postulated in Fig. 2. In an admirable experiment with MNNG, labeled by ^{14}C either at CH$_3$ or at the guanidine group, it has been demonstrated by Sugimura *et al.* (*104*) that alkylation occurs preferably on DNA, and acylation on histones, enzymes, or proteins.

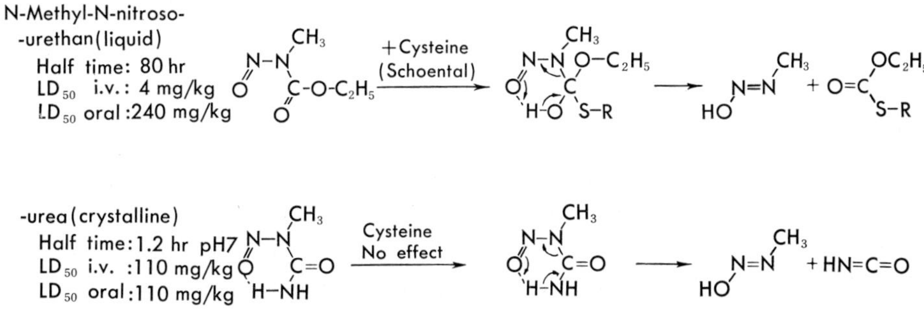

FIG. 2.   Acylalkylnitrosamides
    Differences between structure, reactivity, and breakdown of methylnitroso-urethan (MNUT) and -urea (MNU), both yielding methyldiazohydroxide as the "proximate" alkylating carcinogen (pH 7). i. v.: intravenous injection.

It seemed desirable to present the chemical and biochemical bases, because despite the great number of N-nitroso compounds tested so far, almost 100, there are innumerable other derivatives possible theoretically. Therefore, this group offers the widest opportunities for systematic studies on relationships between chemical structure, reaction mechanisms, and biological actions. Beyond that, N-nitroso compounds can easily be formed by reaction of nitrous acid or nitrogen oxides with alkylamines or -amides, which are widespread in the human environment, as first discussed by Druckrey and Preussmann (*30*). Since then it has been shown by many investigators that such compounds occur in foods and in tobacco smoke (*Lancet*, **1**, 1071 (1968)), as will be reported by Sander in this monograph.

Organotropic Carcinogenicity of Dialkylnitrosamines

According to the formulas in Fig. 1, carcinogenic activity was expected as a general feature of dialkylnitrosamines, liable to αC-hydroxylation. This could be shown in systematic studies with about 60 derivatives by Druckrey et al. (*32*). A review has been published by Magee and Barnes (*75*). Since then, N-nitroso compounds, because of their tremendous variability and the comparative clarity of their mechanism of action, became the preferred models in carcinogenesis research, and numerous new results have been reported. In this paper only the main aspects will be reviewed. The dosages will be indicated not only in mg/kg body weight but also in percentages of the acute LD_{50} for a proper judgement of the "carcinogenic breadth." Our own experiments were usually performed with 10 syngeneic strains of BD rats, the respective genotypes and phenotypes of which, including the relevant biological features, were reported by Druckrey (*15*).

DMN, an excellent solvent, was formerly used in industry. The observation of liver cirrhosis in exposed workers, made by Barnes and Magee (*3*), instigated animal experiments. It proved to be highly toxic. The acute LD_{50} in rats is 40 mg/kg. The carcinogenicity of DMN was discovered by Magee and Barnes (*73*). In chronic experiments on rats at a daily oral dosage of about 1 mg/kg (2.5% LD_{50}), cancer of the liver was observed in all cases and, occasionally, also malignant tumors of the kidneys. The latter is of biochemical interest, because a considerable increase of β-glucuronidase activity after oral administration of nitrosamines was reported by Hoch-Ligeti et al. (*53*). After a single high dose or a short-time exposure, DMN produced nephroblastomas exclusively (*74*), a phenomenon, later observed with various "indirect" carcinogens, requiring α-hydroxylation.

In Syrian hamsters, DMN also proved to be a specific liver carcinogen (*115*). On the other hand, in mice, lung tumors were predominantly observed by Takayama and Oota (*109*). With regard to the high volatility of DMN, inhalation experiments were performed in rats by Druckrey et al. (*32*) at exposures to 100 ppm in the air for 30 min twice a week. Surprisingly, aesthesioneuroblastomas of the olfactory epithelium and carcinomas of the ethmoturbinalia developed exclusively, with no liver cancer. These results indicate that enzymic activation is also possible in the nasal cavity. In this context it is of interest that azo-xymethane (AOM), though isomeric to DMN and after hydroxylation likewise yielding methyldiazonium, proved to be a specific inducer of carcinomas of the colon (*16*), never observed with DMN. Accordingly, the organotropy is independent of the kind of the "ultimate" carcinogen, but depends on the chemical constitution of the parent compound and its enzymic activation (*18*).

DEN, the carcinogenicity of which was first reported by Schmähl *et al.* (*94*), is much less toxic than DMN. The acute LD_{50} in rats is 280 mg/kg. Nevertheless, it proved to be a potent liver carcinogen, even at a daily dosage of less than 0.05% of the LD_{50}. The "carcinogenic breadth" is extraordinarily large. Therefore, DEN was used for extensive quantitative studies by Druckrey *et al.* (*39*), which will be reported later in "Quantitative Evaluations" (p. 118). In the range of small dosages, an increasing proportion of carcinomas of the esophagus was observed, which never occurred with DMN. Hence, the formation of an asymmetric C atom by α-hydroxylation may be responsible for this special effect. The results were independent of the route of administration.

Guinea pigs were selected as another animal species, because at that time they were generally considered to be resistant to chemical carcinogenesis. At a daily dosage of 5 mg/kg, given in the drinking water, DEN produced hepatocellular carcinomas in all treated animals after a medium induction time of 280 ± 25 days, as reported by Druckrey and Steinhoff (*40*). One female became pregnant during the treatment. Its descendant died from liver cancer at the young age of 52 days. This surprising result stimulated systematic studies on transplacental carcinogenesis, as will be reported in "Transplacental Carcinogenesis" (p. 121).

In mice, Clapp and Craig (*11*) obtained a 90% yield of liver cancer associated with carcinomas of the forestomach and, in 18%, of the esophagus, whereas similar experiments by Thomas and Schmähl (*113*) led to hemangioendotheliomas of the liver. After topical application to the skin of mice, Hoffmann and Graffi (*54*) observed exclusively carcinomas of the nasal cavity. Since DEN, like DMN, is highly volatile, this effect may be attributed to the inhalation of the vapors. On the other hand, the induction of such tumors and particularly of olfactory neuroblastomas by subcutaneous (s. c.) injection to hamsters was reported by Herrold (*51*) and by Montesano and Saffiotti (*78*). Oral administration of DEN to hamsters, however, led to lung cancer in experiments by Dontenwill *et al.* (*13*). In rabbits liver cancer exclusively was observed by Thomas and Schmähl (*113*). Of special interest is the induction of hepatocellular carcinomas in monkeys by DEN, reported by Kelly *et al.* (*64*). The dosage was 20 mg/kg given by gavage once to twice every fortnight, and the medium induction time was 24 months.

Theoretically, hydroxylation of DEN is also possible at the βC atom. Therefore, ethyl-2-hydroxyethylnitrosamine was tested in rats. The acute LD_{50} was greater than 7,500 mg/kg. However, a surprisingly high cumulative toxicity was observed, and even a daily dosage of 100 mg/kg had to be interrupted after 29 days, although the total dose administered was only 2,900 mg/kg. This example is of great interest in toxicology. Daily doses of 5 mg/kg produced liver cancer in all treated rats, and 2 out of 20 simultaneously had adenocarcinomas of the pancreas (32). Bis(2-hydroxyethyl)nitrosamine, which has no lipophilic group, showed no acute and no cumulative toxicity. Nevertheless, it proved to be a specific liver carcinogen; this, however, only at the high daily dosage of about 500 mg/kg. The esterified bis(acetoxyethyl)nitrosamine yielded identical results at the lower dosage of 100 mg/kg (32). In contrast to the low efficacy of these compounds, the cyclic ether of diethanolnitrosamine, N-nitrosomorpholine, is a very potent and rapidly acting carcinogen (32). At an oral dosage of 16 mg/kg (5% LD_{50}) it produced liver cancer after an induction time of about 110 days. None of these compounds produced carcinomas of the esophagus.

Dipropylnitrosamine (LD_{50}=480 mg/kg) has been tested only in rats, and similar results were obtained as with DEN. With daily oral administration, the high dosage of 30 mg/kg induced liver cancer exclusively, but with lower dosages down to 0.8% of the LD_{50} an increasing proportion of esophageal carcinomas was observed (32).

The diisopropylnitrosamine seemed to be of special interest for two reasons: (a) α-hydroxylation is impaired by steric hindrance, and (b) the formation of an asymmetric C atom is impossible. As expected, only a 50% yield of liver cancer and no tumors of the esophagus were observed. With the unsaturated diallylnitrosamine at a daily dosage of 20 mg/kg (2.5% LD_{50}) the outcome was negative (32). This may be due either to hydroxylation at the double bond, or to the fact that the resulting propenyldiazonium is less reactive than a saturated alkyldiazonium.

Dibutylnitrosamine (DBN, LD_{50}=1,200 mg/kg) given in the daily diet of rats at the high dosage of 75 mg/kg produced liver cancer exclusively. With lower dosages carcinomas of the esophagus and, surprisingly, of the urinary bladder were also observed (37). The latter prevailed at a low dosage of 20 mg/kg (32), which permits a sufficiently long survival time. In order to circumvent the direct passage through the liver, DBN 200 or 400 mg/kg was given once a week by subcutaneous injections. Under these circumstances, it proved to be a specific bladder carcinogen (33). The organotropic effect was also observed in mice by Bertram and Craig (5) and by Wood et al. (121), and in guinea pigs by Ivankovic and Bücheler (57a).

Analyses of the urine by thin-layer chromatography after subcutaneous injection of DBN to rats revealed the excretion of several water-soluble metabolites at a concentration about 50 times higher than that found in the serum. This indicated that hydroxylation occurred at other C atoms rather than in the α position, probably followed by coupling, for example to glucuronic acid. Biochemically, δ-hydroxylation at a terminal C atom seemed to be the most probable. Therefore, butyl(4-hydroxybutyl)nitrosamine (BOBN) has been synthesized and tested in rats. It proved to be a specific inducer of bladder cancer, even with oral administration. A daily dosage of 20 mg/kg (1% LD_{50}) was highly effective (33). The results were confirmed in rats and mice by Ito et al. (56), Bertram and Craig (4, 5), Okada and Suzuki (86), Akagi et al. (1), and Blattmann and Preussmann (6). BOBN becomes oxidized in the liver to butyl(3-carboxypropyl)nitrosamine, which is not only a major urinary metabolite but also probably the "proximate" carcinogen of DBN and BOBN. Given in the daily drinking water at a concentration of 0.06%, it produced bladder cancer exclusively in all treated rats (*49, 86*).

Further metabolic studies have been performed recently (*6, 67, 89*). According to information from Professor Okada, the carboxylic compound, like fatty acids, partly undergoes β-hydroxylation, and acetic acid is split off, yielding the butyl homolog of nitrososarcosin. This metabolic process is of great interest, because with the 3-hydroxypropyl compound, for example, the breakdown to the highly reactive alkylnitrosocarbamic acid should be expected theoretically. In any case, the number of C atoms, whether it is even or odd, apparently plays an important role.

Diphenylnitrosamine, which is almost insoluble in water, was rather nontoxic (LD_{50}=3,000 mg/kg). Given in the daily diet at a dosage of 100 mg/kg, it nevertheless produced liver cancer in 17 out of 18 treated rats. Six of them simultaneously had multiple carcinomas of the lungs, possibly metastatic; however, one was a primary squamous epithelium cancer. After subcutaneous injections of 500 mg/kg once a week for 6 months, lung cancer was observed almost exclusively (*32*). The complete absence of any tumor in the urinary bladder indicates the relevance of the nature of the alkyl groups to the organotropy of the carcinogenic effect.

Dicyclohexyl- and diphenylnitrosamine were not carcinogenic, although the total dose administered was about 100 g/kg. The negative result is in accordance with our theory, since α-hydroxylation is impaired by steric hindrance in the former, and impossible in the latter compound. Dibenzylnitrosamine, despite its acute toxicity (LD_{50}=900 mg/kg), was not carcinogenic either. Since, according to McMahon (*77*), the benzylamino group is particularly susceptible to α-hydroxylation, another explanation must be sought. As discussed below, the resulting benzyldiazonium may yield the seven-membered ring tropilidene.

The carcinogenic efficacy of the symmetrical nitrosamines varied considerably in the range of 1:100 and decreased with the length of the alkyl chains. The question thus arose whether this is caused by differences in the susceptibility to α-hydroxylation or due to the reactivity of the alkylating intermediate. Therefore, many unsymmetrical dialkylnitrosamines were tested in rats.

Nitrosamines with one methyl group with variation of the second alkyl residue proved to be very effective and the most specific inducers of esophageal cancer, independent of whether the administration was by oral or parenteral route. For example, methylbutylnitrosamine (MBN), which is volatile, exerted this organotropic effect after inhalation of the vapors at a concentration of 25 ppm in the air for 1 hr every week (*28*). At continuous exposure to only 0.05 ppm, however, it produced squamous epithelium carcinomas of the nose (*26*), also observed in mice by Brune and Henning (*10*).

Most of these compounds were tested in rats using oral or subcutaneous application. In general, the greater the second alkyl group was, the higher the efficacy was. For example, the pentyl, benzyl, 2-phenylethyl, isopropyl, and cyclohexyl derivatives produced a high yield of carcinomas of the esophagus (*32*). Since such tumors were never observed with DMN, this organotropic effect probably must be attributed to the higher alkyl residues, which, according to McMahon (77), are particularly susceptible to α-hydroxylation. On the other hand, the occurrence of an asymmetric C atom cannot be crucial, because methyl-cyclohexylnitrosamine proved to be the most potent carcinogen to the esophagus (32). In contrast ethyl-*tert*-butylnitrosamine was neither toxic nor carcinogenic. Two explanations are conceivable. Either hydroxylation occurs first at one βC atom of the *tert*-butyl group, or deethylation does not lead to an alkylating intermediate, but to isobutylene instead. Surprisingly, methylphenylnitrosamine also produced cancer of the esophagus (35), which suggests the possibility of an arylating mechanism. In this context it is of interest that the vinyl derivatives of methyl- and ethylnitrosamine proved to be very potent carcinogens (32).

Furthermore, methyl(2-chloroethyl)nitrosamine, though one of the most toxic derivatives ($LD_{50}=22$ mg/kg), was a rather weak carcinogen. N-nitroso-sarcosine, on the other hand, was practically nontoxic. Nevertheless, it too induced cancer of the esophagus. The ethyl ester was significantly more effective. These examples demonstrate that no relations exist between acute toxicity and carcinogenicity (32).

Cyclic-N-nitroso compounds also revealed organotropic effects. N-nitroso-pyrrolidine produced liver cancer exclusively, whereas with N-nitrosopiperidine mainly carcinomas of the esophagus and of the ethmoturbinalia were observed in rats (20, 32), and in mice cancer of the forestomach and the liver, as reported by Takayama (110). The seven-membered ring N-nitrosohexamethyleneimine, tested by Goodall et al. (46) in rats with oral administration, produced cancer of the liver and esophagus. With N-nitrosopiperazine, given in the drinking water (200 mg/liter), cancer of the snout and nose was observed by Garcia et al. (44), whereas N,N'-dinitrosopiperazine induced cancer of the esophagus and, particularly with s.c. injections, also carcinomas and neuroblastomas of the nasal cavity (20). N-Nitrosomorpholine, the cyclic ether of diethanolnitrosamine, proved to be a fast-acting liver carcinogen (32). At a daily dosage of 8 mg/kg (2% LD_{50}) the median induction time was 165 days. The thio-homolog, studied by Garcia et al. (44) under comparable conditions, produced cancer of the esophagus and the nasal cavity.

The carcinogenicity of N-nitrosopiperidine was the first example suggesting enzymic α-hydroxylation as the initial step of activation (35). The subsequent ring cleavage of cyclic N-nitroso compounds should lead to a corresponding monoalkylnitrosamine with a terminal aldehyde group. However, no explanation can be offered as to the different organotropic effects. Further systematic chemical and biochemical studies are needed to clarify mechanisms of actions in general pharmacology and, beyond that, in planned drug synthesis.

Acylalkylnitrosamides

In contrast to the dialkylnitrosamines, the nitrosamides decompose by hetero-lysis without a metabolic activation, yielding an alkylating intermediate (107), probably the corresponding alkyldiazohydroxide, as discussed previously (p. 111). Accordingly, they are to be considered "directly" acting carcinogens. As expected, the nitrosamides produced local tumors at the site of application, for example sarcomas after s.c. injections in rats (*34*) or topical carcinomas after skin painting in mice, as reported by Graffi *et al.* (*48*). The biological efficacy corresponded clearly to the chemical reactivity. It was the highest with alkylnitrosocarboxylamides, and decreased in the following order: carbamic esters ("urethans"), ureas, biurets, and nitroguanidines (*16*). Within the individual groups, the two properties were more pronounced, the smaller the molecule was, and decreased generally with increasing number of C atoms in both the alkyl and acyl groups (Druckrey *et al.*, unpublished).

After oral administration, various nitrosamides, like methylnitrosoacetamide, -propionylamide, -urethan, -urea, or -nitroguanidine (MNNG) produced carcinomas of the forestomach and, occasionally, also the esophagus in experiments of Druckrey *et al.* (*36*), Schoental and Magee (*97*), and Craddock (*12*) on rats, and of Herrold (*52*) on hamsters. In order to find a model for the induction of adenocarcinomas, guinea pigs were used by Druckrey *et al.* (*19*), since their whole stomach is glandular, like that of men. MNUT proved to be particularly effective and produced gastric carcinomas strikingly resembling human stomach cancer and adenocarcinomas of the pancreas, with multiple metastases in the lungs and liver. The yield of each of the two tumor types was 13/32.

The specific induction of gastric adenocarcinomas in rats by MNNG at low oral dosage for a limited period was then achieved by Sugimura and Fujimura (*103, 105*). The same result was obtained in dogs by Sugimura *et al.* (*106*). Since, from the chemical standpoint, MNNG is an N′-acylated methylnitrosoguanidine, the N′-acetyl-MNU and the N′-carbamoyl-MNU (biuret) were tested in rats using administration in the daily drinking water by Druckrey *et al.* (*22, 29*). The former compound proved to be a specific inducer of gastric carcinomas, whereas with the biuret derivative malignant tumors of the brain were also observed.

In order to study systemic effects, absorption was enforced by intravenous injection. Under these conditions, MNUT proved to be extremely toxic, the acute LD_{50} being only 4 mg/kg. A dosage of 1 mg/kg once every fortnight produced exclusively carcinomas of the lungs in almost all treated rats (*31*). Two explanations are possible for this immediate effect. Either the degradation is catalyzed by thiols, as demonstrated by Schoental and Rive (*98*), or the ester group of MNUT may be split off by esterase in the lungs, yielding the extremely reactive methylnitrosocarbamic acid. Ethylnitrosourethan (ENUT), which is more stable and about 100 times less toxic than MNUT, did not induce lung cancer, but carcinomas of the forestomach instead (*32*).

In contrast to MNUT and MNNG, the heterolysis of MNU is not affected by thiols. Surprisingly, after intravenous injections of MNU to rats at weekly doses of 5 mg/kg (4% LD_{50}) a high yield of neurogenic tumors in the brain and spinal cord was observed by Druckrey *et al.* (*21*). The histological examination revealed iso- or polymorphic gliomas, oligodendrogliomas, ependymomas, and astrocytomas (*24*). Identical results were obtained in rabbits by Jänisch and Schreiber (*60*) and in dogs by Warzok *et al.* (*119*). Since the heterolysis of MNU occurs only at neutral or alkaline pH, it can be stabilized by addition of primary phosphate or citric acid. Under these conditions, the specific induction of brain tumors proved also to be possible with oral administration to rats, as reported by Thomas *et al.* (*114*) and by Strooband and Brucher (*102*). Since almost identical results were obtained with methylnitrosobiuret (*29*), the urea group is probably responsible for the neurotropic effects.

In comparative studies with the homologous series of alkylnitrosoureas in oral administration to rats, the proportion of neurogenic tumors decreased with increasing number of C atoms, and cancer of various other organs, particularly in the digestive tract, was observed (*16*). Surprisingly, the even-numbered derivatives ethyl- and butylnitrosourea (ENU and BNU) simultaneously produced a high yield of leukemias, as reported by Druckrey *et al.* (*32*), Odashima (*83–85*), and Takizawa and Nishihara (*111*).

Benzylnitrosourea, given by s.c. injection to adult rats, was only weakly carcinogenic, probably due to the formation of tropilidene, but after injection to newborn rats, a high yield of neurogenic tumors was observed by Druckrey and Gimmy (unpublished). In order to study whether or not an arylating compound might also be carcinogenic, phenylnitrosourea seemed to be the most suitable example, because phenyldiazonium necessarily occurs by heterolysis. After s.c. injections it produced a low but significant yield of local sarcomas (*91*).

Quantitative Evaluations

As verified in every scientific study, real knowledge is to be expected only if experimental results can be expressed by "measure and number." In carcinogenesis, the N-nitroso compounds are particularly suitable for quantitative studies because most of them are soluble in water, which permits a precise dosage through any route of administration. Beyond that, by use of an appropriate derivative, malignant tumors of almost every organ, closely resembling those of human pathology, can be induced with high selectivity and regularity.

Our experiments were principally performed in a strict quantitative manner with syngeneic BD rats (*15*) at constant dosage (*14, 39*). The evaluation was restricted to those experiments in which at least the majority of rats surviving till the critical age revealed malignant tumors at autopsy. In every dosage (d) group, the induction time (t, days till death) and the total dose administered ($D=dt$) were recorded for each individual rat. At the end of the experiment, the cumulative percentage of rats with malignant tumors was calculated. The individual data, plotted on a logarithmic "probit" scale as a function of D and t, yielded linear regressions of high characteristics, clearly corresponding to "normal distribution" in all individual experiments and dosage groups (*14, 32*). The "standard deviations" (SD) were generally 5 to 15%. This high accuracy obtained in such extreme chronic experiments is astonishing. Surprisingly, different tumor types observed within a certain group also fit fairly well into the linearity, indicating that the mechanism of action involved in the induction of the various tumors by N-nitroso compounds is practically identical. This provides strong support for the "alkylation theory." The only exception was observed with leukemias, which occurred earlier than solid tumors, and the slope of the linear

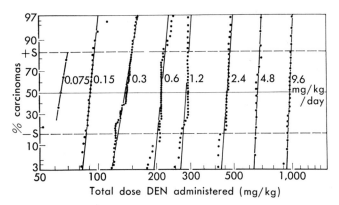

FIG. 3.   Dose-response relationships for the carcinogenic action of DEN given in the daily drinking water to BD-II rats

Eight dosage groups, ranging from 0.075 to 9.6 mg/kg body weight. Each dot corresponds to one individual rat with carcinomas. Decrease of the total dose administered until death from tumors with decreasing dosage.

regression was significantly more flat, probably representing a different mechanism in leukemogenesis than in carcinogenesis (*32*).

Extensive studies have been performed by Druckrey *et al.* (*32*, *39*) with DEN given in the daily drinking water to BD-II rats. The dosages (*d*) of the individual groups decreased from 9.6 mg/kg by the factor of 0.5 to 0.075 mg/kg. The results are presented in Fig. 3. Although the abscissa, indicating the total dose administered (*D*), is 5-fold elongated for better synopsis, the linearity and high accuracy are clearly recognizable. The small SD of 3 to 9% indicates a direct mechanism of the carcinogenic action. At least, indirect processes such as the intermediate induction or activation of a "tumor virus" can be excluded with certainty.

The most important result demonstrated in Fig. 3 is the fact that the total doses *D* required for the production of carcinomas decreased steadily and considerably with decreasing dosage (*d*) from 1,000 to only 64 mg/kg. Since in the last group the induction time was about 900 days, it follows that the carcinogenic primary effects even of the smallest dose are not only irreversible over the whole life span and transmitted to daughter cells (*25*), but also increase far beyond a mere summation. Accordingly, the factor time contributes considerably to carcinogenesis.

The median induction time (*t*) dependent on dosage (*d*) plotted in a double logarithmic system of coordinates showed a definite linear relationship over the whole range (Fig. 4). The slope of the straight line corresponds to an angle of 66.5° and tangent $n=2.3$. Therefore, it is

$$-\log d = 2.3 \log t + \log k$$

or

$$dt^{2.3} = \text{const.} \tag{1}$$

According to Eq. 1, the carcinogenic action of continuous oral administration of DEN proceeds with more than the square of time as an "accelerated process"

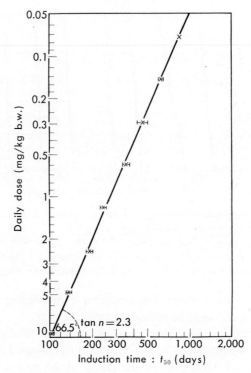

FIG. 4. Linear dependency of the medium induction time (t_{50}) on the daily
dosages of DEN, plotted on log-log coordinates
Results of experiments presented in Fig. 3.

(7) (Verstärkerwirkung) (*32, 39*). The results were confirmed by Rajewsky *et al.*
(*92*) with $n=2.4$. With other N-nitroso derivatives the value of n varied from
1.4 to 4 dependent on the substance used, but proved to be independent of the
organ in which the tumors occurred. As reported by Druckrey (*14*) in numerous
other examples, carcinogenesis corresponds to the simple general equation

$$dt^n = \text{const.} \qquad (2)$$

This mathematical interpretation seems to be rather academic at first sight, but is
of great practical value, because it is accessible to criticism and permits predic-
tions, the validity of which can be tested by planned experiments.

If, according to Eq. 2, carcinogenesis is in fact an "accelerated process,"
then it should be principally possible to "induce" cancer by one single dose
even of very short-lived carcinogens. This has been demonstrated with DMN
(*32, 74*) and various other N-nitroso compounds, particularly with MNU (*41*)
and ENU (*38*), which under physiological conditions decompose within a few
minutes. Hence, the initiating primary effect at the molecular level takes place
very rapidly, and the following processes during the "latent period" until tumor
manifestation develop autonomously.

Transplacental Carcinogenesis

Formerly, cancer was generally thought to be a typical disease of old age. However, there is an increasing frequency of cancer in childhood and youth. In consideration of the long "latent period" (especially observed after exposure to weak carcinogens or to small doses), Peller (*88*) came to the conclusion that the causative process may have occurred already during neonatal or even prenatal development. Since then, transplacental carcinogenesis has become one of the main problems in experimental research. For this purpose N-nitroso compounds, because of their high absorptive efficacy, seemed to be of special interest.

The fact, demonstrated in the section of p. 120, that cancer can principally be induced by one single dose made it possible to study systematically the susceptibility of animals at every stage of prenatal and neonatal development. In BD rats, the duration of pregnancy is 22 days 10 ± 6 hr (*15*).

With dialkylnitrosamines, two aspects should be considered in transplacental studies: appearance of the activating enzyme system in the fetus and the sensitivity of the various organs to malignant transformation. DMN, which is highly fetotoxic, has been tested by Alexandrov (*2*) at a daily dosage of 1 mg per rat during the first, second, and third week of gestation. Only in the last group, 3/94 of the offspring died with renal tumors after more than 600 days. In our experiments, a single dose of 10 mg/kg was not carcinogenic to the fetus, except at the last day before birth, but the tumor yield was rather small (*17, 18*).

DEN proved to be much less toxic to the fetus than DMN, which permits the use of considerably higher doses. After a daily dosage of 4 to 8 mg per rat, Pielsticker *et al.* (*89*) observed only two kidney tumors in an offspring of 91 rats. This almost negative result obviously must be attributed to the fact that the rats were killed at the age of 12 months because, after induction time of 18 to 24 months, an incidence of 14 malignant tumors among 40 descendants was reported by Thomas and Bollmann (*112*). A single dose of 70 mg/kg, when given on the 15th day of gestation, was not carcinogenic to the fetus. Only by treatment on the 22nd (last) day, the high dose of 150 mg/kg produced unequivocally positive results, dependent on route of administration. On i.v. injection, DEN induced olfactory neuroblastomas in 3/15 descendants, but after oral application 14 liver carcinomas and 4 nephroblastomas were observed in an offspring of 23 rats (*18, 57*).

Since DMN and DEN are very potent carcinogens in adult rats, the negative outcome on the 15th day leads to the conclusion that the "proximate" carcinogen formed in the maternal organism is too short-lived to reach the fetus, and, accordingly, that the enzymic activation process must take place in the fetus itself, which is not possible at this stage of development. On the other hand, the positive results observed after treatment at the last day before birth indicate that the relevant enzyme system begins to be operative only then, which is consistent with the biochemical evidence, as reported by Parke and Williams (*87*). In newborn rats, all dialkylnitrosamines tested proved to be carcinogenic, exerting their respective organotropic effects (*18*). The assumption that hydroxylation is the decisive step in activation is strongly supported by observations of

Spatz and Laqueur (*101*), according to which the hydroxylated methylazoxymethanol is carcinogenic to rat fetus already at early stages of development,
whereas AOM, an isomer of DMN, is not (*18*). Surprisingly, hydrazo-, azo-,
and azoxyethane, in contrast to DEN and to AOM, proved to be highly
carcinogenic in extensive transplacental experiments of Druckrey *et al.* (*23*).
From this it follows conclusively that the hydroxylases involved in the
activation of the respective compounds are not only substrate specific, but also
occur at different stages of fetal development. The most striking differences
have been demonstrated between methyl and ethyl derivatives by Druckrey (*18*).

All substances that were carcinogenic to the fetus by application before the
20th day of gestation produced exclusively neurogenic tumors of the brain and
nervous system. The complete absence of cancer in any other organs suggests
that the capability of malignant transformation presupposes a certain degree of
differentiation. In order to test the susceptibility without interference of enzymic
processes, the use of acylalkylnitrosamides is advantageous, provided that they
are sufficiently stable to reach the fetal organs. ENU proved to be the most suitable substance. After administration of one single dose of 80 mg/kg to pregnant
rats on the 15th day of gestation, all offspring developed malignant and mostly
multiple tumors of the brain, spinal cord, trigeminal nerves, and peripheric nervous system (*24*), as first reported by Ivankovic *et al.* (*59*) and Druckrey *et al.*
(*32*).

The surprisingly high transplacental carcinogenicity of ENU stimulated
systematic quantitative studies of single doses administered intravenously to BD-
IX rats on the 15th day of gestation. Again, a great number (292) of neurogenic
tumors in the offspring were observed by Ivankovic and Druckrey (*58*). The
yield clearly corresponded to dose. With 50 mg/kg the median value was 95%,
as confirmed by Druckrey and Landschütz (*27*), Koestner *et al.* (*66*), Jänisch *et
al.* (*61*), and many other authors. Twenty mg/kg yielded 90%, and 5 mg/kg
(2% LD_{50}) still 63%. Plotting the dose-response relations on log-probit coordinates, a linear "normal distribution" was obtained. The medium carcinogenic
dose is about 3 mg/kg. In adult rats, it proved to be 180 mg/kg. Accordingly, the
fetal brain and nervous system at the 15th day is about 60 times more sensitive
than that of adults (*32, 58*).

Like the tumor yield, the length of the median "latent period" (*t*) revealed
a clear dependency on the dose (*d*). If the calculated data are represented in a
double logarithmic network (Fig. 5), a straight linear function resulted with a
slope of 74.5°, and the tangent is $n=3.6$ (*58*). Accordingly, Eq. 2 is also valid in
transplacental carcinogenesis at a single dose. This was confirmed with high accuracy by Swenberg *et al.* (*108*) in analogous experiments on Sprague-Dawley
rats. However, the published value of $n=2.53$ is not correct. By graphic repre-
sentation of the individual data on log-log coordinates, the angle of the slope
was 74°, almost identical to that observed by Ivankovic and Druckrey (*58*).
Therefore, the results of both studies were combined in Fig. 5.

The sensitivity of the fetal brain and nervous system to ENU was then
tested on BD-IX rats during all stages of prenatal and neonatal development
(*38, 58*). Administration before the 12th day of gestation, even at the high dose

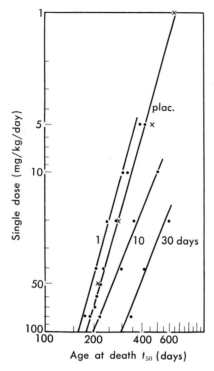

FIG. 5.   Linear dependency of the median latent periods (t_{50}) until death from neurogenic tumors after a single dose of ENU to rats in transplacental experiments, and after administration at the ages of 1, 10, and 30 days
● results of Ivankovic and Druckrey (58) and of Druckrey et al. (38); ✕ data reported by Swenberg et al. (108) in transplacental experiments.

of 60 mg/kg, did not induce any tumors in an offspring of 66 rats. This completely negative result, likewise observed with other potent carcinogens (18, 23), leads to the conclusion that the capability of malignant transformation presupposes a certain stage of differentiation, which occurs later. With the 13th day, the tumor yield increased considerably, and the maximum was reached by treatment on the 18th day. Then it remained constant during the perinatal period.

The sensitivity of BD-IX rats after birth at the ages of 1, 10, and 30 days was tested in quantitative experiments by Druckrey et al. (38). ENU was administered as a single s.c. injection at doses ranging from 5 to 80 mg/kg. On the whole, 242 out of 296 treated rats later died with malignant neurogenic tumors. The sensitivity, judged by the tumor yield and the length of the latent period at comparable doses, was highest in newborn rats. One s.c. injection of 10 mg/kg proved to be the most simple method to produce neurogenic tumors in almost all treated rats, as confirmed by Searle et al. (99) with other strains of rats. At the ages of 10 and 30 days, the equieffective doses were 40 and 80 mg/kg, respectively, and an increasing proportion of extraneural tumors, particularly of nephroblastomas and carcinomas of the female genital tract, was observed.

The median latent periods (t) dependent on doses (d) in all three age groups are represented in Fig. 5. The linearity of the relations is clearly recognizable, confirming the general validity of Eq. 2 also in postnatal carcinogenesis. However, there is a significant shift of the straight lines to longer latent periods with increasing age at treatment, and the values of n decrease from 3.6 to 2.5, demonstrating the steep decrease of susceptibility.

As recognizable in Fig. 5, most rats died from neurogenic tumors within the range of 200 to 400 days, but at low doses, and particularly after treatment at the 30th day, death occurred only at a high age of about 600 days. Corresponding results were obtained in the neonatal induction of various other tumors (18). From this it follows that cancer, even when appearing at old age, can be caused during early life and by very limited exposure.

Conclusions, and the Concept of "Genotoxicology"

According to the results presented, the "proximate" carcinogen of all N-nitroso derivatives most probably is the corresponding alkyldiazonium or diazohydroxide. It is now generally accepted that alkylation of nucleic acids, as convincingly demonstrated by numerous examples with ^{14}C-labeled compounds, is the decisive primary effect at the molecular level responsible for malignant transformation of the affected cells. The "alkylation theory" is strongly supported by the proven carcinogenicity of "direct" alkylating agents such as β-propiolactone, 1,3-propane sultone, dialkyl sulphates, or diazoalkanes (17, 32, 97). However, no correlation can be expected between the extent of alkylation and the yield or localization of tumors, because probably only a very small proportion is really relevant to malignant transformation. Beyond that, the susceptibility of the target organ plays an important role, and that differs considerably, dependent on the stage of differentiation or functional activity (17, 18). For example, in transplacental experiments with ^{14}C-ENU, performed by Goth and Rajewsky (47), the rate of DNA N-7 ethylguanine in the fetal liver was significantly higher than in the brain, although no liver cancer has ever been observed in the offspring. Probably, alkylation of O-6 is more relevant to carcinogenesis (47, 71).

Whatever the decisive target macromolecules may be, they must be genetically active and, therefore, are most probably nucleic acids, because the carcinogenic primary effects are not only irreversible and autonomously progressive, but also transmitted to daughter cells. This conclusion, first drawn from quantitative experiments with 4-dimethylaminoazobenzene by Druckrey and Küpfmüller (25), and later with various other carcinogens (14, 17, 18), followed most convincingly from the regular induction of cancer by a single dose of very short-lived substances, particularly in transplacental experiments. In this respect, the results of pharmacological and biochemical studies are in complete agreement. Accordingly, carcinogens are "genotoxic" and may be defined as "any agent which, by virtue of its physical or chemical properties, can induce or produce heritable changes in those parts of the genetic apparatus of somatic cells, responsible for their homeostatic control and, thereby determining them to malignant transformation" (18). The active forms of almost all carcinogens have proved to be potential mutagens (70, 71). However, the correlations are confined to the primary effects at the molecular level. Carcinogenesis undoubtedly is by far more complex than mutagenesis (*18*). On the other hand, the existence of "genotoxic" substances is beyond dispute. This poses new and very serious problems in both toxicology and pathology.

The differentiation and organospecific function of every somatic cell is governed by nucleic acids, which are the carriers of the genetic code. Therefore, it must be considered probable that "genotoxic" substances may be responsible also for certain disturbances of normal development, as proven by their teratogenicity (*17*, *18*), and for some diseases of unknown etiology. This applies particularly to chronic diseases which, like cancer, become manifest only after long latent periods, then progress autonomously, and are incurable.

The most serious examples are certain disorders of the brain, the causes of which are still completely unknown. Since neuronal cells are unable to divide, the question arose whether or not "genotoxic" substances can induce mental disorders, which may be considered equivalent to "malignant transformation" (*18*). For this reason it was our endeavour to find substances that specifically induced tumors of the brain or impaired its normal development (*21*, *58*). Recently, it has been demonstrated by Kleihues *et al.* (*65*) that after intravenous injection of ^{14}C-methylnitrosourea to rats methylation of neuronal cell nuclear DNA was even more extensive than that of the DNA of the various glial nuclear fractions. It is the brain that makes man what he is. In this connection the exceedingly high vulnerability of the fetal brain and nervous system requires serious consideration.

REFERENCES

1. Akagi, G., Akagi, A., Kimura, M., and Otsuka, H. Comparison of bladder tumors induced in rats and mice with N-butyl-N-(4-hydroxybutyl)-nitrosamine. *Gann*, **64**, 331–336 (1973).
2. Alexandrov, V. A. Blastomogenic effects of dimethylnitrosamine on pregnant rats and their offspring. *Nature*, **218**, 280–281 (1968).
3. Barnes, I. M. and Magee, P. N. Some toxic properties of dimethylnitrosamine. *Brit. J. Ind. Med.*, **11**, 167–174 (1954).
4. Bertram, I. S. and Craig, A. W. Induction of bladder tumours in mice with dibutylnitrosamine. *Brit. J. Cancer*, **24**, 352–359 (1970).
5. Bertram, I. S. and Craig, A. W. Specific induction of bladder cancer in mice by butyl-(4-hydroxybutyl)-nitrosamine and the effects of hormonal modifications on the sex difference in response. *Eur. J. Cancer*, **8**, 587–594 (1972).
6. Blattmann, L. and Preussmann, R. Structure of rat urinary metabolites of carcinogenic dialkylnitrosamines. *Z. Krebsforsch.*, **79**, 3–7 (1973).
7. Blum, H. F. "Carcinogenesis by Ultraviolet Light," Princeton University Press (1959).
8. Boivin, I. L. and Boivin, P. A. Preparation of N-substituted ureas from nitrosomethylurea. *Can. J. Chem.*, **29**, 478–481 (1951).
9. Brodie, B. B., Gilette, I. R., and Ladu, B. N. Enzymatic metabolism of drugs and other foreign compounds. *Annu. Rev. Biochem.*, **27**, 427–454 (1958).
10. Brune, H. and Henning, S. Experimental investigations in mice on the carcinogenic action of several nitrosamines which have been mentioned as possible ingredients

of tobacco smoke. *In* "Chemical Tumor Problems," ed. by W. Nakahara, Japan. Soc. Promot. Sci., pp. 129–138 (1970).

11. Clapp, N. K. and Craig, A. W. Carcinogenic effects of diethylnitrosamine in RF mice. *J. Natl. Cancer Inst.*, **39**, 903–916 (1967).

12. Craddock, V. M. The effect of N'-nitro-N-nitroso-N-methylguanidine on the liver after oral administration to the rat. *Experientia*, **24**, 1148–1149 (1968).

13. Dontenwill, W., Mohr, U., and Zagel, M. Die organotrope Wirkung der Nitrosamine. *Z. Krebsforsch.*, **65**, 166–167 (1962).

14. Druckrey, H. Quantitative aspects in chemical carcinogenesis. *UICC Monogr.*, **7**, 60–77 (1967).

15. Druckrey, H. Genotypes and phenotypes of ten inbred strains of BD-rats. *Arznei-mittel-Forschung*, **21**, 1274–1278 (1971).

16. Druckrey, H. Organospecific carcinogenesis in the digestive tract. *In* "Topics in Chemical Carcinogenesis," ed. by W. Nakahara, S. Takayama, T. Sugimura, and S. Odashima, University of Tokyo Press, Tokyo, pp. 73–120 (1972).

17. Druckrey, H. Chemical structure and action in transplacental carcinogenesis and teratogenesis. *In* "Transplacental Carcinogenesis," IARC Publications No. 4, International Agency for Research on Cancer, Lyon, pp. 45–58 (1973).

18. Druckrey, H. Specific carcinogenic and teratogenic effects of "indirect" alkylating methyl- and ethyl-compounds and their dependency on stages of ontogenic development. *Xenobiotica*, **5**, 271–303 (1973).

19. Druckrey, H., Ivankovic, S., Bücheler, J., Preussmann, R., and Thomas, C. Erzeugung von Magen- und Pankreas-Krebs beim Meerschweinchen durch Methylnitroso-harnstoff und -urethan. *Z. Krebsforsch.*, **71**, 167–182 (1968).

20. Druckrey, H., Ivankovic, S., Mennel, H. D., and Preussmann, R. Selektive Erzeugung von Carcinomen der Nasenhöhle bei Ratten durch N,N'-Di-nitroso-piperazin, Nitrosopiperidin, Nitrosomorpholin, Methyl-allyl-, Dimethyl- und Methyl-vinyl-nitrosamin. *Z. Krebsforsch.*, **66**, 138–150 (1964).

21. Druckrey, H., Ivankovic, S., and Preussmann, R. Selektive Erzeugung maligner Tumoren im Gehirn und Rückenmark von Ratten durch N-Methyl-N-nitroso-harnstoff. *Z. Krebsforsch.*, **66**, 389–408 (1965).

22. Druckrey, H., Ivankovic, S., and Preussmann, R. Selektive Erzeugung von Carcinomen des Drüsenmagens bei Ratten durch orale Gabe von N-Methyl-N-nitroso-N'-acetylharnstoff (AcMNH). *Z. Krebsforsch.*, **75**, 23–33 (1970).

23. Druckrey, H., Ivankovic, S., Preussmann, R., Landschütz, C., Stekar, J., Brunner, U., and Schagen, B. Transplacentar induction of neurogenic malignomas by 1,2-diethyl-hydrazine, azo-, and azoxy-ethane in rats. *Experientia*, **24**, 561–562 (1968).

24. Druckrey, H., Ivankovic, S., Preussmann, R., Zülch, K. J., and Mennel, H. D. Selective induction of malignant tumors of the nervous system by resorptive carcinogens. *In* "The Experimental Biology of Brain Tumors," ed. by W. M. Kirsch, E. Grossi Paoletti, and P. Paoletti, C. C. Thomas, Springfield, pp. 85–147 (1972).

25. Druckrey, H. and Küpfmüller, K. Quantitative Analyse der Krebsentstehung. *Z. Naturforsch.*, **3b**, 254–266 (1948).

26. Druckrey, H. and Landschütz, C. Carcinome der Nase bei Ratten nach chronischer Inhalation von 0.05 ppm Methyl-butylnitrosamin. *Z. Krebsforsch.*, **75**, 221–224 (1971).

27. Druckrey, H., Landschütz, C., and Ivankovic, S. Transplacentare Erzeugung maligner Tumoren des Nervensystems. II. Aethyl-nitrosoharnstoff an 10 genetisch definierten Rattenstämmen. *Z. Krebsforsch.*, **73**, 371–386 (1970).

28. Druckrey, H., Landschütz, C., and Preussmann, R. Oesophagus-Carcinome nach

Inhalation von Methyl-butyl-nitrosamin (MBNA) an Ratten. *Z. Krebsforsch.*, **71**, 135–139 (1968).

29. Druckrey, H., Landschütz, C., Preussmann, R., and Ivankovic, S. Erzeugung von Magenkrebs und neurogenen Malignomen durch orale Gabe von Methyl-nitrosobiuret (MNB) an Ratten. *Z. Krebsforsch.*, **75**, 229–239 (1971).

30. Druckrey, H. and Preussmann, R. Zur Entstehung carcinogener Nitrosamine am Beispiel des Tabakrauchs. *Naturwissenschaften*, **49**, 498–499 (1962).

31. Druckrey, H., Preussmann, R., Afkham, J., and Blum, G. Erzeugung von Lungenkrebs durch Methylnitrosourethan bei intravenöser Gabe an Ratten. *Naturwissenschaften*, **49**, 451–452 (1962).

32. Druckrey, H., Preussmann, R., Ivankovic, S., and Schmähl, D. Organotrope carcinogene Wirkungen bei 65 verschiedenen N-Nitroso-Verbindungen an BD-Ratten. *Z. Krebsforsch.*, **69**, 103–201 (1967).

33. Druckrey, H., Preussmann, R., Ivankovic, S., Schmidt, C. H., Mennel, H. D., and Stahl, K. W. Selektive Erzeugung von Blasenkrebs an Ratten durch Dibutyl- und N-Butyl-N-butanol(4)-nitrosamin. *Z. Krebsforsch.*, **66**, 280–290 (1964).

34. Druckrey, H., Preussmann, R., Ivankovic, S., So, B. T., Schmidt, C. H., and Bücheler, J. Zur Erzeugung subcutaner Sarkome an Ratten carcinogene Wirkung von Hydrazodicarbonsäure-bis-(methylnitrosamid), N-Nitroso-N-*n*-butylharnstoff, N-Methyl-N-nitroso-nitroguanidin und N-Nitroso-imidazolidon. *Z. Krebsforsch.*, **68**, 87–102 (1966).

35. Druckrey, H., Preussmann, R., Schmähl, D., and Müller, M. Chemische Konstitution und carcinogene Wirkung bei Nitrosaminen. *Naturwissenschaften*, **48**, 134 (1961).

36. Druckrey, H., Preussmann, R., Schmähl, D., and Müller, M. Erzeugung von Magenkrebs durch Nitrosamide an Ratten. *Naturwissenschaften*, **48**, 165 (1961).

37. Druckrey, H., Preussmann, R., Schmähl, D., and Müller, M. Erzeugung von Blasenkrebs an Ratten mit N,N-Dibutylnitrosamin. *Naturwissenshaften*, **49**, 19 (1962).

38. Druckrey, H., Schagen, B., and Ivankovic, S. Erzeugung neurogener Malignome durch einmalige Gabe von Äthyl-Nitrosoharnstoff (ÄNH) an neugeborene und junge BD IX-Ratten. *Z. Krebsforsch.*, **74**, 141–161 (1970).

39. Druckrey, H., Schildbach, A., Schmähl, D., Preussmann, R., and Ivankovic, S. Quantitative Analyse der carcinogenen Wirkung von Diäthylnitrosamin. *Arzneimittel-Forschung*, **13**, 841–851 (1963).

40. Druckrey, H. and Steinhoff, D. Erzeugung von Leberkrebs an Meerschweinchen. *Naturwissenschaften*, **49**, 497–498 (1962).

41. Druckrey, H., Steinhoff, D., Preussmann, R., and Ivankovic, S. Erzeugung von Krebs durch eine einmalige Dosis von Methyl-nitroso-harnstoff und verschiedenen Dialkylnitrosaminen an Ratten. *Z. Krebsforsch.*, **66**, 1–10 (1964).

42. Dutton, A. H. and Heath, D. F. Demethylation of dimethylnitrosamine in rats and mice. *Nature*, **178**, 644 (1956).

43. Fahr, E., Kleber, R., and Boebinger, E. Die Einwirkung von UV-Strahlung und von Nitrosaminen auf Nucleinsäurebestandteile. *Angew. Chem.*, **77**, 1019–1020 (1965).

44. Garcia, H., Keefer, L., Lijinsky, W., and Wenyon, C. E. M. Carcinogenicity of nitrosothiomorpholine and 1-nitrosopiperazine in rats. *Z. Krebsforsch.*, **74**, 179–184 (1970).

45. Gilette, I. R. Metabolism of drugs and other foreign compounds by enzymatic mechanisms. *Fortschr. Arzneimittel-Forschung*, **6**, 11–75 (1963).

46. Goodall, C. M., Lijinsky, W., and Tomatis, L. Tumorigenicity of N-Nitroso-
     hexamethyleneimine. *Cancer Res.*, **28**, 1217–1222 (1968).
47. Goth, R. and Rajewsky, M. F. Ethylation of nucleic acids by ethylnitrosourea-1-^{14}C
     in the fetal and adult rat. *Cancer Res.*, **32**, 1501–1505 (1972).
48. Graffi, A., Hoffmann, F., and Schütt, M. N-Methyl-N-nitrosourea as a strong
     topical carcinogen when painted on skin of rodents. *Nature*, **214**, 611 (1967).
49. Hashimoto, Y., Suzuki, E., and Okada, M. Induction of urinary bladder tumors
     in ACI/N-rats by butyl(3-carboxypropyl)nitrosamine, a major urinary metabolite
     of butyl(4-hydroxybutyl)nitrosamine. *Gann*, **63**, 637–638 (1972).
50. Hayaishi, O. and Nozaki, M. Nature and mechanisms of oxygenases. *Science*,
     164, 389–395 (1969).
51. Herrold, K. M. Induction of olfactory neuroepithelial tumors in Syrian hamsters
     by diethylnitrosamine. *Cancer*, **17**, 114–121 (1964).
52. Herrold, K. M. Epidermoid carcinomas of esophagus and forestomach induced
     in Syrian hamsters by N-nitroso-N-methylurethane. *J. Natl. Cancer Inst.*, **37**,
     389–394 (1966).
53. Hoch-Ligeti, C., Lobl, L. T., and Arvin, J. M. Effect of nitrosamine derivatives
     on enzyme concentrations in rat organs during carcinogenesis. *Brit. J. Cancer*, **18**,
     271–284 (1964).
54. Hoffmann, F. and Graffi, A. Nasenhöhlentumoren bei Mäusen nach percutaner
     Diäthylnitrosaminapplikation. *Arch. Geschwulstforsch.*, **23**, 274–288 (1964).
55. Hünig, W., Geldern, L., and Lücke, E. O-Alkylnitroso-immonium-salze, eine
     neue Verbindungsklasse. *Angew. Chem.*, **75**, 476 (1963).
56. Ito, N., Hiasa, Y., Tamai, A., Okajima, E., and Kitamura, H. Histogenesis of
     urinary bladder tumors induced by N-butyl-N-(4-hydroxybutyl)nitrosamine in
     rats. *Gann*, **60**, 401–410 (1969).
57. Ivankovic, S. Prenatal carcinogenesis. *In* "Topics in Chemical Carcinogenesis,"
     ed. by W. Nakahara, S. Takayama, T. Sugimura, and S. Odashima, University
     of Tokyo Press, Tokyo, pp. 463–472 (1972).
57a. Ivankovic, S. and Bücheler, J. Leber- und Blasen-Carcinome beim Meersch-
     weinchen nach Di-*n*-butylnitrosamin. *Z. Krebsforsch.*, **71**, 183–185 (1968).
58. Ivankovic, W., Druckrey, H. Transplacentare Erzeugung maligner Tumoren des
     Nervensystems. I. Aethylnitroso-harnstoff an BD IX Ratten. *Z. Krebsforsch.*, **71**,
     320–360 (1968).
59. Ivankovic, S., Druckrey, H., and Preussmann, R. Erzeugung neurogener Tumoren
     bei den Nachkommen nach einmaliger Injektion von Aethylnitrosoharnstoff an
     schwangeren Ratten. *Naturwissenschaften*, **53**, 410–411 (1966).
60. Jänisch, W. and Schreiber, D. Experimentelle Hirngeschwülste bei Kaninchen
     nach Injektion von Methylnitrosoharnstoff. *Naturwissenschaften*, **54**, 171–172
     (1967).
61. Jänisch, W., Schreiber, D., Varzok, R., and Schneider, J. Die transplazentare In-
     duktion von Geschwülsten des Nervensystems. Vergleichende Untersuchungen
     der Wirksamkeit von Methyl- und Aethylnitrosoharnstoff. *Arch. Geschwulst-
     forsch.*, **39**, 99–105 (1972).
62. Keberle, H., Ries, W., Schmid, K., and Hoffmann, K. Über den Mechanismus der
     biologischen Desalkylierung. *Arch. Int. Pharmacodyn. Ther.*, **142**, 125 (1963).
63. Keefer, L. K. and Fodor, C. H. Facile hydrogen isotope exchange as evidence for
     an α-nitrosamino compound. *J. Am. Chem. Soc.*, 5747–5748 (1970).

64. Kelly, M. G., O'Gara, R. W., Adamson, R. H., Gadekar, K., Botkin, C. C., Reese, W. H., and Kerber, W. T. Induction of hepatic cell carcinomas in monkeys with N-Nitroso diethylamine. *J. Natl. Cancer Inst.*, **36**, 323–351 (1966).

65. Kleihues, P., Magee, P. N., Austoker, I, Cox, D., and Mathias, A. P. Reaction of N-methyl-N-nitrosourea with DNA of neuronal and glial cells *in vivo*. *FEBS Letters*, **32**, 105–108 (1973).

66. Koestner, A., Swenberg, I. A., and Wechsler, W. Transplacental production with ethylnitrosourea of neoplasmas of the nervous system in Sprague-Dawley rats. *Am. J. Pathol.*, **63**, 34–56 (1971).

67. Krüger, F. W. New aspects in metabolism of carcinogenic nitrosamines. *In* "Topics in Chemical Carcinogenesis," ed. by W. Nakahara, S. Takayama, T. Sugimura, and S. Odashima, University of Tokyo Press, Tokyo, pp. 213–232 (1972).

68. Lawley, P. D. and Thatcher, C. I. Methylation of deoxyribonucleic acid in cultured mammalian cells by N-methyl-N′-nitro-N-nitrosoguanidine. The influence of cellular thiol concentrations on the extent of methylation and the 6-oxygen atom of guanine as a site of methylation. *Biochem. J.*, **116**, 693–707 (1970).

69. Lijinsky, W., Loo, I., and Ross, A. E. Mechanism of alkylation of nucleic acids by nitrosodimethylamine. *Nature*, **218**, 1174–1175 (1968).

70. Lingens, F. and Oltmanns, O. Über die mutagene Wirkung von 1-Nitroso-3-nitro-1-methylguanidin auf *Saccharomyces cerevisiae*. *Z. Naturforsch.*, **21b**, 660–661 (1966).

71. Loveless, A. Possible relevance of O-6 alkylation of deoxyguanosine to the mutagenicity and carcinogenicity of nitrosamines and nitrosamides. *Nature*, **223**, 206–207 (1969).

72. Magee, P. N. *In vivo* reactions of nitroso compounds. *Ann. N.Y. Acad. Sci.*, **163**, 717–730 (1969).

73. Magee, P. N. and Barnes, I. M. The production of malignant primary hepatic tumours in the rat by feeding dimethylnitrosamine. *Brit. J. Cancer*, **10**, 114–122 (1956).

74. Magee, P. N. and Barnes, I. M. Induction of kidney tumours in the rat with dimethylnitrosamine. *J. Pathol. Bacteriol.*, **84**, 19–31 (1962).

75. Magee, P. N. and Barnes, I. M. Carcinogenic nitroso compounds. *Adv. Cancer Res.*, **10**, 164–246 (1967).

76. Magee, P. N. and Farber, E. Toxic liver injury and carcinogenesis. Methylation of rat-liver nucleic acids by dimethylnitrosamine *in vivo*. *Biochem. J.*, **83**, 114–124 (1962).

77. McMahon, R. E. Microsomal dealkylation of drugs. *J. Pharm. Sci.*, **55**, 457 (1966).

78. Montesano, R. and Saffiotti, U. Carcinogenic response of the respiratory tract of Syrian golden hamsters to different doses of diethylnitrosamine. *Cancer Res.*, **28**, 2197–2210 (1968).

79. Montgomery, I. A., James, R., McCaleb, G. S., and Johnston, T. P. The modes of decomposition of 1,3-bis (2-chloroethyl)-1-nitrosourea and related compounds. *J. Med. Chem.*, **10**, 668 (1967).

80. Nagata, C. and Imamura, A. Electronic structures and mechanism of carcinogenicity for alkylnitrosamines. *Gann*, **61**, 169–176 (1970).

81. Neunhöffer, O., Lehmann, W., and Lehmann, G. Eine enzymatische Umlagerung cancerogener Nitrosamine. *Z. Naturforsch.*, **25**, 302–307 (1970).

82. O'Connor, P. I., Capps, M. I., Craig, A. W., Lawley, P. D., and Shah, S. A.

Differences in the patterns of methylation in rat liver ribosomal ribonucleic acid after reaction *in vivo* with methylmethanesulfonate and N, N-dimethylnitrosamine. *Biochem. J.*, **129**, 519–528 (1972).

83. Odashima, S. Development of leukemia in rats by oral administration of N-nitrosobutylurea in the drinking water. *Gann*, **60**, 237 (1969).

84. Odashima, S. Leukemogenesis of N-nitrosobutylurea in the rat. I. Effect of various concentrations in the drinking water to female Donryu rats. *Gann*, **61**, 245–253 (1970).

85. Odashima, S. Leukemogenic effect of N-nitroso-N-butylurea in rats. *In* "Topics in Chemical Carcinogenesis," ed. by W. Nakahara, S. Takayama, T. Sugimura, and S. Odashima, University of Tokyo Press, Tokyo, pp. 477–489 (1972).

86. Okada, M. and Suzuki, E. Metabolism of butyl-(4-hydroxybutyl)-nitrosamine in rats. *Gann*, **63**, 391–392 (1972).

87. Parke, D. V. and Williams, R. T. Metabolism of toxic substances. *Brit. Med. Bull.*, **25**, 256–262 (1969).

88. Peller, S. "Cancer in Childhood and Youth," J. Wright & Sons, Ltd., Bristol (1960).

89. Pielsticker, K., Wieser, O., Mohr, U., and Woba, H. Diaplacentar induzierte Nierentumoren bei der Ratte. *Z. Krebsforsch.*, **69**, 345–350 (1967).

90. Preussmann, R. Zum oxydativen Abbau von Nitrosaminen mit Enzym-freien Modell-Systemen. *Arzneimittel-Forschung*, **14**, 769–774 (1964).

91. Preussmann, R., Druckrey, H., and Bücheler, J. Carcinogene Wirkung von Phenyl-nitroso-harnstoff. *Z. Krebsforsch.*, **71**, 63–65 (1968).

92. Rajewsky, M. F., Dauber, W., and Frankenberg, H. Liver carcinogenesis by di-ethylnitrosamine in the rat. *Science*, **152**, 83 (1966).

93. Sasaki, T. and Yoshida, T. Experimentelle Erzeugung des Lebercarcinoms durch Fütterung mit *o*-Amidoazotoluol. *Arch. Pathol. Anat. Physiol.*, **295**, 175 (1935).

94. Schmähl, D., Preussmann, R., and Hamperl, H. Leberkrebs erzeugende Wirkung von Diaethylnitrosamin nach oraler Gabe an Ratten. *Naturwissenschaften*,**47**, 89 (1960).

95. Schoental, R. Lack of correlation between the presence of 7-methylguanine in DNA and RNA of organs and the localisation of tumours after a single carcinogenic dose of N-methyl-N-nitrosourethane. *Biochem. J.*, **114**, 55 (1969).

96. Schoental, R. The mechanism of action of the carcinogenic nitroso and related compounds. *Brit J. Cancer*, **28**, 436–439 (1973).

97. Schoental, R. and Magee, P. N. Induction of squamous carcinoma of the lung and of stomach and oesophagus by diazomethane and N-methyl-N-nitroso-urethane, respectively. *Brit. J. Cancer*, **16**, 92–100 (1962).

98. Schoental, R. and Rive, D. J. Interaction of N-alkyl-N-nitrosourethanes with thiols. *Biochem. J.*, **97**, 466–474 (1965).

99. Searle, C. E., Jones, E. L., and Smith, W. T. Induction of brain tumours in high yield by administration of N-ethyl-N-nitrosourea to newborn rats. *Experientia*, **28** 1452–1453 (1972).

100. Seebach, D. and Enders, D. C-C Verknüpfungen in α-Stellung zum Stickstoff sekundärer Amine. Lithium-dimethylnitrosamin. *Angew. Chem.*, **84**, 350–351 (1972).

101. Spatz, M. and Laqueur, G. L. Transplacental induction of tumours in Sprague-Dawley rats with crude cycad material. *J. Natl. Cancer Inst.*, **38**, 233–245 (1967).

102. Stroobandt, G. and Brucher, J. M. Study of nervous system tumours obtained by methylnitrosourea administration in rats. *Neurochirurgie*, **14**, 515–535 (1968).

103. Sugimura, T. and Fujimura, S. Tumor production in glandular stomach of rat by N-methyl-N-nitro-N-nitrosoguanidine. *Nature*, **216**, 943–944 (1967).

104. Sugimura, T., Fujimura, S., Nagao, M., Yokoshima, T., and Hasegawa, M. Reaction of N-methyl-N-nitro-N-nitrosoguanidine with protein. *Biochim. Biophys. Acta*, **170**, 427–429 (1968).

105. Sugimura, T., Nagao, M., and Okada, Y. Carcinogenic action of N-methyl-N'-nitro-N-nitrosoguanidine. *Nature*, **210**, 962 (1966).

106. Sugimura, T., Tanaka, N., Kawachi, T., Kogure, K., Fujimura, S., and Shimosato, Y. Production of stomach cancer in dogs by N-methyl-N'-nitro-N-nitrosoguanidine. *Gann*, **62**, 67–68 (1971).

107. Swann, P. F. and Magee, P. N. Nitrosoamine induced carcinogenesis. The alkylation of N-7 guanine of nucleic acids of the rat by diethylnitrosamine, ethylnitrosourea and ethyl-methanesulfonate. *Biochem. J.*, **125**, 841–847 (1971).

108. Swenberg, I. A., Koestner, A., Wechsler, W., and Denlinger, R. H. Quantitative aspects of transplacental tumor induction with ethylnitrosourea in rats. *Cancer Res.*, **32**, 2656–2660 (1972).

109. Takayama, S. and Oota, K. Malignant tumours induced in mice fed with N-nitrosodimethylamine. *Gann*, **54**, 465–472 (1963).

110. Takayama, S. Induction of tumours in ICR mice with N-nitrosopiperidine, especially in forestomach. *Naturwissenschaften*, **56**, 142 (1969).

111. Takizawa, S. and Nishihara, H. Induction of tumors in the brain, kidney, and other extra-mammary gland organs by a continuous oral administration of N-nitrosobutylurea in Wistar/Furth rats. *Gann*, **62**, 495–503 (1971).

112. Thomas, C. and Bollmann, R. Untersuchungen zur diaplacentaren krebserzeugenden Wirkung des Diäthylnitrosamins an Ratten. *Z. Krebsforsch.*, **71**, 129–134 (1968).

113. Thomas, C. and Schmähl, D. Vergleichende morphologische und toxikologische Untersuchungen an Maus, Ratte, Meerschweinchen, Kaninchen und Hund zur Prüfung der cancerogenen Wirkung und Organotropie des Diaethylnitrosamins. *Arch. Pathol. Anat. Physiol.*, **340**, 122 (1965).

114. Thomas, C., Sierra, I. L., and Kersting, G. Hirntumoren bei Ratten nach oraler Gabe von N-nitroso-N-methyl-harnstoff. *Naturwissenschaften*, **54**, 228 (1967).

115. Tomatis, L., Magee, P. N., and Shubik, P. Induction of liver tumors in the Syrian hamster by feeding Dimethylnitrosamine. *J. Natl. Cancer Inst.*, **33**, 341–345 (1964).

116. Udenfriend, S., Clark, C. T., Axelrod, J., and Brodie, B. B. Ascorbic acid in aromatic hydroxylation. I. A model system for aromatic hydroxylations. *J. Biol. Chem.*, **208**, 731 (1954).

117. Ullrich, V., Hey, D., Staudinger, H. J., Büch, H., and Rummel, W. Untersuchungenzum Mechanismus der Hydroxylierung und der oxydativen O-Desalkylierung von Phenacetin an Modellsystemen. *Biochem. Pharmacol.*, **16**, 2237 (1967).

118. Warburg, O. "Der Stoffwechsel der Tumoren," Springer Verlag, Berlin, pp. 68–88 (1926).

119. Warzok, R., Schneider, J., Schreiber, D., and Jänisch, W. Experimental brain tumours in dogs. *Experientia*, **26**, 303–304 (1970).

120. Wheeler, G. P. and Bowdon, B. J. Comparison of the effects of cysteine upon the decomposition of nitrosoureas and of 1-methyl-3-nitro-1-nitrosoguanidine. *Biochem. Pharmacol.*, **21**, 265–267 (1972).

121. Wood, M., Flaks, A., and Clayson, D. B. The carcinogenic activity of dibutylnitrosamine in IF×C57 mice. *Eur. J. Cancer*, **6**, 433–440 (1970).

122. Wunderlich, V., Schütt, M., Böttger, M., and Graffi, A. Preferential alkylation of mitochondrial deoxyribonucleic acid by N-methyl-N-nitrosourea. *Biochem. J.*, **118**, 99–109 (1970).

123. Yoshida, T. Histopathologische Untersuchungen mit Amidoazotoluol (*o*-Toluol-azo-*o*-Toluidin). II. Weiteres über die Epithelmetaplasie der Schilddrüse des Meerschweinchens und Fütterungsversuch an Ratten. *Nippon Byōri Gakkai Kaishi (Trans. Japan. Pathol. Soc.)*, **22**, 934–946 (1932).

124. Yoshida, T. Über experimentelle Erzeugung der Geschwulst durch subkutane Injektion von Ölivenöllösung des *o*-Amidotoluols. *Gann*, **28**, 454–457 (1935).

GANN Monograph on Cancer Research 17, 133–143 (1975)

SOME RECENT RESULTS ON THE CHEMISTRY, FORMATION, AND BIOLOGICAL ACTIVITY OF N-NITROSO COMPOUNDS

G. Eisenbrand, S. Ivankovic, R. Preussmann,
D. Schmähl, and M. Wiessler

*German Cancer Research Center, Institute of Toxicology and Chemotherapy**

Recent work performed at the Institute of Toxicology and Chemotherapy of the German Cancer Research Center on various aspects of N-nitroso compounds is reported. The successful synthesis of α-substituted derivatives of nitrosamines opens new possibilities to investigate such compounds, which might be proximate carcinogens. The nitrosation of certain pesticides could be demonstrated by reaction with nitrite; the investigated N-nitrosopesticides are potent mutagens and carcinogens. A summary of transplacental carcinogenic effects of N-nitroso compounds stresses the possible importance of such effects in view of the possible human risk. Finally, testing of diethylnitrosamine in more than 10 animal species including subhuman primates has demonstrated the potent carcinogenicity of this and similar compounds, and the probability of a similar effect in man is discussed.

Synthesis of α-Substituted N-Nitrosamines

Soon after the discovery of the carcinogenic effect of dimethylnitrosamine (DMN) by Magee and Barnes in 1956 (*20*), Dutton and Heath (*2*) suggested that the nitrosamine itself was not the ultimate carcinogen, but that its effect depended on an enzymic activation by drug-metabolizing enzymes of the liver. These findings induced Druckrey *et al.* (*1*) to postulate the "Diazoalkantheorie." In this reaction the enzymically formed α-hydroxylated nitrosamines break down to give an aldehyde and diazohydroxide. The latter substance or the products of its breakdown constitute the ultimate carcinogen. The synthesis of α-hydroxynitrosamines was started only some years ago, due to the fact that they are probably quite unstable. Our attention was therefore given to the synthesis of derivatives that yielded α-hydroxylated nitrosamines under *in vivo* conditions.

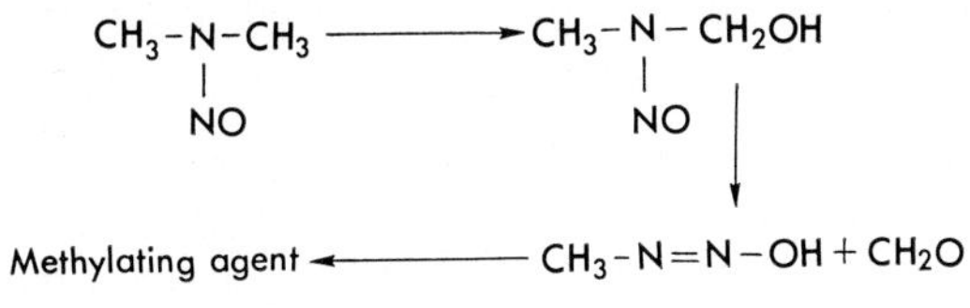

$$CH_3-N-CH_3 \longrightarrow CH_3-N-CH_2OH$$

Methylating agent $\longleftarrow CH_3-N=N-OH + CH_2O$

CHART 1.

* D-69 Heidelberg, West Germany.

The first compound to be synthesized by nitrosation of the easily accessible free base was N-nitrosotetrahydro-1,3-oxazine (I). In the same way N-nitroso-oxazolidine (II) was synthesized. Chemically these compounds can be classified as cyclic ethers of α-hydroxynitrosamines. Both compounds are being tested for their potential carcinogenic activity in rats. In the case of compound I the first tumors have been observed in a long-term feeding study.

A procedure published by Eiter (5) for the synthesis of open-chain ethers of α-hydroxylated nitrosamines (e.g., III) could be extended by us to the synthesis of branched ethers (e.g., IV and V). In that way, α-substituted derivatives of diethylnitrosamine (DEN) can be obtained. It seems likely that long-chain and cyclic α-methoxynitrosamines can also be obtained in this way.

$$CH_3-N-CH_2-OCH_3$$
$$NO$$

(I)   (II)   (III)

$$CH_3-N-\overset{\overset{\displaystyle CH_3}{|}}{CH}-OCH_3 \qquad C_2H_5-N-\overset{\overset{\displaystyle CH_3}{|}}{CH}-OCH_3 \qquad CH_3-N-CH_2Cl$$
$$NO \qquad\qquad NO \qquad\qquad NO$$

(IV)   (V)   (VI)

α-Methoxydimethylnitrosamine (III) furnishes a very good starting material to introduce other functional groups into the α position. The controlled action of acetyl chloride resulted in the synthesis of the labile α-chlorodimethylnitrosamine (VI) by cleavage of the ether linkage. The introduction of the ester function to form α-acetoxydimethylnitrosamine (VII) is accomplished by the action of sodium- or silver-acetate. The corresponding benzoate tends to hydrolyze rapidly, so that a pure product could not yet be obtained. The α-chloro compound (VI) reacts spontaneously with water under evolution of nitrogen, α-hydroxydimethylnitrosamine being probably an intermediate. The synthesis of biologically relevant compounds like α-phosphate, α-sulfate, and α-glucuronide of a nitrosamine seems to be possible in this way.

Another question with which we are concerned is the organo-specificity of the carcinogenic action of nitrosamines. The mode of alkyl substitution is responsible for the induction of liver, esophagus, or bladder cancer (1). The specificity of the metabolizing enzymes might be tested using optically active nitrosamine, for example, N-nitroso-2-methylpiperidine (VIII). The evolution of carcinogenicity experiments showed subtle but not significant differences in the tumor localization.

$$CH_3-N-CH_2-O-COCH_3$$
$$NO$$

(VII)   (VIII)

Testing of N-nitrosotetrahydro-1,2-oxazine (IX) for carcinogenic activity in animal experiments indicated that probably some other mechanisms for the activation of nitrosamines exist besides the proposed alkylation theory. This compound (IX) was found to be a carcinogen without a pronounced organotropy. Enzymic activation in analogy to Chart 1 cannot liberate diazohydroxide, but only a monoester of hyponitrous acid, which might be the ultimate carcinogen. Possibly there might also be a de- or trans-nitrosation as suggested by Sugimura (30). To determine the carcinogenic action of this class of compounds we have synthesized the analogous compounds, X and XI, which are now being investigated in animal experiments for carcinogenicity. The dimethyl derivative (XII) has been tested by Druckrey et al. (1) and found to be noncarcinogenic.

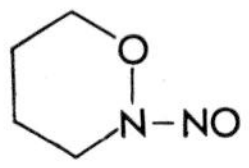

$$C_2H_5-N-OC_2H_5$$
$$|$$
$$NO$$

(IX) 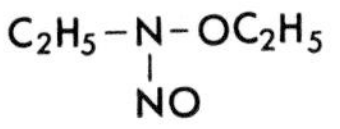   (X)

$$CH_3-N-OCH_3$$
$$|$$
$$NO$$

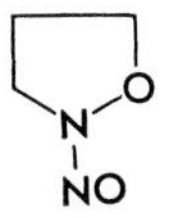

(XI) 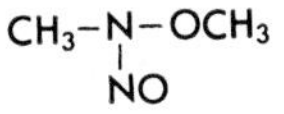   (XII)

Formation of N-Nitroso Compounds from Environmental Chemicals and Nitrite

The role of N-nitroso compounds as one of the most important groups of potential carcinogens in the human environment today is fully recognized. Their presence at low concentrations in various environmental materials, such as foods and tobacco smoke, has been demonstrated by several research groups. The findings that these compounds can also be formed in the alimentary tract from nitrite and nitrosatable substances has caused a great deal of concern. Substances that have been shown to be a potential source for N-nitroso compounds comprise secondary and tertiary amines, including some widely used drugs, alkylureas, amino acids, and some types of agricultural chemicals (4, 6, 7, 18, 19, 21, 22, 24).

The results of our studies on the nitrosation of several pesticides that are potential precursors for the formation of N-nitroso compounds are summarized below.

In a first qualitative experiment some fungicides derived from dithiocarbamic acid were examined. Among bis(dimethyldithiocarbamato)zinc (Ziram), tris(dimethyldithiocarbamato)iron (Ferbam), and dipyrrolidylthiuram disulfide (DPTD), the former two were found to produce DMN and the latter, N-nitrosopyrrolidine, under *in vitro* conditions simulating those in the stomach.

The nitrosation kinetics have been studied in more detail with Ziram as one of the most widely used representatives of this class of compounds (3). The optimum pH for the formation of DMN from Ziram after a 10-min incubation was 1.5–2.0. The acid-catalyzed decomposition of the dithiocarbamate was found to be the rate-limiting process. Dialkyldithiocarbamates are known to decompose under acid conditions into the corresponding dialkylamines (9). However, since substantial amounts of DMN were formed also in strongly acid medium at pH 1, it is not very likely that the nitrosation proceeds via the liberation of dimethylamine. Under the conditions used, the strong base dimethyl-amine (pK_B=3.28) is nitrosated only to a very low extent (21). The reactive intermediate might therefore rather be the unstable free dimethyldithiocarbamic acid. The nitrosamine formation was found to proceed very rapidly; at pH 2.0 the reaction was already complete after 10 min. In 10^{-3} M, 14% of the theoretical yield of DMN was formed after 10-min incubation at pH 2 with 0.1 M nitrite, assuming that two molecules of the carcinogen were formed from one molecule of Ziram. After in vivo reaction of 10^{-4} M Ziram for 15 min in the rat stomach with a 40-fold excess of nitrite, the average yield of DMN in four rats was 126 μg, which corresponds to about 0.9% of the theoretical value.

Further nitrosation studies were carried out with a wider range of different agricultural chemicals at low concentrations (4). The insecticides Carbaryl (1-naphtyl-N-methylcarbamate) and Propoxur (2-isopropoxyphenyl-N-methyl-carbamate), and the herbicides Benzthiazuron (N-(2-benzothiazolyl)-N-methyl-urea), Simazin (2-chloro-4,6-bisethylamino-1,3,5-triazine), and Atrazin (2-chloro-4-ethylamino-6-isopropylamino-1,3,5-triazine) were examined in vitro. The pesticides were nitrosated in concentrations of 10^{-3} and 10^{-4} M, respectively, with a 5-fold molar ratio of nitrite at 37° and pH 1.

All pesticides were found to form N-nitroso products under these conditions. In 10^{-3} M solutions, the yields of N-nitroso compounds after only 15 min of incubation were about 5–6%, with the exception of Carbaryl, which under these conditions was nitrosated only to about 1%. At a 10-fold lower concentration of both the pesticide (20–22 ppm) and nitrite (23 ppm) the yields after 15 min were about 0.3–2.4% of theory.

Under the described conditions, the triazine herbicides formed the mono-nitroso compounds almost exclusively. The respective N-nitroso pesticides were synthesized, and some of them were examined for their biological effects. First evidence for strong biological activity was obtained when N-nitroso-benz-thiazuron, N-nitroso-propoxur, and N-nitroso-carbaryl were examined for their biological effects on yeast cells, using the mitotic gene conversion test system developed by Zimmermann and Schwaier (32). All three substances showed considerable genetic activity, N-nitroso-carbaryl displaying by far the strongest effects (29). This compound can be considered to be one of the strongest known genetically active agents.

N-Nitroso-benzthiazuron was found to be a potent carcinogen in rats. Given orally in single doses of 400–800 mg/kg, it induced mainly carcinomas of the kidney. Repeated oral doses of 50 mg/kg twice a week induced a 100% incidence of squamous cell carcinomas in the forestomach; 25 mg/kg twice a week induced also squamous cell carcinomas in 80% of treated animals, the remaining rats had multiple papillomas of the forestomach. Other malignant tumors were found in the liver, kidney, mediastinum, and uterus. All animals died from tumors (*31*).

The above results show that pesticides with structures that are susceptible to N-nitrosation can be nitrosated at relatively low concentration directly in the stomach or under conditions simulating those in the stomach. The resulting N-nitroso compounds are, as far as they are biologically examined, highly active compounds displaying strong genetic and carcinogenic effects. This suggests a hitherto disregarded aspect to be taken into consideration when establishing tolerance levels for pesticide residues: the possibility that pesticides may undergo N-nitrosation in the human intestinal tract to yield potent carcinogens and mutagens.

Experimental Prenatal Induction of Cancer by N-Nitroso Compounds

Cancer as a biological phenomenon must be considered a result of many

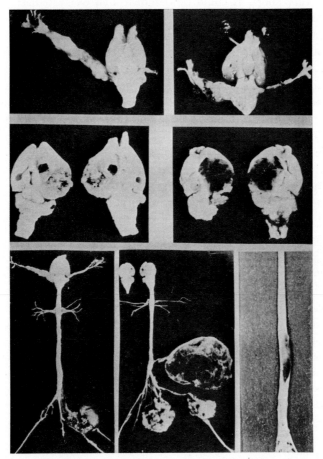

PHOTO 1. Induction of malignant neurogenic tumors in (a) nervous trigeminus, (b) and (c) brain, (d) and (e) peripheral nerves, and (f) spinal cord
Tumors in the offspring of mothers of BD-IX rats, who had been treated with a single dose of 60 mg/kg ethylnitrosourea on the 15th day *post coitus* (p.c.).

different causative factors. Therefore, the etiology of this disease is extremely complicated and at the present moment many aspects are still unknown. Cancer in childhood presents special problems. It is well known that in children up to the age of 15, cancer as a cause of death is second in frequency directly after death by accidents in most industrialized countries.

Since it is known that cancer caused by chemical carcinogens in man has a long latency period, it is probable that the cause of cancer in children can be found in prenatal exposure to carcinogens. Furthermore, an increased sensitivity to carcinogenic stimuli is to be expected in the fetus and embryo. These hypotheses have been presented on several occassions and could be proven in animal experiments (10–13, 14, 16). Model experiments were performed with N-ethyl-N-nitrosourea (ENU). It could be shown that a single treatment of pregnant animals in the second half of pregnancy resulted in a high yield of malignant tumors in the progeny. The predominant tumor localization was the brain and nervous system (Photo 1), and the latency period for tumor induction in the offspring was very short. It could be demonstrated by systematic experimentation that the method of administration of the carcinogen does not influence the result. The rat (BD, Wistar, and Sprague-Dawley strains) was used mainly, but also other rodents. The results obtained with N-nitroso compounds are summarized in Table I.

The main tumor localization in experimental prenatal carcinogens with nitrosoureas is in the nervous system, as can be seen in Table I. The preferential induction of neurogenic tumors by these and other chemical carcinogens, active in prenatal tumor induction (13) indicates a high sensitivity towards carcinogenesis of neurogenic tissue during prenatal development.

DEN is the only carcinogen in the group of N-nitroso compounds so far tested that does not induce neurogenic tumors. Only tumors of the liver and the

TABLE I. Prenatal Induction of Malignant Tumors in the Progeny of Rats by N-Nitroso Compounds (15)

Compound	Active beginning from the day p.c.	Degree of carcinogenicity by prenatal exposure	Main tumor localization
1) Nitrosamides			
Methylnitrosourea	12	+	Nervous system
Ethylnitrosourea	12	⧻	Nervous system
Propylnitrosourea	12	⧻	Nervous system
Butylnitrosourea	12	+	Nervous system
Pentylnitrosourea	—	—	—
Benzylnitrosourea	—	—	—
2) Nitrosamines			
Dimethylnitrosamine	—	—	—
Diethylnitrosamine	22	⧺	Liver, kidney
Methylbutylnitrosamine	22	+	Bulbus olfactorius
Ethylvinylnitrosamine	22	⧺	Forestomach, nervous system

+ weakly active; ⧺ clearly active; ⧻ very active.

kidney were induced with this compound; it is also remarkable that DEN is only active when given at the end of pregnancy (22nd day of gestation). A similar effect is observed with other nitrosamines, such as N-methyl-N-butyl- and N-ethyl-N-vinylnitrosamine (Table I). Another interesting fact is that remarkable differences exist with different alkyl-substituted nitrosoureas (Table I): a maximum of transplacental carcinogenic effectiveness has been found with N-ethyl- and N-propyl-N-nitrosourea. The corresponding methyl and butyl derivatives only showed weak activity under the same experimental conditions, and the N-pentyl- and N-benzyl-N-nitrosoureas were absolutely ineffective, even when given during the most sensitive periods of prenatal development.

Therefore, prenatal effects of nitrosoureas are mainly governed by reaction of the carcinogen with embryonic or fetal tissue and by the stage of development of the target tissue. Nitrosamines like DEN, on the other hand, are typical indirect carcinogens requiring enzymic activation by hydroxylating mixed-function oxidases. In such cases the presence of such activating enzyme systems might be a prerequisite for carcinogenic activity in transplacental carcinogenesis. The fact that DEN, for example, is only active in the late stages of fetal development (see Table I) indicates that activating enzymes are not present in earlier stages.

Recent results, however, have indicated that human fetal tissue in very early stages of development already has enzymic activity to dealkylate DMN *in vitro* (*17*). This is in contrast to the situation found in the rat, and it indicates a risk for man also in the first week of fetal development by such compounds.

The possible importance of prenatal carcinogenesis in man has recently been demonstrated by Herbst *et al.* (*8*). Adenosarcomas of the vagina were reported in young girls whose mothers had been treated with diethylstilbestrol during the first three months of pregnancy. Such vaginal tumors are very rare, especially among young girls, and therefore it seems very likely to discuss their origin in connection with the transplacental effects of diethylstilbestrol treatment.

Nitroso Compounds as Carcinogens in Man

The widespread presence of nitroso compounds in our environment and the fact that these compounds are taken with food as well as formed in the stomach from precursors require special attention to potential carcinogenic hazards in man. Because of the lack of epidemiological data, conclusions must be drawn from animal experiments. In our group an attempt was made to elucidate this question by (1) comparative testing of nitroso compounds in as many animal species as possible and (2) investigation of syncarcinogenic effects of various nitrosamines.

We were able to establish the hepatocarcinogenic effect of DEN in many species, such as mouse, rat, guinea pig, rabbit, dog, pig, and parakeet (*25*); its liver carcinogenic effect could also be proved in hedgehogs (Graw and Berg, unpublished). Other investigators reported carcinogenic effects of DEN (and also DMN) in the hamster, mink, monkey, duck, trout, *Brachydanio rerio*, and guppy. In these species mainly liver tumors were seen, with the exception of the hamster, which predominantly reacted with tumors of the respiratory system and less frequently developed tumors of the liver. The effective single and total doses of these carcinogens were in the same order of magnitude (25). In rats, guinea pigs, and rabbits mainly liver malignomas of epithelial origin occurred, but in other species tumors of the mesenchyma (hemangioendotheliomas in mouse) or of the fibrous tissue (sarcomas in dog) were predominant.

Simply built nitrosamines have been extensively studied regarding their carcinogenicity in various animal species. In not fewer than 15 species the carcinogenic potency of these compounds could be proved. Fish, birds, and mammalians reacted in the same manner, so that it may be permissible to assume that man in this respect is no exception. This suggestion is supported by the findings of Montesano and Magee who were able to demonstrate *in vitro* that the metabolism of DEN is virtually the same in rat and man.

The organotropy of the carcinogenic effect of these compounds obviously depends not only on its chemical structure, but also on the applied single dose and the animal species used. This can be demonstrated by some examples.

If DEN is given to rats in a single dose of 200 mg/kg (70% of the LD_{50}) the surviving animals develop carcinomas of the kidney in a high percentage. Chronic oral application of 3 mg/kg/day of this substance (1% of the LD_{50}) results in liver tumors exclusively. If the daily dose is reduced to 0.5 mg/kg (0.15% of the LD_{50}) in 60% liver tumors and in 40% tumors of the esophagus are produced. The latter tumors do not occur if a higher dose is applied (25). In these cases the organotropy is also influenced by the applied dose.

DEN leads predominantly to liver tumors in various species, but other nitrosamines may have different effects. We observed (27) that ethylbutylnitrosamine, which in rats selectively induces esophagus cancer, in mice caused tumors of the stomach; N,N'-dinitrosopiperazine in rats produces carcinomas of the paranasal sinus, but in mice induces malignomas of the liver and lung (28). This shows that also in closely related species, such as the rat and mouse, the organotropy of the carcinogenic effect must not be the same. It is, therefore, extremely difficult to associate a certain organotropy with a certain substance, if both dosage and species play a decisive role. The complexity that arises is obvious if we are concerned with the explanation of certain organotropic effects and their assignment to human conditions. It seems certain that man is susceptible to the carcinogenic effects of nitroso compounds. The organotropy of these effects, however, is not foreseeable.

Nitroso compounds are probably taken daily or formed in the body of man. The quantities are very small and may lie within the ppb or at most ppm range. It was, therefore, interesting to investigate whether minute dosages of nitrosamines are able to produce tumors. For this purpose rats were given simultaneously four liver carcinogens, namely DMN, DEN, 4-dimethylaminoazobenzene, and nitroso morpholine. The applied doses of these substances were not effective when given alone (26). By addition of the carcinogenic effects of these compounds liver tumors were expected after 600 days. After 700 ± 110 days in 34% (29/86) of the rats malignant tumors occurred, 10% of the animals developed benign tumors of the liver (adenomas). Twelve rats (14%) died from extrahepatic malignomas. The total yield of malignant carcinomas amounted to 44% (41/86). In the control series only 3 of 100 animals showed malignant tumors.

These results show evidently that the effects of minute carcinogenic doses can sum up if the organotropy of the carcinogenic effect is the same. We have, therefore, reason to believe that even minimum doses of nitrosamines suffice to cause cancer in man. This is supported by the finding that in rats even a single intravenous injection of 1 mg/kg of DEN is sufficient to induce malignant tumors of the kidney (23).

In conclusion, from the present results and reflections it appears likely that nitroso compounds are carcinogens to man even when taken in minimum dosages. The elimination of these compounds from the environment and the prevention of their formation in the human body would be an important step towards an effective cancer prophylaxis.

REFERENCES

1. Druckrey, H., Preussmann, R., Schmähl, D., and Ivankovic, S. Organotrope carcinogene Wirkungen bei 65 verschiedenen N-Nitroso-Verbindungen an BD-Ratten. *Z. Krebsforsch.*, **69**, 103–201 (1967).

2. Dutton, A. H. and Heath, D. F. Demethylation of dimethylnitrosamine in rats and mice. *Nature*, **178**, 644–645 (1956).

3. Eisenbrand, G., Ungerer, O., and Preussman, R. Rapid formation of carcinogenic N-nitrosamines by interaction of nitrite with fungicides derived from dithiocarbamic acid *in vitro* under simulated stomach conditions and *in vivo* in the rat stomach. *Food Cosmet. Toxicol.*, **12**, 229–232 (1974).

4. Eisenbrand, G., Ungerer, O., and Preussmann, R. Formation of N-nitroso compounds from agricultural chemicals and nitrite. *In* "N-Nitroso Compounds in the Environment" IARC Scientific Publications No. 9, International Agency for Research on Cancer, Lyon (1974).

5. Eiter, K., Hebenbrock, K. F., and Kabbe, H. J. Neue offenkettige und cyclische α-Nitrosaminalkyläther. *Ann. Chem.*, **765**, 55–77 (1972).

6. Elespuru, R. K. and Lijinsky, W. The formation of carcinogenic nitroso compounds from nitrite and some types of agricultural chemicals. *Food Cosmet. Toxicol.*, **11**, 807–817 (1973).

7. Friedmann, M. A. Nitrosation of sarcosine: Chemical kinetics and gastric assay. *Bull. Environ. Contam. Toxicol.*, **8**, 375–382 (1972).

8. Herbst, A. L., Ulfelder, H., and Poskanzer, D. Adenocarcinoma of the vagina: association of maternal stilbestrol therapy with tumor appearance in young women. *New Engl. J. Med.*, **284**, 878–881 (1971).

9. Houben-Weyl " Methoden der Organischen Chemie," Band IX, 4. Aufl., 824–826 (1955).

10. Ivankovic, S. "Selektive Erzeugung von Geschwülsten im Gehirn und Nervensystem," Deutscher Krebskongress, München, (Feb. 1966).

11. Ivankovic, S. Erzeugung maligner Tumoren im Gehirn, Rückenmark und Nervensystem bei den Nachkommen von Ratten und Hamstern durch transplazentare Einwirkung von Aethyl-nitrosoharnstoff. Habils Schrift, Freiburg/Brsg. (1968).

12. Ivankovic, S. Erzeugung von Malignomen bei Ratten nach transplazentarer

Einwirkung von N-Isopropyl-α-2-(methylhydrazino)-*p*-toluamid. HCl (Natulan). *Arzneimittel-Forschung*, **22**, 905–907 (1972).

13. Ivankovic, S. Praenatal carcinogenesis. *In* "Topics in Chemical Carcinogenesis," ed. by W. Nakahara, S. Takayama, T. Sugimura, and S. Odashima, University of Tokyo Press, Tokyo, pp. 463–475 (1972).

14. Ivankovic, S. and Druckrey, H. Transplazentare Erzeugung maligner Tumoren des Nervensystems. I. Äthylnitrosoharnstoff (ÄNH) an BD-IX-Ratten. *Z. Krebsforsch.*, **71**, 320–360 (1968).

15. Ivankovic, S. and Zeller, W. J. Transplazentare blastomogene Wirkung von N-Propyl-nitrosoharnstoff an BD-Ratten. *Arch. Geschwulstforsch.*, **40**, 99–102 (1972).

16. Ivankovic, S., Druckrey, H., and Preussmann, R. Erzeugung neurogener Tumoren bei den Nachkommen nach einmaliger Injektion von Äthylnitrosoharnstoff an schwangeren Ratten. *Naturwissenschaften*, **53**, 410 (1966).

17. Ivankovic, S., Schmähl, D. and Zeller, W. J. N-Demethylierung des carcinogenen Dimethylnitrosamin durch embryonales menschliches Gewebe. *Z. Krebsforsch.*, **81**, 269–272 (1974).

18. Lijinsky, W., Keefer, L., Conrad, E., and van de Bogart, R. Nitrosation of tertiary amines and some biological implications. *J. Natl. Cancer Inst.*, **49**, 1239–1249 (1972 a).

19. Lijinsky, W., Conrad, E., and van de Bogart, R. Carcinogenic nitrosamines formed by drug-nitrite interactions. *Nature*, **239**, 165–167 (1972 b).

20. Magee, P. N. and Barnes, J. M. The production of malignant primary hepatic tumors in the rat by feeding dimethylnitrosamine. *Brit. J. Cancer*, **10**, 114–122 (1956).

21. Mirvish, S. S. Kinetics of dimethylamine nitrosation in relation to nitrosamine carcinogenesis. *J. Natl. Cancer Inst.*, **44**, 633–639 (1970).

22. Mirvish, S. S. Kinetics of nitrosamine formation from alkylureas, N-alkylurethans and alkylguanidines: Possible implications for the etiology of human gastric cancer. *J. Natl. Cancer Inst.*, **46**, 1183–1193 (1972).

23. Mohr, U. and Hilfrich, J. Effect of a single dose of N-diethylnitrosamine on the rat kidney. *J. Natl. Cancer Inst.*, **49**, 1729–1731 (1972).

24. Sander, J., Schweinsberg, F., and Menz, H. P. Untersuchungen über die Entstehung cancerogener Nitrosamine im Magen. *Z. Physiol. Chem.*, **349**, 1691–1697 (1968).

25. Schmähl, D. "Entstehung, Wachstum und Chemotherapie maligner Tumoren," Editio Cantor, Aulendorf (1969).

26. Schmähl, D. Addition minimaler Dosen von vier verschiedenen hepatotropen Carcinogenen bei der Leberkrebserzeugung bei Ratten. *Z. Krebsforsch.*, **74**, 457–466 (1970).

27. Schmähl, D., Thomas, C., and Schold, G. Carcinogene Wirkung von Äthyl-butyl-nitrosamin bei Mäusen. *Naturwissenschaften*, **50**, 717–718 (1963).

28. Schmähl, D. and Thomas, C. Erzeugung von Lungen- und Lebertumoren bei Mäusen mit N, N'-Dinitrosopiperazin. *Z. Krebsforsch.*, **67**, 11–15 (1965).

29. Siebert, D. and Eisenbrand, G. Induction of mitotic gene conversion in *Saccharomyces cerevisiae* by N-nitrosated pesticides. *Mutat. Res.*, **22**, 121–126 (1974).

30. Sugimura, T., Kawachi, T., Kogure, K., Nagao, M., Tanaka, N., Fujimura, S., Takayama, S., Shimosato, S., Noguchi, M., Kuwabara, N., and Yamada, T. Induction of stomach cancer by N-methyl-N'-nitro-N-nitrosoguanidine: Experi-

ments on dogs as clinical models and the metabolism of this carcinogen. *In* "Topics in Chemical Carcinogenesis," ed. by W. Nakahara, S. Takayama, T. Sugimura, and S. Odashima, University of Tokyo Press, Tokyo, pp. 105–119 (1972).

31. Ungerer, O., Eisenbrand, G., and Preussmann, R. Zur Reaktion von Nitrit mit Pestiziden: Bildung, chemische Eigenschaften und cancerogene Wirkung der N-Nitrosoverbindung des Herbizids N-methyl-N'-(2-benzothiazolyl)-harnstoff (Benzthiazuron). *Z. Krebsforsch.*, **81**, 217–224 (1974).

32. Zimmermann, F. K. and Schwaier, R. Induction of mitotic gene conversion with nitrous acid, 1-methyl-3-nitro-1-nitrosoguanidine and other alkylating agents in *Saccharomyces cerevisiae*. *Mol. Genet.*, **100**, 63–76 (1967).

GANN Monograph on Cancer Research 17, 145–160 (1975)

NITRITE AND NITROSABLE AMINO COMPOUNDS IN CARCINOGENESIS

J. Sander, F. Schweinsberg, J. LaBar, G. Bürkle,
and E. Schweinsberg

*Hygiene-Institut der Universität Tübingen**

Carcinogenic N-nitroso compounds may be synthesized in the environment or *in vivo*. It was demonstrated that the nitrosation of amino compounds *in vitro* can be accelerated by halide ions, *e.g.*, thiocyanate, and by certain aldehydes. In the presence of ascorbic acid or phenolic compounds the nitrosation is prevented for the most part.

Concurrent application in high doses of amino compounds of low or moderate basicity and nitrite to experimental animals resulted in the same tumors that were obtained with the corresponding N-nitroso compounds. For the quantitative determination of N-nitroso compounds formed *in vivo*, four different factors were considered; tumor induction time, typical toxic reactions, analysis of gastric contents, analysis of urine.

A nitrosation in the human body could be demonstrated with the noncarcinogenic diphenylamine. Nitrosonornicotine, the most likely nitroso derivative to be formed *in vivo* from the precursors occurring in tobacco smoke, could not be detected in gastric juice of smokers. *In vitro* experiments with gastric juice, ham, and amidopyrine under physiological conditions yielded up to 1.5 mg N-nitrosodimethylamine.

Experiments with plants showed that nitrosamines, which might be formed in the soil, are readily absorbed. In the plants tested they were not detectable for more than a few days. Nitroso compounds could not be detected in surface water. More experiments will be necessary to prove whether with the concentrations of the precursors occurring in the environment or which are ingested by man, sufficient amounts of N-nitroso compounds are formed to induce cancer in man.

The impressive results on the carcinogenic activity of a great number of N-nitroso compounds in laboratory animals (*9, 28, 45*) have led us to question whether these compounds might well be a major cause of human cancer.

On the first analysis, this seemed to be quite possible since many nitrosamines and nitrosamides are easily formed and because the precursors—amines, amides, and nitrite—are widespread throughout the environment.

In recent years a number of scientists have concentrated their efforts toward

---

* D-74 Tübingen, West Germany.

understanding the nitrosation reaction and investigating the conditions under which carcinogenic nitroso compounds may be formed in the environment or within the human body. A compact review of the pertinent data available to date follows.

Two Principles of the Reaction of Nitrite with Amino Compounds

The first step of the nitrosation mechanism of amino compounds is an electrophilic attack of the nitrosating agent on the free pair of electrons of the nitrogen atom (Fig. 1). This holds true for the nitrosation of primary, secondary, and tertiary amines, as well as for amides and enamines. The reaction with primary amines does not yield any stable N-nitroso compounds (Fig. 1a). The nitrosation of secondary amines can be represented by the substitution of hydrogen by NO (b). To obtain N-nitroso compounds from tertiary amines—a reaction which has been "discovered" at least 3 times in the past 100 years (*18*)—one of the alkyl groups first has to be split off oxidatively by the assistance of NO (*57*) to yield the secondary amine, which then in turn is nitrosated (c). Enamines are nitrosated in a similar fashion, except that the group to be removed is in a higher oxidation state and therefore can be split off by hydrolysis without being previously activated (d).

If the nitrosation is carried out in at least 50% perchloric acid, NO⁺ is the nitrosating agent (*56*). This nitrosyl cation—which often is incorrectly believed to be responsible for all nitrosation reactions—is a very reactive electrophile. It is the only species that is able to nitrosate protonated amino compounds.

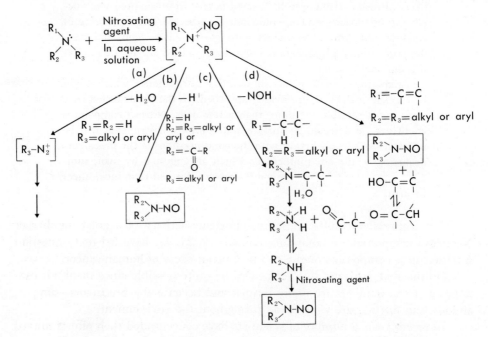

FIG. 1.   Schema for the different reactions of amino compounds with nitrosating agent

The nitrosating agent in intermediate acidities (1–6 N strong acid solutions) is $H_2NO_2^+$, whereas in the pH range 1–4, N_2O_3 is the reactive molecule. In biological systems, which are of interest in this connection, only mildly acidic conditions are to be expected. It is therefore sufficient to confine the discussion to N_2O_3.

Protonation and nitrosation compete at the basic center of the amino compound. Because of these concurrent reactions a pH maximum for the nitrosation of secondary amines, *e.g.*, dimethylamine (*29*) or morpholine (*13*) , of pH 3.4 is obtained. A correlation between basicity of the secondary amine and the yield of nitrosamine can also be demonstrated. With increasing basicity the formation of nitrosamine decreases (*48*).

Kinetic experiments (*29*) on the nitrosation of the strongly basic secondary amine, dimethylamine (pK_a 10.7 (25°)) showed that at pH 3.4 the reaction rate is proportional to the concentration of the amine and to the square of the nitrite concentration (Eq. 1).

$$\text{rate} \sim [\text{amine}][\text{nitrite}]^2 \tag{1}$$

The reaction rate of the nitrosation of the weakly basic secondary amine, N-methylaniline (pK_a 4.8 (25°)), at pH 2.7, however, is independent of the amine concentration (Eq. 2) (*23*).

$$\text{rate} \sim [\text{nitrite}]^2 \tag{2}$$

These two results can be explained by the following two equations:

$$2HNO_2 \underset{V_{-1}}{\overset{V_1}{\rightleftharpoons}} N_2O_3 + H_2O \tag{3}$$

$$N_2O_3 + \underset{R}{\overset{R}{>}}NH \overset{V_2}{\longrightarrow} \underset{R}{\overset{R}{>}}N\text{–}NO + HNO_2 \tag{4}$$

The nitrous anhydride is formed in a rapid preequilibrium step, and attacks the unprotonated amine. At lower acidities strongly basic amines exist only to a very small extent in the unprotonated state and $V_{-1} \gg V_2$, whereas the unprotonated weakly basic amines are present in higher concentrations and remove N_2O_3 from the equilibrium as soon as it is formed ($V_2 \gg V_{-1}$).

The nitrosation of amides (*e.g.*, alkylureas, alkylurethans) follows the kinetics of the nitrous acidium ion ($H_2NO_2^+$) reaction. The reaction rate does not show a maximum at any pH (*30*).

$$\text{rate} \sim [\text{amide}][H_2NO_2^+] \tag{5}$$

The nitrosation rate of simple aliphatic tertiary amines at 100° was found to be dependent on the amine concentration and on the cube of the nitrite concentration (*52*).

$$\text{rate} \sim [\text{amine}][\text{nitrite}]^3 \tag{6}$$

Because the amount of N-nitrosodiethylamine (diethylnitrosamine, DEN) found in the nitrosation of triethylamine at 100° was 200 times smaller than in the reaction with diethylamine, it should be emphasized that simple aliphatic tertiary amines do not play an important role as precursors of N-nitroso compounds.

Enamines, which are not readily hydrolyzed in aqueous solution, are nitrosated and subsequently dealkylated much better than tertiary amines. The nitrosation of amidopyrine produced N-nitrosodimethylamine (dimethylnitrosamine, DMN) in high yield (26).

The nitrosation rate in organic solvents increases with increasing basicity of a secondary amine; a high electron density at the nitrogen atom facilitates the attack of the electrophilic nitrosating agent.

In the presence of halide ions the nitrosation of secondary amines is accelerated (21, 50). Thiocyanate, which occurs in human saliva, similarly influences the reaction rate (3, 4, 58).

Kinetic studies of the nitrosation of morpholine in the presence of thiocyanate at pH values below 2 resulted in a first-order dependence of the reaction rate with respect to nitrous acid, amine, and thiocyanate (13). This can be explained by Eqs. 7 and 8:

$$HNO_2 + H_3O^+ + SCN^- \underset{V_{-1}}{\overset{V_1}{\rightleftharpoons}} NOSCN + 2H_2O \qquad (7)$$

$$\underset{R}{\overset{R}{>}}NH + NOSCN \overset{V_2}{\longrightarrow} \underset{R}{\overset{R}{>}}N-NO + HSCN \qquad (8)$$

Under these conditions NOSCN acts as the nitrosating agent, which is rapidly formed and then attacks the unprotonated amine $(V_{-1} \gg V_2)$.

$$\text{rate} \sim [HNO_2][H_3O^+][SCN^-][\text{sec. amine}] \qquad (9)$$

The nitrosation reaction of secondary amines can also be facilitated by the presence of some aldehydes, e.g., formaldehyde or chloral (34). Here, in the first step, an unstable intermediate is formed which subsequently can be attacked directly by nitrite.

The nitrosation reaction of amines can also be inhibited (7). Vitamin C, for instance, reacts faster than secondary amines with nitrous acid. Therefore, in the presence of sufficient amounts of ascorbic acid only small quantities of N-nitroso compounds are formed (32).

Also the nitrosation of phenolic compounds is much easier than that of most secondary amines. In an acidic medium, amines are predominantly present in the unreactive protonated form, whereas phenols undergo nitrosation readily by a pH independent pathway at pH values of 1 to 5 (5).

Nitrosamine Formation in the Environment

1. In water and waste water

In addition to nitrite, which is generally used as an indicator of water pollution, amines and amides are also known to occur in water, waste water, or in water-bearing soil strata. Therefore, we analyzed surface water and the effluents of sewage treatment plants to test the likelihood of nitrosamine formation. The dichloromethane-extractable total Kjeldahl nitrogen of the samples varied between 0.6 ppb and 4.3 ppb N, and ranged up to 10 ppb in the effluents. Nitrite concentrations reached 1 ppm in rivers and exceeded 80 ppm in the effluents of an experimental sewage treatment plant. The effluent of a galvanizing factory contained amounts greater than 500 ppm nitrite. The nitrosable amines, dimethylamine, diethylamine, pyrrolidine, and piperidine, were found in concentrations up to 2 ppb, but with a detection limit of 0.5 ppb, none of their respective N-nitroso derivatives were detected (46).

It can be calculated from the known reaction kinetics and the concentrations of the precursors that in rivers with average pollution levels, only 10^{-14} to 10^{-16} moles/liter of a nitrosamine can be formed in 1 hr by chemical reactions. In addition, nitrosamines are highly susceptible to light. A concentration of 333 ppb DEN was reduced to about one-third within 2-hr exposure to sunlight in one experiment, and 16 hr of daylight under partly cloudy conditions was sufficient to decompose the nitrosamine almost completely. Water plants were not effective in the degradation of nitrosamines (46).

In interpreting our results it should be kept in mind that only a small group of N-nitroso compounds has been examined. Nonvolatile nitrosamines have not been investigated, nor have nitrosamides. Also, biosynthesis was not taken into consideration. It has been suggested (2, 6, 17, 25, 35) that bacteria might contribute to nitrosamine synthesis other than solely by the production of nitrite. More experiments are necessary to demonstrate or to exclude a health risk due to carcinogenic N-nitroso compounds in water.

2. In the soil and edible plants

Nitrite, an important intermediary product in the nitrogen cycle, could possibly react with amines and amides also present in the soil (often in the form of pesticides). It is known that nitrosamines can be absorbed from the soil by plants (39, 45). However, when wheat was harvested from fields that had been treated several times during the growth period with dimethylamine, N-methylbenzylamine, or N-methylaniline along with a heavy dose of nitrogen fertilizers, none of the corresponding nitrosamines could be detected (40). These negative results may be partially clarified by a later series of experiments with cress plants (Lepidium sativum). Of a nitrosamine supplied in aqueous solution (20 mg/5 liters) to the roots for 17–20 hr, 0.5–13% could be detected in the green plant material. These concentrations fell rapidly (within 24 hr for DMN and within 3–4 days for N-nitrosomorpholine and N,N'-dinitrosopiperazine) to trace levels when the nitrosamine supply was removed and replaced by fresh water (44). Thus it seems that absorbed nitrosamines do not accumulate in the green plant material, but nothing is yet known about the breakdown of these compounds in the plants or of the toxicological significance of the metabolites. Nor has it been investigated whether nitrosamides, e.g., nitrosated pesticides, can be transported into the plants through the roots, and it must be examined whether nitrosamines are accumulated in other parts of plants, e.g., fruits, bulbs, oil seed. More experiments in this direction are urgently needed, as several nitroso derivatives of pesticides have proven to be highly carcinogenic or mutagenic (*11*, *55*, *59*).

Nitrosamine Formation in the Mammalian Body

1. Experiments with laboratory animals

From the results of the *in vitro* experiments nitrosamine synthesis in the mammalian body can be expected. In fact, the feeding of certain amines, the N-nitroso derivatives of which were known carcinogens, and nitrite to laboratory animals has led to the development of tumors (*37*).

Of the many amino compounds tested, the secondary amines of low or moderate basicity, which react well *in vitro*, have proven successful in the induction of tumors when fed concurrently with nitrite to rats or mice. To this group belong N-methylaniline (esophagus carcinomas), N-methylbenzylamine (esophagus and forestomach carcinomas), and morpholine (liver carcinomas) (*41*). Greenblatt *et al.* (*16*) have reported a considerable increase in the number of spontaneous lung adenomas in mice that had received piperazine plus nitrite. Diethylamine, a secondary amine of high basicity, failed to induce tumors when administered with nitrite to rats even in high doses (*10*, *41*), although it was possible to demonstrate by analysis of gastric contents that this amine, too, is nitrosated to a small extent in the animal stomach (*54*). Another secondary amine of high basicity, piperidine, also caused no tumors when applied with nitrite (*37*).

Similarly, no tumors have, as yet, been induced from tertiary amines and nitrite, even in high doses (*52*). Quaternary ammonium bases have not been tested; *in vitro* only small amounts of N-nitroso compounds are obtained (*14*).

The enamine, amidopyrine, caused tumors of the kidneys when rats received a diet containing 2,000 ppm of this compound simultaneously with drinking water containing 5,000 ppm sodium nitrite for 126 days (*45*). Liver tumors resulted when drinking water with 1,000 ppm nitrite and 1,000 ppm amidopyrine was administered for 50 weeks (*27*).

The alkylamides showed a similar correspondence between the *in vitro* and *in vivo* experiments. Methyl-, ethyl-, and ethyleneurea, which racted very easily *in vitro* (*30*, *42*), also effectively produced tumors in rats when applied together with nitrite, but other less reactive amides yielded no cancer (*36*, *37*). The same holds true for some amino acids (*15*).

The earlier experiments described above, although very helpful in demonstrating which amino compounds react effectively with nitrite *in vivo*, were all performed using doses much higher than seems to be realistic when considering amounts that might be ingested by man. More data are also necessary with respect to the lowest doses that can cause cancer. For example, when rats were fed diets containing 2,500 ppm N-methylbenzylamine concurrently with drinking water containing 800 and more ppm sodium nitrite, all animals developed tumors. However, when the nitrite concentration was 600 ppm and below, no tumors were found, demonstrating clearly the important influence of the nitrite concentration. Using ethyleneurea and nitrite, the lowest concentrations producing tumors were 500 ppm in the feed and 500 ppm in the drinking water, respectively (*37*).

Besides the dose, there are other chemical and biological factors that influence the nitrosation reaction *in vivo*. The method of administration of the amines and nitrite in feeding experiments is also decisive. Since it is known that the concentrations of these compounds decrease rapidly in the stomach, the nitrosamine yield will be lower with increasing time intervals between ingestion of the amines and the ingestion of nitrite. Nitrite is especially rapidly degraded due to chemical reactions in the acidic gastric juice (*12*), although when consumed with the food, residual amounts could be still detected after 2 hr (*43*).

Simultaneous ingestion of the precursors would provide an optimal, but less realistic, situation for the nitrosation reaction *in vivo*. The latter method has in fact yielded more tumors and toxic reactions than the separate administration of amino compounds and nitrite (*12*).

As mentioned previously, there are certain compounds that enhance the nitrosation reaction. Thiocyanate is known to occur in saliva and in gastric juice. Experiments *in vitro* with gastric juice and feeding experiments demonstrated that acceleration does take place. Addition of thiocyanate to the diet or drinking water, however, did not further increase the nitrosamine yield (*51*).

Perhaps even more important is the inhibition of the nitrosation reaction *in vivo*. Ascorbic acid reduces the yield of nitroso products not only *in vitro*, but in the stomach as well. Thus rats, when treated with high doses of amidopyrine and nitrite, did not develop severe liver damage when protected by ascorbic acid, but did so when ascorbic acid was not supplied (*25*). Malformations of the brain (hydrocephalus) occurred in young rats when the mothers were treated during pregnancy with either N-nitrosoethylurea or with ethylurea and nitrite, whereas no hydrocephali were observed in cases where ascorbic acid had been given concurrently with the nitrosation precursors (*22, 23*). Even so, the inhibition afforded by ascorbic acid is not complete; in analysis of the stomach contents of rats that had received piperazine, nitrite, and ascorbic acid, small amounts of dinitrosopiperazine were still detectable, although these values were much lower than those obtained without addition of the inhibitor (*43*). In gastric juice, glutathione also proved to be an effective inhibitor of nitrosamine formation (*53*).

The different factors influencing the nitrosation reaction *in vivo* made it highly desirable to develop methods that allow a quantitative determination of the formation of N-nitroso compounds. Very different methods have been applied, each having its measurable degree of success and failure.

1) It is, in principle, possible to estimate the total amount of a nitrosamine formed *in vivo* from the tumor induction time when the effect of the corresponding carcinogen is known. The induction of tumors, however, can last years, and a great number of animals is necessary when low, realistic concentrations, of the precursors are tested.

2) The observation of typical toxic reactions has been used by several authors as a short-term test (*12, 25*). This method has the disadvantage of requiring high doses.

3) Various attempts have been made to analyze the gastric content and to cal-

J. SANDER ET AL.

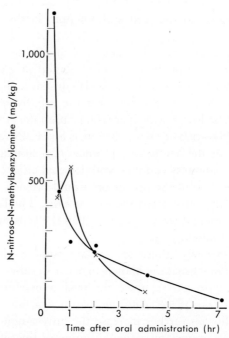

FIG. 2. Determination of N-nitroso-N-methylbenzylamine in the stomach and body tissues after oral administration of 4 mg/kg

● N-nitroso-N-methylbenzylamine in the stomach; × N-nitroso-N-methyl-benzylamine in the body tissues.

culate the amount of N-nitroso compound formed from the amount present at the time of analysis (*32*). However, as our analyses on the resorption of nitrosamines from the stomach and on the degradation in the organ tissues show, these measurements are very time-dependent, and reproducibility can be obtained only with great difficulty (*43*) (Fig. 2).

4) Many nitrosamines are easily soluble in water. A certain proportion of the nitrosamine formed and thereafter resorbed can thus be expected to be excreted unchanged with the urine. The analysis of the urine was therefore applied to measure the amount of dinitrosopiperazine formed from piperazine and nitrite in rats (*43*) and was used to demonstrate that boiled ham and piperazine yield measurable amounts of dinitrosopiperazine in the dog (*47*). (The maximum dose of piperazine in these experiments was 150 mg/kg, a dose corresponding to that used for treatment of helminthoses in children). While investigation of the urine seems to offer an improvement over other quantitative methods, being of short duration and of reasonable reproducibility, it must be noted that only small percentages (max. 4.2% for dinitrosopiperazine in the dog) are excreted (Fig. 3).

Only a few animal experiments have been conducted with respect to nitrosamine formation in organs other than the stomach. Hill and Hawksworth (*19*) have described the formation of nitrosopiperidine from dietary piperidine and nitrate in rats having a chronic *Escherichia coli* infection of the urinary bladder. A possible production of nitrosamines in the human vaginal vault by *Trichomonas vaginalis* has also been suggested (*1*).

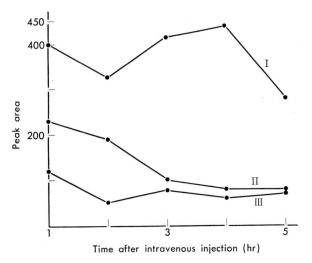

FIG. 3.   Excretion of 1,4-dinitrosopiperazine after intravenous injection of dinitrosopiperazine (experiment with dogs)
    I, 5 mg/kg; II, 1 mg/kg; III, 0.2 mg/kg.

2.   *Applications to man*

Besides the possible ingestion by man of nitroso compounds already formed in the environment it is reasonable from the results obtained with experimental animals to assume that a nitrosation reaction can also occur in the human stomach. Among the different amines and amides that readily react with nitrite to form carcinogenic nitroso compounds, several may be ingested by man. Some are natural constituents of foods (*e.g.*, dimethylamine in fish) and others are contaminants (*e.g.*, pesticides). Nitrite is plentifully available either as a natural constituent (*e.g.*, in spinach and lettuce after bacterial reduction of nitrate) or as a food additive (*e.g.*, in meats).

A further important source of nitrosable amino compounds is represented by drugs. It has been suggested that a major proportion of amidopyrine might be converted to DMN in the human stomach under suitable conditions (*27*). In reality, however, none of the drugs that are easily nitrosated is known to induce cancer in man, nor have they produced toxic reactions that might be attributed to an N-nitroso compound. The actual demonstration of nitrosamine synthesis in the human stomach and the seemingly contradictory failure to observe reactions typical for nitrosamines may perhaps be explained if one accepts the following ideas:

1)   Nitrosamines, although probably carcinogenic in man, will not necessarily induce specific tumors. It is not unlikely that, if at all, tumors will be developed that also could have been caused by a number of other factors. If this is true, a correlation between the ingestion of a nitrosable amine and the growth of a tumor (probably several tens of years later) would easily be overlooked.

2)   One has to keep in mind that, at least in the laboratory animals, typical toxic reactions, *e.g.*, severe liver damage, occur only when considerably high doses of a nitrosamine are administered or formed. The LD_{50} for DMN, for example,

was found to be 40 mg/kg, and for dinitrosopiperazine the dose was still greater (160 mg/kg) (9).

To produce a significant increase of liver-specific enzymes (serum-glutamate-oxalacetate-transaminase and serum-glutamate-pyruvate-transaminase) in the blood serum of rats, we had to inject at least 10 mg/kg of DMN (unpublished). It is nearly impossible to synthesize such amounts of DMN in the human stomach from a drug ingested in a therapeutic dose even if a meal rich in nitrite is consumed concurrently. In *in vitro* experiments with gastric juice and boiled ham containing up to 60 ppm sodium nitrite, maximal 1.5 mg of DMN was found per 100 mg amidopyrine (one tablet of a commercially available product). The mixture—boiled ham, or an aqueous extract of the ham, gastric juice, and amidopyrine—was allowed to react at 37° for 25 min, after which time both the nitrite and the amidopyrine would no longer be present in the stomach except for residual amounts. The latter was demonstrated by sampling the stomach juice every 5–10 min after ingestion of one or the other precursor (unpublished).

There is no doubt that in principle nitrosamines can be synthesized in the human stomach. That was demonstrated by analyzing the gastric content of 31 persons who had received 300 mg sodium nitrate, 1,000 mg glucose, and 10 mg diphenylamine, which is nontoxic in this dose. In this experiment no nitrite was given, but a microbial nitrate reduction allowed a small proportion (up to 0.1%) of the very easily nitrosable amine to be converted to the noncarcinogenic N-nitrosodiphenylamine (49).

3. Nitrosamine formation in the human stomach from constituents of tobacco smoke?

Tobacco smoke is known to be carcinogenic. It was suggested (8) that this may be partly due to the formation of N-nitroso compounds in the gaseous phase from nitrogen oxides and amines. If an artifactual reaction is excluded, DMN and N-nitrosonornicotine are found in the main-stream smoke in the range of 100 ng per cigarette (20). Because dimethylamine, pyrrolidine, and nornicotine, which are present in tobacco smoke, are water-soluble, it is also possible that these nitrosable amines together with nitrite, thiocyanate, and aldehydes reach the stomach, where favorable conditions for nitrosation prevail.

In experiments with volunteers, about 10% of the nornicotine in the main-stream smoke could be recovered in the saliva (unpublished). Because not all of the saliva produced during smoking could be collected for this sample, the actual amount of dissolved nornicotine must be still greater. When the nitrosation of nornicotine was compared to that of N-methylbenzylamine, which is more easily nitrosated than either dimethylamine or pyrrolidine (48), nornicotine was found to be even more reactive. The tertiary amine, nicotine, which is also present in high concentration in tobacco smoke, yields about 100 times less nitrosonornicotine than was found with nornicotine (unpublished).

From tobacco smoke nornicotine is therefore the most likely precursor of nitrosamine synthesis in the stomach. In order to investigate the possible nitrosamine formation in the stomach, gastric juice was drawn off from smokers. In this experiment 280 cigarettes were smoked, and 6-liter samples of gastric juice collected. After isolation by extraction with dichloromethane, purification by thin-layer chromatography, and identification by gas chromatography with a nitrogen-specific detector, no nitrosonornicotine could be detected (detection limit 5–10 ppb). From this negative result, it should not be concluded that nitrosamine formation in the stomach of smokers does not play a role in the carcinogenesis caused by smoking.

CONCLUDING REMARKS

In the last decade the nitrosation of amino compounds has been more and more extensively investigated. This was triggered by the fact that most N-nitroso compounds proved to be strong carcinogens and because tumors could be induced as well by the concurrent application of the precursors of N-nitroso compounds.

Recently, however, it has turned out to be extremely difficult to prove that the minute amounts of carcinogenic nitroso derivatives formed from precursors found in the environment are in part responsible for the induction of human cancer.

Although one cannot at present draw a direct correlation between environmental N-nitroso compounds and cancer in man, the necessity of continued research in this field must be emphasized for a number of reasons:

1) It is commonly accepted that chemical carcinogens, which include a great number of N-nitroso compounds, play a major part in the etiology of human cancer.

2) There are a number of nitrosable substances, including pesticides and drugs, for which the reactivity with nitrite and the carcinogenesis of the N-nitroso derivative is still unknown.

3) Very little is known about the influence of chemical substances on the nitrosation reaction and on the carcinogenic activity of nitroso compounds within the complex systems that occur in the environment and *in vivo*.

4) There is a great lack of imformation on the exact amounts of N-nitroso compounds formed under varying conditions *in vivo*. More sensitive quantitative methods have to be developed. Such methods should be applicable to man, as it is highly desirable to measure possible nitrosamine formation, for example, in people who have to take certain medications or who have certain food preferences. One possibility in this direction is the analysis of excreted metabolites of N-nitroso compounds.

5) Lastly, although it is inconvenient, more long-term, low-dose tumor induction experiments with the necessary large number of experimental animals are needed if we are to evaluate at all realistically the probability of actual carcinogenesis in man due to N-nitroso compounds.

REFERENCES

1. Allsobrook, A. J. R., du Plessis, L. S., Harington, J. S., Nunn A. J., and Nunn, J. R. N-Nitrosamines in the human vaginal vault. *In* "N-Nitroso Compounds: Analysis and Formation," IARC Scientific Publications No. 9, International Agency for Research on Cancer, Lyon, 197–199 (1975).

2. Ayanaba, A., Verstraete, W., and Alexander, M. Possible microbial contribution to nitrosamine formation in sewage and soil. *J. Natl. Cancer Inst.*, **50**, 811–813 (1973).

3. Boyland, E. The effect of some ions of physiological interest on nitrosamine synthesis. *In* "N-Nitroso Compounds: Analysis and Formation," IARC Scientific Publications No. 3, International Agency for Research on Cancer, Lyon, pp. 124–126 (1972).

4. Boyland, E., Nice, E., and Williams, K. The catalysis of nitrosation by thiocyanate from saliva. *Food Cosmet. Toxicol.*, **9**, 639–643 (1971).

5. Challis, B. Rapid nitrosation of phenols and its implications for health hazards from dietary nitrites. *Nature*, **244**, 466 (1973).

6. Collins-Thomson, D. L., Sen, N. P., Aris, B., and Swinghamer, L. Non-enzymatic *in vitro* formation of nitrosamines by bacteria isolated from meat products. *Can. J. Microbiol.*, **18**, 1968–1971 (1972).

7. Dahn, H., Loewe, L., and Bunton, C. A. Über die Oxidation von Ascorbinsäure durch salpetrige Säure. VI. Übersicht und Diskussion der Ergebnisse. *Helv. Chim. Acta*, **43**, 320–333 (1960).

8. Druckrey, H. and Preussmann, R. Zur Entstehung carcinogener Nitrosamine am Beispiel des Tabakrauchs. *Naturwissenschaften*, **49**, 498 (1962).

9. Druckrey, H., Preussmann, R., Ivankovic, S., and Schmähl, D. Organotrope carcinogene Wirkung bei 65 verschiedenen N-Nitroso-Verbindungen an BD-Ratten. *Z. Krebsforsch.*, **69**, 103–201 (1967).

10. Druckrey, H., Steinhoff, D., Beuthner, H., Schneider, H., and Klärner, P. Prüfung von Nitrit auf chronisch toxische Wirkung an Ratten. *Arzneimittel-Forschung*, **13**, 320–323 (1963).

11. Eisenbrand, G., Ungerer, O., and Preussmann, R. Rapid formation of carcinogenic N-nitrosamines by interaction of nitrite with fungicides derived from dithiocarbamic acid *in vitro* under simulated gastric conditions and *in vivo* in the rat stomach. *Food Cosmet. Toxicol.*, **12**, in press (1974).

12. Epstein, S. S. *In vivo* studies on interactions between secondary amines and nitrites and nitrates. *In* "N-Nitroso Compounds: Analysis and Formation," IARC Scientific Publications No. 3, International Agency for Research on Cancer, Lyon, pp. 109–115 (1972).

13. Fan, T. Y. and Tannenbaum, S. R. Factors influencing the rate of formation of nitroso morpholine from morpholine and nitrite: Acceleration by thiocyanate and other anions. *J. Agr. Food Chem.*, **21**, 237–240 (1973).

14. Fiddler, W., Pensabene, J. W., Doerr, R. C., and Wasserman, A. E. Formation of N-nitrosodimethylamine from naturally occurring quaternary ammonium compounds and tertiary amines. *Nature*, **236**, 307 (1972).

15. Greenblatt, M. and Lijinsky, W. Failure to induce tumors in Swiss mice after concurrent administration of amino acids and sodium nitrite. *J. Natl. Cancer Inst.*, **48**, 1389–1392 (1972).

16. Greenblatt, M., Mirvish, S. S., and So, B. T. Nitrosamine studies: Induction of lung adenomas by concurrent administration of sodium nitrite and secondary amines in Swiss mice. *J. Natl. Cancer Inst.*, **46**, 1029–1034 (1971).

17. Hawksworth, G. M. and Hill, M. J. Bacteria and the N-nitrosation of secondary amines. *Brit. J. Cancer*, **25**, 520–526 (1971).

18. Hein, G. E. The reaction of tertiary amines with nitrous acid. *J. Chem. Educ.*, **40**, 181–184 (1963).

19. Hill, M. J. and Hawksworth, G. Some studies on the production of N-nitrosamines

in the urinary bladder and their subsequent effects. *In* "N-Nitroso Compounds: Analysis and Formation," IARC Scientific Publications No. 9, International Agency for Research on Cancer, Lyon, 220–222 (1975).

20. Hoffmann, D., Rathkamp, G., and Lin, Y. Y. Chemical studies on tobacco smoke. XXVI. On the isolation and identification of volatile and nonvolatile N-nitrosamines and hydrazines in cigarette smoke. *In* "N-Nitroso Compounds: Analysis and Formation," IARC Scientific Publications No. 9, International Agency for Research on Cancer, Lyon, 159–165 (1975).

21. Hughes, E. D. and Ridd, J. H. Nitrosation diazotisation and deamination. V. Catalysis by anions of strong acids in the diazotisation of aniline and *o*-chloroaniline. *J. Chem. Soc.*, 82–88 (1958).

22. Ivankovic, S., Preussmann, R., Schmähl, D., and Zeller, J. Verhütung von Nitrosamid-bedingtem Hydrocephalus durch Ascorbinsäure nach pränataler Gabe von Äthylharnstoff und Nitrit und Ratten. *Z. Krebsforsch.*, **79**, 145–147 (1973).

23. Ivankovic, S., Preussmann, R., Schmähl, D., and Zeller, J. Prevention by ascorbic acid of *in vivo* formation of N-nitroso compounds. *In* "N-Nitroso Compounds: Analysis and Formation," IARC Scientific Publications No. 9, International Agency for Research on Cancer, Lyon, 101–102 (1975).

24. Kalatzis, E. and Ridd, J. H. The kinetics of N-nitrosation of N-methylaniline. *J. Chem. Soc. B*, 529–533 (1966).

25. Kamm, J. J., Dashman, T., Conney, A. H., and Burns, J. J. Protective effect of ascorbic acid on hepatotoxicity caused by sodium nitrite plus aminopyrine. *Proc. Natl. Acad. Sci. U.S.*, **70**, 747–749 (1973).

26. Klubes, P. and Jondorf, W. R. Dimethylnitrosamine formation from sodium nitrite and dimethylamine by bacterial flora of rat intestine. *Res. Commun. Chem. Pathol. Pharmacol.*, **2**, 24 (1971).

27. Lijinsky, W., Conrad, E., and van de Bogart, R. Carcinogenic nitrosamines formed by drug/nitrite interactions. *Nature*, **239**, 165–167 (1972).

28. Lijinsky, W., Taylor, H. W., Snyder, C., and Nettesheim, P. Malignant tumors of liver and lung in rats fed amidopyrine or heptamethyleneimine together with nitrite. *Nature*, **244**, 176–178 (1973).

29. Magee, P. N. and Barnes, J. M. Carcinogenic nitroso compounds. *Adv. Cancer Res.*, **11**, 163–264 (1967).

30. Mirvish, S. S. Kinetics of dimethylamine nitrosation in relation to nitrosamine carcinogenesis. *J. Natl. Cancer Inst.*, **44**, 633–639 (1970).

31. Mirvish, S. S. Kinetics of nitrosamide formation from alkylureas, N-alkylurethans, and alkylguanidines: Possible implications for the etiology of human gastric cancer. *J. Natl. Cancer Inst.*, **46**, 1183–1193 (1971).

32. Mirvish, S. S. and Chu, C. Chemical determination of methylnitrosourea (MNU) in the rat stomach after giving methylurea (MU) plus sodium nitrite. *Proc. Am. Assoc. Cancer Res.*, **13**, 108 (1972).

33. Mirvish, S. S., Wallcave, L., Eagen, M., and Shubik, P. Ascorbate-nitrite reaction: possible means of blocking the formation of carcinogenic N-nitroso compounds. *Science*, **177**, 65–68 (1972).

34. Roller, P. P. and Keefer, L. K. Catalysis of nitrosation reactions. *In* "N-Nitroso Compounds: Analysis and Formation," IARC Scientific Publications No. 9, International Agency for Research on Cancer, Lyon, 86–89 (1975).

35. Sander, J. Nitrosaminsynthese durch Bakterien. *Hoppe-Seyler's Z. Physiol. Chem.*, **349**, 429–432 (1968).

36. Sander, J. Induktion maligner Tumoren bei Ratten durch orale Gabe von

N, N'-Dimethylharnstoff und Nitrit. *Arzneimittel-Forschung*, **20**, 418–419 (1970).

37. Sander, J. Untersuchungen über die Entstehung kanzerogener Nitrosoverbindungen im Magen von Versuchstieren und ihre Bedeutung für den Menschen. *Arzneimittel-Forschung*, **21**, 1572–1580, 1707–1713, 2034–2039 (1971).

38. Sander, J. Weitere Versuche zur Tumorinduktion durch orale Applikation niederer Dosen von N-Methylbenzylamin und Nitrit. *Z. Krebsforsch.*, **76**, 93–96 (1971).

39. Sander, J. Formation of carcinogenic nitroso compounds under biological conditions. *In* "Environment and Cancer" (A collection of papers presented at the 24th Annual Symposium on Fundamental Cancer Research, Houston, Texas, 1971), Williams and Wilkins Corp., Baltimore (1972).

40. Sander, J., Aeikens, B., Schweinsberg, F., and Eisenbrand, G. Untersuchungen zur Frage einer Nitrosaminakkumulation in Weizen nach gleichzeitiger Gabe hoher Dosen eines Nitratdüngers und sekundärer Amine. *Z. Krebsforsch.*, **80**, 11–15 (1973).

41. Sander, J. and Bürkle, G. Induktion maligner Tumoren bei Ratten durch gleichzeitige Verfütterung von Nitrit und sekundären Aminen. *Z. Krebsforsch.*, **13**, 54–66 (1969).

42. Sander, J., Bürkle, G., Flohé, L., and Aeikens, B. *In-vitro*-Untersuchungen über die Möglichkeit einer Bildung kanzerogener Nitrosamide im Magen. *Arzneimittel-Forschung*, **21**, 411–414 (1971).

43. Sander, J., LaBar, J., Ladenstein, M., and Schweinsberg, F. Quantitative analysis of the nitrosamine formation *in vivo*. *In* "N-Nitroso Compounds: Analysis and Formation," IARC Scientific Publications No. 9, International Agency for Research on Cancer, Lyon, 123–131 (1975).

44. Sander, J., Ladenstein, M., LaBar, J., and Schweinsberg, F. Experiments on the degradation of N-nitrosamines by plants. *In* "N-Nitroso Compounds: Analysis and Formation," IARC Scientific Publications No. 9, International Agency for Research on Cancer, Lyon, 205–210 (1975).

45. Sander, J. and Schweinsberg, F. Wechselbeziehungen zwischen Nitrat, Nitrit und kanzerogenen N-Nitrosoverbindungen. *Zentr. Bakteriol. Parasitenk. Abt. I. Orig. B.*, **156**, 299–340 (1972).

46. Sander, J., Schweinsberg, E., Ladenstein, M., and Schweinsberg, F. Toxikologische Beurteilung einiger aktueller stickstoffhaltiger Substanzen im Wasser. *Zentr. Bakteriol. Parasitenk. Abt. I. Orig. B.*, in press (1974).

47. Sander, J., Schweinsberg, F., Ladenstein, M., Benzing, H., and Wahl, S. Messung der renalen Nitrosaminausscheidung am Hund zum Nachweis einer Nitrosaminbildung *in vivo*. *Hoppe-Seyler's Z. Physiol. Chem.*, **354**, 384–390 (1973).

48. Sander, J., Schweinsberg, F., and Menz, H.-P. Untersuchungen über die Entstehung cancerogener Nitrosamine im Magen. *Hoppe-Seyler's Z. Physiol. Chem.*, **349**, 1691–1697 (1968).

49. Sander, J. and Seif, F. Bakterielle Reduktion von Nitrat im Magen des Menschen als Ursache einer Nitrosaminbildung. *Arzneimittel-Forschung*, **19**, 1091–1093 (1969).

50. Schmid, H. Über "katalytisch-polare" Stoffe. *Z. Elektrochem.*, **43**, 626–629 (1937).

51. Schweinsberg, F. Catalysis of nitrosamine synthesis. *In* "N-Nitroso Compounds: Analysis and Formation," IARC Scientific Publications No. 9, International Agency for Research on Cancer, Lyon, 80–85 (1975).

52. Schweinsberg, F. and Sander, J. Cancerogene Nitrosamine aus einfachen aliphatischen tertiären Aminen und Nitrit. *Hoppe-Seyler's Z. Physiol. Chem.*, **353**, 1671–1676 (1972).

53. Sen, N. P. and Donaldson, B. The effect of ascorbic acid on the formation of

nitrosopiperazines from piperazine and nitrite. *In* "N-Nitroso Compounds: Analysis and Formation," IARC Scientific Publications No. 9, International Agency for Research on Cancer, Lyon, 103–106 (1975).

54. Sen, N. P., Smith, C. D., and Schwinghamer, L. Formation of N-nitrosamines from secondary amines and nitrite in human and animal gastric juice. *Food Cosmet. Toxicol.*, **7**, 301–307 (1969).

55. Siebert, D. and Eisenbrand, G. Induction of mitotic gene conversion in *Saccharomyces cerevisiae*, by N-nitrosated pesticides. *Mutat. Res.*, **22**, 121–126 (1974).

56. Singer, K. and Vamplew, P. A. Spectroscopic investigation of the equilibrium between NO^+ and nitrous acid in aqueous perchloric acid. *J. Chem. Soc.*, 3971–3974 (1956).

57. Smith, P. A. and Loeppky, R. H. Nitrosative cleavage of tertiary amines. *J. Am. Chem. Soc.*, **89**, 1147–1157 (1967).

58. Stedman, G. and Whincup, P. A. E. The equilibrium constant for the formation of nitrosyl thiocyanate in aqueous solution. *J. Chem. Soc.*, 5796–5797 (1963).

59. Ungerer, O., Eisenbrand, G., and Preussmann, R. Zur Reaktion von Nitrit mit Pestiziden: Bildung, chemische Eigenschaften und cancerogene Wirkung der N-Nitrosoverbindungen des Herbizids N-methyl-N'(2-benzo-thiazolyl)-harnstoff (Benzthiazuron). *Z. Krebsforsch.*, in press (1974).

EXPLANATION OF PHOTOS

PHOTO 1.   Cerebellopontile-angle tumor of a rat after application of methylurea and nitrite. Histologically neuroblastoma.

PHOTO 2.   Papillomatosis in the middle third and predominantly exophytically growing carcinoma of the squamous cells in the distal third of the esophagus of a rat after application of N-methylbenzylamine and nitrite.

PHOTO 3.   Multicentral hepatocellular tumors in the liver of a rat after application of morpholine and nitrite.

PHOTO 4a.   Angiograph of a nephroblastoma in a rat after application of amidopyrine and nitrite.

PHOTO 4b.   Pathological anatomic substrate to Photo 4a.

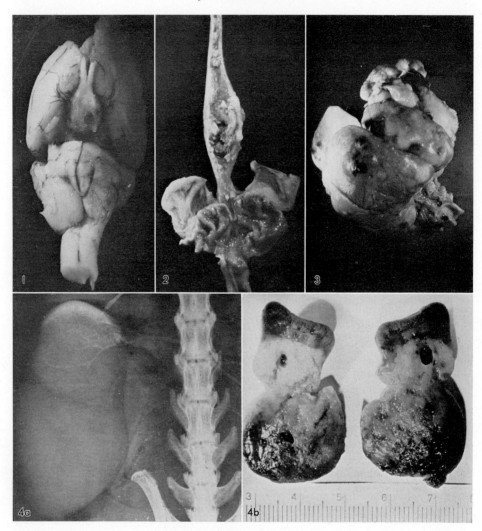

GANN Monograph on Cancer Research 17, 161–176 (1975)

METABOLISM AND CARCINOGENICITY OF N-BUTYL-N-(4-HYDROXYBUTYL)NITROSAMINE AND RELATED COMPOUNDS, WITH SPECIAL REFERENCE TO INDUCTION OF URINARY BLADDER TUMORS

Masashi OKADA, Emako SUZUKI, Junko AOKI, Minoru IIYOSHI,
and Yoshiyuki HASHIMOTO

*Tokyo Biochemical Research Institute**

Metabolic fate of N-butyl-N-(4-hydroxybutyl)nitrosamine (BBN) and N,N-dibutylnitrosamine (DBN) was investigated in the rat, guinea pig, and other animal species in order to elucidate a possible relationship between metabolism and organotropic carcinogenicity to the urinary bladder of these N-nitrosamines. The principal urinary metabolite of BBN in rats was identified as N-butyl-N-(3-carboxypropyl)nitrosamine (BCPN). Several minor metabolites characterized were subsequent transformation products of BCPN formed by β-oxidation according to the Knoop mechanism and glucuronic acid conjugates of BBN or BCPN. DBN underwent ω-oxidation as well as (ω-1)-oxidation giving also BCPN as the principal urinary metabolite in rats. Bladder cancer was selectively induced in rats by the oral administration of BCPN. The species difference in response to BBN and DBN was discussed on the basis of the urinary excretion rate of BCPN which could be regarded as the common proximate form of these N-nitrosamines as urinary bladder carcinogens.

In vivo metabolism and carcinogenicity of a number of N-nitrosamines related to DBN and BBN were investigated in rats after oral administration. A general scheme for biotransformations of N,N-dialkylnitrosamines and/or N-alkyl-N-(ω-hydroxyalkyl)-nitrosamines is given, and a possible correlation of structure and metabolism with organotropic carcinogenicity of N,N-dialkylnitrosamines is discussed, with special reference to selective induction of urinary bladder tumors.

Druckrey and his colleagues (*9*) have reported a comprehensive study on the carcinogenicity and target organs of numerous N-nitroso compounds in rats. An intriguing finding by these workers was that of all the compounds investigated, only two, namely N,N-dibutylnitrosamine (DBN) and its ω-hydroxylated derivative, N-butyl-N-(4-hydroxybutyl)nitrosamine (butyl-butanol-(4)-nitrosamine) (BBN), induced tumors of the urinary bladder. Especially, BBN had a

---

* Takada 3-41-8, Toshima-ku, Tokyo 171, Japan (岡田正志, 鈴木恵眞子, 青木純子, 飯吉　稔, 橋本嘉幸).

potent and selective action on the bladder after oral administration, as reported by Druckrey *et al.* (*8*) and Ito *et al.* (*16*).

Already in 1964, several polar metabolites which retained the nitrosamino moiety had been detected by Druckrey *et al.* (*8*) in the urine of rats given a large dose of DBN. On the other hand, it was demonstrated by Ito *et al.* (*17*) that unilateral ligation of the ureter resulted in a marked increase in the incidence of carcinoma in the renal pelvis and ureter of rats treated with BBN. These findings strongly suggested that the urinary metabolite(s) of BBN or DBN might take the leading role in the induction of cancer of the urinary bladder. In order to elucidate a possible relationship between metabolism and organotropic effect of BBN or DBN, the metabolic fate of these compounds in rats was investigated.

Metabolic Fate of BBN and DBN in Rats

A large dose (*ca.* 800 mg/kg body weight) of BBN was given orally to male Wistar rats and 48-hr urine was collected, which was processed according to the scheme shown in Chart 1. It was found by the quantitative determination using the colorimetric method reported by Eisenbrand and Preussmann (*11*) that urinary excretion in 48 hr of metabolites retaining the nitrosamino moiety amounted to nearly 80% of the dose and after that almost none were excreted into the urine (*31*). Chromatographic separation of each extract indicated in Chart 1

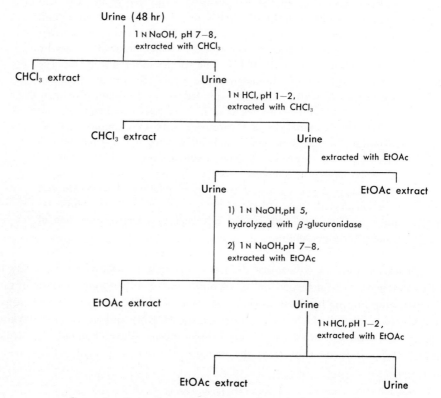

CHART 1.   Extraction and separation of metabolites from urine

using silica gel column or thin-layer plate gave several metabolites. Separation of the extract containing acidic metabolites was performed after methylation with diazomethane. The structure of the metabolites was definitely established either by direct comparison with the respective authentic specimen synthesized or on the basis of their various analytical data including infrared, nuclear magnetic resonance, and mass spectra, if the authentic sample was not available.

Thus, based on the urinary metabolites characterized, the metabolic pathway of BBN (II) in the rat has been revealed by Okada and his co-workers (*23, 31*), as shown in Chart 2. The principal urinary metabolite obtained in about 40% of the dose was N-butyl-N-(3-carboxypropyl)nitrosamine (BCPN) (V) which was formed by the oxidation of the alcoholic hydroxyl group of BBN to the carboxylic group. Besides BCPN, several compounds were characterized as minor metabolites*; glucuronic acid conjugates of BBN and BCPN (III and VI); subsequent transformation products of BCPN formed by β-oxidation according to the Knoop-mechanism, *i.e.*, N-butyl-N-(2-hydroxy-3-carboxypropyl)-nitrosamine (VIII), N-butyl-N-(carboxymethyl)nitrosamine (BCMN) (IX), N-butyl-N-(2-oxopropyl)nitrosamine (BOPN) (X). While no BBN could be detected in the urine, urinary excretion rates of these metabolites approximately estimated, are given in Table I.

Similarly, metabolic fate of DBN in the rat was investigated. Oral adminis-

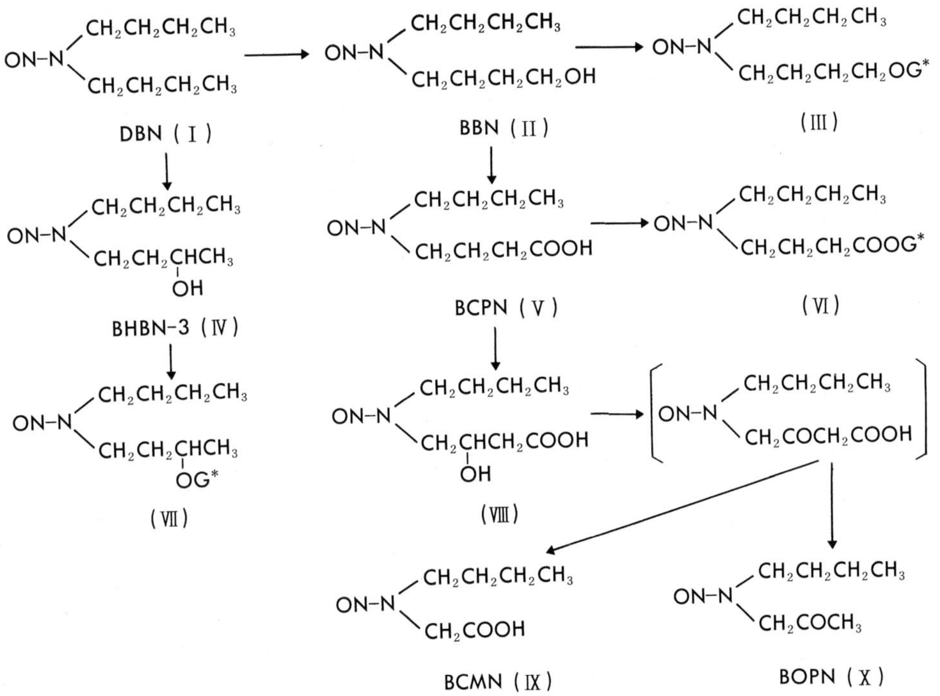

CHART 2.   Metabolism of BBN and DBN
G*: β-D-glucopyranosiduronic acid residue.

* In the present work, urinary metabolites, if any, which did not retain the nitrosamino moiety were not pursued.

TABLE I. Urinary Metabolites and Their Excretion Rates in Animals after Oral Administration of BBN, DBN, and BCPN[a]

Animal	Compound	Metabolite (% of the dose)							
		III[b]	IV (BHBN-3)	V (BCPN)	VI	VII[b]	VIII	IX (BCMN)	X (BOPN)
Rat	BBN	2	—	43	Trace	—	3	4	1
	DBN	—	1	10	—	3	Trace	2	—
	DBN (s.c.)	~[c]	~	25	~	~	1	5	~
	BCPN	—	—	40	Trace	—	2	4	1
Guinea pig	BBN	9	—	6	—	—	1	8	1
	DBN	—	1	4	—	12	Trace	5	1
	BCPN	—	—	9	Trace	—	1	11	1
Mouse	BBN	~	~	8	~	~	~	8	~
	DBN	~	~	5	~	~	~	4	~
	BCPN	~	~	9	~	~	~	16	~
Hamster	BBN	~	~	6	~	~	~	5	~
	DBN	~	~	8	~	~	~	6	~
Dog	BBN	~	~	7	~	~	~	36	~
	DBN	~	~	6	~	~	~	15	~

s.c.: subcutaneous. [a] Rats and guinea pigs weighing 300–400 g and 350–500 g, respectively, received about 800 mg/kg body weight of BBN, DBN, or BCPN, and the combined 48-hr urine of 3 animals was analyzed according to Chart 1. Mice, hamsters, and dogs weighing 25–40 g, 100–130 g, and 9.5–10.5 kg, respectively, received 5 mg, 10 mg, and 1 g/head of BBN, DBN, or BCPN, respectively, and the 48-hr urine was collected. In these animals, of all the metabolites, only BCPN and BCMN were determined by the colorimetric method after separation by thin-layer chromatography. [b] Calculated on the basis of the amount of compounds liberated after β-glucuronidase hydrolysis. [c] Not estimated.

tration of DBN to rats resulted also in a considerable urinary excretion of metabolites retaining the nitrosamino moiety which amounted to about 30% of the dose as determined by the colorimetric method. As shown in Chart 2, DBN (I) was metabolized in two ways (5, 6, 31). First, it was metabolized via BBN (II), whereby DBN underwent ω-oxidation of the one butyl group, giving also BCPN (V) as the major urinary metabolite which was estimated to be about 10% of the dose (ca. 800 mg/kg body weight). Secondly, DBN underwent (ω-1)-oxidation of the alkyl group to produce N-butyl-N-(3-hydroxybutyl)nitrosamine (BHBN-3) (IV) which in turn was conjugated with glucuronic acid to form the glucuronide (VII). Urinary excretion rates of the metabolites characterized of DBN are also given in Table I.

BCPN, the Common Proximate Form of BBN and DBN, as Urinary Bladder Carcinogen

In view of the findings that the principal urinary metabolite of BBN as well as of DBN was BCPN, and more than 40% of the dose was recovered unchanged from the 48-hr urine when BCPN was given orally to rats (23), the carcinogenicity of BCPN itself was examined in rats. It was demonstrated definitely by Hashimoto *et al.* (*12*) that BCPN was a selective and potent bladder carcinogen as BBN in rats. Histological type of tumors induced by BCPN and BBN was entirely similar. Urinary metabolites so far tested of BBN and DBN other than BCPN did not induce bladder tumors in rats by their oral administration, as described below. It seems quite reasonable to presume, therefore, that the induction of urinary bladder tumors by BBN or DBN may be attributable to their common major urinary metabolite, BCPN. While about 10% of the dose was recovered as urinary BCPN after oral administration of DBN to rats, the recovery was found to be about 25% with the subcutaneous injection, as indicated in Table I. This result may elucidate the earlier finding described by Druckrey *et al.* (*8*) that a much higher incidence of bladder cancer was observed with the subcutaneous injection of DBN in rats than with the oral route.

Hashimoto *et al.* (*14*) studied the direct carcinogenic action of BCPN on the urinary bladder epithelium by the intravesicular instillation of BCPN in female rats. Induction of papillomas and carcinomas of the urinary bladder was demonstrated by this treatment not only with BCPN but also with BBN. In this connection, there is a possibility that BBN is converted into BCPN by epithelial cells of the urinary bladder which may act as a more proximate carcinogen (*13*). Simultaneous calculus formation was observed in these experiments, however, it would be irrelevant at present to conclude that the tumor induction was due to the direct action of BCPN on the bladder epithelium.

Species Difference in the Metabolism of BBN and DBN

The metabolic fate of BBN and DBN was also investigated in other animal species, namely guinea pig, mouse, hamster, and dog. All the urinary metabolites were separated and characterized in case of the guinea pig, but only urinary BCPN and BCMN were determined colorimetrically in other animals. These results are also given in Table I (*25*). The urinary excretion of BCPN in the guinea pig was found to be much lower than that in the rat, while that of BCMN in the former was higher than that in the latter. Moreover, an increased urinary excretion of the glucuronide of BBN and BHBN-3 (III and VII in Chart 2) was observed with BBN and DBN, respectively, demonstrating a higher glucuronylation activity in the guinea pig than in the rat. As for the urinary excretion of BCPN and BCMN, essentially similar results were obtained with mice, hamsters, and dogs, as shown in Table I. Oral administration of BCMN, BOPN, and BHBN-3 did not induce bladder tumors in rats as described below, while carcinogenic effect on the bladder would not be expected with the above glucuronides. Accordingly, previous observations concerning the species difference in response to BBN or DBN may be explained on the basis of the different urinary excretion of BCPN after administration of BBN or DBN to animals. (1) Guinea pigs and hamsters were much less sensitive than rats to the induction of bladder cancer by BBN (*18*). (2) Induction of bladder tumors in guinea pigs with DBN required a much longer latent period than in rats (*19*). (3) A long induction time should be necessary for the development of bladder tumors in dogs with BBN and DBN (*29, 30*). On the contrary, this explanation does not seem to be applicable to mice, because BBN- (*1, 4*) as well as DBN (*3, 34*)-induced bladder cancer rather readily in this species. An acidic metabolite*[1] other than BCPN, N-butyl-N-(2-hydroxy-3-carboxypropyl)nitrosamine (VIII) and BCMN, which was found in fairly large amount only in the urine of mice given BBN or DBN, may play an important role in the induction of bladder cancer in mice.

Metabolism of N-Nitrosamines Related to DBN and BBN in Rats

It was assumed by Druckrey *et al.* (*8*) that the whole molecule of DBN was responsible for the induction of bladder cancer, because neither symmetric N, N-dialkylnitrosamines other than DBN nor asymmetric N, N-dialkylnitrosamines having a butyl group such as N-ethyl-N-butylnitrosamine (EBN)-induced bladder cancer.

In order to elucidate a possible relationship among chemical constitution, *in vivo* metabolism, and striking organotropic specificity to the urinary bladder of BBN or DBN, the following N-nitrosamines which were divided into four groups were synthesized and their metabolic fate in rats was investigated in the same way as BBN and DBN.

1) Symmetric N,N-dialkylnitrosamines: N,N-dipropylnitrosamine (DPN), N,N-diamylnitrosamine (DAN)

2) Asymmetric N,N-dialkylnitrosamines having a butyl group: N-ethyl-N-butylnitrosamine, N-propyl-N-butylnitrosamine (PBN), N-butyl-N-amylnitrosamine (BAN)

3) N-Alkyl-N-(ω-hydroxyalkyl)nitrosamines: N-methyl-N-(4-hydroxybutyl)nitrosamine (MHBN), N-ethyl-N-(4-hydroxybutyl)nitrosamine (EHBN), N-propyl-N-(4-hydroxybutyl)nitrosamine(PHBN), N-amyl-N-(4-hydroxybutyl)nitrosamine (AHBN), N-butyl-N-(2-hydroxyethyl)nitrosamine (BHEN), N-butyl-N-(3-hydroxypropyl)nitrosamine (BHPN)

4) Urinary metabolites of BBN and DBN: BCPN, BCMN, BOPN, BHBN-3

Prior to separating and characterizing the urinary metabolites of these compounds, urinary excretion of total metabolites retaining the nitrosamino moiety was determined colorimetrically with 48-hr urine which was collected after giving a dose of each compound equivalent to 50 mg of BCPN orally to rats. The results including DBN and BBN were as follows*[2]: DPN (11 ± 1), DBN (29 ± 1), DAN (38 ± 5), EBN (9 ± 1), PBN (29 ± 2), BAN (41 ± 3), MHBN (85 ± 5), EHBN (87 ± 0), PHBN (76 ± 7), BBN (76 ± 3), AHBN (61 ± 2), BHPN (72 ± 2), BHEN (67 ± 4), BCPN (78 ± 4), BCMN (76 ± 2), BOPN (45 ± 4), BHBN-3 (61 ± 4). These results suggest that the induction of bladder cancer was not simply ascribable to the urinary excretion of a large amount of metabolites retaining the nitrosamino moiety, since DAN, BAN, AHBN, BHPN, BHEN, BCMN, *etc.*, did not induce any bladder tumors in rats, as reported previously or described below.

---

*[1] Recently this metabolite has been characterized as a glycine conjugate of BCPN, and its carcinogenicity has not yet been examined.

*[2] Value in parentheses indicates the urinary excretion (%) of the dose (mean$\pm$SE in three determinations).

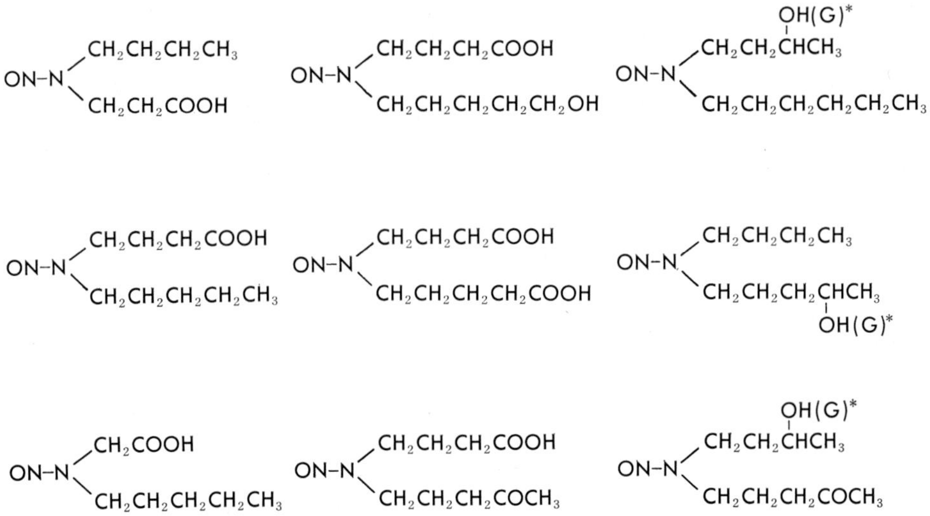

ON–N⟨ CH₂CH₂CH₂CH₃ / CH₂CH₂COOH

ON–N⟨ CH₂CH₂CH₂COOH / CH₂CH₂CH₂CH₂CH₂OH

ON–N⟨ CH₂CH₂CHCH₃ (OH(G)*) / CH₂CH₂CH₂CH₂CH₂CH₃

ON–N⟨ CH₂CH₂CH₂COOH / CH₂CH₂CH₂CH₂CH₃

ON–N⟨ CH₂CH₂CH₂COOH / CH₂CH₂CH₂CH₂COOH

ON–N⟨ CH₂CH₂CH₂CH₃ / CH₂CH₂CH₂CHCH₃ (OH(G)*)

ON–N⟨ CH₂COOH / CH₂CH₂CH₂CH₂CH₃

ON–N⟨ CH₂CH₂CH₂COOH / CH₂CH₂CH₂COCH₃

ON–N⟨ CH₂CH₂CHCH₃ (OH(G)*) / CH₂CH₂CH₂COCH₃

CHART 3. Urinary metabolites of BAN in rats
(G)*: The glucuronide was characterized together with free compound.

The metabolic fate of both symmetric and asymmetric N,N-dialkylnitro-samines in rats was essentially similar to that of DBN. The urinary metabolites were oxidation products with hydroxy-, oxo-, and/or carboxy groups usually in the one alkyl chain formed by ω- and β-oxidation or by (ω-1)-oxidation. Besides (ω-1)-oxidation, (ω-2)- as well as (ω-3)-oxidation was demonstrated with DAN. Moreover, both alkyl chains were attacked in DAN and BAN. Generally, the hydroxyl group was glucuronylated to some extent. All the urinary metabolites of BAN characterized are given in Chart 3 as a typical example (*33*).

The metabolic fate of N-alkyl-N-(ω-hydroxyalkyl)nitrosamines, on the other hand, was substantially the same as that of BBN. The principal metabolites were the corresponding N-alkyl-N-(ω-carboxyalkyl)nitrosamines or their sub-sequent degrdaation products formed by β-oxidation according to the Knoop

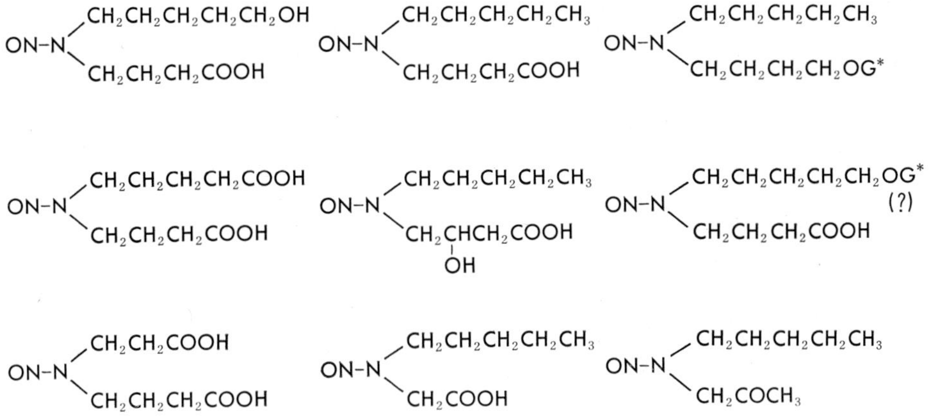

ON–N⟨ CH₂CH₂CH₂CH₂CH₂OH / CH₂CH₂CH₂COOH

ON–N⟨ CH₂CH₂CH₂CH₂CH₃ / CH₂CH₂CH₂COOH

ON–N⟨ CH₂CH₂CH₂CH₂CH₃ / CH₂CH₂CH₂CH₂OG*

ON–N⟨ CH₂CH₂CH₂CH₂COOH / CH₂CH₂CH₂COOH

ON–N⟨ CH₂CH₂CH₂CH₂CH₃ / CH₂CHCH₂COOH (OH)

ON–N⟨ CH₂CH₂CH₂CH₂CH₂OG* (?) / CH₂CH₂CH₂COOH

ON–N⟨ CH₂CH₂COOH / CH₂CH₂CH₂COOH

ON–N⟨ CH₂CH₂CH₂CH₂CH₃ / CH₂COOH

ON–N⟨ CH₂CH₂CH₂CH₂CH₃ / CH₂COCH₃

CHART 4. Urinary metabolites of AHBN in rats
G*: β-D-glucopyranosiduronic acid residue.

M. OKADA ET AL.

TABLE II. Urinary Metabolites, Carcinogenicity, and Target Organs of
N-Nitrosamines Related to BBN and DBN in Rats

Compound	No. of metabolites characterized	Principal metabolite	Carcinogenicity and target organs (oral administration)
DPN (5, 32) $ON-N\begin{cases}CH_2CH_2CH_3\\CH_2CH_2CH_3\end{cases}$	5	$ON-N\begin{cases}CH_2CH_2CH_3\\CH_2CH_2COOH\end{cases}$	+ L, E (9)
DBN (5, 6, 31) $ON-N\begin{cases}CH_2CH_2CH_2CH_3\\CH_2CH_2CH_2CH_3\end{cases}$	7	$ON-N\begin{cases}CH_2CH_2CH_2CH_3\\CH_2CH_2CH_2COOH\end{cases}$	+ L, E, B (9)
DAN (5, 6, 32) $ON-N\begin{cases}CH_2CH_2CH_2CH_2CH_3\\CH_2CH_2CH_2CH_2CH_3\end{cases}$	13	$ON-N\begin{cases}CH_2CH_2CH_2CH_2CH_3\\CH_2CH_2COOH\end{cases}$	+ L (9)
EBN (33) $ON-N\begin{cases}CH_2CH_3\\CH_2CH_2CH_2CH_3\end{cases}$	4	$ON-N\begin{cases}CH_2CH_3\\CH_2CH_2CH_2COOH\end{cases}$	+ E, L (9)
PBN (33) $ON-N\begin{cases}CH_2CH_2CH_3\\CH_2CH_2CH_2CH_3\end{cases}$	7	$ON-N\begin{cases}CH_2CH_2CH_3\\CH_2CH_2CH_2COOH\end{cases}$	+ L, E (28)
BAN (33) $ON-N\begin{cases}CH_2CH_2CH_2CH_3\\CH_2CH_2CH_2CH_2CH_3\end{cases}$	12	$ON-N\begin{cases}CH_2CH_2CH_2CH_3\\CH_2CH_2COOH\end{cases}$	+ L (s.c.) (9)
MHBN (15) $ON-N\begin{cases}CH_3\\CH_2CH_2CH_2CH_2OH\end{cases}$	6	$ON-N\begin{cases}CH_3\\CH_2CH_2CH_2COOH\end{cases}$	+ B (28)
EHBN (15) $ON-N\begin{cases}CH_2CH_3\\CH_2CH_2CH_2CH_2OH\end{cases}$	7	$ON-N\begin{cases}CH_2CH_3\\CH_2CH_2CH_2COOH\end{cases}$	+ B (28)
PHBN (24) $ON-N\begin{cases}CH_2CH_2CH_3\\CH_2CH_2CH_2CH_2OH\end{cases}$	6	$ON-N\begin{cases}CH_2CH_2CH_3\\CH_2CH_2CH_2COOH\end{cases}$	+ B (26)
BBN (23, 31) $ON-N\begin{cases}CH_2CH_2CH_2CH_3\\CH_2CH_2CH_2CH_2OH\end{cases}$	6	$ON-N\begin{cases}CH_2CH_2CH_2CH_3\\CH_2CH_2CH_2COOH\end{cases}$	+ B (8)
AHBN (15) $ON-N\begin{cases}CH_2CH_2CH_2CH_2CH_3\\CH_2CH_2CH_2CH_2OH\end{cases}$	9	$ON-N\begin{cases}CH_2CH_2CH_2CH_2CH_3\\CH_2COOH\end{cases}$	− (28)
BHPN (24) $ON-N\begin{cases}CH_2CH_2CH_2CH_3\\CH_2CH_2CH_2OH\end{cases}$	2	$ON-N\begin{cases}CH_2CH_2CH_2CH_3\\CH_2CH_2COOH\end{cases}$	− (26)
BHEN (24) $ON-N\begin{cases}CH_2CH_2CH_2CH_3\\CH_2CH_2OH\end{cases}$	2	$ON-N\begin{cases}CH_2CH_2CH_2CH_3\\CH_2COOH\end{cases}$	+ L, E (26)

Continued . . .

TABLE II

Compound	No. of metabolites characterized	Principal metabolite	Carcinogenicity and target organs (oral administration)
BCPN (*31*) ON–N$\diagup$CH$_2$CH$_2$CH$_2$CH$_3$ $\diagdown$CH$_2$CH$_2$CH$_2$COOH	5	ON–N$\diagup$CH$_2$CH$_2$CH$_2$CH$_3$ $\diagdown$CH$_2$CH$_2$CH$_2$COOH	+ B (*12*)
BCMN (*25*) ON–N$\diagup$CH$_2$CH$_2$CH$_2$CH$_3$ $\diagdown$CH$_2$COOH	2	ON–N$\diagup$CH$_2$CH$_2$CH$_2$CH$_3$ $\diagdown$CH$_2$COOH	− (*28*)
BOPN (*24*) ON–N$\diagup$CH$_2$CH$_2$CH$_2$CH$_3$ $\diagdown$CH$_2$COCH$_3$	4	ON–N$\diagup$CH$_2$CH$_2$CH$_2$CH$_3$ $\diagdown$CH$_2$CHCH$_3$ $\,$ OG	+ L (*26*)
BHBN-3 (*27*) ON–N$\diagup$CH$_2$CH$_2$CH$_2$CH$_3$ $\diagdown$CH$_2$CH$_2$CHCH$_3$ $\,$ OH	10	ON–N$\diagup$CH$_2$CH$_2$CH$_2$CH$_3$ $\diagdown$CH$_2$CH$_2$CHCH$_3$ $\,$ OG	− (*28*)

L: liver. E: esophagus. B: urinary bladder. G: β-D-glucopyranosiduronic acid residue.

mechanism. Both amyl and 4-hydroxybutyl chains of AHBN underwent metabolic transformations like BAN or DAN. Formation of the glucuronides of the N-alkyl-N-(ω-hydroxyalkyl)nitrosamines as well as of the corresponding carboxylic acids was usually demonstrated. All the urinary metabolites of AHBN characterized are listed in Chart 4 as a model of the N-alkyl-N-(ω-hydroxyalkyl)-nitrosamines and for the comparison with those of BAN (Chart 3) (*15*).

Numbers of the urinary metabolites characterized and the principal one are given in Table II together with those of DBN and BBN (*25*). Carcinogenicity and target organs of the compounds on their oral administration are also indicated in the same table.

Carcinogenic Effect of N-Nitrosamines Related to BBN and DBN in Rats

Carcinogenic effect of the compounds other than those reported by Druckrey *et al.* (*9*) was investigated in rats and the results are summarized in Table III (*12, 26, 28*). Carcinogenicity test was carried out in the following way. A group of 8–10 ACI/N male rats, 10 weeks old, received the compounds in the drinking water. The concentration of BBN as the control was 0.5 mg/ml and those of other compounds were equivalent to BBN. The compounds dissolved in distilled water were administered to rats daily in the dose of 20 ml per rat for 20 weeks, and subsequently the rats were maintained on tap water. Some of the rats of each group were sacrificed after 20 weeks and all the rest after 30 weeks for histological examinations.

DISCUSSION

Among the N-alkyl-N-(ω-hydroxyalkyl)nitrosamines, PHBN, BHPN, and BHEN were investigated first for their metabolism and carcinogenicity in rats. The principal urinary metabolites of these compounds were identified by Okada *et al.* (*24*) as the corresponding carboxylic acids, namely N-propyl-N-(3-carboxypropyl)nitrosamine, N-butyl-N-(2-carboxyethyl)nitrosamine, and BCMN, as shown in Table II, and the urinary excretion was estimated to be about 40, 70, and 40% of the dose, respectively. Bladder cancer was selectively induced by PHBN as did BBN, while BHPN, the counterpart of PHBN, induced neither bladder tumors nor any tumors in other organs in our experimental conditions. BHEN induced hepatoma as well as papilloma in the esophagus, but not bladder cancer (Table III). Consequently, of these three N-alkyl-N-(ω-hydroxyalkyl)-nitrosamines only PHBN which has a 4-hydroxybutyl group like BBN induced bladder cancer in rats. The principal metabolite of PHBN, N-propyl-N-(3-carboxypropyl)nitrosamine, is a homolog of BCPN, the principal urinary metabolite of BBN. It seemed reasonable, therefore, to suppose that an essential structural requirement of the N-nitrosamine for the selective induction of the urinary bladder cancer may be to possess a 4-hydroxybutyl group which undergoes metabolic transformation to a 3-carboxypropyl group, although carcinogenic effect of N-propyl-N-(3-carboxypropyl)nitrosamine on the urinary bladder has not yet been demonstrated.

In order to verify this assumption, metabolism and carcinogenicity of other N-alkyl-N-(4-hydroxybutyl)nitrosamines such as MHBN, EHBN, and AHBN were studied (*15, 28*). The principal urinary metabolites of MHBN and EHBN in rats were again the corresponding carboxylic acids, N-methyl-N-(3-carboxypropyl)nitrosamine and N-ethyl-N-(3-carboxypropyl)nitrosamine (Table II),

TABLE III. Induction of Tumors in Rats with N-Nitrosamines Related to BBN or DBN and Their Histological Findings

Compound	Period for drinking water (weeks) With compound	Period for drinking water (weeks) Without compound	Effective No. of rats	Urinary bladder Papilloma No. (%)	Urinary bladder Cancer No. (%)	Liver Hepatoma No. (%)	Esophagus Papilloma No. (%)
BBN	20	10	7	7 (100)	7 (100)	0	0
BCPN	20	10	5	5 (100)	5 (100)	0	0
MHBN	20	10	5	5 (100)	5 (100)	0	0
EHBN	20	0	10	10 (100)	10 (100)	0	0
PHBN	20	10	7	7 (100)	7 (100)	0	0
AHBN	20	10	7	3 (43)	0	0	0
BHPN	20	10	7	0	0	0	0
BHEN	20	0	9	0	0	8 (90)	9 (100)
BCMN	20	10	7	0	0	0	0
BOPN	10–17	10	5	0	0	3 (60)	0
PBN	16–19	0	9	0	0	9 (100)	6 (67)
BHBN-3	20	10	7	0	0	0	0

and the urinary excretion was found to be *ca.* 42% and *ca.* 48% of the dose, respectively, while that of AHBN was not the corresponding carboxylic acid, N-amyl-N-(3-carboxypropyl)nitrosamine, but N-amyl-N-(carboxymethyl)nitrosamine, a further degradation product of the former formed by metabolic β-oxidation (Chart 4) (*15*). Moreover, the urinary excretion rate of N-amyl-N-(3-carboxypropyl)nitrosamine was estimated to be only about 2%. In accordance with the metabolic studies, MHBN and EHBN selectively induced bladder cancer in rats as BBN and PHBN did, while AHBN induced neither bladder tumors nor any tumors in other organs in our experimental conditions (Table III) (*28*).

The presence of a 4-hydroxybutyl chain in the N-alkyl-N-(ω-hydroxyalkyl)-nitrosamines was thus essential as presumed but not sufficient enough for the selective induction of bladder cancer. As illustrated with AHBN, the metabolic transformation of the 4-hydroxybutyl group was affected by the other alkyl chain, giving a compound with carboxymethyl group (N-nitrososarcosine type) instead of 3-carboxypropyl group as the principal urinary metabolite. On the contrary, with BBN, PHBN, and EHBN, only a small percent of the dose was excreted into the urine as N-nitrososarcosine-type metabolite. Furthermore, simultaneous metabolic changes in the amyl chain of AHBN (Chart 4) might be concerned with its noncarcinogenicity.

In the case of MHBN, nearly 20% of the dose was recovered as urinary N-methyl-N-(carboxymethyl)nitrosamine(=N-nitrososarcosine) besides the principal metabolite having a 3-carboxypropyl group. N-Nitrososarcosine was reported by Druckrey *et al.* (*9*) to induce esophageal tumors only at a very high dose. In this connection, BCMN, a homolog of N-nitrososarcosine, was not carcinogenic in our experimental conditions (Table III) (*28*), whereby more than 50% of the dose was recovered unchanged from the urine. BCMN was first obtained as one of several minor urinary metabolites of BBN or DBN in rats, and then as the principal metabolite of BHEN, as described above. BHEN-induced hepatoma as well as papilloma in the esophagus but did not induce any bladder tumors in spite of excreting a large quantity of BCMN into the urine. Consequently, the carcinogenic effect of BCMN on the urinary bladder had not been anticipated. In relation to the carcinogenicity and target organs of BHEN, it should be noted that N-ethyl-N-(2-hydroxyethyl)nitrosamine also induced hepatoma and papilloma in the esophagus as reported by Druckrey *et al.* (*9*).

It was very surprising as well as interesting that BHPN did not induce any tumors in any organs in our experimental conditions. In view of the finding that a very large amount of N-butyl-N-(2-carboxyethyl)nitrosamine was excreted into the urine after oral administration of BHPN, the principal metabolite or structurally related compounds expressed by N-alkyl-N-(2-carboxyethyl)nitrosamines should not be involved in the induction of bladder cancer in rats. By analogy of the relationship between BBN and BCPN, moreover, carcinogenic action on the urinary bladder may not be expected with N-alkyl-N-(3-hydroxypropyl)nitrosamines. Anyhow, carcinogenicity of other N-alkyl-N-(3-hydroxypropyl)nitrosamines such as N-propyl- and N-ethyl-N-(3-hydroxypropyl)-nitrosamines should be examined.

A considerable significance is to be attached to the metabolism and car-

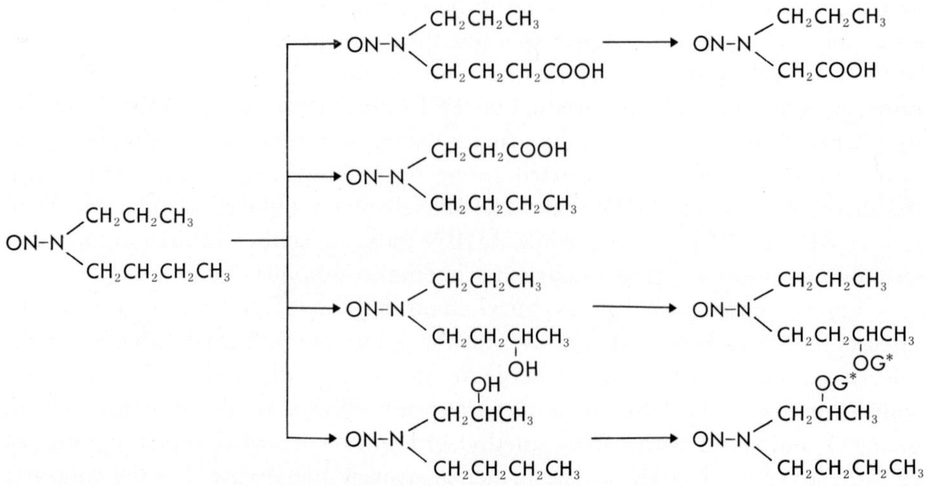

CH₂CH₂CH₃ — represented below as chemical structures:

ON-N⟨ $CH_2CH_2CH_3$ / $CH_2CH_2CH_2COOH$ ⟩ → ON-N⟨ $CH_2CH_2CH_3$ / CH_2COOH ⟩

ON-N⟨ CH_2CH_2COOH / $CH_2CH_2CH_2CH_3$ ⟩

ON-N⟨ $CH_2CH_2CH_3$ / $CH_2CH_2CH_2CH_3$ ⟩

ON-N⟨ $CH_2CH_2CH_3$ / $CH_2CH_2CHCH_3$ (OH) ⟩ → ON-N⟨ $CH_2CH_2CH_3$ / $CH_2CH_2CHCH_3$ (OG*) ⟩

ON-N⟨ CH_2CHCH_3 (OH) / $CH_2CH_2CH_2CH_3$ ⟩ → ON-N⟨ CH_2CHCH_3 (OG*) / $CH_2CH_2CH_2CH_3$ ⟩

CHART 5. Metabolism of PBN in rats
G*: β-D-glucopyranosiduronic acid residue.

cinogenicity of PBN in rats, because ω-oxidation of PBN gives rise to either PHBN or BHPN while (ω-1)-oxidation of the propyl group of PBN results in the formation of N-butyl-N-(2-hydroxypropyl)nitrosamine which is closely related to BOPN and to N-propyl-N-(2-hydroxypropyl)nitrosamine or N-propyl-N-(2-oxopropyl)nitrosamine as described below. Based on its urinary metabolites characterized the metabolic fate of PBN is indicated in Chart 5 (33). The carcinogenicity of PBN, on the other hand, had not been examined by Druckrey et al. (9) who had investigated the carcinogenicity of asymmetric N,N-dialkyl-nitrosamines having a butyl group such as N-methylbutylnitrosamine (MBN) (10), EBN, and BAN in rats. The principal metabolite of PBN was identified as N-propyl-N-(3-carboxypropyl)nitrosamine, and the urinary excretion was estimated to be about 5% of the dose. Nearly similar amount of N-butyl-N-(2-carboxyethyl)nitrosamine was excreted simultaneously into the urine. These metabolites are identical with the principal urinary metabolite of PHBN and BHPN, respectively. Their urinary excretion rate, however, was much higher with PHBN and BHPN than with PBN. In our experimental conditions, PBN induced hepatoma as well as papilloma in the esophagus (Table III) (28). From the metabolic point of view, it seemed likely, therefore, that the urinary excretion of N-propyl-N-(3-carboxypropyl)nitrosamine was not sufficient enough to induce bladder cancer with PBN, resulting in the death of rats due to hepatoma prior to the production of bladder tumors, with whose induction (ω-1)-oxidation of PBN could be concerned. It might be explained analogously that MBN, EBN, and BAN all having a butyl chain did not induce bladder cancer: the urinary excretion of the principal metabolite, N-ethyl-N-(3-carboxypropyl)nitro-samine, was only ca. 3% of the dose with EBN (33) whereas it was about 42% with EHBN which induced bladder cancer. The principal urinary metabolite of BAN (33) was N-butyl-N-(2-carboxyethyl)nitrosamine identical with that of BHPN which did not induce any bladder tumors in spite of excreting a very large

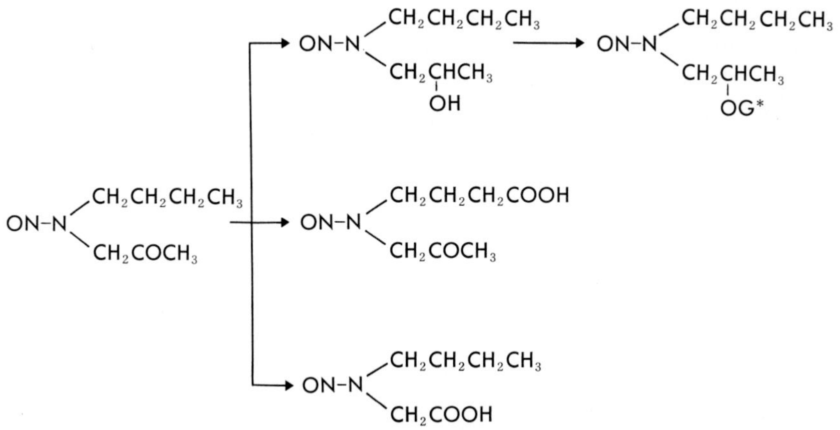

$$\text{ON-N} \begin{cases} CH_2CH_2CH_2CH_3 \\ CH_2CHCH_3 \\ \quad\;\; OH \end{cases} \longrightarrow \text{ON-N} \begin{cases} CH_2CH_2CH_2CH_3 \\ CH_2CHCH_3 \\ \quad\;\; OG^* \end{cases}$$

$$\text{ON-N} \begin{cases} CH_2CH_2CH_2CH_3 \\ CH_2COCH_3 \end{cases} \longrightarrow \text{ON-N} \begin{cases} CH_2CH_2CH_2COOH \\ CH_2COCH_3 \end{cases}$$

$$\text{ON-N} \begin{cases} CH_2CH_2CH_2CH_3 \\ CH_2COOH \end{cases}$$

CHART 6.   Metabolism of BOPN in rats
G*: β-D-glucopyranosiduronic acid residue.

amount of this metabolite into the urine, as described above. In the case of MBN, urinary metabolites were characterized recently by Blattmann *et al.* (7) but their urinary excretion rate was not reported. Probably, the urinary excretion of N-methyl-N-(3-carboxypropyl)nitrosamine was not sufficient for inducing bladder tumors, while its urinary excretion with MHBN was estimated to be about 40% of the dose, or the principal urinary metabolite of MBN was not the 3-carboxy-propyl compound but the carboxymethyl compound, *i.e.*, N-nitrososarcosine.

The metabolic fate of BOPN, a minor urinary metabolite of BBN (Chart 2), in rats is indicated in Chart 6 (24). The principal urinary metabolite was charac-terized as the glucuronide of N-butyl-N-(2-hydroxypropyl)nitrosamine which was also found as a minor urinary metabolite of PBN (Chart 5). Urinary excretion of the glucuronide amounted to about 10% of the dose. BOPN ex-erted a detrimental effect on the liver and induced only hepatomas in rats (26). Carcinogenicity of this type of N-nitrosamine having an oxo group had never been tested (9). Very recently, Althoff *et al.* (2) reported that subcutaneous in-jection of DPN, N-propyl-N-(2-hydroxypropyl)nitrosamine (a metabolite of DPN (5, 32)), and the corresponding oxo compound, N-propyl-N-(2-oxopropyl)-nitrosamine, induced only hepatomas in rats, while oral administration of DPN had been reported to induce hepatomas as well as esophageal tumors (9). The oxo derivative of DPN is a homolog of BOPN and, therefore, its metabolic fate in rats is expected to be essentially similar to that of BOPN.

Among a number of N,N-dialkylnitrosamines only DBN-induced tumors of the urinary bladder as well as tumors of the liver and esophagus by its oral administration (9). Other N,N-dialkylnitrosamines so far examined induced principally tumors in the liver or esophagus. From the metabolic point of view, it seems quite reasonable to assume that ω-oxidation of DBN is responsible for the induction of bladder cancer, while (ω-1)-oxidation of DBN may be respon-sible for inducing tumors of the liver and esophagus. The former part of this assumption was clearly demonstrated with BBN, the ω-hydroxylated derivative of DBN, which selectively induced bladder cancer. In order to substantiate the latter part of the assumption, carcinogenic effect of BHBN-3, the (ω-1)-hydroxylated derivative of DBN, was examined in rats by the oral administration. However, it did not induce any tumors in our experimental conditions, although degenerative changes in the liver were observed histologically in a few rats treated with BHBN-3 (Table III) (28). The principal urinary metabolite of BHBN-3, on the other hand, was found to be its glucuronide and 4 out of 10 metabolites characterized were proved to have a 3-oxobutyl group (27). In the light of the potent carcinogenic effect of BOPN and N-propyl-N-(2-oxopropyl)nitrosamine on the liver carcinogenicity of N-butyl-(3-oxobutyl)nitrosamine should be examined. Moreover, in connection with the β-oxidation* hypothesis concerning metabolic degradation leading to carcinogenesis of the N, N-dialkylnitrosamines, which was developed by Krüger (20–22) with DPN, metabolism and carcinogenicity of N-butyl-N-(2-hydroxybutyl)nitrosamine and N-butyl-N-(2-oxobutyl)nitrosamine should also be investigated, although these compounds have not been detected so far in the urine as metabolites.

Acknowledgments

The authors are grateful to Dr. S. Odashima, National Institute of Hygienic Sciences, Tokyo, and Dr. N. Ito, Cancer Center Institute, Nara Medical University, for histological examinations. They are also indebted to Mr. K. Suzuki for his assistance in animal experiments. Works reported in this paper were supported in part by a Grant-in-Aid for Scientific Research from the Ministry of Education, Japan.

REFERENCES

1. Akagi, G., Akagi, A., and Kimura, M. Tumors of urinary bladder induced by N-butyl-N-butanol-(4)-nitrosamine (BBN) in mice and rats. *Proc. Japan. Cancer Assoc., 29th Annu. Meet.*, 65 (1970) (in Japanese); Akagi, G., Akagi, A., Kimura, M., and Otsuka, H. Comparison of bladder tumors induced in rats and mice with N-butyl-N-(4-hydroxybutyl)nitrosamine. *Gann*, **64**, 331–336 (1973).
2. Althoff, J., Krüger, F. W., Hilfrich, J., Schmähl, D., and Mohr, U. Carcinogenicity of β-hydroxylated dipropylnitrosamine. *Naturwissenshaften*, **60**, 55 (1973).
3. Bertram, J. S. and Craig, A. W. Induction of bladder tumors in mice with dibutylnitrosamine. *Brit. J. Cancer*, **24**, 352–359 (1970).
4. Bertram, J. S. and Craig, A. W. Specific induction of bladder cancer in mice by butyl(4-hydroxybutyl)nitrosamine and the effects of hormonal modifications on the sex difference in response. *Eur. J. Cancer*, **8**, 587–594 (1972).
5. Blattmann, L. and Preussmann, R. Struktur von Metaboliten carcinogener Dialkylnitrosamine im Rattenurin. *Z. Krebsforsch.*, **79**, 3–5 (1973).
6. Blattmann, L. and Preussmann, R. Biotransformation von carcinogenen Dialkylnitrosaminen. Weitere Urinmetaboliten von Di-*n*-butyl- und Di-*n*-pentyl-nitrosamin. *Z. Krebsforsch.*, in press.
7. Blattmann, L., Joswig, N., and Preussmann, R. Struktur von Metaboliten des carcinogenen Methyl-*n*-butyl-nitrosamins im Rattenurin. *Z. Krebsforsch.*, in press.
8. Druckrey, H., Preussmann, R., Ivankovic, S., Schmidt, C. H., Mennel, H. D.,

---

* β-Oxidation means (ω-1)-oxidation in DPN, while it means (ω-2)-oxidation with DBN.

and Stahl, K. W. Selektive Erzeugung von Blasenkrebs an Ratten durch Dibutyl- und N-Butyl-N-butanol-(4)-nitrosamin. *Z. Krebsforsch.*, **66**, 280–290 (1964).

9. Druckrey, H., Preussmann, R., Ivankovic, S., and Schmähl, D. Organotrope carcinogene Wirkungen bei 65 verschiedenen N-Nitroso-Verbindungen an BD-Ratten. *Z. Krebsforsch.*, **69**, 103–201 (1967).

10. Druckrey, H., Landschütz, Ch., and Preussmann, R. Oesophagus-Carcinome nach Inhalation von Methyl-butyl-nitrosamin (MBNA) an Ratten. *Z. Krebsforsch.*, **71**, 135–139 (1968).

11. Eisenbrand, G. and Preussmann, R. Eine neue Methode zur kolorimetrischen Bestimmung von Nitrosaminen nach Spaltung der N-Nitrosogruppe mit Bromwasserstoff in Eisessig. *Arzneimittel-Forschung*, **20**, 1513–1517 (1970).

12. Hashimoto, Y., Suzuki, E., and Okada, M. Induction of urinary bladder tumors in ACI/N rats by butyl(3-carboxypropyl)nitrosamine, a major urinary metabolite of butyl(4-hydroxybutyl)nitrosamine. *Gann*, **63**, 637–638 (1972).

13. Hashimoto, Y., Kurashima, C., and Okada, M. Metabolic transformation of a urinary bladder carcinogen butyl(4-hydroxybutyl)nitrosamine and its analogs *in vitro*. *Proc. Japan. Cancer Assoc., 32nd Annu. Meet.*, 171 (1973) (in Japanese).

14. Hashimoto, Y., Suzuki, K., and Okada, M. Induction of urinary bladder tumors by intravesicular instillation of butyl(4-hydroxybutyl)nitrosamine and its principal urinary metabolite, butyl(3-carboxypropyl)nitrosamine in rats. *Gann*, **65**, 69–73 (1974).

15. Iiyoshi, M. and Okada, M. Metabolism of N-methyl-N-(4-hydroxybutyl)nitrosamine, N-ethyl-N-(4-hydroxybutyl)nitrosamine and N-*n*-amyl-N-(4-hydroxybutyl)nitrosamine in the rat. *Abstr. 94th Annu. Meet., Pharm. Soc. Japan*, **III**, 20 (1974) (in Japanese).

16. Ito, N., Hiasa, Y., Tamai, A., Okajima, E., and Kitamura, H. Histogenesis of urinary bladder tumors induced by N-butyl-N-(4-hydroxybutyl)nitrosamine in rats. *Gann*, **60**, 401–410 (1969).

17. Ito, N., Makiura, S., Yokota, Y., Kamamoto, Y., Hiasa, Y., and Sugihara, S. Effect of unilateral ureter ligation on development of tumors in the urinary system of rats treated with N-butyl-N-(4-hydroxybutyl)nitrosamine. *Gann*, **62**, 359–365 (1971).

18. Ito, N., Matayoshi, K., Arai, M., Yoshioka, Y., Kamamoto, Y., Makiura, S., and Sugihara, S. Effect of various factors on induction of urinary bladder tumors in animals by N-butyl-N-(4-hydroxybutyl)nitrosamine. *Gann*, **64**, 151–159 (1973).

19. Ivankovic, S. and Bücheler, J. Leber- und Blasen-Carcinome beim Meerschweinchen nach Di-*n*-butylnitrosamin. *Z. Krebsforsch.*, **71**, 183–185 (1968).

20. Krüger, F. W. Metabolismus von Nitrosaminen *in vivo*. I. Über die β-Oxidation aliphatischer Di-*n*-alkylnitrosamine: Die Bildung von 7-Methylguanin neben 7-Propyl-bez. 7-Butylguanin nach Applikation von Di-*n*-propyl- oder Di-*n*-butylnitrosamin. *Z. Krebsforsch.*, **76**, 145–154 (1971).

21. Krüger, F. W. Metabolism of nitrosamines *in vivo*. II. On the methylation of nucleic acids by aliphatic di-*n*-alkyl-nitrosamines *in vivo*, caused by β-oxidation: The increased formation of 7-methylguanine after application of β-hydroxypropyl-propyl-nitrosamine compared to that after application of di-*n*-propyl-nitrosamine. *Z. Krebsforsch.*, **79**, 90–97 (1973).

22. Krüger, F. W. and Bertram, B. Metabolism of nitrosamines *in vivo*. III. On the methylation of nucleic acids by aliphatic di-*n*-alkyl-nitrosamines *in vivo* resulting from β-oxidation: The formation of 7-methylguanine after application of 2-oxo-

propyl-nitrosamine and methyl-propyl-nitrosamine. *Z. Krebsforsch.*, **80**, 189–196 (1973).

23. Okada, M. and Suzuki, E. Metabolism of butyl(4-hydroxybutyl)nitrosamine in rats. *Gann*, **63**, 391–392 (1972).

24. Okada, M., Suzuki, E., and Aoki, J. Metabolism and carcinogenicity of N-nitrosamines related to butyl(4-hydroxybutyl)nitrosamine in the rat. *Proc. Japan. Cancer Assoc., 32nd Annu. Meet.*, 136 (1973) (in Japanese).

25. Okada, M., Suzuki, E., Aoki, J., Iiyoshi, M., Kurashima, C., Miyajima, K., Suzuki, K., and Hashimoto, Y. Studies on the correlation of structure and metabolism with organotropic carcinogenicity to the urinary bladder of N, N-dialkyl-nitrosamines. *Proc. 5th Symp. on Drug Metabolism and Action*, 89–92 (1973) (in Japanese).

26. Okada, M. and Hashimoto, Y. Carcinogenic effect of N-nitrosamines related to butyl(4-hydroxybutyl)nitrosamine in ACI/N rats, with special reference to induction of urinary bladder tumors. *Gann*, **65**, 13–19 (1974).

27. Okada, M. and Suzuki, E. Unpublished.

28. Okada, M. and Hashimoto, Y. Unpublished.

29. Okajima, E., Hiramatsu, T., Motomiya, Y., Iriya, K., Ijuin, M., Kondo, T., Hirao, Y., and Matsushima, S. Studies on the development of urinary bladder tumors in dogs treated with N-nitrosodibutylamine (DBN) and N-butyl-N-(4-hydroxybutyl)nitrosamine (BBN). *Proc. Japan. Cancer Assoc., 31st Annu. Meet.*, 10 (1972) (in Japanese).

30. Okajima, E., Hiramatsu, T., Motomiya, Y., Iriya, K., Ijuin, M., Kondo, T., Hirao, Y., Matsushima, S., Ikuma, S., Yamada, K., and Sugihara, S. Development of urinary bladder tumors in dogs induced by N-nitrosodibutylamine (DBN) and N-butyl-N-(4-hydroxybutyl)nitrosamine (BBN). *Proc. Japan. Cancer Assoc., 32nd Annu. Meet.*, 134 (1973) (in Japanese).

31. Suzuki, E., Aoki, J., and Okada, M. Metabolism of butyl(4-hydroxybutyl)nitrosamine (BBN) and dibutylnitrosamine (DBN). *Proc. Japan. Cancer Assoc., 31st Annu. Meet.*, 9 (1972) (in Japanese).

32. Suzuki, E., Aoki, J., and Okada, M. Metabolism of N, N-di-*n*-propylnitrosamine and N, N-di-*n*-amylnitrosamine in the rat. *Abstr. 93rd Annu. Meet., Pharm. Soc. Japan*, **III**, 208 (1973) (in Japanese).

33. Suzuki, E., Aoki, J., Sugano, R., and Okada, M. Metabolism of N-ethyl-N-*n*-butylnitrosamine, N-*n*-propyl-N-*n*-butylnitrosamine and N-*n*-butyl-N-*n*-amyl-nitrosamine in the rat. *Abstr. 94th Annu. Meet., Pharm. Soc. Japan*, **III**, 20 (1974) (in Japanese).

34. Wood, M., Flaks, A., and Clayson, D. B. The carcinogenic activity of dibutyl-nitrosamine in IF × C57 mice. *Eur. J. Cancer*, **6**, 433–440 (1970).

ENVIRONMENTAL CARCINOGENESIS

GANN Monograph on Cancer Research 17, 179–187 (1975)

CIRCULATION OF CARCINOGENIC SUBSTANCES IN THE ENVIRONMENT: FROM LABORATORY EXPERIMENTS TO FIELD INVESTIGATIONS

L. M. Shabad

Department of Carcinogenic Agents, The Institute of Experimental and Clinical Oncology*

During the last 20 years the author and his collaborators detected some sources of carcinogenic substances, evaluated the level of these substances in the environment, and elaborated some measures of prevention. Some new facts were discovered, which are described in this paper. A peculiar circulation of blastomogenic substances is noted; from air to soil and water, then to the vegetation, with the vegetables into fodder and (directly or indirectly) to the food. On the other hand, some carcinogenic substances can be destroyed by environmental factors, for example, by soil microorganisms.

The contribution of the Japanese school to cancer research is especially great. The modern era of experimental oncology had its beginning with the pioneer work of Yamagiwa and Ichikawa who opened the way to the systematic induction of skin cancer in rabbit ear by painting it with coal tar (*30*). Applied by Tsutsui (1918) to mice, this method has received worldwide recognition. The study of carcinogenicity of different tar fractions led to the discovery of chemically pure carcinogenic hydrocarbons (*5*). At about the same time, chemically pure carcinogens were discovered by Japanese investigators in another class of substances. Thus, at the beginning of 1930s metaplasia and epithelial growth induced by *o*-aminoazotoluene (OAT) in the thyroid were observed by Yoshida. In 1935, Sasaki and Yoshida published their vast work on the induction of liver tumors in rats with OAT (*18*). These results were confirmed in different laboratories as well as in our studies by Morosenskaja (1936–1938). Finally, in 1937 the hepatotropic carcinogenic action of another aminoazo dye, 4-dimethylaminoazobenzene (DAB), was discovered by Kinosita (*10*).

The first results of the work with chemical carcinogens seemed to be purely of theoretical interest, but considering their importance, from the beginning they had implications beyond the framework of laboratory studies. With discovery of the carcinogenic properties of some tars comes the problem of their hazards for the workers involved in highway construction or in coke chemical plants and oil refineries. It must be emphasized that various tars have different carcinogenicity, and in order to prevent cancer some of them can be substituted for others, as was shown for U.S.S.R. shale tars by Larionov *et al.* (*13*).

The discovery of the carcinogenicity of some aminoazo compounds (*10, 18*)

---

* Novopeecheneja-str., 3 ap., 64 Moscow 125057, U.S.S.R.

suggested questions about the use of these substances as dyes in the food industry. The technical name of DAB was Butter Yellow in English or Buttergelb in German, and this substance was used to color not only butter, but margarine, flour, macaroni, *etc.*

Lung Cancer and Polycyclic Aromatic Hydrocarbons (PAH)

In spite of all this, for many years the data on chemical carcinogens were underestimated by epidemiologists and hygienists. The situation has changed only during the last 20–25 years. This change was incited by the enormous increase of lung cancer during the last 50 years. The sad priority in the rate of lung cancer belonged to England, which was the first industrialized country. Lung cancer morbidity is higher in cities than in villages and in big cities than in small towns. As was shown by the statistics from the world-famous Japanese epidemiologist Segi (*19*), the incidence of lung cancer continues to increase. It must be pointed out that the lung cancer rate is higher in the cohorts of persons born later; those who reached 60 years in 1960 or 1970 have much more chance to have this illness than those who reached this age in 1920 or 1930.

All these observations show that at least one of the causes of lung cancer is the inhalation of polluted atmospheric air. The fact that the lung cancer rate is so high in heavy cigarette smokers does not contradict this.

Thus, the attention of investigators was called to the search for carcinogens in inhaled air.

PAH in the Air

Such investigations were carried out on a large scale only after spectral fluorescent methods were developed that permitted evaluation of PAH and especially a powerful carcinogenic compound—benzo(a)pyrene (BP)—in air pollution. Such work was first undertaken in 1949 in the U.S.S.R. by Gurinov *et al.* (*8*). With similar methods, BP was found in the atmospheric pollution of London, England (*29*), and Los Angeles, in the U.S.A. (*12*). After these first communications, a great number of analogous investigations were performed in many cities in various countries. For example, in 1959, the results of 250 investigations of the air pollution in 18 cities and towns of the U.S.S.R. were published (*23*). In the following years similar work was carried out in some large cities of various countries. In Tokyo, for example, investigations of the atmospheric air are performed by special sanitary centers in various districts of this enormous city.

The methods of selecting samples from atmospheric pollution and of their physical and chemical investigation were systematically improved. Aspiration is the main way of obtaining air pollutants but sedimentation and especially snow samples are also used. The spectral-fluorescent analysis used in our laboratory is based on the so-called Shpolski effect, *i.e.*, on the appearance of the quasilinear spectra of PAH in normal paraffin solutions by Kelvin temperature (77°K). These methods make it possible to obtain not only qualitative but also quantitative evaluation of PAH.

The main sources of PAH in air pollution are (1) heating systems, (2) industrial plants, especially coke-chemical and oil refining factories, and (3) exhausts of internal combustion engines. The importance of the last source is becoming more prominent because of the increase of the number of automobile cars. Recently a new source of carcinogenic air pollution was discovered; aircraft engines, that is, plane exhausts (25).

The maximal quantity of PAH and especially of BP was found in the air pollution of big cities and industrialized areas. In the north, more PAH and BP were registered in winter than in summer, this being due to the heating systems. But recently these seasonal differences have leveled off as shown by our work in Berlin, G.D.R. (21), because of the increasing role of automobile exhaust in the pollution of the atmosphere.

The wide distribution of PAH and especially of BP far from the sources of their exhaust must be emphasized. In our investigations, for example, an increased level of these substances was found at 15–25 km from big coke-chemical or oil refining factories. However, the level of carcinogens depends also on the capacity and technology of the plant, on the wind direction, etc.

Nevertheless, the exhausts of industrial plants and heating systems are in principle local ones, but the exhaust gases of automobiles and especially those of aircraft engines are polluting the atmosphere at an enormous distance. It is not surprising, therefore, that the contamination of the environment with carcinogenic substances increases from year to year and has reached global significance.

PAH in the Soil

What is the fate of the carcinogenic PAH in air pollution? A part of it can probably be destroyed by ultraviolet rays and by ozone. But the major part must sediment on the earth with rain and snow, and pollute the soil. BP was discovered in samples of soil in a large city for the first time in 1959 by Shabad and Dikun (23). These data were confirmed in the following years in many other countries; U.S.A. (2), F.R.G. (3), France (14), and Czechoslovakia (31). Systematic investigations of PAH and especially of BP content in soil samples from various areas of the U.S.S.R. were performed in our laboratory during the last 10 years.

The highest levels of BP and other PAH have been found in soil samples from the territory of an oil refining plant. Its level there reached 200 mg/kg of dried soil. This was 400–500 times more than in the soil of a habitation area of a large city. In the old districts of the city the level of BP in the soil was 2–3 times higher than in the new ones. Thus, this substance probably accumulates in the soil. On the other hand, the quantity of BP in the soil can decrease also, showing seasonal fluctuations; at the end of summer its level is, as a rule, less than in the middle of winter. Not only seasonal variations of air pollution are reflected here. The BP content of the soil depends on other processes that take place in the soil itself.

In order to fight soil erosion caused by wind it was proposed to cover fields in some districts of the U.S.S.R. with shale tars. These tars, of course, contain

PAH. The level of BP was 80–100 mg/kg. Skin painting with these tars induced papillomas and carcinomas in mice. Soil samples taken within various intervals after the tar treatment (1,500 kg/hr) were studied. Many hundreds of micrograms of BP/kg of dried soil were recorded in the first week after treatment, but the content of this substance during the following months decreased. Not only the passage of BP into the deep layers of the soil was recorded, but also its true disappearance. About 12–15 months after the tarring, the amount of BP returned to its normal level, *i.e.*, to 5–10 μg/kg.

The decrease of BP in the soil can be the consequence of its transition to plants. Such a possibility was proved in direct experiments in our laboratory by Shcherbak (*27, 28*). Flowers were cultivated in a soil heavily polluted with BP, and its presence was proved by spectral-fluorescent analyses. Recently we observed BP transition from polluted soil into some agricultural plants and crops (*11, 12*). Differences between various plants must be emphasized. For example, BP is accumulated by sunflower and especially by sunflower seeds but not by the cotton plant or cereals; its content is much higher in potatoes than in pumpkins, *etc.*

In the upper layers of the soil, BP can be destroyed by ultraviolet rays, and from the lower layers it can pass to water. But the main cause of the disappearance of BP from the soil is the activity of some soil microorganisms. Recently we selected bacteria from the soil samples and obtained cultures, for example, *B. sphericus*, that are able to destroy BP (*16, 17*). This proved both in bacterial cultures in which BP was added and in soil samples highly polluted with BP in which bacteria cultures were introduced. Our work showed that the flora of various kinds of soil and sewage also possess the capacity of destroying BP, and this process can be increased by addition of the cultivated bacteria. The mechanism of BP degradation consists probably in the induction by this substance of oxidative enzymes in the bacteria. The endmetabolites are not carcinogenic; they were found to induce no tumors in mice injected subcutaneously.

Many hundreds of soil samples from various districts of the U.S.S.R. were analyzed in our laboratory, and all of them contained BP. But in the majority of the samples taken in agricultural areas, far from cities, industrial plants, and highways, the quantity of BP was not more than 1–2 μg/kg of dried soil and in rare cases, 5–10 μg/kg. This level of BP pollution is the consequence of its spreading all over the world from the sources and especially from the exhaust gases of the aircraft engines. This level of BP could be recorded as the background of this substance in the environment. Higher levels indicate local sources of pollution, which must be detected in each case.

PAH in the Water and Sea Food

In some cases carcinogenic PAH, and especially BP, can pass from soil to water. But the most serious sources of carcinogenic water pollution are (1) industrial sewage, especially of coke-chemical and oil refining plants, (2) internal combustion engines of ships and boats, and (3) sewage of big cities. In addition, bodies of water and especially seas and oceans can be polluted immediately by oil and oil products from tankers. Sedimentation of carcinogens from air pollution could also play a role.

The first suggestions of ocean pollution with carcinogenic PAH were the observations of Shimkin *et al.* (*25*) who found them in barnacles and of Cahnman and Kuratsune (*4*) who found BP in oysters. The latter study proves the possibility of the contamination of sea food with carcinogens. In recent years much attention has been paid by Kuratsune to the study of carcinogenic ingredients in some other kinds of food.

In the sewage of shale processing, oil refining, and coke-chemical plants, large quantities of PAH and especially of BP can be found, as shown by systematic investigations by Soviet authors, beginning in 1958 (G. M. Gortalum, P. P. Dikun, A. P. Ilnitzki, L. M. Shabad, N. Ja. Janysheva *et al.*). These substances can be spread over great distance, far from their sources, by rivers and other bodies of water. For example, the BP pollution of water, bottom sediments, and aquatic plants from a river downstream from a big city was found to be much heavier than upstream (*24*). In water samples upstream it was 0.001 μg/liter, and downstream, 0.04, *i.e.*, 40 times more, and in the aquatic plants and bottom sediments it was even 200 times more.

Motorboats play an important role in the pollution of water bodies with carcinogenic PAH. It was shown in our laboratory (*9*) that during 1 hr of work a hanging motor of a boat gives out in the water about 500 μg of BP. A carburetor motor exhausts 10 times more BP than a diesel engine. Mouse skin was painted with benzene extracts of soot from boat motors, and as a result practically all animals developed papillomas and then carcinomas.

A large number of investigations of water in the U.S.S.R. (*9*) showed that in industrial areas they are much more polluted with BP than in agricultural areas. In the latter and aquatic plants, little quantities of BP, not more than 1–2 μg/kg, can be found, and this is a peculiar background of this substance.

The investigations carried out by Gortalum (*7*) on the seacoasts of the U.S.S.R. have shown that BP content in sand, algae, mollusks, and fish can vary. It is of interest that the highest levels of BP were found in jellyfish (71.7 μg/kg of dried sample). These results are analogous to the data of French authors (*15*) who found especially large quantities of BP in midias and oysters.

This short paper cannot survey all the investigations devoted to the carcinogenic pollution of the human environment and especially of food products. The results of our work in this field were recently summarized in a book (*20*). The facts recorded here seem to be sufficient to outline a peculiar circulation of carcinogenic substances and especially of PAH in the human environment. Some sources pour them out into the atmospheric air, from which they are sedimented and pollute the soil and then can pass to the plants and, consequently, to fodder and food. In the process of circulation, under some conditions they can accumulate and under others, undergo a degradation and be destroyed. This is the general scheme of carcinogen circulation.

At the same time, we observed in each sphere of the environment a separate circulation of carcinogens governed by distinct rules. In the soil, for example, the carcinogens penetrate into deep layers and can reach the subsoil waters.

Passing to the plants they can accumulate in them in various quantities depending on the species of the plant and, perhaps, on the character of the soil. It is
possible that in the plants the carcinogens can undergo degradation, but if not,
they return to the soil with the faded plants. Finally, simultaneously with accumulation of carcinogens, an opposite process takes place; the decrease of the
quantity of carcinogens in the soil due to their degradation. In the upper layers
of the soil this depends on the ultraviolet rays of the sun. But the main role in
the degradation of carcinogens is played by soil bacteria.

A peculiar circulation of BP occurs also in bodies of water. Carcinogens can
accumulate in the bottom sediments, and in the aquatic plants, they can also be
suspended or to some extent dissolved in water. From there they can reach living
organisms, microplankton, mollusks, fish, *etc*. From all these objects they
can get into food. Together with accumulation, a reduction of the quantity of
carcinogens in water takes place due to the degradation of these substances by
microorganisms and in the organisms of higher plants and animals.

Degradation of PAH

The possibility of PAH and BP degradation by soil microorganisms shown
in our investigations demonstrates a very interesting and promising natural
phenomenon, which could occur in human organisms as well.

The study of the BP level in the atmosphere and in the inhaled air made it
possible for many authors (and for us as well) to calculate the quantity of BP
that could get into the human lungs during the whole of man's life. This quantity reaches 12–16 mg and perhaps can be higher. However, we found in the lung
tissue of inhabitants of a big city 1,000 times less BP than was expected from the
calculated quantity (*23*). Human embryo fibroblast monolayers were found to
destroy about 50% of BP introduced in the culture during 3 days (*1*). After feeding cows with fodder containing BP (about 10 mg daily) this substance can be
detected in small amounts in the milk, but was not found in the muscles (meat)
of these animals, neither was it found in the muscles of pigs, rabbits, and fowl
(*6*). It is evident that BP can be metabolized and disappears from the human
and animal organisms.

The processes of the degradation of carcinogenic substances depend on many
factors, but the most important one is probably the quantity. An extremely important fact, proved by numerous observations on occupational cancers in man
and by all the data of experimental oncology, is the dose-effect relationship in
carcinogenesis. A decrease of the dose leads to the decrease of the number of
induced tumors and to the delay of their appearance. On this basis, the possibility
of decreasing the level of carcinogens in the human environment seems to be
quite feasible. The question arises of hygienic limits for carcinogenic substances
in various spheres of the environment.

The problem of maximum allowable concentration (MAC) for carcinogens
has a long history. In the first period, for about 10 years (1956–1966), the possibility of establishing them was unanimously denied, but recently the opinion
has changed. The main cause of this change is the ubiquitous presence of some

carcinogens in the environment. The results of our investigations presented above showed the global distribution of the carcinogenic PAH and especially of BP and the formation of a peculiar background of these substances. The recent data on the naturally occurring carcinogens, for example, aflatoxins, also be borne in mind. The results obtained in our laboratory indicated that BP is "irremediable" in the environment and in this case the second part of the FAO-WHO Recommendations (Technical Reports, 1961, N 220, p. 23, Summary, point 10) must be applied: "Nevertheless, the Committee points out that permissible levels for some carcinogenic agents are unavoidable, as, for example, with naturally occurring substances or *carcinogens of ubiquitous distribution*" (my italics).

DISCUSSION

We are firmly convinced that the tolerance level must be elaborated for each carcinogenic substance separately. This standardization must be started from the most studied PAH, first of all with BP, which should be regarded as an indicator of other PAH. After many investigations, calculations, and discussions, the following limits for BP were proposed in the U.S.S.R.: 15 μg/100 m³ for the air of industrial working zones (legislated by the Ministry of Health, November, 1972) and 0.1 μg/100 m³ in the atmospheric air (legislated by the Ministry of Health, February, 1973).

These first suggestions need further development. Hygienic limits can be determined on the basis of (1) studies of carcinogen distribution and circulation in the environment, (2) epidemiological data and studies on occupational tumors, and (3) experimental investigations of dose-response relationship.

The above-mentioned facts and the associated problems show that the study of carcinogenic substances, starting with the classic work of Yamagiwa and Ichikawa, has come a long way from single and isolated laboratory experiments in animals to wide hygienic investigations that put forward and solve problems in which all humanity is involved. In the pollution of the environment carcinogenic substances are present. Decreasing the amount and preventing contact with them are steps toward cancer prevention.

REFERENCES

1. Andrianov, L. A., Belitsky, G. A., and Vasiliev, Yu. M. The interactions of carcinogenic hydrocarbons with normal and tumor cells. Moscow (1971) (in Russian).
2. Blumer, M. Benzpyrenes in soil. *Science*, **134**, 414 (1961).
3. Borneff, I. and Kunte, H. Kanzerogene Substanzen in Wasser und Boden. XI. Polyzyklische aromatische Kohlenwasserstoffe im Walderde. *Arch. Hyg. Bakteriol.*, **146**, 430 (1962).
4. Cahnman, H. and Kuratsune, M. Determination of polycyclic aromatic hydrocarbons in oysters collected in polluted water. *Ann. Chem.*, **29**, 1312 (1957).
5. Cook, J. W., Hieger, I., Kennaway, E. L., and Mayneord, W. V. The production of cancer by pure hydrocarbons. *Proc. Roy. Soc. Biol.*, **111**, 455 (1932).
6. Gorelova, N. D. and Cherepanova, A. I. On the possibility of accumulation of 3, 4-benzopyrene in tissues and organs of cows and calves, as well as in milk in

case of presence of this carcinogen in fodder. *Vopr. Onkol.*, **16**, 69 (1970) (in Russian).

7. Gortalum, G. M. On the circulation of polycyclic aromatic hydrocarbons in the seas. *In* "Problems of Prevention of the Pollution of Human Environment with Carcinogenic Substances," Tallinn, pp. 87–91 (1972) (in Russian).

8. Gurinov, B. P., Zore, V. A., Iljina, A. A., and Shabad, L. M. On content of polycyclic aromatic hydrocarbons in atmospheric pollutions and smoke exhausts. *Gygiena Sanit.*, **2**, 10–16 (1953) (in Russian).

9. Iljnitsky, A. P., Klubkov, V. G., and Shabad, L. M. Navigation as one of sources of pollution of water basins by carcinogenic hydrocarbons. *Vopr. Onkol.*, **18** (1), 49–54 (1972) (in Russian).

10. Kinosita, R. Studies on the carcinogenic chemical substances. *Nippon Byōri Gakkai Kaishi (Trans. Japan. Pathol. Soc.)*, **27**, 665 (1937) (in Japanese).

11. Cohan, J. L. The fate of benz(a)pyrene by treatment of the cotton plant fields by nerosine. *Khlopkovodstvo*, **11**, 39 (1971) (in Russian).

12. Kotin, P., Falk, H. L., Mader, P., and Thomas, M. Aromatic hydrocarbons. 1. Presence in the Los Angeles atmosphere and the carcinogenicity of atmospheric extracts. *Arch. Ind. Hyg. Occup. Med.*, **9**, 153 (1954).

13. Larionov, L. F., Soboleva, N. G., and Shabad, L. M. On the carcinogenic action of some shale tars. *Vestn. Rentgen.*, **13**, 131 (1934) (in Russian).

14. Mallet, L. and Héros, M. Polution des terres végétales par les hydrocarbures polybenzéniques du type benzo-3, 4-pyrene. *C. R. Acad. Sci.*, **254**, 953 (1962).

15. Mallet, L. and Priou, M. L. Sur la rétention des hydrocarbures polybenzéniques du type benzo-3, 4-pyrene par les sédiments, la faune et la flore marines de la baie de Saint-Malo. *C.R. Acad. Sci.*, **264**, 969 (1967).

16. Poglasova, M. N., Fedoseeva, G. E., and Chesina, A. J. On possible benz(a) pyrene metabolism by soil bacteria. *Dokl. Akad. Nauk SSSR*, **198**, 1211 (1971) (in Russian).

17. Poglasova, M. N., Chesina, A. J., and Fedoseeva, G. E. On the degradation of benz(a)pyrene by microorganisms in sewage. *Dokl. Akad. Nauk SSSR*, **204**, 222 (1972) (in Russian).

18. Sasaki, T. and Yoshida, T. Experimentelle Erzeugung des Lebercarcinoma durch Fütterung mit *o*-Aminoazotoluol. *Arch. Pathol. Anat. Physiol.*, **295**, 175 (1935).

19. Segi, M. Cancer mortality for selected sites in 24 countries. No. 5. Tohoku Univ. School of Medicine, Sendai (1969).

20. Shabad, L. M. "On the Circulation of Carcinogens in the Environment," Medizina, Moscow, pp. 367 (1973).

21. Shabad, L. M., Chesina, A. J., and Wettig, K. Lufthygiene-Krebsprophylaxe. *Wiss. Fortsch.*, **23**, 386 (1973).

22. Shabad, L. M. and Cohan, J. L. The contents of benzo(a)pyrene in some crops. *Arch. Geschwulstforsch.*, **40**, 237 (1972).

23. Shabad, L. M. and Dikun, P. P. "Air Pollution by Carcinogenic Hydrocarbon—Benzo(a)pyrene," Medgiz, Moscow/Leningrad, pp. 218 (1959) (in Russian).

24. Shabad, L. M. and Iljnitsky, A. P. The aspects of the problem of water pollution with carcinogenic substances. *Gygiena Sanit.*, **8**, 84 (1970) (in Russian).

25. Shabad, L. M. and Smirnov, G. A. 3,4-Benzpyrene containing in the soot and exhaust gases of turbo-jet and turbo-prop engines. *Gygiena Sanit.*, **2**, 98–99 (1969) (in Russian).

26. Shimkin, M. B., Keneth, B., and Zechmeister, L. An instance of the occurrence of carcinogenic substances in certain barnacles. *Science*, **113**, 650 (1951).

27. Shcherbak, N. P. and Cohan, J. L. Investigation of benz(a)pyrene in the soil of different industrialized districts. *Trans. Perm Med. Inst.* (1970).

28. Shcherback, N. P. and Cohan, J. L. Carcinogenic substances in soil and in plants. *In* "Carcinogenic Substances in the Environment" (1971).

29. Waller, R. The benzpyrene of town air. *Brit. J. Cancer*, **6**, 8 (1952).

30. Yamagiwa, K. and Ichikawa, K. *Mitt. Mediz. Fakultät. Kaiserlich Universität Tokyo*, **15**, 295 (1916).

31. Zdrazil, J. and Picha, F. The occurrence of the carcinogenic compounds 3,4-benzpyrene and arsenic in the soil. *Neoplasma*, **13**, 49 (1966).

GANN Monograph on Cancer Research 17, 189-204 (1975)

ONCOGENICITY OF CYCASIN AND METHYLAZOXYMETHANOL

Gert L. Laqueur and Maria Spatz

*Laboratory of Experimental Pathology, National Institute of Arthritis, Metabolism and Digestive Diseases, and Laboratory of Neuropathology and Neuroanatomical Sciences, National Institute of Neurological Diseases and Stroke, National Institutes of Health[*1]*

Toxic properties of the naturally occurring aliphatic azoxyglycosides which include the β-glucoside cycasin have been recognized for several decades. Their ability to also induce cancer was established more recently in our laboratory when tumors developed in liver, kidneys, and colon as single or multiple primary neoplasms in rats fed cycasin. The paper reviews these studies and those of others which indicated that the oncogenic effect of cycasin depended on enzymatic hydrolysis of the azoxyglycoside to the aglycone, methylazoxymethanol (MAM), and the respective sugar. MAM was, therefore, the proximate oncogen of cycasin.

The circumstances under which cycasin hydrolysis occurs *in vivo* thus become of central importance to cycasin oncogenesis. They are different in neonatal and postweanling rodents and the pertinent investigations are cited in greater detail. In postweanling rats, cycasin hydrolysis and oncogenicity depend (1) on enteric administration and (2) on an intestinal microflora providing the enzymes for the hydrolysis of cycasin. In neonatal and very young rats, parenteral injections of cycasin result in subsequent tumor development, and enzymic activity can be demonstrated in extracts of various tissues including skin, small intestines, liver, and kidneys.

In addition to rats, oncogenic effects of cycasin and MAM have been demonstrated in mice, guinea pigs, and hamsters. In general, predominant tumor sites are dependent on the duration of exposure and are influenced by age and sex, and by the species.

MAM readily crosses the placenta and reacts with fetal tissue components by virtue of its alkylating and mutagenic properties. Toxicity and oncogenicity are expressed in fetal malformations and in neoplasms in the progenies under these conditions.

The uncovering of an oncogenic[*2] substance in seeds, stems, and tubers of plants of the family of Cycadaceae came about incident to studies undertaken in a search for a neurotoxin in this plant. This endeavor appeared justified after reports indicated that flour prepared from the seeds of *Cycas circinalis* growing on

---

[*1] Bethesda, Maryland 20014, U.S.A.

[*2] Throughout this paper, we have used the word oncogen and its derivatives to include benign and malignant epithelial and mesenchymal tumors.

the Pacific island of Guam, where a high incidence of amyotrophic lateral scle-
rosis (ALS) prevailed, was poisonous unless carefully prepared. The possibility
existed therefore that a relationship might be found between eating improperly
prepared cycad material and the development of ALS. There were additional
reports which linked an irreversible hindleg paralysis of cattle observed in several parts of the world to the presence of cycads on grazing lands. Much of the
then available information on the toxicology of cycads was published by Whiting (45). In the following sections we shall limit this review to work dealing with
the oncogenicity of components in cycads. A more general review of the toxicology
of cycasin was published in 1968 (17).

Isolation of Cycad Toxins

Cooper (1) is credited with having first isolated a crystalline toxic substance from *Macrozamia spiralis* in 1941 which she named macrozamin. Its
chemical structure as an azoxyglycoside was determined in 1949 and 1951 in
Professor Lythgoe's laboratory in England (11, 20). Macrozamin was also found
by Lythgoe in one of the African cycads, *Encephalartos barkeri* CATRUTH as
quoted in a footnote in a paper by Riggs (34). Cycasin was first identified in
seeds of *Cycas revoluta* THUNB. in 1955 by Nishida *et al.* in Japan (31) and subsequently by Riggs in *C. circinalis* L. from Guam (35). Macrozamin and cycasin
share the basic aliphatic azoxy structure but they differ in the sugar moiety,
macrozamin having primeverose, whereas cycasin has glucose attached in β
linkage. Several additional glycosides, referred to as neocycasins have been isolated from seeds of *C. revoluta* THUNB. (26, 30) but they also have an aglycone
part identical with that of macrozamin and cycasin. From this we may expect
that these azoxyglycosides will produce similar effects *in vivo* under conditions
in which hydrolysis of the glycosides occurs yielding the aglycone common to
all and sugars of different kinds.

Oncogenicity of Cycasin in Rats

For the "pilot" study, seeds of *C. circinalis* L. were obtained from Guam,
and the inner white fleshy part (endosperm) was ground into a coarse meal.
This was thoroughly mixed with a basal diet consisting of commercially available
Startena chicken feed and given to groups of weanling male Osborne-Mendel
rats in concentrations varying from 0.25 to 10%. The diets were fed until the
animals died or became ill.

Beginning 5 months after the start of feeding crude cycad meal at a concentration of 1 and 2%, 18 of 34 rats were found to have hepatocellular carcinomas. In 5, metastases were seen in lungs and lymph nodes. In addition, all
rats with hepatic carcinomas had one or several kidney tumors, often involving
both kidneys. The renal tumors were epithelial or mesenchymal in type but
metastases were observed in only one animal which had a renal sarcoma. Two
rats had primary intestinal carcinomas and one a pulmonary adenoma. No lesions were found in the brain which would have suggested a neurotoxic effect.

TABLE I. Summary of Experiment Demonstrating Oncogenicity of
Cycasin Contained in Crude Cycad Meal

Strain	Sex	Age at start (days)	No. of rats	Compound fed	Duration of feeding	Surviving 6 months	Tumor sites in % of survivors		
							Liver	Kidney	Colon
A. Chronic exposure									
S. D.[a]	F and M	30	80	Crude cycad meal[b]	6–9 months	76	71	49	17
S. D.	F and M	30	80	Cycasin	6–9 months	68	59	43	35
B. Short exposure									
O. M.[c]	M	30	45	Crude cycad meal	13–21 days	40	12	88	33
O. M.	M	30	140	Cycasin	13–21 days	62	27	87	26
Total			345			246			

[a] S. D.: Sprague-Dawley.   [b] Crude cycad meal containing 2.3% cycasin.   [c] O. M.: Osborne-Mendel.

Crude cycad meal, therefore, contained a substance with general oncogenic properties and the nature of this substance required investigation (16).

The simultaneous occurrence of tumors in liver and kidneys of rats fed crude cycad meal resembled the response of rats to dimethylnitrosamine (DMN) (21). Moreover, a chemical similarity between the synthetic DMN and the naturally occurring azoxyglycosides existed and it now remained to be determined whether cycasin was the oncogen in the crude cycad material.

As crystalline cycasin* became available, acute toxicity experiments showed that cycasin was a hepatotoxin, and its degree was dose-related. Subsequently, collaborative studies with Olaf Mickelsen were undertaken in which the oncogenicity of cycasin was compared with that of crude cycad meal in two strains of rats. The results are summarized in abbreviated form in Table I. They showed that oncogenic effects were demonstrable with crystalline cycasin similar to those obtained with the crude meal. Moreover, when cycasin had been removed from the crude cycad meal, tumors did not develop even after prolonged periods of feeding (46). Hence, the oncogenicity of crude cycad material apparently depended on its content in cycasin. Chronic feeding (6–9 months) was strongly hepatocarcinogenic whereas short-term exposure (13–21 days) preferentially induced renal neoplasms of both the epithelial and mesenchymal types. Tumors of the liver in contrast were found infrequently after brief exposure. This difference in relative frequency of hepatic and renal neoplasms as being related to the duration of exposure had already been observed with DMN (21).

Colonic tumors which were the third most frequently observed neoplasms developed independent of the duration of exposure. Analysis of a possible influence of sex on the development of colonic neoplasms showed a ratio of female to male of 1: 2 in favor of the male sex (13).

---

* Cycasin, methylazoxymethyl-β-D-glucoside, was generously supplied by Dr. A. Kobayashi of Kagoshima University and by Dr. H. Matsumoto of the University of Hawaii in whose laboratories it had been extracted from seeds of C. revoluta and C. circinalis, respectively.

Among the 246 rats surviving 6 months listed in Table I, 31 rats or 12.6% were found free of tumors at necropsy. In 10 of these 31 rats, the cycasin intake was well within the tumor-inducing range. A search for an explanation for this finding appeared to us worthy of pursuit, and the ensuing paragraphs deal with studies looking for biological variables which might explain the noted absence of the oncogenic effect.

Hydrolysis of Cycasin in Vivo

Macrozamin and cycasin were toxic only after enteric administration and these effects appeared after a lag period of about 12 hr (*1, 32*). The latter fact suggested that a metabolite of the azoxyglycosides was the toxic compound. The likely metabolite was the aglycone of the azoxyglycosides, methylazoxymethanol (MAM), which resulted from enzymic hydrolysis of the glycosides (*9*). Recent studies not only confirmed these observations but also showed that MAM itself was highly toxic (*25*). Our interest centered on the gastrointestinal tract as a likely site for finding the biological variable which might explain the absence of oncogenic effects in several of our rats.

Two main sites for the elaboration of hydrolytic enzymes were considered. They might be provided by the intraluminal contents particularly by microorganisms of the lower bowel or by the cellular components of the bowel wall. As will be shown below, both sources for the hydrolytic enzyme could be demonstrated under certain conditions.

Importance of the Intestinal Bacterial Flora

The availability of a germ-free unit in our Institute allowed us to explore, first of all, the importance of an intestinal microflora as a possible source for β-glucosidase activity. Technique had become available to measure cycasin excretion in urine and feces, and a comparative study of cycasin excretion between conventional and germ-free rats appeared eminently appropriate for answering this first question.

When large doses of cycasin (200 mg%) were fed in the basal diet to small groups of conventional and germ-free rats, the mortality among the conventional rats was high, approaching 100% by the 20th day whereas germ-free rats uniformly remained healthy (*12*). This difference in handling cycasin is best illustrated in Fig. 1 (*15*) which shows the body weight gains in the two groups. Microscopic study of the liver showed severe, diffuse, centrilobular hemorrhagic necrosis often involving the midzonal areas in the conventional rats, whereas the liver of the germ-free rats was normal. Cycasin apparently was nontoxic to germ-free rats. To demonstrate that cycasin was also non-oncogenic under these conditions an additional group of germ-free rats identically treated were set aside for long-term observations lasting up to 2 years. None developed neoplasms which could be considered to have been induced by cycasin.

The fate of the ingested cycasin in germ-free and conventional rats was then investigated by measuring cycasin intake and its fecal and urinary excretion.

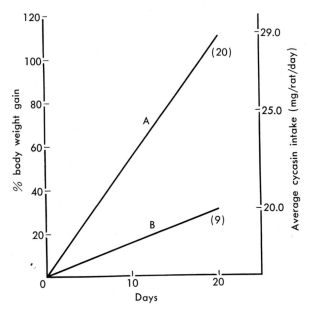

FIG. 1.   Cycasin (200 mg%) in germ-free diet fed *ad libitum* to germ-free (A) and conventional (B) S.D. rats

Initial number of rats per group: 20. Numerals in parentheses show No. of rats alive after 20 days.

When this was done, the germ-free rats were found to have excreted 97% of the intake, whereas the corresponding figure in conventional rats was 26% (*43*). Thus germ-free rats excreted nearly quantitatively the ingested cycasin and thus were similar to adult rats into which cycasin had been parenterally injected (*10*). These observations strongly suggested that intestinal microorganisms played an important role, providing the enzyme for cycasin hydrolysis *in vivo*.

It lastly remained to be demonstrated, however, that contamination of germ-free rats with microorganisms of the intestinal flora would restore in such animals the ability to hydrolyze cycasin. We decided to monocontaminate germ-free rats with a few selected strains of microorganisms on which information was available as to their ability to produce β-glucosidase. The cultures were assayed before use to obtain information about the levels of enzymic activity. Good agreement was found between the enzymic activity of the microorganisms, the extent of cycasin hydrolysis as measured by the amount of the excreted, unhydrolyzed cycasin, severity of hepatic injury, and survival time (*44*).

We can summarize these observations by noting that the hydrolysis of cycasin when enterically administered to rats depends on a bacterial intestinal flora containing organisms which possess a sufficiently high level of β-glucosidase activity.

Importance of the Intestinal Wall

The other possibility that the hydrolytic enzyme may be produced by components of the intestinal wall has only recently been demonstrated when possible sites for cycasin hydrolysis during neonatal life were investigated. By comparing liver, kidneys, skin, and small intestine for their ability to hydrolyze β-glycosides, the highest activity was found in the small intestine reaching its peak about the 16th day of neonatal life after which the activity dropped sharply, stabilizing at a low level between the 24th and 28th days and remaining at that level up to 90 days after birth when the last determinations were made (24).

Returning to the observation that individual rats failed to respond with tumor formation after ingestion of amounts of cycasin sufficient to induce neoplasms in the majority of similarly treated rats, it is conceivable that the tumor-free rats for reasons still unknown may have had an intestinal bacterial flora deficient in microorganisms capable of providing the hydrolytic enzyme for β-glycosides. Although we cannot state in retrospect that this had been the case in our tumor-free rats, this remains a definite possibility.

Oncogenicity of MAM

Investigations into the toxicology of cycasin had demonstrated that its aglycone, MAM, produced severe toxic effects independent of the route of administration (10). MAM had been obtained in one of the fractions during the extraction of cycasin from cycad seeds and subsequently after enzymic hydrolysis of cycasin. It became clear, however, that the techniques involving the isolation of cycasin were time-consuming and cumbersome; yet continuation of studies with cycasin and its aglycone depended on an available supply. At this critical time, the synthesis of the aglycone was successfully undertaken by Matsumoto *et al.* (23), and continuation of investigations into the biological activities of this naturally occurring oncogen was assured. It is of interest that this synthesis started from 1,2-dimethylhydrazine (DMH) and proceeded through azomethane to azoxymethane and finally to methylazoxymethyl acetate (MAMA). In the meantime DMH and azoxymethane each have proven to be potent carcinogens for colon and rectum (3). MAMA is now available from several commercial sources.

The oncogenicity of MAM and of the synthetic MAMA was subsequently demonstrated under a variety of experimental conditions. The results of these experiments can be summarized as follows: benign and malignant tumors of liver, kidneys, colon, and rectum were found and the microscopic findings were similar to those observed previously with cycasin in feeding experiments. The neoplasms developed, however, independent of the route of administration in conventional and germ-free animals. Repeated intraperitoneal administration of MAM or MAMA produced in addition carcinomas of the duodenum in 11 of 28 rats. This type of neoplasm had only once been seen in previous feeding experiments. The localization of these carcinomas in the middle third of the duodenum suggested the possibility that small amounts of the carcinogen may have been excreted with the bile (14, 15). It has recently been reported that intrarectal instillations of MAMA were also particularly effective in inducing colon cancer and that the number of tumors was dose-related (29).

Experiments in Teratology and Transplacental Oncogenesis

Once the oncogenic properties of cycasin and MAM had been recognized, it appeared important to know whether the active component might cross the placenta and thus induce malformations in the fetuses and neoplasia in the progeny.

The pertinent experiments were performed in rats and hamsters in which it was shown, first, that cycasin and MAM had crossed the placenta and were demonstrable by thin-layer chromatography in the fetuses of rats and of MAM in the fetuses of hamsters (*42*). These compounds were considered, therefore, as acting directly on the fetuses. Subsequent studies not only confirmed the transplacental passage of MAM into the fetuses but, additionally demonstrated that MAM had reacted with fetal nucleic acids and protein (*28*).

Using the method of Ferm (*4*), pregnant female golden hamsters received various doses of MAM in saline intravenously on the 8th day of gestation. At laparotomy on day 12, sites of implantation, living fetuses as determined by a pulsating heart, dead fetuses, and sites of resorption were counted. The living fetuses were grossly examined for malformation. The optimal dose which resulted in survival and in malformation of brain, spinal cord, eyes, and extremities of the fetuses was in the neighborhood of 20 mg/kg body weight (*40*). Slightly larger doses resulted in fetal death and many sites of fetal resorption, whereas smaller doses failed to induce malformations in the majority of living fetuses.

The first evidence for transplacental tumor induction was obtained in Sprague-Dawley rats who had been fed a diet mixed with various concentrations of crude cycad meal. This lot of cycad meal contained 3% cycasin. Details of the experiment have been published (*41*). Among 81 rats surviving 6 months, 15 (18.5%) had tumors which were found at various sites such as colon, kidney, lung, leg muscle, chest wall, brain, and jejunum. The jejunal tumors were histologically identical and occurred in 4 of 6 litter mates. They were mesenchymal in nature, being polypoid or sessile, and composed of plump cytoplasm-rich cells. Their appearance suggested the possibility of an origin from smooth muscle.

Although tumor induction by the transplacental route was possible, many questions remained unanswered. The fact that only 18.5% of the rats developed tumors was surprising but could be explained on the basis of insufficient amounts of the active oncogen having been absorbed and crossed the placenta. Except for the jejunal tumors there was also no evidence that particular tumor sites were related to the period of fetal development at which the oncogen had been administered.

The experiment was repeated, therefore, and pregnant Fischer rats received intraperitoneally or intravenously a single dose of MAM or MAMA at differing periods of gestation. In the majority of the rats this dose was 20 mg/kg body weight. The results of this study are presented here, a preliminary report having been made on a previous occasion (*18*).

The present summary is based on pathological studies of 340 rats all of which had been exposed *in utero* to MAM or MAMA at various days of fetal

TABLE II. Transplacental Tumor Induction after a Single Dose
(20 mg/kg Body Weight) of MAM

| | Weeks of pregnancy | | | Total |
	First	Second	Third	
No. of litters	7	8	44	59
No. of progeny surviving 6 months	49	49	242	340
No. of progeny with tumors	4	3	35	42
No. of progeny with multiple primaries	—	2	5	—
Tumor sites				
Lungs	1	2	13	16
Brain	1	—	6	7
Kidney	1	1	8	10
Colon	—	1	3	4
Small intestine	—	—	2	2
Miscellaneous	1	1	9	11
Total	4	5	41	50

development. There were 42 rats with tumors or 12.3% and of them, 19 (45%) were found among the progeny of 9 mothers who had received the oncogen on the 21st day of pregnancy. Details of the experimental findings are shown in Table II. Multiple primary sites were noted in several rats raising the total number of primary neoplasms induced with MAM by the transplacental route to 50. None of these tumors was found in the offsprings of saline-treated or -untreated dams.

When primary tumor sites were related to the day of exposure during fetal development, it was found that 10 of 16 pulmonary tumors and 6 of the 7 gliomas had occurred in rats exposed on the 21st day. Hence, the last day of intrauterine life not only was the most sensitive period for later tumor development but also reflected a heightened sensitivity of pulmonary and cerebral tissue to the oncogenic action of MAM.

This increased sensitivity appears to extend to the first day of life in Fischer rats as previously demonstrated in an experiment with Hirono in which neonatal rats of the same strain had received a single subcutaneous dose of cycasin (0.5 mg/ g body weight) (6). Among 46 long-term survivors, 12 had pulmonary and 5 cerebral tumors. Hence it would appear that the "perinatal" period extending from the day before to the day after birth is particularly suitable for tumor induction with MAM in lungs and brain in the Fischer strain of rats.

Summarizing the results of these 2 experiments on transplacental carcinogenesis, it is evident that crude cycad material and MAM can induce tumors in the progeny by this route. The tumor yield was low, however. Nevertheless, we observed 3 instances in which an unusual aggregation of certain neoplasms occurred. The first example of this was noted when in a litter of 6 rats, 4 had histologically identical tumors in the jejunum. Whether this event resulted from a combination of factors peculiar to this particular pregnancy or whether the oncogen had played a role, we do not know. The frequent occurrence of pulmonary and intracerebral tumors in rats exposed to MAM on the 21st day of fetal development must, we believe, be ascribed to the activity of MAM. The reasons for pulmonary and cerebral tumors to occur with increased frequency during the "perinatal" period were not clear. There was first of all an increase of all tumors in rats exposed during the late period of fetal life when compared with earlier periods. This would suggest the possibility that there might have been a change in the responsiveness of tissues to the carcinogen related in some way to their degree of metabolic maturation. Secondly, whereas MAM has been established as the "proximate" carcinogen of cycasin, it is not definitely cartain that it is also the "ultimate" carcinogen. There is evidence from the studies of Nagasawa et al. (27) that methylcarbonium ion is the likely methylating intermediate in the metabolic breakdown of MAM, a process previously suggested by Druckrey (3). If methylation of nucleic acids which has been repeatedly demonstrated with MAM both in in vitro (22) and in in vivo (36) is causally related to the initiation of carcinogenesis, the metabolic situation in lungs and brain around the day of birth may be preferentially suitable for the interaction between the ultimate carcinogen and cellular constituents.

Our observations of a relatively high frequency of pulmonary tumors during the "perinatal" period in rats exposed to MAM are comparable to those in mice transplacentally exposed to urethan as reported by several investigators (2, 8, 19). In mice, incidence and number of pulmonary neoplasms significantly increased as the interval between the administration of urethan and birth was shortened, reaching a peak when the injections were made within hours before birth. Several physiological adjustments in the respiratory and circulatory systems incident to birth which might contribute to a higher concentration of the oncogen at particular sites have been suggested as possible contributory factors. A measurable potentiating effect of induced hyperoxemia on the incidence of pulmonary tumors over that found in mice at room environment after urethan injections has been reported (8). To what extent any of these factors might have contributed to the aggregation of pulmonary tumors in our rats exposed to MAM within the "perinatal" period is not known.

Hydrolysis of Cycasin during the "Perinatal" Period

It was repeatedly stressed that toxic and oncogenic effects of cycasin were observable only in feeding experiments, in which hydrolysis of cycasin to MAM was facilitated by bacterial enzymes. This holds for animals, 1 month old and older. That a different mechanism for the conversion of cycasin to MAM must be operating in rats younger than 1 month became apparent when tumors developed in 83% of the rats which had received subcutaneously a single dose of cycasin within 24 hr after birth (6).

In order to explain this difference between neonatal and older rats we first considered the possibility that (1) the cycasin which had been injected into the newborns was excreted in the urine, (2) that the dams in the process of cleaning their young had swallowed the cycasin-containing urine and hydrolyzed it to MAM in the intestinal tract, and (3) that the newborns received the MAM through the maternal milk. Evidence for passage of MAM into the mammary gland had been described (*42, 47*). To test the likelihood of this sequence of events, the experiment was repeated in germ-free rats in which the second step, namely the conversion of cycasin to MAM in the maternal intestinal tract was excluded. The young of the germ-free mothers responded to the subcutaneous administration of cycasin the same way as those of the conventional rats. The conclusion to be drawn was that the newborn rats themselves possessed the mechanism for hydrolyzing cycasin and that it was independent of the mother rats.

Evidence for hydrolysis of cycasin in newborns in skin and subcutaneous tissue of conventional and germ-free Sprague-Dawley rats and in conventional Fischer rats during the "perinatal" period was reported by Spatz (*38*) and in the small intestine, kidney, liver, and skin in Wistar albino rats by Matsumoto *et al.* (*24*). In both studies overall enzyme activity markedly decreased by the end of the first month of postnatal life. In the study of Spatz high enzyme activity in the skin preceded birth and started to drop by the 4th to 6th day postpartum, whereas Matsumoto observed the greatest activity in the small intestine with the peak of activity at the 16th day of life. This peak in enzyme activity also coincided with the highest yield in tumors later in life. No tumors were observed when cycasin injections were made on the 25th day even though low levels of β-glucosidase activity were found in small intestines and kidneys as late as 90 days after birth (*24*).

The prolonged persistence of low enzymatic activity may very well be significant in view of observations in germ-free rats in which malignant tumors were induced after intraperitoneal (i.p.) and subcutaneous (s.c.) administration of cycasin (1 mg/g body weight) in 50% of the rats treated as late as 35 days after birth. The overall results of this unpublished experiment are presented in Table III which also indicates the localization of the tumors. The most frequent site was the kidney followed in frequency by colon, liver, and duodenum. The greater total number of primary tumors when compared with the total number of rats was due to the development of multiple primary tumor sites. Two primaries

TABLE III. Frequency of Tumor Sites in Germ-free Sprague-Dawley Rats after Receiving One s.c. or i.p. Injection of Cycasin at Designated Days Postpartum

Age at injection (days)	No. of rats	No. of rats with tumor/ No. of rats	No. of rats with tumors at specific sites				
			Kidney	Colon	Liver	Duodenum	Miscel.
5	18	16/18	16	4 (2)[a]	5	—	—
9	9	9/ 9	9 (1)	3	1 (1)	—	—
16	19	17/19	15	4 (3)	4 (1)	2	—
25	22	8/22	3	2 (2)	2	—	2
35	12	6/12	1	3	1	—	1
Total	80		44	16	13	2	3[b]

[a] No. in parentheses indicates number of tumors with metastases. [b] Two fibrosarcomas of anterior chest wall and one transitional cell papilloma of bladder.

were found in 21 rats and 3 primaries in 3 rats. The most frequent combination of 2 primary sites involved kidney and colon, whereas independent tumors in liver, kidney, and colon accounted for all with 3 primary sites.

The overall results of the studies just cited indicate that neonatal rats for certain periods of time are capable of hydrolyzing β-glucosides after parenteral administration and that this enzymic ability was demonstrable in the absence of microorganisms. The physiological role of this enzyme is presently unknown. The combined evidence presented in various papers referred to indicates, however, that the enzyme was not induced with cycasin.

Oncogenicity of Cycasin and MAM in Guinea Pigs, Hamsters, and Mice

The review of the oncogenicity of cycasin and MAM would be incomplete without citing several observations made in animals other than the rat. Induction of hepatomas in guinea pigs with crude cycad meal was first accomplished by Spatz in experiments in which effects of dietary deficiences were also explored (37). Liver tumors were found in 9 of 27 guinea pigs of which 4 were hepatocellular carcinomas and 5 were diagnosed as intrahepatic bile duct carcinomas. Because of the dietary factors which might have contributed to the development of the liver tumors, the experiment was repeated with a basal guinea pig diet and, instead of crude cycad meal, injections of MAM and MAMA were given by the subcutaneous or intraperitoneal route, respectively. The results of these studies published in abstract form (39) are summarized in Table IV. Hepatocellular carcinomas were found in 30 of 45 guinea pigs surviving 6 months or longer

TABLE IV. Tumor Induction in 6-Week-old Guinea Pigs after Repeated i.p. or s.c. Injections of MAM or MAMA[a]

No. of guinea pigs 6 mos. after start	Sex	Compound used and route of admin.	Total dose[b] (mg)	No. with tumor	Primary liver tumors			Other tumor sites
					Hepatocell. carcinoma	Bile duct carcinoma	Vascular tumors	
20	M	MAM i.p.	9–19.5	14	5 (5)[c]	2	3	1 jejunal adenocarcinoma 3 squamous cell carcinoma of anterior nasal cavity 2 pulmonary adenoma 1 hemangiosarcoma of nose
6	M	MAMA i.p.	57–73	6	6 (4)	—	3	
6	F	MAMA i.p.	49–64	6	6 (6)	—	4	1 carcinoma of breast
7	M	MAMA s.c.	47–70	7	7 (4)	—	3	
6	F	MAMA s.c.	44–59	6	6 (4)	—	4	
47	M	Saline i.p./s.c.	—	0	—	—	—	
12	F	Saline i.p./s.c.	—	0	—	—	—	

[a] M. Spatz, unpublished data. [b] Individual dose: 6 mg/kg body weight. [c] No. in parentheses indicates number of tumors with metastases.

after onset of treatment at 6 weeks of age. In addition 2 intrahepatic bile duct carcinomas were noted and a few neoplasms at other sites including one adenocarcinoma of the jejunum.

Studies in hamsters by Hirono *et al.* (*5*) and by Spatz (*39*) have shown that cycasin, MAM, and MAMA are oncogenic for this species as well. Using cycasin in newborn and 2-month-old animals, it was noted that hepatocellular carcinomas developed only in the group of newborn hamsters, whereas intrahepatic bile duct carcinomas were found with about equal frequency in newborn and young adult animals. Intestinal tumors occurred more frequently in adult hamsters receiving single or multiple doses of cycasin by stomach tube (8/78) than in the newborns which had recieved cycasin subcutaneously at different dose levels (1/73) (*5*). In our laboratory, MAM was employed as the oncogen and administered either in a single intravenous (i.v.) dose or in multiple intraperitoneally given injections. The results of these experiments are summarized in Table V. Although proliferative changes of the intrahepatic bile ducts occurred with considerable frequency, a carcinoma of the intrahepatic bile duct with metastases to lung and over the splenic peritoneum was seen only in one hamster. Hyperplasia of the epithelium lining the gall bladder was common and adenocarcinomas arising from the gall bladder mucosa were seen in two hamsters. The relatively high incidence of both colonic adenomas and adenocarcinomas, the latter with local extensions and distant metastases were the most striking findings. These tumors occurred as single or multiple separate lesions.

TABLE V.   Tumor Induction with MAM in Male and Female
Golden Hamsters[a]

| | Experimental groups | | | | Controls |
	I	II	III	IV	V
No. of hamsters	36	5	8	15	56
No. of injections	Single	3×	4×–5×	4×–5×	Single or multiple
Route of administration	i.v.	i.p.	i.p.	i.p.	i.v. or i.p.
Dose of carcinogen (mg/kg body weight)	20	20	15	10	Saline
Liver					
Cystadenomas and cystic lesions	34	4	8	15	—
Vascular tumors	8	—	5	10	—
Hepatocellular carcinomas	3 (1)[b]	—	2	3	—
Adenocarcinomas	1 (1)	—	—	—	—
Gallbladders					
Hyperplasias	24	5	6	4	—
Adenocarcinomas	—	2 (2)	—	—	—
Large intestines					
Adenomas	16	—	3	2	—
Adenocarcinomas	15	2 (2)	8 (4)	15 (5)	—
Miscellaneous					
Infraorbital carcinoma	—	—	—	3	—

[a] M. Spatz, unpublished data.   [b] No. in parentheses indicates number of tumors with metastases.

The first description of an oncogenic effect of cycads in mice was given by O'Gara *et al.* (*33*) who observed tumors in liver and kidneys in C57BL/6 male mice after topical application of an aqueous emulsion of endosperm of *C. circinalis* to skin ulcers previously induced with 10% croton oil. The incidence and localization of tumors in newborn and adult mice of the C57BL/6 strain which had been given cycasin by the subcutaneous or intragastric routes, respectively, was reported by Hirono *et al.* (*7*). Among 26 mice treated as newborns and surviving longer than 50 days, they found 4 reticulum cell neoplasms, 4 liver cell adenomas, 9 hepatomas with metastases in 4, one pulmonary adenoma, and one leukemia. In contrast only two hepatomas, one pulmonary adenoma, one kidney adenoma, and one fibroma of the subcutis were observed among the surviving 35 adult mice.

The results of studies just reviewed indicate that cycasin and MAM induce tumors in a variety of laboratory animals which include rats, mice, guinea pigs, and hamsters. Sites of tumor development varied among different species. Renal tumors which in their manyfold forms and high frequency had been observed in rats were nearly absent in the other species.

REFERENCES

1. Cooper, J. M. Isolation of a toxic principle from the seeds of *Macrozamia spiralis*. *Proc. Roy. Soc. New South Wales*, **74**, 450–454 (1941).
2. DiPaolo, J. A. Effects of oxygen concentration on carcinogenesis induced by transplacental exposure to urethan. *Cancer Res.*, **22**, 299–304 (1962).
3. Druckrey, H. Production of colonic carcinomas by 1,2-dialkylhydrazines and azoxyalkanes. *In* "Carcinoma of the Colon and Antecedent Epithelium," ed. by W. J. Burdette, Charles C. Thomas, Springfield, Ill., pp. 267–279 (1970).
4. Ferm, V. H. The rapid detection of teratogenic activity. *Lab. Invest.*, **14**, 1500–1505 (1965).
5. Hirono, I., Hayashi, K., Mori, H., and Miwa, T. Carcinogenic effects of cycasin in Syrian golden hamsters and the transplantability of induced tumors. *Cancer Res.*, **31**, 283–287 (1971).
6. Hirono, I., Laqueur, G. L., and Spatz, M. Tumor induction in Fischer and Osborne-Mendel rats by a single administration of cycasin. *J. Natl. Cancer Inst.*, **40**, 1003–1010 (1968).
7. Hirono, I., Shibuya, Ch., and Fushimi, K. Tumor induction in C57BL/6 mice by a single administration of cycasin. *Cancer Res.*, **29**, 1658–1662 (1969).
8. Klein, M. The transplacental effect of urethan on lung tumorigenesis in mice. *J. Natl. Cancer Inst.*, **12**, 1003–1010 (1952).
9. Kobayashi, A. Biochemical studies on cycasin. II. Existence of free aglycone of cycasin in its enzymatic hydrolysis. *Agr. Biol. Chem. (Tokyo)*, **26**, 208–212 (1962).
10. Kobayashi, A. and Matsumoto, H. Studies on methylazoxymethanol, the aglycone of cycasin isolation, biological and chemical properties. *Arch. Biochem. Biophys.*, **110**, 373–380 (1965).
11. Langley, B. W., Lythgoe, B., and Riggs, N. V. Macrozamin. Part II. The aliphatic azoxy structure of the aglycone part. *J. Chem. Soc.*, **46**, 2309–2316 (1951).
12. Laqueur, G. L. Carcinogenic effects of cycad meal and cycasin, methylazoxymethanol glycoside, in rats and effects of cycasin in germfree rats. *Fed. Proc.*, **23**, 1386–1387 (1964).

13. Laqueur, G. L. The induction of intestinal neoplasms in rats with the glycoside cycasin and its aglycone. *Arch. Pathol. Anat. Physiol.*, **340**, 151–163 (1965).

14. Laqueur, G. L. and Matsumoto, H. Neoplasms in female Fischer rats following intraperitoneal injection of methylazoxymethanol. *J. Natl. Cancer Inst.*, **37**, 217–232 (1966).

15. Laqueur, G. L., McDaniel, E. G., and Matsumoto, H. Tumor induction in germ-free rats with methylazoxymethanol (MAM) and synthetic MAM acetate. *J. Natl. Cancer Inst.*, **39**, 355–371 (1967).

16. Laqueur, G. L., Mickelsen, O., Whiting, M .G., and Kurland, L. T. Carcinogenic properties of nuts from *Cycas circinalis* L. indigenous to Guam. *J. Natl. Cancer Inst.*, **31**, 919–951 (1963).

17. Laqueur, G. L. and Spatz, M. Toxicology of cycasin. *Cancer Res.*, **28**, 2262–2267 (1968).

18. Laqueur, G. L. and Spatz, M. Transplacental induction of tumors and malformations in rats with cycasin and methylazoxymethanol. *In* "Transplacental Carcinogenesis," IARC Scientific Publications No. 4, International Agency for Research on Cancer, Lyon, pp. 59–64 (1973).

19. Larsen, C. D. Pulmonary-tumor induction by transplacental exposure to urethane. *J. Natl. Cancer Inst.*, **8**, 63–70 (1947).

20. Lythgoe, B. and Riggs, N. V. Macrozamin. Part I. The identity of the carbohydrate component. *J. Chem. Soc.*, **4**, 2716–2718 (1949).

21. Magee, P. N. and Barnes, J. M. The Experimental production of tumors in the rat by dimethylnitrosamine (N-nitrosodimethylamine). *Acta Unio Int. Cancrum*, **15**, 187–190 (1959).

22. Matsumoto, H. and Higa, H. H. Studies on methylazoxymethanol, the aglycone of cycasin: Methylation of nucleic acids *in vitro. Biochem. J.*, **98**, 20c–22c (1966).

23. Matsumoto, H., Nagahama, T., and Larson, H. O. Studies on methylazoxymethanol, the aglycone of cycasin: A synthesis of methylazoxymethyl acetate. *Biochem. J.*, **95**, 13c–14c (1965).

24. Matsumoto, H., Nagata, Y., Nishimura, E. T., Bristol, R., and Haber, M. β-Glucosidase modulation in preweanling rats and its association with tumor induction by cycasin. *J. Natl. Cancer Inst.*, **49**, 423–433 (1972).

25. Matsumoto, H. and Strong, F. M. The occurrence of methylazoxymethanol in *Cycas circinalis* L. *Arch. Biochem. Biophys.*, **101**, 299–310 (1963).

26. Nagahama, T. Studies on neocycasin, new glycosides of cycads. *Bull. Fac. Agr. Kagoshima Univ.*, No. 14, 1–50 (1964).

27. Nagasawa, H. T., Shirota, F. N., and Matsumoto, H. Decomposition of methylazoxymethanol, the aglycone of cycasin, in D_2O. *Nature*, **236**, 234–235 (1972).

28. Nagata, Y. and Matsumoto, H. Studies on methylazoxymethanol: Methylation of nucleic acids in the fetal rat brain. *Proc. Soc. Exp. Biol. Med.*, **132**, 383–385 (1969).

29. Narisawa, T. and Nakano, H. Carcinoma of the large intestine of rats induced by rectal infusion of methylazoxymethanol. *Gann*, **64**, 93–95 (1973).

30. Nishida, K. Azoxyglucosides (from *Cycas revoluta* THUNB.). *Japan. J. Chem.*, **13**, 730–737 (1959).

31. Nishida, K., Kobayashi, A., and Nagahama, T. Studies on cycasin, a new toxic glycoside of *Cycas revoluta* THUNB.: Part I. Isolation and the structure of cycasin. *Bull. Agr. Chem. Soc. Japan*, **19**, 77–83 (1955).

32. Nishida, K., Kobayashi, A., Nagahama, T., Kojima, K., and Yamane, M. Studies on cycasin, a new toxic glycoside of *Cycas revoluta* THUNB. IV. Pharmacological

study of cycasin. *Seikagaku* (*J. Japan. Biochem. Soc.*), **28**, 218–223 (1956) (in Japanese).

33. O'Gara, R. W., Brown, J. M., and Whiting, M. G. Induction of hepatic and renal tumors by topical application of aqueous extract of cycad nut to artificial skin ulcers in mice. *Fed. Proc.*, **23**, 1383 (1964).

34. Riggs, N. V. The occurrence of macrozamin in the seeds of cycads. *Austr. J. Chem.*, **7**, 123–124 (1954).

35. Riggs, N. V. Glucosyloxyazoxymethane, a constituent of the seeds of *Cycas circinalis* L. *Chem. Ind.*, 926 (1956).

36. Shank, R. C. and Magee, P. N. Similarities between the biochemical actions of cycasin and dimethylnitrosamine. *Biochem. J.*, **105**, 521–527 (1967).

37. Spatz, M. Carcinogenic effect of cycad meal in guinea pigs. *Fed. Proc.*, **23**, 1384–1385 (1964).

38. Spatz, M. Hydrolysis of cycasin by β-D-glucosidase in skin of newborn rats. *Proc. Soc. Exp. Biol. Med.*, **128**, 1005–1008 (1968).

39. Spatz, M. Carcinogenicity of methylazoxymethanol (MAM) in guinea pigs and hamsters. *Abstr. Xth. Int. Cancer Congr.* (*Houston*), 24–25 (1970).

40. Spatz, M., Dougherty, W. J., and Smith, D. W. E. Teratogenic effects of methylazoxymethanol. *Proc. Soc. Exp. Biol. Med.*, **124**, 476–478 (1967).

41. Spatz, M. and Laqueur, G. L. Transplacental induction of tumors in Sprague-Dawley rats with crude cycad material. *J. Natl. Cancer Inst.*, **38**, 233–245 (1967).

42. Spatz, M. and Laqueur, G. L. Evidence for transplacental passage of the natural carcinogen cycasin and its aglycone. *Proc. Soc. Exp. Biol. Med.*, **127**, 281–286 (1968).

43. Spatz, M., McDaniel, E. G., and Laqueur, G. L. Cycasin excretion in conventional and germ-free rats. *Proc. Soc. Exp. Biol. Med.*, **121**, 417–422 (1966).

44. Spatz, M., Smith, D. W. E., McDaniel, E. G., and Laqueur, G. L. Role of intestinal microorganisms in determining cycasin toxicity. *Proc. Soc. Exp. Biol. Med.*, **124**, 691–697 (1967).

45. Whiting, M. G. Toxicity of cycads. *Econ. Botany*, **17**, 269–302 (1963).

46. Yang, M. G., Mickelsen, O., Campbell, M. E., Laqueur, G. L., and Keresztesy, J. C. Cycad flour used by Guamanians: Effects produced by long-term feeding. *J. Nutr.*, **90**, 153–156 (1966).

47. Yang, M. G., Mickelsen, O., and Sanger, V. L. Cycling of cycasin from newborn rats to their mother and back to the newborn. *Proc. Soc. Exp. Biol. Med.*, **131**, 135–137 (1969).

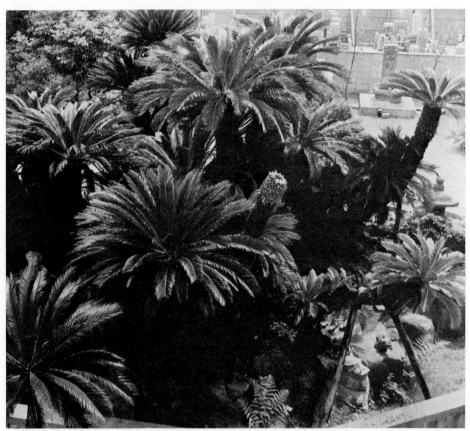

⇑ The enormous 400-year-old sago
palm (*Cycas revoluta*) in the gardens
of Myokoku temple in Osaka, now
a part of City of Osaka (Courtesy
of Sankei Shimbun Co., Ltd.)

⇨ How chill the morning seems
    as I visit the Sago Palm
        at Myokokuji

                    Masaoka Shiki
                     (1867–1902)

Poem written by Kimiko Yoshida,
the widow of Prof. Tomizo Yoshida;
English version by Dorothy Britton

GANN Monograph on Cancer Research 17, 205–217 (1975)

NATURAL CARCINOGENIC PRODUCTS
OF PLANT ORIGIN

Iwao Hirono,[*1] Ikuo Sasaoka,[*1] Chiken Shibuya,[*1] Masaru Shimizu,[*1]
Katsumasa Fushimi,[*1] Hideki Mori,[*1] Kazuo Kato,[*1]
and Masanobu Haga[*2]

*Department of Pathology, Gifu University School of Medicine,[*1] and
Faculty of Pharmaceutical Science, Nagoya City University[*2]*

Carcinogenicity of bracken (*Pteridium aquilinum*) and petasites (*Petasites japonicus* Maxim.) was studied. Rats fed bracken developed tumors mainly in the ileum, and these tumors were not only epithelial, such as adenoma and adenocarcinoma, but also sarcomas. Carcinogenicity of bracken could be reduced to some extent by its treatment with boiling water and most remarkably by treatment with wood ash, sodium hydrogen carbonate, or sodium chloride. In comparing the carcinogenicity in each part of bracken, the curled tops of the young fronds had stronger activity than the stalks, and the rhizomes had stronger activity than young fronds. In addition, it was also revealed that the carcinogenicity of the immature young bracken was stronger than that of mature bracken, and it was influenced by geographic conditions. Carcinogenicity of pterolactam, 5-methoxy-2-pyrrolidone, which is a new compound isolated from bracken was studied by implantation into the urinary bladder and by oral administration, but its carcinogenic activity was not proved. The carcinogenicity of young flower stalks of both wild and cultivated petasites and that of mature terrestrial part of cultivated petasites were studied. Rats fed diets containing the flower stalks of wild petasites developed hemangioendothelial sarcomas in the liver. Hepatocellular carcinomas were also infrequently observed. On the other hand, as to the flower stalks of cultivated petasites, carcinogenicity was much weaker than that of the wild type. Further, mature terrestrial part of cultivated petasites did not show carcinogenic activity.

The most representative naturally occurring carcinogens of plant origin are pyrrolizidine alkaloids (*1, 16, 22*), cycasin (*14*), and bracken carcinogen (*2, 3*). We have reported the carcinogenic activity of cycasin in different species of animals (*4, 6–9*) and that of young bracken used as a human food (*5, 10, 11*). In Japan, especially in rural areas, various kinds of wild plants have long been accepted as human food or herbal remedy. Thus, carcinogenicity of artemisia, horsetail, and osmund, which were in the same stage of growth as they are used

---

[*1] Tsukasa-machi 40, Gifu 500, Japan (広野　巌, 笹岡郁乎, 渋谷智顕, 清水　勝, 伏見勝正, 森　秀樹, 加藤一夫).
[*2] Tanabe-dōri 3, Mizuho-ku, Nagoya 467, Japan (羽賀正信).

as human food, was also studied. However, any significant results suggesting the carcinogenicity were not obtained (*12*). Recently, we found that the young flower stalks of *Petasites japonicus* MAXIM. (Japanese name "Fuki-no-toh"), a kind of coltsfoot, which is bitter as bracken and has long been used as a food or a herbal remedy, such as a cough cure, expectorant, or stomachic, has a potent carcinogenic activity (*13*). The experimental results obtained in our laboratory concerning the carcinogenic properties of bracken and petasites are summarized.

Bracken

The carcinogenicity of bracken (*Pteridium aquilinum*) was first evidenced by the experiments of Evans and Mason (*3*) who found that rats fed bracken developed multiple intestinal adenocarcinomas. Pamukcu *et al.* (*17, 19*) and Price and Pamukcu (*21*) also confirmed that bracken was carcinogenic to cows and rats. In Japan, the young bracken frond in the fiddlehead or crosier stage of growth is used as a human food. Our laboratory has been working to assess the carcinogenic role of bracken in the etiology of human cancer and also to contribute to the study of the nature of the bracken carcinogen. Some of the results are reported in this paper. Each experiment was terminated in 480 days, unless otherwise stated.

1. Carcinogenic activity of young unprocessed bracken and processed bracken treated with boiling water (*10*)

Young bracken was collected in Hokkaido, in the northern part of Japan, from May through June and the carcinogenic activity was studied in inbred strain ACI rats, 1 month old, of both sexes. Group I: for 4 months, 26 rats received bracken-containing pellets. To prepare the pellets, the fresh bracken was dried, milled, and then mixed with the rat basal diet CE-2 (CLEA Japan Inc., Tokyo) in the proportion by weight of 1 part bracken to 2 parts basal diet and made into pellets. The composition of the basal diet CE-2 was described previously (*10*). Group II: for 4 months, 12 rats received the pellets containing the following processed bracken (1:2 by weight as those in Group I). Fresh bracken was immersed in boiling water for 5–10 min, dried, and made into pellets. After the termination of bracken feeding, rats were returned to the normal diet. Another group of 13 rats fed the normal diet served as controls.

In Group I, 2 out of 26 rats died of pneumonia within 7 months and 19 rats died of multiple ileal tumors within 11 months after the start of feeding. Remaining 5 rats also died of tumor within 14 months. Thus, all the rats surviving beyond 7 months after the start of the experiment had ileal tumors (24/24). In addition, 6 developed concomitantly tumors in the cecum. Only 1 rat had a urinary bladder tumor. Histological types of tumors induced by bracken are summarized in Table I. The ileal tumors were histologically adenomas, adenocarcinomas (Photo 1), and sarcomas (Photo 2). Tumors of the cecum were mainly adenomas. One urinary bladder tumor in this group was a papilloma. In Group II, tumors developed later than in Group I. The first tumor was observed 10 months after the start of the experiment. The incidence of the intestinal tumor

TABLE I. Sites and Histological Types of Tumors Induced in Rats of Each Group

Tumor site and histological type	No. of rats with tumors		
	Group I	Group II	Control
Ileum			
Adenoma	16	7	0
Adenocarcinoma	18	3	0
Sarcoma	12	0	0
Cecum			
Adenoma	6	0	0
Sarcoma	1	0	0
Rectum			
Adenocarcinoma	0	1	0
Urinary bladder			
Papilloma	1	3	1
Carcinoma	0	3	0
Lung			
Adenoma	0	1	0

in Group II was lower than that in Group I, *i.e.*, in Group II it was 75%, 9 of 12 rats, whereas in Group I it was 100% (24/24). Furthermore, neither the cecal tumors nor ileal sarcomas were found in Group II. However, the incidence of urinary bladder tumors in Group II was much higher than that in the control group (Table I). From these results, it may be evident that the carcinogen in bracken could be removed to some extent by boiling water.

2. Carcinogenic activity of processed bracken used as human food (11)

In Japan, bracken is usually used as a human food after the harshness is removed as follows: (1) after fresh bracken is immersed in boiling water containing wood ash or sodium hydrogen carbonate, it is seasoned. Sometimes, however, bracken treated with plain boiling water alone is also eaten, and (2) fresh bracken is pickled in salt and immersed in boiling water before use. The carcinogenic activity of bracken thus prepared for human use was compared with that of fresh bracken. Young bracken used in this study was collected in Okumyogata District, Gifu Prefecture, Japan, from the end of April through June. ACI rats, 1–1.5 months old, of both sexes were divided into 4 groups and treated as follows. Group I: for 4 months, 14 rats received the unprocessed bracken-containing pellets (1:2 by weight). Group II: for 4 months, 12 rats received the pellets containing the processed bracken treated with wood ash (1:2 by weight as those in Group I). Group III: for 4 months, 10 rats received the pellets containing the processed bracken treated with sodium hydrogen carbonate. Group IV: pellets containing salted bracken were given for 4 months to 10 rats and for 9 months to 11 rats. Control group: 12 rats were fed the normal diet without bracken material. Eleven out of 14 rats in Group I developed tumors and most tumors were observed in the ileum. The terminal 3-centimeter section of the ileum was the most preferred site of bracken-induced multiple tumors in the intestinal canal. The latent period of tumors in Group II was longer than in

Group I, and the tumor incidence was much lower compared with that in Group I, *i.e.*, in Group II it was 25.0% (3/12), whereas in Group I it was 78.5% (11/14). In Group III, only 1 of 10 rats developed an adenocarcinoma at the end of the ileum. Of 10 rats in Group IV fed salted bracken-containing pellets for 4 months, 1 animal developed an ileal multiple adenoma. In the Group fed salted bracken pellets for 9 months, however, tumor was not induced, except for 1 rat with a reticulum cell sarcoma of the mesenteric lymph nodes. No tumors were observed in the control group. These results suggest that the content of carcinogen in processed bracken was much less compared with unprocessed bracken. However, it is of importance that bracken thus prepared still retained carcinogenic activity.

In rats fed unprocessed bracken for 4 months, which was collected in Hokkaido, the latent period of tumor was about 8–11 months, but it was more than 12 months in rats fed unprocessed bracken collected in Gifu Prefecture, used in this study. Furthermore, as to the Gifu bracken group, the intestinal tumors were restricted to the ileum and most tumors were adenomas, whereas both epithelial tumors and sarcomas developed in the ileum and cecum in rats fed Hokkaido bracken. Thus, it may be inferred that bracken collected in Hokkaido has stronger carcinogenicity and that the carcinogenic activity of bracken is influenced by geographic locations.

3. *Carcinogenic activity in each part of bracken* (5)

The carcinogenic activity of the curled tops and stalks of the young bracken fronds, and also of the fronds and rhizomes was compared in ACI rats. For 2 months, rats received the pellets of 6 different compositions; containing the curled tops or the stalks of bracken fronds in the proportion of 1: 2, 1: 4, and 1: 8 by weight. In another experiment, rats were fed the pellets containing bracken fronds or rhizomes (1: 2) for 4 months. Carcinogenic activity was observed in each part of the bracken, and tumors were most frequently induced in the ileum. In rats given the curled tops, the incidence and multiplicity of the intestinal tumors were higher than in those receiving the stalks. Furthermore, in rats fed the pellets containing the bracken rhizome, the latent period of the tumor was shorter and the multiplicity was much higher than in those given the fronds. However, starch from the bracken rhizomes was not carcinogenic. Conceivably the bracken carcinogen was water-soluble and washed away in the preparation process. These results showed that the carcinogenic activity of the curled tops of young bracken fronds was stronger than that of the stalks and that the carcinogenic activity of the bracken rhizomes was stronger than that of young fronds.

4. *Relationship between the stage of maturation of bracken and the carcinogenic activity*

To compare the carcinogenic activity of mature bracken with that of immature young bracken with curled tops, the following experiment was undertaken. The mature bracken used in this experiment was collected in September in the same area of Hokkaido, where the immature bracken had been collected.

ACI rats, 1–1.5 months old, of both sexes were divided into 3 groups. Group I: for 4 months, 17 rats received pellets containing the mature bracken in pro-

TABLE II. Time at Which Rats Fed Mature Bracken Died or Were Killed, and the Corresponding Incidence of Tumor

Time after initiation of feeding (months)	Group I					Group II		
	No. of deaths	No. of rats with tumors of				No. of deaths	No. of rats with tumors of	
		Ileum	Colon	Bladder	Miscell.		Ileum	Bladder
0– 3	3					1		
9–10	1	1		1		1		
10–11						2	2	
11–12	1	1				3	3	1
12–13						3	3	1
13–14	3	1		2	1[a]	1	1	1
14–15						4	4	2
15–16	9	7	1	1	1[b]	2	2	
Total	17	10	1	4	2	17	15	5

[a] Mammary carcinoma. [b] Hemangioendothelial sarcoma of the mesentery.

portion by weight of 1 part bracken to 2 parts basal diet. Group II: for 8 months, 17 rats received the same pellets as in Group I. Another group of 20 rats served as controls; they were fed the normal diet. All the rats in both Groups I and II survived beyond 9 months, except for a few animals which died within 3 months after the start of feeding (Table II). Comparing the results obtained in this study with those in the previous experiment, in which rats were fed pellets containing the young bracken for 4 months, it was evident that the latent period of the tumor in rats fed pellets containing mature bracken was longer than in those fed pellets containing immature young bracken, i.e., although the majority of animals fed young bracken died of tumor within 11 months and all the animals died within 14 months after the start of feeding, the majority of rats fed mature bracken were still alive even 16 months after the start of experiment. In the incidence of the intestinal tumors, there was a significant difference between the two groups (24/24 and 10/14). As to the incidence of urinary bladder tumors, tendency of slightly higher carcinogenicity was noticed in the group fed mature bracken (4/14) than that fed bracken (1/24). Although the histological types of the intestinal tumors were mainly adenocarcinomas in the group fed young bracken, the majority of intestinal tumors in the group fed mature bracken were adenomas rather than adenocarcinomas. In the control group, there were no tumors except for 1 rat with an adrenal tumor. Thus, it was evident that even the mature bracken retained a relatively potent carcinogenic activity, though it was weak compared with the young bracken. The latent period for ileal tumors was shorter in rats fed mature bracken pellets for 8 months than in those fed the same bracken pellets for 4 months (Table II).

5. *Carcinogenic activity of young bracken in mice*
Thirty-four mice of C57BL/6 strain and 20 mice of dd strain, 1 month old, of both sexes were used. For 4 months they received the same pellets containing

the young bracken (1 : 2) as used in rats. The tumor incidence was lower in mice than in rats. Although intestinal tumors developed in 11 mice of C57BL/6 strain, unlike in rats, the location of the tumors was restricted to the terminal jejunum. On the other hand, intestinal tumors were not induced in dd strain, whereas lung adenomas were encountered in 7 of 10 mice which survived beyond 9 months after the start of experiment. In control mice of each strain, neither intestinal tumors nor lung adenomas were observed. Evans (2) also reported the development of lung adenomas in mice fed bracken, but no intestinal tumors. Urinary bladder tumors were not induced in mice.

6. Carcinogenicity of pterolactam isolated from bracken

We have successfully isolated a 5-membered lactam, 5-methoxy-2-pyrrolidone, from bracken, which was named pterolactam (23). Carcinogenicity of this compound was studied with the following three experiments. Experiment I: pterolactam was mixed with 4 times its weight of cholesterol by grinding thoroughly in a mortar. The mixture was compressed into columnar pellets, 0.5 cm in diameter and weighing 22 to 26 mg. Pellets of comparable mass were also prepared from cholesterol. The pterolactam-cholesterol pellets were surgically implanted into the urinary bladder of 30 female, 7- or 8-week-old Swiss mice. Another 30 mice serving as a control group were implanted with cholesterol pellets. Experiment II: ACI rats, 1.5 months old, of both sexes received the experimental diet for 64 days, in which pterolactam was mixed with the basal diet to 0.07% of the total. The concentration of pterolactam used was derived from the previous bracken feeding experiments, and was assumed to be sufficient for producing tumors, considering this compound is carcinogenic. Experiment III: 8 newborn rats of ACI strain received the intragastric dose of aqueous solution of pterolactam 1 mg/g body weight within 24 hr after birth and another dose 1 week later. Experiment I was terminated after 365 days and Experiments II and III were terminated 480 days after the start of administration of pterolactam. There was no significant difference in results obtained between experimental groups and controls. Thus, the carcinogenic activity of pterolactam could not be proved.

Petasites japonicus MAXIM.

The carcinogenicity of young flower stalks of wild petasites, which were collected in Gifu Prefecture from the end of March to April, and of cultivated young flower stalks and also that of cultivated mature terrestrial part of petasites were studied in ACI rats of both sexes. The fresh plant material was dried, milled, and mixed with the rat basal diet CE-2 in various ratios and administered to rats according to the dietary regimens shown in Tables III and V. The experiments were terminated 480 days after the start of feeding.

1. Carcinogenic activity of flower stalks of wild petasites (13)

In rats fed 33–8% diet of young flower stalks of wild petasites (Groups 1–7 in Table III), the most remarkable changes were observed in the liver. Although

TABLE III. Experimental Groups Administered the Flower
Stalks of Wild Petasites

Group No.	Age of ACI rats (months)	Number			Treatment: concentration of flower stalks and period of administration
1	2	13	M	6	33% diet for 3 weeks, subsequently 26.6% diet for 180 days
			F	7	
2	1.5	19	M	10	32% diet for 1 week and a normal diet for 3 weeks alternately, until the termination of experiment
			F	9	
3	2	13	M	7	16.6% diet for 134 days, followed by 8.3% diet for 86 days
			F	6	
4	1.5	23	M	10	16% diet for 1 week and a normal diet for 2 weeks alternately
			F	13	
5	1.5	36	M	21	12% diet for 1 week and a normal diet for 1 week alternately
			F	15	
6	1	14	M	6	8% diet until the termination of experiment
			F	8	
7	1	30	M	15	8% diet for 180 days, then two cycles of 5 days of 32% diet and 10 days of normal diet; thereafter followed by 5 days of 8% and 10 days of normal diets alternately
			F	15	
8	1.5	30	M	15	8% diet for 1 week and a normal diet for 1 week alternately
			F	15	
9	1	19	M	11	4% diet until the termination of experiment
			F	8	
10	1	27	M	12	4% diet for 180 days, subsequently 8% diet for 1 week and a normal diet for 1 week alternately
			F	15	
11	1	30	M	15	1% diet until the termination of experiment
			F	15	

TABLE IV. Time at Which Rats in Groups 9 and 10 Died or Were Killed and
the Corresponding Incidence of Tumor

Time after initiation of feeding (months)	Group 9				Group 10			
	No. of deaths	No. of rats with			No. of deaths	No. of rats with		
		Hemangio-endothelial sarcoma	Hepato-cellular adenoma	Hepato-cellular carcinoma		Hemangio-endothelial sarcoma	Hepato-cellular adenoma	Hepato-cellular carcinoma
0– 7					2			
7– 8	2							
12–13	2	2						
13–14	1	1						
14–15	1	1			1			
15–16	13	4	4	1	24	3	6	2
Total	19	8	4	1	27	3	6	2

microscopic findings of liver sections in these rats varied with the concentration of the plant material in diet and the period of administration, megalocytosis, proliferation of the bile duct, and nodular hyperplasia were the most prominent findings. These changes finally resulted in cirrhosis without tumors. In Groups 8, 9, and 10, hemangioendothelial sarcomas (Photos 3–5) were induced in the liver

Table V.   Experimental Groups Administered
the Cultivated Mature Petasites

Group No.	Age of ACI rats (months)	Number			Treatment: concentration of petasites and period of administration
1	1.5	20	M F	11 9	32% diet for 190 days
2	1	10	M F	5 5	32% diet for 10 days and a normal diet for 10 days alternately during 365 days
3	1	15	M F	7 8	16% diet until the termination of experiment
4	1	15	M F	7 8	16% diet for 120 days and then a normal diet for 75 days, subsequently 32% diet for 10 days and a normal diet for 10 days alternately

in 3/30, 8/19, and 3/27, respectively. Thus, the incidence was the highest, 42%, in Group 9 which continuously received the 4% diet (Tables III and IV). In addition to the hemangioendothelial sarcoma, hepatocellular adenomas and hepatocellular carcinomas (Photo 6) were also observed in relatively low incidence. In Group 11, which continuously received the 1% diet, no particular changes were observed.

2.   Carcinogenic activity of flower stalks of cultivated petasites

One group of 16 rats, 1 month old, received the 8% diet of flower stalks of cultivated petasites for 120 days. Another group of 30 rats received alternately the 8% diet for 1 week and a normal diet for 1 week, until the termination of this experiment. The flower stalks of cultivated petasites had much weaker hepatotoxicity compared with the wild type, and almost all the animals did not show any particular changes in their liver, except that 1 of 16 animals which received the 8% diet for 120 days had hemangioendothelial sarcoma.

3.   Carcinogenic activity of cultivated mature petasites

The carcinogenicity of the mature terrestrial part of cultivated petasites, Japanese name "Fuki," was studied in 4 dietary regimens as shown in Table V. The hepatotoxicity was very slight and only proliferation of bile ducts was observed even in rats fed 32% diet. Thus, it was inferred that the hepatotoxicity of mature petasites is weaker than that of the flower stalks.

DISCUSSION

Evans and Mason (3) and Pamukcu and Price (19, 21) found that intestinal tumors induced in rats fed bracken were only epithelial. But our rats fed unprocessed young bracken had a high incidence of sarcoma in addition to that of epithelial tumors. Such a difference may be attributed to the fact that rats in our experiment received the younger bracken which contained probably more carcinogen for a longer period than those used by Evans and Mason. This speculation was supported by our experimental finding that the carcinogenic activity of mature bracken was weaker than that of immature young bracken.

Pamukcu and Price (*19*) suggested that the high incidence of human stomach cancer in Japan could be partially the result of bracken, since significant quantities of this plant have long been accepted as a human food. In Japan, bracken is usually used as a human food after the harshness is removed by treatment with wood ash, sodium hydrogen carbonate, or sodium chloride. The present study revealed that carcinogenicity of bracken could be reduced remarkably by such a process. These facts should be taken into consideration in the evaluation of carcinogenic risk of bracken to man. The high incidence of urinary bladder tumors in rats fed processed bracken treated with boiling water or mature bracken suggests that urinary bladder tumors develop in rats when a relatively small amount of bracken carcinogen is given for a long period.

The nature of the carcinogen in bracken and petasites has not yet been elucidated. Pamukcu *et al.* (*18*) divided urine from cattle fed bracken into nonacidic and acidic fractions, and implanted the pellets containing each fraction into the urinary bladder of mice. Tumor incidence was significantly higher in the group of animals exposed to the acidic fraction. Furthermore, they implanted the pellets containing the methanol extract of bracken into the urinary bladder of mice and suggested that the carcinogenic substance is soluble in methanol (*20*). Leach *et al.* (*15*) reported the isolation of an active principle, $C_7H_8O_4$, from the bracken fern that is mutagenic, carcinogenic, and lethal to mice. However, detailed data have not yet been published. The carcinogenicity of pterolactam, a new compound isolated from bracken, was not proved. It seems to be of utmost importance to establish a screening test for the carcinogenicity of each fraction processed from bracken.

Acknowledgments

The authors are indebted to Dr. K. Takatori, Pharmacy of Nagoya University Hospital, Nagoya, for the isolation of pterolactam. This investigation was supported by Grants-in-Aid for Scientific Research from the Ministry of Education and from the Japan-U.S. Cooperative Medical Science Program.

REFERENCES

1. Bull, L. B., Culvenor, C. C. J., and Dick, A. T. "The Pyrrolizidine Alkaloids," North-Holland Publ. Co., Amsterdam (1968).
2. Evans, I. A. The radiomimetic nature of bracken toxin. *Cancer Res.*, **28**, 2252–2261 (1968).
3. Evans, I. A. and Mason, J. Carcinogenic activity of bracken. *Nature*, **208**, 913–914 (1965).
4. Hirono, I. Carcinogenicity and neurotoxicity of cycasin with special reference to species difference. *Fed. Proc.*, **31**, 1493–1497 (1972).
5. Hirono, I., Fushimi, K., Mori, H., Miwa, T., and Haga, M. Comparative study of carcinogenic activity in each part of bracken. *J. Natl. Cancer Inst.*, **50**, 1367–1371 (1973).
6. Hirono, I., Hayashi, K., Mori, H., and Miwa, T. Carcinogenic effects of cycasin in Syrian golden hamsters and the transplantability of induced tumors. *Cancer Res.*, **31**, 283–287 (1971).
7. Hirono, I., Laqueur, G. L., and Spatz, M. Tumor induction in Fischer and

Osborne-Mendel rats by a single administration of cycasin. *J. Natl. Cancer Inst.*, **40**, 1003–1010 (1968).

8. Hirono, I. and Shibuya, C. High incidence of pulmonary tumors in dd mice by a single injection of cycasin. *Gann*, **61**, 403–407 (1970).

9. Hirono, I., Shibuya, C., and Fushimi, K. Tumor induction in C57BL/6 mice by a single administration of cycasin. *Cancer Res.*, **29**, 1658–1662 (1969).

10. Hirono, I., Shibuya, C., Fushimi, K., and Haga, M. Studies on carcinogenic properties of bracken, *Pteridium aquilinum*. *J. Natl. Cancer Inst.*, **45**, 179–188 (1970).

11. Hirono, I., Shibuya, C., Shimizu, M., and Fushimi, K. Carcinogenic activity of processed bracken used as human food. *J. Natl. Cancer Inst.*, **48**, 1245–1250 (1972).

12. Hirono, I., Shibuya, C., Shimizu, M., Fushimi, K., Mori, H., and Miwa, T. Carcinogenicity examination of some edible plants. *Gann*, **63**, 383–386 (1972).

13. Hirono, I., Shimizu, M., Fushimi, K., Mori, H., and Kato, K. Carcinogenic activity of *Petasites japonicus* MAXIM., a kind of coltsfoot. *Gann*, **64**, 527–528 (1973).

14. Laqueur, G. L. and Spatz, M. Toxicology of cycasin. *Cancer Res.*, **28**, 2262–2267 (1968).

15. Leach, H., Barber, G. D., Evans, I. A., and Evans, W. C. Isolation of an active principle from the bracken fern that is mutagenic, carcinogenic and lethal to mice on intraperitoneal injection. *Biochem. J.*, **124**, 13–14 (1971).

16. McLean, E. K. The toxic actions of pyrrolizidine (senecio) alkaloids. *Pharmacol. Rev.*, **22**, 429–483 (1970).

17. Pamukcu, A. M., Göksoy, S. K., and Price, J. M. Urinary bladder neoplasms induced by feeding bracken fern (*Pteris aquilina*) to cows. *Cancer Res.*, **27**, 917–924 (1967).

18. Pamukcu, A. M., Olson, C., and Price, J. M. Assay of fractions of bovine urine for carcinogenic activity after feeding bracken fern (*Pteris aquilina*). *Cancer Res.*, **26**, 1745–1753 (1966).

19. Pamukcu, A. M. and Price, J. M. Induction of intestinal and urinary bladder cancer in rats by feeding bracken fern (*Pteris aquilina*). *J. Natl. Cancer Inst.*, **43**, 275–281 (1969).

20. Pamukcu, A. M., Price, J. M., and Bryan, G. T. Assay of fractions of bracken fern (*Pteris aquilina*) for carcinogenic activity. *Cancer Res.*, **30**, 902–905 (1970).

21. Price, J. M. and Pamukcu, A. M. The induction of neoplasms of the urinary bladder of the cow and the small intestine of the rat by feeding bracken fern (*Pteris aquilina*). *Cancer Res.*, **28**, 2247–2251 (1968).

22. Schoental, R. Toxicology and carcinogenic action of pyrrolizidine alkaloids. *Cancer Res.*, **28**, 2237–2246 (1968).

23. Takatori, K., Nakano, S., Nagata, S., Okumura, K., Hirono, I., and Shimizu, M. Pterolactam, a new compound isolated from bracken. *Chem. Pharm. Bull. (Tokyo)*, **20**, 1087 (1972).

EXPLANATION OF PHOTOS

PHOTO 1.   Adenocarcinoma of the ileum. ×45.

PHOTO 2.   Spindle cell fibrosarcoma of the ileum. ×280.

PHOTO 3.   Hemangioendothelial sarcoma of the liver inarat which continuously received the 4% diet of young flower stalks of wild petasites. 372 days after the start of experiment.

PHOTO 4.   Microscopic findings of hemangioendothelial sarcoma. Tumor cells form a complex vascular network. ×260.

PHOTO 5.   Hemangioendothelial sarcoma. Anaplastic endothelial cells are of a giant cell type. ×520.

PHOTO 6.   Hepatocellular carcinoma. ×260.

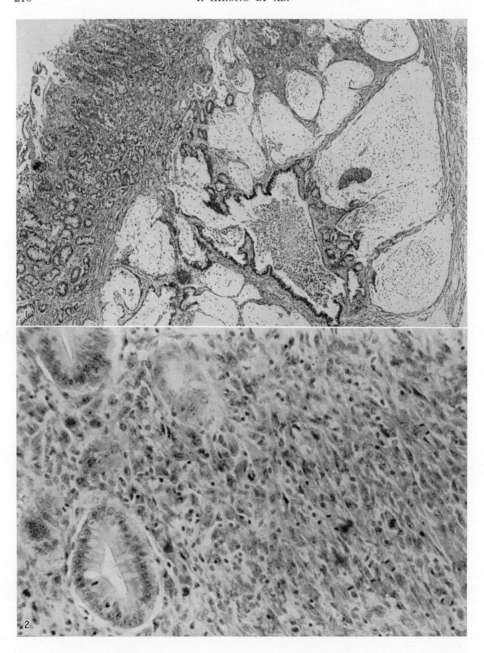

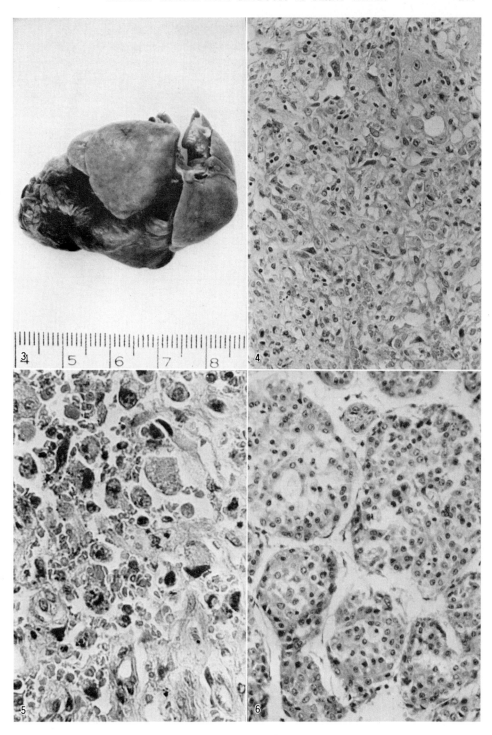

GANN Monograph on Cancer Research 17, 219–241 (1975)

STUDIES ON THE CARCINOGENICITY OF DDT

Lorenzo TOMATIS and Vladimir TURUSOV

International Agency for Research on Cancer*

The experimental studies on the possible carcinogenicity of $1,1,1$-trichloro-2, 2-bis (p-chlorophenyl) ethane (DDT) in mice indicate that (1) lifetime exposure to technical DDT results in a high incidence of hepatomas in males at concentrations of 2, 10, 50, and 250 ppm, and in females at a concentration of 250 ppm; (2) DDT-induced hepatomas rarely metastasize and in many instances do not show obvious signs of invasiveness; in mice exposed to 250 ppm DDT, however, they could be related to a considerable shortening of the life span; (3) the capacity of DDT to induce liver tumors is related to the dose administered, as well as to the duration of the administration; (4) the persistence of DDT-induced hepatomas does not depend on the continuous administration of DDT; DDT-induced hepatomas do not regress but continue to grow after cessation of the treatment; and (5) with lifetime exposure, one of the two main metabolites of DDT, p,p'-1, 1-dichloro-2, 2-bis (p-chlorophenyl) ethylene (DDE), caused a high incidence of hepatomas in both sexes and the other, p,p'-1, 1-dichloro-2, 2-bis (p-chlorophenyl) ethane (DDD), caused a high incidence of lung tumors. The results of long-term studies carried out in other animal species indicate a borderline carcinogenic effect of DDT in rats, which has not been confirmed, however, by more recent studies, and no effect in hamsters. The few available studies in man refer to a small number of individuals and for too limited an observation period to allow any conclusion regarding a possible carcinogenic effect of DDT in man.

Among the pesticides used at present, some are acutely toxic but are rapidly biodegradable, and current good practice can assure their residues in food within acceptable levels, and others are much less acutely toxic but persist in the environment and accumulate in the food chain. Most of the organochlorine pesticides (OCIs) are in this latter category. They are generally only slightly soluble in water and very soluble in fatty substances. For this reason, they tend to be stored in animal fat tissue, including that of man, at levels which depend on the intake and metabolic capacities of the species concerned (*25*).

The results of investigations carried out in a laboratory model ecosystem indicate that OCIs accumulate in the tissues of fish and snails at levels from 200 to 84,000 times greater than in water of the model system. OCIs therefore undergo a pronounced ecological magnification, which is inversely correlated to their

---

* 150 cours Albert Thomas, Lyon 69008, France.

water solubility, and have instead low biodegradability indices (30). These laboratory investigations confirm environmental observations that fish can build up concentrations of 1, 1, 1-trichloro-2, 2-bis (p-chlorophenyl) ethane (DDT) at mg/kg levels from ng/liter concentrations in the water (25, 34).

OCIs are stored in tissues of adult animals and also in fetal tissues. Man is no exception, and OCIs have been found in human fetal tissues as well as in human milk (17, 58).

The main reasons for concern regarding the potential hazard for human health represented by OCIs, and by DDT in particular, are based on (a) their ubiquity, (b) their persistence in the environment, (c) their capacity to accumulate in living organisms, including man, and their capacity to accumulate in the fetus and in mothers' milk, and (d) the experimental evidence that some of them increase tumor incidence in laboratory animals.

A few OCIs have been used for public health purposes and in agriculture and forestry. The most widely used is undoubtedly DDT, which was initially employed to control body lice, and therefore typhus, and later used to fight against various disease carriers. It has been the most successful of all pesticides used in malaria control, and has also reduced the cost of operations by 20 times. Although massively used in the fight against disease carriers, its use has progressively expanded in agriculture and forestry, to the point that only a minor part of the total world production in 1971 was employed for public health purposes.

In 1967, at a joint FAO/WHO Committee Meeting on Pesticide Residues, a recommendation was made to the International Agency for Research on Cancer (IARC) to carry out an experimental investigation on the possible carcinogenicity of DDT. At that time the experimental evidence of carcinogenicity of DDT was based on the results obtained in three experiments. The first was by Fitzhugh and Nelson in 1947 (11) in which 192 rats were exposed to dietary concentrations of DDT ranging from 100–800 ppm. Of these, 83 survived at least 18 months, and of these, 4 had hepatic cell tumors and 11 had nodular adenomatoid hyperplasia of the liver. The results of an experiment by Kemény and Tarján were published in a preliminary report in 1966 (26) and indicated a progressively increased occurrence of tumors—mainly leukemias, reticulum cell sarcomas, and lung tumors—in BALB/c mice exposed to dietary concentrations of 2.8 to 3.0 ppm of DDT (crystalline p, p'-DDT). A third report (14) indicated the occurrence of hepatomas in rainbow trout fed a diet containing 18 or 75 ppm of DDT.

In 1968 the IARC initiated a large collaborative study, partly carried out in Lyon and partly at three other national laboratories, namely, the Research Institute of Oncology in Leningrad, the Institute of Experimental and Clinical Oncology in Moscow, and the Istituto Nazionale per lo Studio e la Cura dei Tumori in Milan. At the IARC laboratory in Lyon, the experiment was carried out on CF-1 minimal inbred mice (48, 50), in Milan on BALB/c mice (42), in Moscow on Strain A mice (38), and in Leningrad on white rats (23).

In Lyon, Moscow, and Leningrad, technical DDT from the same source (Ugine Kuhlmann, Jarrie, France) was used. Its average composition was 73–

78% p, p'-DDT, 20% o, p'-DDT, 1% m, p'-DDT, 0.5–1.5% p, p'-1, 1-dichloro-2, 2-bis (p-chlorophenyl) ethane (DDD), and 0.5% p, p'-1, 1-dichloro-2, 2-bis (p-chlorophenyl) ethylene (DDE). For the experiment carried out in Milan, technical DDT obtained by Geigy, Milan, had an average composition of 70–75% p, p'-DDT, 20% o, p'-DDT, and 0.2–4% p, p'-DDD. The results of the experiments carried out at the IARC laboratories in Lyon will be reviewed here in detail, and the other studies will be mentioned only for comparison or to discuss discordant results. An ample review of the DDT studies is available in a recent IARC publication (*25*).

Experimental Results

1. Multigeneration study

The largest experimental investigation carried out at the IARC laboratory in Lyon consisted of a multigeneration study in which the parents and five consecutive generations of CF-1 mice were exposed to DDT mixed into the diet for the lifetime. The concentrations of DDT used were 2, 10, 50, and 250 ppm, and these were fed to groups of 60 males and 60 females. Two groups of the same size served as controls, one fed a control diet was a negative control, and one given urethan at a concentration of 0.01% in the drinking water serving as positive control. Details of materials and methods have been reported previously (*48, 50*). The acute oral LD_{50} in CF-1 mice was 251.3 mg/kg in females and 237.0 mg/kg in males. (In a parallel experiment carried out by Terracini *et al.* (*41, 42*), the acute oral LD_{50} in BALB/c mice was found to be 160 mg/kg in both sexes.)

There were minor differences in the breeding records of the various experimental groups, but fertility and fecundity did not appear to be impaired by DDT, even in the group given the highest dose. Preweaning mortality was similar in all experimental groups, except in the group receiving 250 ppm of DDT, in which it was higher than in any other group (Table I). No differences in survival rates were observed between the untreated control and the 2, 10, and 50 ppm DDT groups up to the 90th week, at which time over 50% of the animals were alive. After the 90th week, mortality was higher in the DDT-treated groups

TABLE I. Breeding Record and Preweaning Mortality in CF-1 Mice Untreated
or Exposed to Various Dose Levels of DDT or to Urethan
(Cumulative Data for Generations F_1–F_5) (*50*)

Group	No. of females		No. of newborns	Aver. No. of newborns per litter	Dead before weaning	
	Mated	Fertile			No.	%
Control	152	143	1,376	9.5	185	13.4
DDT 2 ppm	139	137	1,384	10.1	131	9.4
DDT 10 ppm	146	134	1,253	9.3	135	10.7
DDT 50 ppm	112	104	1,077	10.0	100	9.2
DDT 250 ppm	189	177	1,598	10.2	482	30.1
Urethan	111	110	1,107	10.0	148	13.3

TABLE II. Cumulative Percentages of Animals Surviving by Treatment
Group, Sex, and Age (4)

Treatment	Sex	No. of animals	% alive at age (weeks)				
			0	70	90	110	130
Control	M	348	100	80.7	63.5	32.5	13.8
	F	363	100	79.1	60.0	35.0	14.0
DDT 2	M	362	100	83.7	57.2	22.4	3.0
	F	354	100	77.4	55.1	23.7	5.6
DDT 10	M	367	100	81.7	57.2	25.1	8.2
	F	370	100	83.8	64.9	42.4	15.4
DDT 50	M	396	100	84.6	52.8	21.5	3.5
	F	349	100	80.2	56.4	26.9	6.3
DDT 250	M	372	100	72.3	28.5	1.3	0.0
	F	334	100	66.5	41.3	9.9	1.5
Urethan	M	315	100	72.1	39.7	8.9	0.1
	F	248	100	72.2	40.7	12.1	1.2

than in untreated controls. Mortality was highest in the 250 ppm DDT and
urethan-treated groups, beginning from the 60th week (Table II). The percentage of tumor-bearing animals (TBA) was slightly higher in DDT and urethan-
treated mice than in untreated controls, and this was more evident in mice exposed to the highest level of DDT (48, 50). The average number of tumors per
mouse was higher in males of all DDT groups than in controls, but in DDT-
treated females it was only higher in the groups exposed to 50 and 250 ppm.
CF-1 mice have a rather high incidence of tumors occurring in untreated animals, the most common types being lymphomas, lung tumors, and osteomas in
both sexes and hepatomas in males. With the exception of hepatomas, the incidences of these tumors were not consistently affected by DDT treatment.

The incidence of hepatomas was increased in male mice in all DDT groups

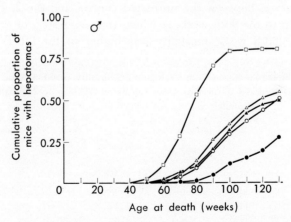

FIG. 1. Cumulative proportion of mice with hepatomas dying at different time
periods (males) (50)

● control; ▲ DDT 2 ppm; ○ 10 ppm; △ 50 ppm; ☐ 250 ppm.

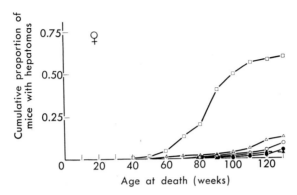

F<small>IG</small>. 2. Cumulative proportion of mice with hepatomas dying at different time periods (females) (*50*)
     See Fig. 1 for symbol key.

compared to negative controls, and was significant (*P*<0.001) even at the lowest level of exposure, *i.e.*, 2 ppm. It was similar in the 2-, 10-, and 50-ppm groups. In females, the incidence of hepatomas was not increased in the 2 ppm group. It was slightly higher than controls in the 10-ppm group and significantly increased (*P*<0.01) in the 50-ppm group. The incidences of hepatomas were greatly elevated in mice of both sexes exposed to 250 ppm (Figs. 1 and 2).

Macroscopically, the liver tumors were solitary, multiple, or confluent nodules, ranging from 2 to 20 mm in diameter. The nodules were pink or pinkish yellow with, in some instances, hemorrhagic areas. Microscopically, the tumors could be divided into three histological types (1) well-differentiated nodular growth, compressing but not obviously infiltrating the surrounding parenchyma, (2) nodular growth in which the normal architecture of the liver was disrupted and with frequent trabecular or glandular patterns, and (3) nodular growth consisting of poorly differentiated cells arranged in rows or rosettes and with a conspicuous vascular component. Transitional forms between (1) and (2), which could be described as hepatomas with different degrees of malignancy, were often seen. The tumors indicated in (3) have been described in detail as hepatoblastomas by Turusov *et al.* (*51*). The incidence of hepatomas giving rise to metastasis was low and not consistently different in DDT-treated and control mice. The incidence of metastasizing hepatoblastomas was relatively more elevated.

2. *Regression study*

Following the results obtained in the study described above, indicating that lifetime exposure of CF-1 mice to DDT results in a high incidence of liver tumors, an investigation was started in which mice were exposed to DDT for limited periods and sacrificed at different time intervals. The purpose of this study was to investigate (a) the effect of exposure of mice to DDT for limited periods of time and (b) whether the persistence and progression of the liver tumors that might result from DDT exposure for limited periods depended on the continuous administration of DDT, or, in other words, if the tumors would regress after cessation of DDT administration (*47*).

TABLE III.　Storage Levels of DDT and Metabolites in the Liver and in Various Tumors of CF-1 Mice Exposed to DDT for 15 or 30 Weeks and Killed at Different Time Intervals (47)

Group No.	Treatment	Time of killing[a] (weeks)	Sex	Liver					Tumors				
				p,p'-DDE (ppm)	o,p'-DDT (ppm)	p,p'-DDD (ppm)	p,p'-DDT (ppm)	Total (ppm)	p,p'-DDE (ppm)	o,p'-DDT (ppm)	p,p'-DDD (ppm)	p,p'-DDT (ppm)	Total (ppm)
1	15 wk DDT	15	F	4.08	0.60	10.13	5.52	20.33					
			F	15.60	3.71	26.65	34.60	79.56					
			F	7.47	0.34	18.32	16.91	43.04					
			F	7.50	0.23	27.20	29.55	64.48					
			M	2.92	0.32	9.93	11.63	24.80					
			M	3.76	0.61	8.47	20.25	33.09					
			M	6.40	1.78	16.90	19.50	44.58					
			M	13.93	0.98	22.01	19.25	56.17					
2	15 wk DDT	65	F	0.46	0.67	0.74	0.38	2.25	0.10	0.55	0.49	0.23	1.37[b]
			F	Lost					0.07	0.17	0.24	0.13	0.61[b]
			M	0.24	0.47	0.51	0.40	1.62	0.11	0.26	0.19	0.16	0.72[b]
			M	0.22	0.31	0.29	0.30	1.12	0.06	0.32	0.29	0.27	0.94[b]
4	15 wk DDT	120	F	0.04	0.16	0.13	0.03	0.36	0.03	0.05	0.05	0.04	0.17[c]
			F	0.02	0.04	0.02	0.03	0.11					
			M	0.03	0.02	0.06	0.26	0.37	0.20	0.02	0.05	0.07	0.34[c]
			M	0.02	0.03	0.02	0.03	0.10					
5	30 wk DDT	30	F	7.98	0.17	36.20	29.20	73.52					
			F	11.20	1.60	28.01	33.60	74.41					
			F	13.01	1.22	39.40	26.55	80.18					
			F	3.23	0.06	2.66	3.43	9.38					

Continued...

TABLE III

Group No.	Treatment	Time of killing[a] (weeks)	Sex	Liver					Tumors				
				p,p'-DDE (ppm)	o,p'-DDT (ppm)	p,p'-DDD (ppm)	p,p'-DDT (ppm)	Total (ppm)	p,p'-DDE (ppm)	o,p'-DDT (ppm)	p,p'-DDD (ppm)	p,p'-DDT (ppm)	Total (ppm)
6	30 wk DDT	65	M	6.25	1.18	37.80	22.10	67.33					
			M	4.86	1.31	30.50	12.80	49.47					
			M	3.84	0.24	17.78	21.55	43.41					
			M	4.33	0.33	28.15	29.75	62.56					
			F	0.10	0.08	0.22	0.59	0.99					
			F	0.06	0.05	0.09	0.27	0.47					
			F	0.52	0.31	0.37	0.33	1.53	0.65	0.75	1.22	1.12	3.74[b]
			F	1.72	0.31	9.08	0.33	11.44	0.70	1.11	3.74	0.93	2.74[b]
7	30 wk DDT	95	M	0.24	0.04	0.11	0.06	0.45	0.03	0.02	0.05	0.17	0.27[b]
			M	Lost	0.20	0.44	2.50	5.25	0.21	0.30	0.61	0.56	1.68[b]
			M	2.11	0.31	7.58	0.81	10.21	1.51	0.34	9.78	0.38	12.01[b]
			M	1.51	0.25	0.47	0.23	0.98	0.03	0.12	0.33	0.35	0.83[b]
			F	0.03	0.13	0.51	0.49	1.18	0.04	0.03	0.09	0.13	0.29[d]
			F	0.05					0.06	0.04	0.09	0.11	0.30[d]
									0.06	0.11	0.62	0.21	1.00[b]
			M	0.03	0.07	0.21	0.22	0.53	0.07	0.04	0.07	0.02	0.20[b]
									0.02	0.08	0.17	0.04	0.31[b]
			M	0.03	0.27	0.57	0.40	1.27	0.12	0.04	0.31	0.09	0.56[b]
									0.02	0.04	0.60	0.09	0.75[b]
8	30 wk DDT	120	F	0.05	0.07	0.12	0.16	0.40	0.05	0.05	0.16	0.11	0.37[b]
			F	0.05	0.10	0.09	0.16	0.40	0.05	0.05	0.09	0.09	0.26[b]
			M	0.05	0.09	0.09	0.13	0.36	0.03	0.05		0.09	
			M	0.05	0.23	0.13	0.17	0.58	0.09	0.16	0.23	0.26	0.74[b]

[a] Weeks from the beginning of the experiment. [b] Tumor of the liver. [c] Lung adenoma. [d] Tumor of the kidney.

Table IV. Storage Levels of DDT and Metabolites in the Interscapular
and Killed at Different

Group No.	Treatment	Time of killing (weeks)	Sex	Interscapular fat				
				p,p'-DDE (ppm)	o,p'-DDT (ppm)	p,p'-DDD (ppm)	p,p'-DDT (ppm)	Total (ppm)
1	15 wk DDT	15	F	91.60	12.40	72.10	402.50	578.60
			F	79.25	6.59	30.30	271.00	387.14
			F	50.30	12.70	32.80	171.50	267.30
			F	62.90	13.15	35.90	248.00	359.95
			M	45.25	15.80	37.45	343.50	442.00
			M	46.00	22.40	47.40	441.00	511.26
			M	48.00	6.87	35.80	282.00	372.67
			M	27.80	5.74	19.00	207.00	259.54
2	15 wk DDT	65	F	1.26	1.85	1.52	1.06	5.69
			F	1.15	2.03	2.20	1.21	6.59
			M	2.03	2.98	4.88	1.71	11.60
			M	0.49	0.88	0.87	1.56	3.80
4	15 wk DDT	120	F	0.03	0.02	0.25	0.17	0.47
			F	0.09	0.02	0.19	0.97	1.27
			M	0.05	0.04	0.23	0.24	0.56
			M	0.04	0.01	0.32	0.25	0.62
5	30 wk DDT	30	F	45.20	13.10	35.85	183.50	277.65
			F	65.30	9.41	32.50	495.00	602.21
			F	84.50	5.87	37.70	612.00	740.07
			F	3.44	4.38	8.87	50.08	66.77
			M	43.10	15.20	45.30	658.00	761.60
			M	49.60	14.70	70.70	616.50	751.50
			M	44.00	18.80	53.80	266.00	382.60
			M	29.35	56.35	34.80	157.00	277.50
6	30 wk DDT	65	F	0.45	0.33	0.77	0.53	2.08
			F	0.39	0.12	0.37	0.45	1.33
			F	12.10	1.36	2.85	11.70	28.01
			F	4.17	2.71	22.75	3.59	33.22
			M	0.19	0.14	0.48	0.55	1.36
			M	0.14	0.08	0.30	0.12	0.64
			M	0.83	2.48	2.51	5.20	11.02
			M	12.62	6.65	75.50	8.95	103.72
7	30 wk DDT	95	F	1.03	0.25	0.66	7.75	9.69
			F	0.10	0.63	0.96	3.27	4.96
			M	0.60	0.18	0.92	2.66	4.36
			M	1.03	0.34	2.29	17.45	21.11
8	30 wk DDT	120	F	0.28	0.29	0.45	0.28	1.30
			F	0.20	0.18	0.48	0.33	1.19
			M	0.25	0.41	0.90	0.62	2.18
			M	0.12	0.17	0.23	0.22	0.74

[a] ND : not detected.

Fat, Kidney, and Brain of CF-1 Mice Exposed to DDT for 15 or 30 Weeks Time Intervals (47)

	Kidney					Brain				
p,p'-DDE (ppm)	o,p'-DDT (ppm)	p,p'-DDD (ppm)	p,p'-DDT (ppm)	Total (ppm)		p,p'-DDE (ppm)	o,p'-DDT (ppm)	p,p'-DDD (ppm)	p,p'-DDT (ppm)	Total (ppm)
ND[a]						ND				
ND						ND				
6.45	0.76	7.08	21.20	35.49		4.26	0.83	4.69	11.70	21.48
5.85	0.87	6.64	25.20	38.56		2.96	0.61	2.87	11.70	18.13
2.04	0.90	4.05	20.80	27.79		1.73	1.13	3.44	16.15	22.45
4.82	2.13	7.07	37.13	51.15		2.91	0.93	3.95	2.27	10.06
ND						ND				
ND						ND				
0.48	0.73	0.56	0.47	2.24		0.66	0.80	1.05	1.11	3.62
0.43	0.84	0.91	0.50	2.68		0.48	0.94	0.77	0.84	3.03
0.49	0.96	0.52	0.55	2.52		0.65	0.96	1.39	1.09	4.09
0.30	0.44	0.65	0.34	1.73		0.36	0.54	0.40	0.62	1.92
ND						ND				
ND						ND				
ND						ND				
ND						ND				
4.76	0.59	5.42	38.20	48.97		20.15	0.45	4.81	15.40	40.81
ND						ND				
ND						ND				
5.41	0.54	2.28	5.96	14.19		8.57	0.71	3.52	8.35	21.15
ND						ND				
ND						ND				
4.20	1.20	5.29	33.40	44.09		2.59	0.91	4.41	17.75	25.66
2.47	1.13	30.00	23.20	56.80		1.32	0.68	3.52	8.20	13.72
0.09	0.10	0.25	0.16	0.60		0.10	0.12	0.23	0.15	0.60
0.06	0.07	0.35	0.11	0.59		0.14	0.23	0.31	0.20	0.88
0.72	0.52	0.82	0.76	2.82		0.58	0.51	1.07	1.86	4.02
1.45	0.52	6.10	0.96	9.03		1.59	0.62	4.62	1.36	8.19
0.07	0.06	0.16	1.07	1.36		0.10	0.16	0.28	0.20	0.74
0.02	0.04	0.08	0.55	0.69		0.04	0.04	0.08	0.12	0.28
0.18	0.36	0.98	3.80	5.32		0.73	0.46	0.98	3.87	6.04
2.31	0.51	5.95	7.65	16.42		1.84	1.00	4.28	2.08	9.20
0.02	0.15	0.22	0.29	0.68		0.04	0.23	0.40	0.15	0.82
0.23	0.03	0.14	0.18	0.58		0.03	0.09	0.28	0.46	0.86
0.02	0.10	0.18	0.11	0.41		0.04	0.05	0.22	0.98	1.29
0.04	0.22	0.47	0.23	0.96		0.04	0.39	0.75	0.66	1.84
0.09	0.15	0.15	0.44	0.83		0.12	0.13	0.15	0.37	0.77
0.08	0.08	0.19	0.28	0.63		0.06	0.15	0.11	0.20	0.52
0.05	0.14	0.18	0.29	0.66		0.09	0.14	0.25	0.24	0.72
0.08	0.13	0.12	0.31	0.64		0.14	0.24	0.24	0.29	0.91

TABLE V. Storage Levels of DDT and Metabolites in the Liver and Interscapular Fat of CF-1 Control Mice Killed at Different Time Intervals (47)

Group No.	Treatment	Time of killing (weeks)	Sex	Liver					Tumors				
				p,p'-DDE (ppm)	o,p'-DDT (ppm)	p,p'-DDD (ppm)	p,p'-DDT (ppm)	Total (ppm)	p,p'-DDE (ppm)	o,p'-DDT (ppm)	p,p'-DDD (ppm)	p,p'-DDT (ppm)	Total (ppm)
9	Control	15	F	0.026	<0.004	<0.005	0.007	0.033	0.010	<0.009	0.030	0.008	0.048
			F	0.005	0.006	0.006	0.012	0.029	0.007	<0.009	0.173	0.009	0.189
			M	0.216	0.445	0.173	<0.003	0.834	0.007	<0.009	0.021	0.017	0.045
			M	0.008	0.010	0.006	0.008	0.032	0.016	0.018	0.036	0.026	0.096
10	Control	30	F	0.008	<0.004	0.006	0.008	0.022	0.308	0.376	0.071	0.562	1.317
			F	0.006	<0.004	0.012	<0.003	0.018	0.050	<0.009	0.038	0.016	0.104
			M	0.008	0.022	0.003	0.005	0.038	0.065	0.030	0.044	0.022	0.161
			M	0.015	0.011	0.223	0.051	0.300	0.088	0.093	0.080	0.043	0.304
11	Control	65	F	0.011	0.011	0.022	0.003	0.047	0.013	0.049	0.056	0.008	0.126
			F	0.003	0.004	0.014	0.002	0.023	0.047	0.008	0.145	0.006	0.206
			M	0.028	0.003	0.020	0.010	0.061	0.010	0.007	0.063	0.009	0.089
			M	Lost					Lost				
12	Control	120	F	0.005	0.004	0.008	0.007	0.024	0.040	0.006	0.070	0.020	0.136
			F	0.006	0.007	0.017	0.003	0.033	0.015	0.005	0.034	0.008	0.062

Eight groups of 120 ten-week-old CF-1 mice, equally divided by sex, were exposed to technical DDT mixed into the diet at a concentration of 250 ppm, either for 15 or 30 weeks. Following 15 weeks of exposure, group 1 was killed at 15 weeks, that is, at the cessation of the treatment, group 2 at 65 weeks, group 3 at 95 weeks, and group 4 at 120 weeks. Following 30 weeks of exposure, group 5 was killed at 30 weeks, that is, at cessasion of the treatment, group 6 at 65 weeks, group 7 at 95 weeks, and group 8 at 120 weeks. Five additional groups (groups 9 to 13), given a normal diet, served as controls and were killed at 15, 30, 65, 95, and 120 weeks, respectively.

The evaluation of storage levels of DDT was carried out at the time DDT exposure was discontinued. In addition, in the groups exposed for 15 weeks, an evaluation was carried out 50 and 105 weeks later, and in the groups exposed for 30 weeks, 35, 65, and 90 weeks later. The analyses were carried out on fresh tissue of the following organs: liver, brain, kidney, interscapular fat, and some tumors. The results are given in Tables III, IV, and V. Storage levels following 15 and 30 weeks of exposure were similar, indicating that a saturation level was already reached after 15 weeks. Storage levels dropped more rapidly and intensively in the animals that were exposed for 15 weeks than in those exposed for 30 weeks. These findings indicate that mice can eliminate a large proportion of the DDT accumulated during the administration period, but indicate also that the cessation of administration of DDT does not mean cessation of exposure. Sixty-five weeks after 30 weeks of exposure, the storage levels in fat tissue and liver were of the same order as those found in tissues of mice exposed to 2 ppm of DDT (*49*).

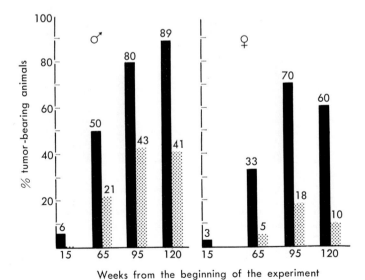

FIG. 3.   Percentage of mice bearing tumors at all sites and of mice bearing hepatomas among CF-1 mice exposed to DDT for 15 weeks and killed or dying at different time intervals (*47*)

■ all tumors; ▨ hepatomas.

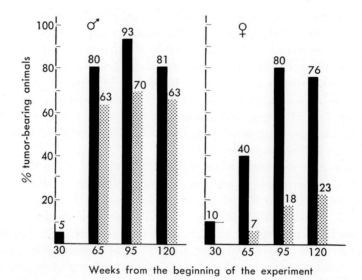

FIG. 4. Percentage of mice bearing tumors at all sites and of mice bearing hepatomas among CF-1 mice exposed to DDT for 30 weeks and killed or dying at different time intervals (47)

See Fig. 3 for symbol key.

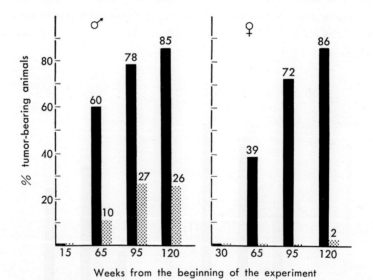

FIG. 5. Percentage of mice bearing tumors at all sites and of mice bearing hepatomas among untreated CF-1 mice killed or dying at different time intervals (47)

See Fig. 3 for symbol key.

Figures 3, 4, and 5 summarize data on animals bearing tumors at all sites and on animals bearing hepatomas, and Figs. 6, 7, and 8 summarize mortality data and hepatoma incidences. Tables VI, VII, and VIII summarize data on the size and multiplicity of hepatomas. Thirty weeks of exposure resulted in a high

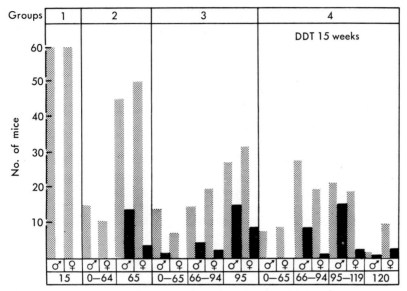

FIG. 6. Number of mice killed, dead, or killed moribund at different time intervals among CF-1 mice exposed to DDT for 15 weeks (experimental groups 1–4)

All mice were 9–10 weeks old at the beginning of the experiment. ⊠ No. of mice; ■ No. of mice with hepatomas.

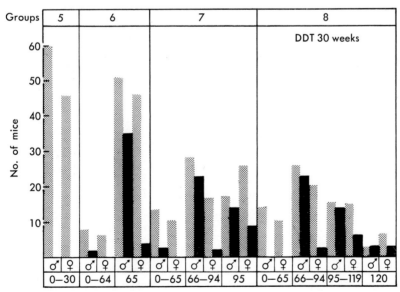

FIG. 7. Number of mice killed, dead, or killed moribund at different time intervals among CF-1 mice exposed to DDT for 30 weeks (experimental groups 5–8)

All mice were 9–10 weeks old at the beginning of the experiment. See Fig. 6 for symbol key.

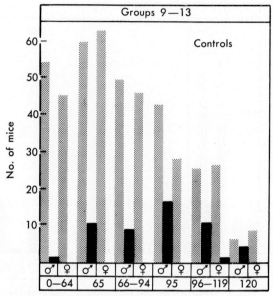

FIG. 8. Number of mice killed, dead, or killed moribund at different time intervals among untreated CF-1 mice (experimental groups 9–13)

All mice were 9–10 weeks old at the beginning of the experiment. See Fig. 6 for symbol key.

TABLE VI. Size and Multiplicity of Hepatomas in CF-1 Mice Exposed to DDT for 15 Weeks and Killed at Different Times (47)

No. at start	Killed at (weeks)[a]	Mice with hepatomas	Size of nodules (mm)[b]			Multiplicity		
			<5	6–10	>10	Single	Multiple	No. of nodules per mouse
60 M	15	—	—	—	—	—	—	—
60 F		—	—	—	—	—	—	—
60 M	65	13	7	3	3	6	7	2.7
60 F		3	2	1	—	2	1	1.3
60 M	95	25	4	4	17	10	15	2.5
60 F		11	9	2	—	8	3	1.3
60 M	120	25	4	5	16	11	14	2.6
60 F		5	2	3	—	5	—	1.0

[a] All mice were between 9 and 10 weeks old at the beginning of the experiment. [b] Number of mice with a nodule of a given size. In the case of multiple nodules, only the largest is considered.

incidence of hepatomas in males, which was consistently the same at 35, 65, and 90 weeks after cessation of exposure. In females, an increase in the incidence of hepatomas was observed from the 65th to the 120th week. In both sexes hepatomas larger than 10 mm were more frequent at 95 and 120 weeks than at 65

TABLE VII. Size and Multiplicity of Hepatomas in CF-1 Mice Exposed for 30 Weeks to DDT and Killed at Different Times (47)

No. at start	Killed at (weeks)[a]	Hepatomas						
		Mice with hepatomas	Size of nodules (mm)[b]			Multiplicity		
			<5	6–10	>10	Single	Multiple	No. of nodules per mouse
60 M	30	—	—	—	—	—	—	—
48 F		—	—	—	—	—	—	—
60 M	65	38	8	12	18	8	30	3.1
54 F		4	3	1	—	3	1	1.2
60 M	95	41	3	3	35	4	37	<4
55 F		11	4	3	4	4	7	2.7
60 M	120	37	6	4	27	6	31	2.6
54 F		11	4	2	5	7	4	1.5

[a] All mice were between 9 and 10 weeks old at the beginning of the experiment. [b] Number of mice with a nodule of a given size. In the case of muliple nodules, only the largest is considered.

TABLE VIII. Size and Multiplicity of Hepatomas in Untreated CF-1 Mice Killed at Different Times (47)

No. at start	Killed at (weeks)[a]	Hepatomas						
		Mice with hepatomas	Size of nodules (mm)[b]			Multiplicity		
			<5	6–10	>10	Single	Multiple	No. of nodules per mouse
10 M	15	—	—	—	—	—	—	—
10 F								
10 M	30	—	—	—	—	—	—	—
10 F								
70 M	65	12	6	4	2	9	3	1.2
69 F		—	—	—	—	—	—	—
83 M	95	24	9	7	8	13	11	1.6
72 F		—	—	—	—	—	—	—
98 M	120	33	9	10	14	15	18	1.9
90 F		1	1	—	—	—	—	—

[a] All mice were between 9 and 10 weeks old at the beginning of the experiment. [b] Number of mice with a nodule of a given size. In the case of multiple nodules, only the largest is considered.

weeks. Similar results were observed in mice exposed to DDT for 15 weeks, but the incidence of hepatomas was lower than after 30 weeks of exposure.

3. Long-term exposure to DDT metabolites

The biotransformation of DDT in various mammalian species is believed to first give rise to the two major metabolites, p, p'-DDE and p, p'-DDD (46).

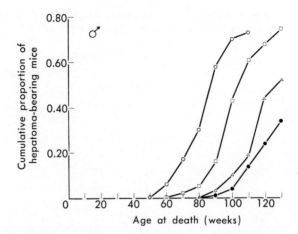

FIG. 9.   Cumulative proportion of male mice with hepatomas dying at different time periods (*46*)

● control;   △ DDD 250 ppm;   ○ DDE 250 ppm;   □ DDD 125 ppm
plus DDE 125 ppm.

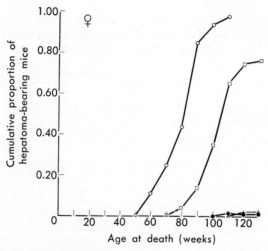

FIG. 10.   Cumulative proportion of female mice with hepatomas dying at
different time periods (*46*)

See Fig. 9 for symbol key.

It has been shown that in mice exposed to technical DDT, p, p'-DDE represents
about 15% of the total DDT stored in the liver and 3–10% in the fat tissue, and
p, p'-DDD represents 39% in the liver and 10% in the fat tissue (*49*). In contrast,
in man most of the total DDT stored in fat tissue is represented by p, p'-DDE
(*19, 28*). With the purpose of investigating the possible carcinogenicity of these
two main metabolites, CF-1 mice were exposed for the life span to dietary concentrations of 250 ppm of either p, p'-DDE or p, p'-DDD, or dietary concentrations of 125 ppm of p, p'-DDE plus 125 ppm of p, p'-DDD.

As can be seen in Figs. 9 and 10, lifetime exposure to p, p'-DDE, and to a
lesser extent to the mixture of p, p'-DDE plus p, p'-DDD, resulted in a high in-

cidence and early appearance of liver tumors. Exposure to p, p'-DDD alone resulted in a moderate increase in the incidence of hepatomas in males and in a pronounced increase in lung tumors in both sexes.

Human Evidence

A general scarcity of epidemiological studies has often been noticed, and the case of DDT is no exception. Compared to the rather large number of experimental studies, there have been only very few studies in man, involving a limited number of people and for a limited period of time. The largest controlled exposure for man is that of "volunteers" from a penitentiary, who received daily doses of 3.5 or 35 mg/man/day of p, p'-DDT for 21.5 months (18). These volunteers (in total 24) were followed for a few years, and no information relevant to the possible carcinogenicity of DDT was provided. Two studies in 1958 (32) and 1967 (28) on workers occupationally exposed to DDT involved a total of 75 people for too short a period to draw any useful conclusions relevant to an assessment of the carcinogenicity of DDT (25). Laws et al. (29) investigated the liver function of 31 of the 35 men involved in the 1967 study, and with the exception of a slight elevation in alkaline phosphatases and transaminases found in 4 workers, no alterations of the liver were reported. Data on storage levels of DDT and metabolites in human tissues, mainly fat tissue, are available from studies carried out in several countries (25, 49, 57). Marked individual variations in storage levels were noted in all studies, and conspicuous variations in the average storage levels were found in different countries. In no instance, however, was a sample of human fat tissue ever found to be DDT-free. Storage levels of 2.47, 18.1, 2.5, and 4.5 ppm were found, for example, in fat tissue samples from, respectively, Japan, Israel, U.K., and Kenya (1, 2, 7, 56, 58).

Recent studies do not indicate that restrictions in the widespread and indiscriminate use of DDT have been consistently followed by a reduction of DDT storage levels. Although in the U.K., for instance, a decrease in the level of DDT storage in fat tissue was observed in successive years (1, 2, 9), an apparent increase in the level of DDT was found in human milk in the U.S.A. from 1964 to 1973 (15).

Several studies have been carried out on the levels of DDT and other chlorinated hydrocarbons in various tissues of patients with cancer and other chronic diseases, and two of these studies indicate that DDT residues were higher in cancer patients than in controls (6, 21, 33). However, no conclusions can be made from these studies concerning a possible causal relationship.

DISCUSSION AND CONCLUSION

The three experimental studies on the possible carcinogenicity of DDT in mice summarized here indicate that (1) lifetime exposure to technical DDT results in a high incidence of hepatomas in males at concentrations of 2, 10, 50, and 250 ppm, and in females at a concentration of 250 ppm, (2) DDT-induced hepatomas rarely metastasize and in many instances do not show obvious signs of invasiveness; in mice exposed to 250 ppm DDT, however, they could be related to a considerable shortening of the life span, (3) the capacity of DDT to induce liver tumors is related to the dose administered, as well as to the duration of the administration, (4) the persistence of DDT-induced hepatomas does not depend on the continuous administration of DDT; DDT-induced hepatomas do not regress, but continue to grow after cessation of the treatment (as mentioned previously in the text, with a chemical like DDT, cessation of treatment does not, however, mean cessation of exposure), and (5) with lifetime exposure, one of the two main metabolites of DDT, p, p'-DDE, caused a high incidence of hepatomas in both sexes and the other, p, p'-DDD, caused a high incidence of lung tumors.

The hepatocarcinogenic effect of DDT in mice has been confirmed in different studies carried out in several laboratories and on several strains of mice (*22, 42, 44, 55*). DDT exposure in mice has been reported to influence the incidence of tumors in organs other than the liver (*38, 40*), but this has not been confirmed (*41, 42, 48, 50*). An apparent low incidence of lymphomas in mice exposed to a high level of DDT, compared to untreated controls or mice exposed to low levels of DDT has been reported (*41, 42*). A negative association between lymphomas and hepatomas was found in another study (*4*) and awaits confirmation from a serial sacrifice experiment.

The results of long-term studies carried out in other animal species indicate a borderline carcinogenic effect of DDT in rats (*11*), which has not been confirmed, however, by more recent studies (*24, 31*), and no effect in hamsters (*3*).

The few available studies in man referred to a small number of individuals and for too limited an observation period to allow any conclusion regarding a possible carcinogenic effect of DDT in man. In the absence of objective criteria to extrapolate from experimental data to man, the lack of epidemiological studies or case reports does not allow any conclusions to be drawn from animal studies in terms of a possible carcinogenic hazard to man. In fact, the use of DDT has been restricted in several countries because of its impact on the environment and not because of the carcinogenic effect observed in mice.

Prevention of cancer is largely based on a somewhat arbitrary and uneven interpretation of experimental results. In general, a positive carcinogenic test carried out in rodents is sufficient to recommend a zero tolerance for a substance that may be an intentional or unintentional food additive. This procedure implies that experimental evidence *per se* is sufficient to predict a carcinogenic effect in man and amounts *de facto* to an extrapolation carried out for public health purposes.

While such a cautious procedure appears on the whole more than justified, no similar precaution is adopted when exposure, even at high levels, may occur in circumstances other than through food intake, as for instance, with occupational exposure.

The case of DDT is complicated by the co-existence of several factors: (1) DDT has already been used for over 25 years; it is a chemical with a very low and slow biodegradability, which, to a great extent, is the reason for its efficacy, and it is therefore here to stay for many years to come, whatever measures we may take today, (2) it has been extremely useful in almost every part of the world and is still indispensable in the fight against malaria, (3) it is of low acute toxicity, and (4) in mice, the only species in which a definite carcinogenic effect has been shown and confirmed, it produced only liver tumors.

It has been claimed that the induction of liver tumors in the mouse is not a significant index of carcinogenicity (13). Moreover, there is no consensus among pathologists on the interpretation of some of the liver lesions observed in long-term experiments with mice; in particular, the morphological resemblance between hepatomas and hyperplastic nodules has made the tracing of a borderline between these two lesions very difficult (5, 48).

From a recent review, it appears that a correlation exists between the capacity of a chemical to induce parenchymal liver tumors in the mouse and its capacity to induce tumors at any site in the rat and hamster (45). This finding indicated that neither the mouse in general nor the liver of the mouse in particular is necessarily a less reliable experimental model for demonstrating the carcinogenicity of a chemical than the rat and the hamster.

There are several examples showing that results obtained in experimental tests may predict similar results in man. Stilbestrol was known to be carcinogenic in experimental animals in the early 1950s (16, 39) at a time when it was used in human therapy, and not for life-saving reasons. However, measures concerning its indiscriminate use were not taken until 1971, when the first report by Herbst et al. (20) indicated the increased risk of cancer in daughters of women exposed to stilbestrol during pregnancy. The experimental evidence of carcinogenicity of bis(chloromethyl) ether was published in 1968, confirmed in 1969, and reconfirmed in 1971 (12, 27, 52, 53). It was 2 years later that measures were taken following the evidence obtained in retrospective studies in man (10, 43). The carcinogenicity of vinyl chloride in rats was shown in 1970 (54), but it was only in 1974, following the evidence of an excessive risk of angiosarcoma of the liver in workers exposed to vinyl chloride (8, 35), that measures were taken to reduce the maximum acceptable concentration to 50 ppm and then to reduce it even further.

The case of DDT is different from the three cases mentioned above, if for nothing else, at least for its different level of toxicity. Acute and subacute toxic effects of DDT have been very rarely reported, even following high levels of exposure, and the studies of Hayes et al. (18) and Laws et al. (29) seem to confirm the relatively low toxicity of DDT. The report of Schüttman (37), however, helps to remind us that DDT is certainly not free from toxic effects. Taking all this into account, and adding the capital fact that DDT has helped one billion people to live free from malaria and therefore saved millions of lives, it seems obvious to conclude that the benefits obtained from the usage of DDT have surpassed its possible risk (36). This conclusion is based on a risk versus benefit evaluation made a posteriori, that is, after almost 30 years of worldwide usage of DDT, and it is certainly not to be recommended as a standard procedure. We are, in fact, still unable to predict with certainty that DDT will not have any carcinogenic effect in man.

It is quite clear from all these considerations that additional efforts in developing criteria for evaluating experimental data in terms of possible human risk are both necessary and urgent. Everyone will probably agree that it is better to prevent the occurrence of cancer in man by preventing exposure to a chemical for which we can predict the carcinogenic effect in man, than by demonstrating that it has already produced a carcinogenic effect in man.

Acknowledgment

The authors gratefully acknowledge the excellent help of Elspeth Perez in the preparation of the manuscript and the tables.

REFERENCES

1. Abbott, D. C., Collins, G. B., and Goulding, R. Organochlorine pesticide residues in human fat in the United Kingdom, 1969–71. *Brit. Med. J.*, **2**, 553–556 (1972).

2. Abbott, D. C., Goulding, R., and Tatton, J. O'G. Organochlorine pesticide residues in human fat in Great Britain. *Brit. Med. J.*, **3**, 146–149 (1968).

3. Agthe, C., Garcia, H., Shubik, P., Tomatis, L., and Wenyon, E. Study of the potential carcinogenicity of DDT in the Syrian golden hamster. *Proc. Soc. Exp. Biol. Med.*, **134**, 113–116 (1970).

4. Breslow, N. E., Day, N. E., Tomatis, L., and Turusov, V. S. Associations between tumor types in a large-scale carcinogenesis study of CF-1 mice. *J. Natl. Cancer Inst.*, **52**, 233–239 (1974).

5. Butler, W. Pathology of liver cancer in experimental animals. *In* "Liver Cancer," IARC Scientific Publications No. 1, International Agency for Research on Cancer, Lyon, pp. 30–41 (1971).

6. Casarett, L. J., Fryer, G. C., Yauger, W. L., Jr., and Klemmer, H. Organochlorine pesticide residues in human tissue—Hawaii. *Arch. Environ. Health*, **17**, 306–311 (1968).

7. Curley, A., Burse, V. W., Jennings, R. W., Villanueva, E. C., Tomatis, L., and Akazaki, K. Chlorinated hydrocarbon pesticides and related compounds in adipose tissue from people of Japan. *Nature*, **242**, 338–340 (1973).

8. Editorial. Cancer deaths among PVC workers cause concern. *Chem. Eng. News*, p. 6, January 28 (1974).

9. Egan, H., Goulding, R., Roburn, G., and Tatton, J.O'G. Organochlorine pesticide residues in human fat and human milk. *Brit. Med. J.*, **2**, 66–69 (1965).

10. Figueroa, W. G., Raszkowski, R., and Weiss, W. Lung cancer in chloromethyl ether workers. *New Engl. J. Med.*, **288**, 1096–1097 (1973).

11. Fitzhugh, O. G. and Nelson, A. A. The chronic oral toxicity of DDT (2, 2-bis-(*p*-chlorophenyl)-1, 1, 1-trichlorethane). *J. Pharmacol. Exp. Ther.*, **89**, 18–30 (1947).

12. Gargus, J. L., Reese, W. H., Jr., and Rutter, H. A. Induction of lung adenomas in newborn mice by bis(chloromethyl) ether. *Toxicol. Appl. Pharmacol.*, **15**, 92–96 (1969).

13. Grasso, P. and Crampton, R. F. The value of the mouse in carcinogenicity testing. *Food Cosmet. Toxicol.*, **10**, 418–426 (1972).

14. Halver, J. E. Crystalline aflatoxin and other factors for trout hepatoma. Trout Hepatoma Research Conference Papers, Bureau of Sport Fisheries and Wild Life, Research Report No. 70, pp. 78–102 (1967).

15. Hagyard, S. B., Brown, W. H., Stull, J. W., Whiting, F. M., and Kemberling,

S. R. DDT and DDE content in human milk in Arizona. *Bull. Environ. Contam. Toxicol.*, **9**, 169–172 (1973).

16. Hartwell, J. L. Survey of compounds which have been tested for carcinogenic activity. Public Health Publ. No. 469, US Government Printing Office, Washington (1951).

17. Hayes, W. H., Jr. Monitoring food and people for pesticide content; scientific aspects of pest control. NAS-NRC Publ. No. 1402, pp. 314–332 (1966).

18. Hayes, W. J., Jr., Dale, W. E., and Pirkle, C. I. Evidence of safety of long-term, high, oral doses of DDT for man. *Arch. Environ. Health*, **22**, 119–135 (1971).

19. Hayes, W. J., Jr., Quinby, G. E., Walker, K. C., Elliott, J. W., and Upholt, W. M. Storage of DDT and DDE in people with different degrees of exposure to DDT. *Arch. Ind. Health*, **18**, 398–406 (1958).

20. Herbst, A. L., Ulfelder, H., and Poskanzer, D. C. Adenocarcinoma of the vagina: association of maternal stilbestrol therapy with tumour appearance in young women. *New Engl. J. Med.*, **284**, 878–881 (1971).

21. Hoffman, W. S., Adler, H., Fishbein, W. I., and Bauer, F. C. Relation of pesticide concentrations in fat to pathological changes in tissues. *Arch. Environ. Health*, **15**, 758–765 (1967).

22. Innes, J. R. M., Ulland, B. M., Valerio, M. G., Petrucelli, L., Fishbein, L., Hart, E. R., Pallotta, A. J., Bates, R. R., Falk, H. L., Gart, J. J., Klein, M., Mitchell, I., and Peters, J. Bioassay of pesticides and industrial chemicals for tumorigenicity in mice. A preliminary note. *J. Natl. Cancer Inst.*, **42**, 1101–1114 (1969).

23. International Agency for Research on Cancer. Annu. Rep., 1971, Lyon, p. 75 (1972).

24. International Agency for Research on Cancer. Annu. Rep., 1972–1973, Lyon, p. 69 (1973).

25. International Agency for Research on Cancer. "Evaluation of Carcinogenic Risk of Chemicals to Man: Some Organochlorine Pesticides," IARC Monograph, No. 5 (1974).

26. Kemény, T. and Tarján, R. Investigations on the effects of chronically administered small amounts of DDT in mice. *Experientia*, **22**, 748–749 (1966).

27. Laskin, S., Kuschner, M., Drew, R. T., Cappiello, V. P., and Nelson, N. Tumors of the respiratory tract induced by inhalation of bis(chloromethyl) ether. *Arch. Environ. Health*, **23**, 135–136 (1971).

28. Laws, E. R., Curley, A., and Biros, F. J. Men with intensive occupational exposure to DDT. *Arch. Environ. Health*, **15**, 766–775 (1967).

29. Laws, E. R., Jr., Maddrey, W. C., Curley, A., and Burse, V. W. Long-term occupational exposure to DDT. *Arch. Environ. Health*, **27**, 318–321 (1973).

30. Metcalf, R. L., Kapoor, I. P., Lu, P. Y., Schuth, C. K., and Sherman, P. Model ecosystem studies of the environmental fate of six organochlorine pesticides. *Environ. Health Perspect.*, No. 4, 35–44 (1973).

31. Napalkov, N. P. Personal communication.

32. Ortelee, M. F. Study of men with prolonged intensive occupational exposure to DDT. *A.M.A. Arch. Ind. Health*, **18**, 433–440 (1958).

33. Radomski, J. L., Deichmann, W. B., and Clizer, E. E. Pesticide concentrations in the liver, brain and adipose tissue of terminal hospital patients. *Food Cosmet. Toxicol.*, **6**, 209–220 (1968).

34. Reinert, R. E. Pesticide concentrations in Great Lakes fish. *Pestic. Monit. J.*, **3**, 233–240 (1970).

35. Rules and Regulations: Occupational Safety and Health Standards. *Fed. Regist.*, **39**, No. 67, 12342–12345 (1974).

36. Safe Use of Pesticides. WHO Tech. Rep. Ser., No. 513 (1973).

37. Schüttman, U. Chronische Lebererkrankungen nach beruflicher Einwirkung von Dichlordiphenyltrichloräthan (DDT) und Hexachlorcyclohexan (HCH). *Int. Arch. Gewerbepathol. Gewerbehyg.*, **24**, 193–210 (1968).

38. Shabad, L. M., Kolesnichenko, T. S., and Nikonova, T. V. Transplacental and combined long-term effect of DDT in five generations of A-strain mice. *Int. J. Cancer*, **11**, 688–693 (1973).

39. Shubik, P. and Hartwell, J. C. Survey of compounds which have been tested for carcinogenic activity. US Government Printing Office, Washington, Suppl. I (1957).

40. Tarján, R. and Kemény, T. Multigeneration studies on DDT in mice. *Food Cosmet. Toxicol.*, **7**, 215–222 (1969).

41. Terracini, B., Cabral, R. J., and Testa, M. C. A multigeneration study of the effects of continuous administration of DDT to BALB/c mice. *In* "Pesticides and the Environment, a Continuing Controversy" (Proc. 8th Interam. Conf. Toxicol. Miami, Fla., 1973), ed. by W. B. Deichmann, Intercontinental Medical Book Corp., New York/London, p. 77 (1973).

42. Terracini, B., Testa, M. C., Cabral, J. R., and Day, N. The effects of long-term feeding of DDT to BALB/c mice. *Int. J. Cancer*, **11**, 747–764 (1973).

43. Thiess, A. M., Hey, W., and Zeller, H. Zur Toxikologie von Dichlorodimethyläther —Verdacht auf kanzerogene Wirkung auch beim Menschen. *Z. Arbeitsmed.*, **23**, 97–102 (1973).

44. Thorpe, E. and Walker, A. I. T. The toxicology of dieldrin (HEOD). II. Comparative long-term oral toxicity studies in mice with dieldrin, DDT, phenobarbitone, β-BHC and γ-BHC. *Food Cosmet. Toxicol.*, **11**, 433–442 (1973).

45. Tomatis, L., Partensky, C., and Montesano, R. The predictive value of mouse liver tumour induction in carcinogenicity testing—A literature survey. *Int. J. Cancer*, **12**, 1–20 (1973).

46. Tomatis, L., Turusov, V., Charles, R. T., and Boiocchi, M. Effect of long-term exposure to 1,1-dichloro-2,2-bis(p-chlorophenyl)ethylene, to 1,1-dichloro-2,2-bis(p-chlorophenyl)ethane, and to the two chemicals combined on CF-1 mice. *J. Natl. Cancer Inst.*, **52**, 883–891 (1974).

47. Tomatis, L., Turusov, V., Charles, R. T., Boiocchi, M., and Gati, E. Liver tumours in CF-1 mice exposed for limited periods to technical DDT. *Z. Krebsforsch.*, in press (1974).

48. Tomatis, L., Turusov, V., Day, N., and Charles, R. T. The effect of long-term exposure to DDT on CF-1 mice. *Int. J. Cancer*, **10**, 489–506 (1972).

49. Tomatis, L., Turusov, V., Terracini, B., Day, N., Barthel, W., Charles, R. T., Collins, G. B., and Boiocchi, M. Storage levels of DDT metabolites in mouse tissues following long term exposure to technical DDT. *Tumori*, **57**, 377–396 (1971).

50. Turusov, V. S., Day, N. E., Tomatis, L., Gati, E., and Charles, R. T. Tumors in CF-1 mice exposed for six consecutive generations to DDT. *J. Natl. Cancer Inst.*, **51**, 983–997 (1973).

51. Turusov, V. S., Deringer, M. K., Dunn, T. B., and Stewart, H. L. Malignant mouse-liver tumors resembling human hepatoblastomas. *J. Natl. Cancer Inst.*, **51**, 1689–1695 (1973).

52. Van Duuren, B. L., Goldschmidt, B. M., Katz, C., Langseth, L., Mercado, G.,

and Sivak, A. Alpha-haloethers: A new type of alkylating carcinogen. *Arch. Environ. Health*, **16**, 472–476 (1968).

53. Van Duuren, B. L., Sivak, A., Goldschmidt, B. M., Katz, C., and Melchionne, S. Carcinogenicity of halo-ethers. *J. Natl. Cancer Inst.*, **43**, 481–486 (1969).

54. Viola, P. L., Bigotti, A., and Caputo, A. Oncogenic response of rat skin, lungs, and bones to vinyl chloride. *Cancer Res.*, **31**, 516–522 (1971).

55. Walker, A. I. T., Thorpe, E., and Stevenson, D. E. The toxicology of dieldrin (HEOD). I. Long-term oral toxicity studies in mice. *Food Cosmet. Toxicol.*, **11**, 415–432 (1973).

56. Wassermann, M., Rogoff, M. G., Tomatis, L., Day, N. E., Wassermann, D., Djavaherian, M., and Guttel, C. Storage of organochlorine insecticides in the adipose tissue of people in Kenya. *Ann. Soc. Belge Med. Trop.*, **52**, 509–514 (1972).

57. Wassermann, M., Tomatis, L., and Wassermann, D. Storage map of organochlorine compounds (OCC) in humans. Epidemiological deductions for further monitoring. Int. Symp. on Recent Advances in the Assessment of the Health Effects of Environmental Pollution, Paris, in press (1974).

58. Wassermann, M., Wassermann, D., Zellermayer, L., and Con, M. Pesticides in people. *Pestic. Monit. J.*, **1**, 15–20 (1967).

GANN Monograph on Cancer Research 17, 243–252 (1975)

INDUCTION OF TUMORS IN MICE WITH SYNTHETIC SEX HORMONES

G. Rudali

*Department of Genetics, Fondation Curie**

Three contraceptives (Enovid, Ovulen, and C-Quens) and their gestagens have been studied as possible carcinogenic agents for the mammary glands of mice. Intact and/or castrated females with the MTV (RIII, C3H, and (C3H×RIII)F₁ hybrids), and intact and castrated (C3H×RIII)F₁ hybrid males received the drugs mixed with the diet in lifetime experiments. The different hormones did not enhance mammary carcinogenesis in intact females. The two contraceptives norethynodrel and ethynodiol diacetate (but not chlormadinone acetate) shortened the latencies and raised the frequencies of mammary tumors in castrates of both sexes.

These results and in particular their possible significance for the hormonal etiology of human breast cancer are discussed.

The prevention of pregnancies with a chronic hormonal treatment was imagined nearly 20 years ago after the description by Pincus *et al.* of the anti-ovulatory activity of nor-steroids (*19*). Some years later contraceptive pills were introduced for human use, but their diffusion on a large scale started in fact only in 1966 and 1967. Now over 150 different preparations are available on the market. Most of them are mixtures of a gestagen and a small proportion (5 to 10%) of an estrogen. The estrogens in the "pills" are practically always the same in the commercial drugs; either mestranol or ethynylestradiol. The difference between the preparations arises from the progestin components.

The carcinogenic activity of natural estrogens in mice has been a well-established fact for four decades (*14*). After the discovery of synthetic estrogens, it appeared that all those tested in suitable animal material produced mammary gland cancers (*15, 21, 22, 24*). Furthermore, it appeared that the genetic constitution of the animals plays an important role as well in mice (*11, 16, 17, 26*) as in rats (*6, 7, 12*). Some animals are susceptible and others are resistant to the production of adenocarcinomas. The susceptibility of human beings to mammary cancer induction by hormones is, of course, unknown. But, it is highly probable that genetic variations, as in animals, also play an important role in man. In fact, the information in the literature concerning this problem is of questionable value. The statement that long-term administration of estrogens represents a carcinogenic risk for humans has never been clearly demonstrated. However, such a risk seems to be probable, or at least possible, although its degree cannot be estimated. It should be mentioned that Fechner could not confirm such a hypothesis (*9, 10*).

---

* 26, rue d'Ulm, 75005 Paris, France.

Because in 1966 no information was available about possible carcinogenic activity of progestins in mice or rats, a relatively large research program on this question was thought to be advisable. Its goal was to determine whether gestagens of various structures may have different biological activities, especially on the mammary gland. But the main interest of work in this field is, of course, to establish whether the commercial pills represent potential carcinogenic risks for the human population.

Several thousands of mice were used in our work. They belonged mostly to well-known pure strains or were F_1 hybrids of pure strain parents. A part of this work has already been reported (4, 23–25), but some of these experiments are unpublished.

Testing of Mice

In a preliminary stage of our research we had to establish what kind of mice to use for testing the hormones. It is well known that many strains, or substrains, of mice are resistant to the carcinogenic action of hormones on the mammary gland, whatever the doses used. Furthermore, in some other strains, virgin females have a very high spontaneous frequency of mammary tumors. In these animals hormonal administration does not raise the frequency or shorten the latencies. This appeared clearly in two different experiments with RIII and (C3H ×RIII)F_1 females. Table I shows the results obtained in these experiments in which intact females received a diet containing either 0.25 μg (RIII) or 2.5 μg of mestranol/mouse/day [(C3H ×RIII)F_1].

As shown, mestranol did not accelerate the normal spontaneous carcinogenesis of intact RIII and (C3H ×RIII)F_1 females, but accelerated the appearance of mammary tumors in castrated females and males. Mammary tumor virus (MTV)-free C57BL, XVII/G, and C3H/f castrated males or intact females

TABLE I. Mammary Carcinogenesis in Female and Male Mice Receiving a Diet Containing Mestranol

Groups	Strains	Number of mice	Number with tumors	Frequency (%)	Mean latency in days
Intact control females	RIII	15	12	80.0	358
Intact females receiving mestranol		40	26	65.0	379
Intact control females	(C3H × RIII)F_1	167	161	96.3	213
Intact females receiving mestranol		34	30	88.2	254
Castrated females		34	28	82.3	345
Castrated females receiving mestranol		34	32	94.1	221
Castrated males		41	7	17.1	480
Castrated females receiving mestranol		26	24	92.3	198
Intact males receiving mestranol		27	23	85.1	323

that received either a diet containing mestranol or a subcutaneous implantation with a paraffin pellet containing 10% estradiol did not develop mammary cancers.

It was accordingly decided to test the carcinogenic activity of gestagens and of contraceptive mixtures in castrated (C3H ×RIII)F$_1$ mice of both sexes, in intact (C3H ×RIII)F$_1$ males, and in intact C3H, RIII, and (C3H ×RIII)F$_1$ females also, the latter animals being considered as controls.

Testing of Hormones

Three complete contraceptives have been tested, Enovid, Ovulen, and Lutestral* as well as the gestagens of these mixtures, norethynodrel, ethynodiol diacetate, and chlormadinone acetate.

The hormones were mixed with the diet of the animals. The average intake/ mouse/ day was 2.5 g. Administration of the drugs started at the age of 3.5 weeks and was continued throughout life.

1) Enovid

Enovid is the first contraceptive that appeared for commercial diffusion. In many countries, it is now removed from the market. The preparation contains 99% norethynodrel and 1% mestranol. It was mixed in a proportion of 15 ppm with the diet of the mice. The average daily intake of the drug has been estimated at 30–40 μg/mouse. Enovid has been tested in intact RIII females, in castrated (C3H ×RIII)F$_1$ females, and in castrated (C3H ×RIII)F$_1$ males.

As expected, this contraceptive did not modify spontaneous carcinogenesis in intact RIII females. However, in (C3H ×RIII)F$_1$ castrates of both sexes the mixture considerably shortened the latencies (Table II).

TABLE II. Mammary Carcinogenesis in Mice Receiving Enovid Mixed with the Diet

Groups	Strains	Number of mice	Number with tumors	Frequency (%)	Mean latency in days
Control females	RIII	73	50	68.5	339
Females receiving Enovid		21	12	57.1	340
Castrated control females	(C3H× RIII)F$_1$	34	28	82.3	446
Castrated females receiving Enovid		33	24	72.7	178
Castrated control males		61	10	16.4	576
Castrated males receiving Enovid		23	20	86.9	242

2) Ovulen

Ovulen is still widely used as a contraceptive in many countries. It is a mixture of 90% ethynodiol diacetate and 10% mestranol. Its eventual carcinogenic

---

* Lutestral is the French commercial name for C-Quens.

TABLE III. Mammary Carcinogenesis in Intact and Castrated (C3H × RIII)F$_1$
Female and Male Mice Receiving Ovulen

Groups	Number of mice	Number with tumors	Frequency (%)	Mean latency in days
Intact females (controls)	167	161	96.3	213
Intact females receiving Ovulen	38	37	97.5	233
Castrated females (controls)	34	28	82.3	345
Castrated females receiving Ovulen	26	20	76.9	180
Intact males (controls)	76	0	—	—
Intact males receiving Ovulen	25	14	56	535
Castrated males (controls)	61	10	16.4	576
Castrated males receiving Ovulen	28	21	75	302

activity for the mammary gland was tested in castrated and intact (C3H ×RIII)
F$_1$ males and females. It was mixed with the diet in a proportion of 3 ppm.
The daily hormone intake/mouse was estimated at 7.5–10 μg. The results of these
experiments are shown in Table III. Like Enovid, Ovulen seems to promote
mammary carcinogenesis in the castrated males and females, but is without
effect in intact females (4).

3) Lutestral

Lutestral is a mixture of chlormadinone acetate (97.5%) and ethynylestradiol
(2.5%), known in the United States under the commercial name C-Quens. Contraceptives containing chlormadinone acetate have been removed from the market
in some countries. Lutestral is still widely used in other countries, as in France.
Lutestral was tested in intact RIII, C3H, and (C3H ×RIII)F$_1$ females and
in intact and castrated (C3H ×RIII)F$_1$ males. Eight ppm of Lutestral was incorporated in the diet. The daily intake/mouse was estimated at 20–30 μg.

TABLE IV. Mammary Carcinogenesis in Mice Receiving Lutestral

Groups	Strains	Number of mice	Number with tumors	Frequency (%)	Mean latency in days
Intact females (controls)	RIII	73	50	68.5	339
Intact females receiving Lutestral		40	31	77.5	359
Intact females (controls)	C3H	92	54	58.7	386
Intact females receiving Lutestral		30	20	66.6	427
Intact females (controls)	(C3H× RIII)F$_1$	167	161	96.3	213
Intact females receiving Lutestral		31	28	90.3	290
Castrated males (controls)		61	10	16.4	576
Castrated males receiving Lutestral		28	23	82.1	348
Intact males (controls)		76	0	—	—
Intact males receiving Lutestral		32	10	31.2	651

Table IV shows that this contraceptive, which contains like the two others a small proportion of an estrogen, has for some mice a promoting activity. This is the case especially with intact or castrated males. In intact females, however, a significant inhibitory activity was observed.

In summary, it appears that in some animal models the three different contraceptives tested induce mammary cancers with a high frequency. But if in a given model, as, for example, the castrated $(C3H \times RIII)F_1$ male, the frequencies and the latencies of the tumors are compared, it seems that the carcinogenic activity of the contraceptives depends on their structure. Enovid seems to be more active than Lutestral.

Such a difference does not result, obviously, from the chemical structure or the dose of the estrogen. It seemed to us more probable that it can be explained by the gestagens of the contraceptives. Experiments with these hormones confirmed our suspicion.

4) Norethynodrel

Norethynodrel, 13.5 ppm, was mixed with the diet. The daily hormone intake/mouse was 25 to 35 μg. The activity of the compound was studied in intact RIII, C3H, and $(C3H \times RIII)F_1$ females and in castrated $(C3H \times RIII)F_1$ females and males. Mammary carcinogenesis in these mice is shown in Table V. It appears that in at least one of the experimental models, the $(C3H \times RIII)F_1$ castrated male, norethynodrel is a potent carcinogenic agent.

TABLE V. Mammary Carcinogenesis in Mice Receiving Norethynodrel

Groups	Strains	Number of mice	Number with tumors	Frequency (%)	Mean latency in days
Intact females (controls)	RIII	73	50	68.5	339
Intact females receiving norethynodrel		31	19	61.3	444
Intact females (controls)	C3H	92	54	58.7	386
Intact females receiving norethynodrel		77	45	58.4	457
Intact females (controls)	$(C3H \times RIII)F_1$	167	161	96.3	213
Intact females receiving norethynodrel		49	48	98	213
Castrated females (controls)		34	28	82.3	345
Castrated females receiving norethynodrel		37	32	86.1	310
Castrated males (controls)		61	10	86.4	576
Castrated males receiving norethynodrel		29	29	100	262

5) Ethynodiol diacetate

Ethynodiol diacetate is the gestagen of Ovulen. It has been tested with several doses but only one of the experiments will be reported here. Ethynodiol diacetate has been studied with a particularly low dose, 0.075 ppm in diet. The

TABLE VI. Mammary Carcinogenesis in (C3H×RIII)F$_1$ Mice Receiving
Very Low Doses of Ethynodiol Diacetate in the Diet

Groups	Number of mice	Number with tumors	Frequency (%)	Mean latency in days
Intact females (controls)	167	161	96.3	213
Intact females receiving ethynodiol diacetate	32	30	94	253
Castrated males (controls)	61	10	16.4	576
Castrated males receiving ethynodiol diacetate	26	11	42.3	569

estimated daily intake of hormone/mouse was 1.50 to 2.50 μg. This is approximately the same as the human dose/kg. The aim of this experiment was to investigate whether such a small quantity of hormone can have any activity on mammary carcinogenesis. Intact female and castrated male (C3H ×RIII)F$_1$ mice have been used. The results are reported in Table VI.

6) Chlormadinone acetate

Particular attention was paid to chlormadinone acetate because Lutestral seemed to have less activity than Enovid or Ovulen. Accordingly, it may be imagined that chlormadinone acetate is lacking in carcinogenic activity.

The compound was tested at several doses. Two of these experiments will be reported here; one with 0.8 ppm of hormone mixed with the diet and the other with 8 ppm. With the first dose the daily intake/mouse was estimated to be 2 to 3 μg, and in the second experiment, 20 to 30 μg. Table VII shows that the low dose seems lacking in activity. The diet containing 8 ppm of hormone did not induce cancers in the castrated male and did not accelerate their appearance in spayed (C3H ×RIII)F$_1$ females.

TABLE VII. Mammary Carcinogenesis in Mice Receiving a Diet Containing
0.8 ppm of Chlormadinone Acetate

Groups	Strains	Number of mice	Number with tumors	Frequency (%)	Mean latency in days
Intact females (controls)	RIII	73	50	68.5	339
Females receiving chlormadinone acetate		19	10	52.6	444
Intact females (controls)	C3H	92	54	58.7	386
Females receiving chlormadinone acetate		43	28	65.1	390
Intact females (controls)	(C3H× RIII)F$_1$	167	161	96.3	213
Intact females receiving chlormadinone acetate		46	45	97.8	215
Castrated males (controls)		61	10	16.4	576
Castrated males receiving chlormadinone acetate		26	7	26.9	617

TABLE VIII. Mammary Carcinogenesis in Mice Receiving a Diet Containing
8 ppm of Chlormadinone Acetate

Groups	Strains	Number of mice	Number with tumors	Frequency (%)	Mean latency in days
Intact females (controls)	RIII	73	50	68.5	339
Females receiving chlormadinone acetate		30	18	60	459
Intact females (controls)	C3H	92	54	58.7	386
Females receiving chlormadinone acetate		36	24	66.6	453
Intact females (controls)	(C3H× RIII)F$_1$	167	161	96.3	213
Intact females receiving chlormadinone acetate		40	34	85	255
Castrated females (controls)		34	28	82.3	446
Castrated females receiving chlormadinone acetate		35	26	74.3	457
Castrated males (controls)		61	10	16.4	576
Castrated males receiving chlormadinone acetate		28	2	7.1	560

DISCUSSION

For 60 years, mice, especially of inbred strains, have been the most commonly used animals for research on mammary tumors. In 1916, Lathrop and Loeb (18) confirmed the clinical observations of Beatson (1) that ovarian secretions play a role in the course of these cancers. In 1932, Lacassagne (14) induced an adenocarcinoma in a male mouse with pure estrone.

The morphological similarity between mouse and human adenocarcinomas, as well as the experiments of Lathrop and Loeb suggested that the mouse is a convenient animal for comparative pathological research on human breast cancer and in particular on the role of hormones in the etiology of these tumors. It is, however, questionable whether direct transposition of results obtained in mice to human beings is always possible.

The role of endogenous or exogenous hormones in the etiology of mammary cancers in mice is one of the best known facts in cancer research. Such a role has never been clearly demonstrated in women. Estrogens have been used for 40 years in therapeutics. Several million women have been treated, sometimes for long periods and with large doses. There is practically no information available in the literature on breast cancers occurring in patients treated with these hormones.

A large number of male patients with prostatic cancer have been treated with estrogens, mostly stilboestrol, during the last three decades. In spite of the difficulty of performing statistical studies in usually elderly patients, there seem to be few observations of breast cancer occurring after such treatments (2). Symmers (27) observed two cases of breast cancer in trans-sexual males who had estrogens for several years.

The results reported here demonstrate some interesting facts. Complete contraceptives that contain estrogens enhance the development of mammary cancers in some animal models in which these tumors are infrequent and appear late in life, *i.e.*, castrated (C3H ×RIII)F_1 females and males. For intact females with a high incidence of spontaneous mammary cancers, *i.e.*, RIII, C3H, and (C3H ×RIII)F_1 virgins, the contraceptives have a mild but significant inhibitory activity.

The same phenomenon has been observed with two gestagens, norethynodrel and ethynodiol diacetate. Chlormadinone acetate, although an inhibitor of mammary carcinogenesis in intact females, did not shorten the latencies nor raise the frequencies in castrated animals. It can be supposed, accordingly, that a gestagen with progesterone-like anti-ovulatory activity is not necessarily carcinogenic for the mammary glands of castrated mice. We have at present no explanation for the cancer-promoting activity of some hormones in castrates and their inhibitory activity in intact females.

These experiments, furthermore, did not clearly answer the main question at the origin of this research; do contraceptive pills represent a potential carcinogenic risk for the mammary gland of women? Fechner (8) in a statistical study on patients with fibroadenomas of the breast before (1956) and after (1958) the "pill era" could not demonstrate an increase of frequency during the last 15 years. The frequency of breast cancer in young women (under 35 years of age) is actually the same as 5% which was observed before 1958 (9). Chemama *et al.* (3) have treated young women operated for breast cancer with estrogen-progestin mixtures for 2–5 years and did not observe increased recurrences in such patients, supposed to be liable to develop tumors.

The induction or the enhancement, of mammary carcinogenesis in castrates shows that, in at least one experimental system, the hormones accelerate the appearance of tumors. But the significance of this model for the human users is questionable.

In a recent work (5) by an important group of British pathologists with nearly 7,000 mice and rats of both sexes, a careful study was made not only of the mammary glands but also of the uterus, liver, lungs, pituitary, adrenals, gonads, and lymphoid system. Very few tumors were obtained after administration of various doses of gestagens or contraceptive mixtures. The final conclusion of the authors was that, considering their experimental conditions, there is no evidence that the hormones investigated can be suspected as potential carcinogenic agents for women using contraceptive pills. Rieche (20) in Germany did not obtain with Anovlar an enhancement of mammary carcinogenesis in C3H intact virgin females. Welsh and Meites (29), and Weisburger *et al.* (28) observed with high doses of Enovid an inhibition of mammary carcinogenesis in 7,12-dimethylbenz(a)anthracene-treated rats. Heston *et al.* (13) have recently published a study of the action of Enovid on mice of five strains and found, as in our group, a mild inhibitory effect of this drug on spontaneous mammary carcinogenesis in C3H females. Our negative results obtained in intact female mice are accordingly similar to those observed by other authors in mice and rats.

If small rodents are still considered acceptable material for such research, it appears that contraceptive mixtures are probably not carcinogenic for intact women.

For some years beagle bitches have been proposed for testing the eventual activity of these hormones in women. It is doubtful whether such animals, as different from women as mice are, from the point of view of their ovarian cycle and their general hormonal balance, can provide better results than rodents. The value of primates is certainly better. But the systematic use of such animals would probably produce technical problems that will be difficult to resolve.

Acknowledgments

It is obvious that the reported experiments required the active collaboration of several scientists and of well-qualified technicians. Mrs. E. Coezy, D. Sc., and Mr. R. Chemama, M. D. have realized an important part of this work. Mrs. F. Apiou, Miss F. Frederic, and Mrs. M. Guggiari have provided appreciated technical assistance. Mr. L. Aussepe, our chief animal technician for many years, supplied us with the mice in excellent condition. We are highly indebted to him for his continuous help.

The hormones used in these experiments were offered to our laboratory by Dr. V. A. Drill from G. D. Searle and Co. (Enovid and norethynodrel); Dr. C. Lafaurie from Cassenne-France Co. (Lutestral and chlormadinone acetate); Dr. M. Brunaud from Clin-Byla-Laboratory, France (Ovulen, mestranol, and ethynodiol diacetate).

REFERENCES

1. Beatson, G. T. On the treatment of inoperable cases of carcinoma of the mamma: suggestions for a new method of treatment with illustrative cases. *Lancet*, **2**, 104–106 (1896).
2. Benson, W. R. Carcinoma of the prostate with metastases to breasts and testis. *Cancer*, **10**, 1235–1245 (1957).
3. Chemama, R., Jayle, M. F., Ennuyer, A., Bataini, P., and Dhermain, P. Remarques au sujet de quelques malades encore jeunes soumises à l'association gestagène—oestrogène immédiatement après traitement radical de tumeurs malignes du sein. *Bull. Cancer*, **57**, 239–250 (1970).
4. Coezy, E. and Rudali, G. Action d'un contraceptif (Ovulène) sur la carcinogenèse mammaire des souris. *Rev. Eur. Etud. Clin. Biol.*, **15**, 205–209 (1970).
5. Committee on Safety of Medicines. "Carcinogenicity Tests of Oral Contraceptives," Her Majesty's Stationery Office, London (1972).
6. Dunning, W. F., Curtis, M. R., and Segaloff, A. Strain differences in response to diethylstilboestrol and the induction of mammary gland and bladder cancer in the rat. *Cancer Res.*, **7**, 511–521 (1947).
7. Dunning, W. F. and Curtis, M. R. The incidence of diethylstilboestrol-induced cancer in reciprocal F_1 hybrids obtained from crosses between rats of inbred lines that are susceptible and resistant to the induction of mammary cancer by this agent. *Cancer Res.*, **12**, 702–706 (1952).
8. Fechner, R. E. Fibroadenomas in patients receiving oral contraceptives. A clinical and pathological study. *Am. J. Clin. Pathol.*, **53**, 857–864 (1970).
9. Fechner, R. E. Breast cancer during oral contraceptive therapy. *Cancer*, **26**, 1204–1211 (1970).
10. Fechner, R. E. Carcinoma of the breast during estrogen replacement therapy. *Cancer*, **29**, 566–573 (1972).

11. Gardner, W. U. Estrogens in carcinogenesis. *Arch. Pathol.*, **27**, 138–170 (1939).

12. Geschickter, C. F. Mammary carcinoma in the rat with metastasis induced by estrogen. *Science*, **89**, 35–37 (1939).

13. Heston, W. E., Vlahakis, G., and Desmukes, B. Effects of the antifertility drug Enovid in five strains of mice, with particular regard to carcinogenesis. *J. Natl. Cancer Inst.*, **51**, 209–222 (1973).

14. Lacassagne, A. Apparition de cancers de la mamelle chez la souris mâle soumise à des injections de folliculine. *Compt. Rend.*, **195**, 630–632 (1932).

15. Lacassagne, A. Apparition d'adenocarcinomes mammaires chez des souris mâles traitées par une substance oestrogène synthétique. *C. R. Soc. Biol.*, **129**, 641–643 (1938).

16. Lacassagne, A. A comparative study of the carcinogenic action of certain oestrogenic hormones. *Am. J. Cancer*, **28**, 735–740 (1936).

17. Lacassagne, A. Influence d'un facteur familial dans la production par la folliculine de cancers mammaires de la souris. *C.R. Soc. Biol.*, **114**, 427–429 (1933).

18. Lathrop, A. E. C. and Loeb, L. Further investigations on the origin of tumors in mice. III. On the part played by internal secretion in the spontaneous development of tumors. *J. Cancer Res.*, **1**, 1–19 (1916).

19. Pincus, G., Chang, M. C., Zarron, N. X., Hafez, E. S. E., and Merrill, A. Studies of the biological activity of certain 19-norsteroids in female animals. *Endocrinology*, **59**, 695–707 (1956).

20. Rieche, K. Perorale Langzeitbehandlung mit "Anovlar" bei mammakarzinom-belastenen Inzuchtmäuse. *Abh. Dtsch. Akad. Wiss. Berlin Kl. Med.*, **1**, 35–38 (1967).

21. Robson, J. M. and Bonser, G. M. Production of mammary carcinomas in mice of a susceptible strain by the synthetic oestrogen, triphenylethylene. *Nature*, **142**, 836–883 (1938).

22. Rudali, G. Production de tumours mammaires à l'aide d'un dérivé de l'acide allènolique chez des souris mâles. *C.R. Soc. Biol.*, **146**, 916–918 (1952).

23. Rudali, G., Coezy, E., and Gourdon, A. C. Action d'un anticonceptionnel de synthèse sur la carcinogenèse mammaire de la souris RIII. *Rev. Fr. Etud. Clin. Biol.*, **12**, 1010–1014 (1967).

24. Rudali, G., Coezy, E., Frederic, F., and Apiou, F. Susceptibility of mice of different strains to the mammary carcinogenic action of natural and synthetic oestrogens. *Rev. Eur. Etud. Clin. Biol.*, **16**, 425–429 (1971).

25. Rudali, G., Coezy, E., and Chemama, R. Mammary carcinogenesis in female and male mice receiving contraceptives or gestagens. *J. Natl. Cancer Inst.*, **49**, 813–819 (1972).

26. Suntzeff, V., Kirtz, M. M., Blumenthal, H. T., and Loeb, L. The incidence of mammary gland carcinoma and cancer age in mice injected with estrogen and in non-injected mice of different strains. *Cancer Res.*, **1**, 446–456 (1941).

27. Symmers, W. S. C. Carcinoma of the breast in trans-sexual individuals after surgical and hormonal interference with the primary and secondary sex characteristics. *Brit. Med. J.*, **2**, 83–87 (1968).

28. Weisburger, J. H., Weisburger, E. K., and Griswold, D. P., Jr. Reduction of carcinogen induced breast cancer in rats. *Life Sci.*, **5**, 259–266 (1964).

29. Welsch, W. and Meites, J. Effects of norethynodrel-mestranol combination (Enovid) on development and growth of carcinogen-induced mammary tumors in female rats. *Cancer*, **23**, 601–607 (1969).

EXPERIMENTAL MODEL
OF TUMORS IN
VARIOUS ORGANS

GANN Monograph on Cancer Research 17, 255-267 (1975)

INDUCTION OF UNDIFFERENTIATED ADENO-CARCINOMA IN THE STOMACH OF RATS BY N-METHYL-N'-NITRO-N-NITROSO-GUANIDINE WITH VARIOUS KINDS OF SURFACTANT[*1]

Michihito Takahashi, Shoji Fukushima, and Motoo Hananouchi

First Department of Pathology, Nagoya City University Medical School[*2]

Undifferentiated adenocarcinoma of the glandular stomach in rats was induced by N-methyl-N'-nitro-N-nitrosoguanidine (MNNG) with various kinds of surfactant as a vehicle. Surfactants employed were polyoxyethylene sorbitan monostearate, polyoxyethylene nonyl-phenyl ether, and two types of alkylbenzenesulfonate.

Diagnostic criteria of undifferentiated adenocarcinoma were based on the absence of glandular structures. Undifferentiated adenocarcinomas consisting of anaplastic glandular cells were induced in a high incidence in the experimental groups (administered MNNG combined with the surfactant). Lymphatic invasion of cancer cells was found in 6 cases and one metastasized to intestinal lymph nodes. However, the control group (administered MNNG alone) revealed well-differentiated adenocarcinomas in many cases and neither lymphatic invasion nor metastasis was found.

Electron-microscopic examination of the undifferentiated adenocarcinoma which showed signet-ring cells, revealed two types. One type of tumor cells was closely packed with mucin, pushing the nucleus to one side and forming a signet-ring appearance. The mucin granules were pale, large, and mutually fused. The other type revealed a small cystic luminal structure in the cytoplasm. The wall was lined with microvilli projecting into the lumen. The microcyst became distended and the nucleus was pushed to one side of the cell.

The morphological characteristics and the biological behavior of undifferentiated adenocarcinomas of the glandular stomach in rats resemble those of human gastric cancer.

N-Methyl-N'-nitro-N-nitrosoguanidine (MNNG), which is an alkylating agent, is known to be a potent mutagen (*12*). The antitumor, antileukemic, antimicrobial, and antimalarial properties have been described by many investigators (*6*). Druckrey *et al.* (*4*), Schoental (*18*), and Sugimura *et al.* (*22*) reported the

[*1] This work was supported in part by a Grant-in-Aid for Cancer Research from the Ministry of Education and from the Ministry of Health and Welfare, Japan.

[*2] Kawasumi 1, Mizuho-cho, Mizuho-ku, Nagoya 467, Japan (高橋道人, 福島昭治, 花之内基夫).

carcinogenic properties of MNNG. Sugimura *et al.* (*23–25*) succeeded in producing a high incidence of adenocarcinomas in the glandular stomach of rats administered MNNG in the drinking water (*7*).

Previous papers (*27, 28*) from this laboratory reported that when 4-nitroquinoline 1-oxide in diluted ethanol combined with alkylbenzenesulfonate, one of the strongest surfactants, was administered to rats by esophageal intubation, undifferentiated adenocarcinoma was produced in the glandular stomach with metastasis. This evidence may support the penetration of the carcinogen through the protective mucus barrier in the stomach by virtue of the surfactants.

This paper describes the carcinogenic effect of MNNG combined with four kinds of surfactant. Electron-microscopic examination of the undifferentiated adenocarcinoma was made.

Production of Stomach Cancer in Rats

Sixty-eight male rats of Wistar strain were used. They ranged from 140 to 155 g in weight at the beginning of the experiment. They were fed commercial pellet food, Oriental MF (Oriental Yeast Ind., Tokyo) freely during the experiment. MNNG was obtained as a commercial chemical (Aldrich Chemical Company, Inc., Milwaukee, U.S.A.). Both hard and soft types of sodium alkylbenzenesulfonate were prepared by sulfonation of the commercial alkylbenzenes at Nitto Whaling Co., Ltd. (Tokyo). Polyoxyethylene sorbitan monostearate (Tween 60) was purchased (Katayama Chemical, Osaka). Polyoxyethylene nonylphenyl ether (Nonipol) was supplied by Sanyo Chemical, Osaka.

The rats were divided into four experimental groups (Groups I, II, III, and IV) and one control group (Group V). Group I: 13 male rats received MNNG at a concentration of 100 mg/liter containing 0.4% Tween 60 in the drinking water freely for 36 weeks. Group II: 16 rats were given MNNG at a concentration of 100 mg/liter containing 0.2% Nonipol in the drinking water in the same way as in Group I. Groups III and IV: 15 rats and 10 rats were administered MNNG at a concentration of 100 mg/liter containing 0.1% hard type alkylbenzenesulfonate and 0.1% soft type alkylbenzenesulfonate in the same way for 63 weeks. Group V (control): 14 rats were given MNNG solution alone without a surfactant at a concentration of 100 mg/liter for 63 weeks.

Thereafter, all the rats received ordinary tap water until the termination of the experiment. The rats which survived more than 18 weeks after the beginning of the experiment were considered to be effective. The body weight was measured weekly. All the rats which died or were killed were autopsied. The stomach was opened along the greater curvature and other organs were carefully examined. Tissues were fixed in 10% formalin solution. The specimens were sent for routine histological examination and selected tissues were stained by special staining methods.

For electron microscopy, small pieces of tumor tissue obtained from Group II rats were fixed for 1 hr at 4° in 2.5% glutaraldehyde buffered at pH 7.4 with cacodylate, then post fixed in 1% osmium tetroxide in the same buffer at 4° for 1 hr, dehydrated in graded ethanol and acetone, and embedded in Epon 812.

TABLE I. Induction of Tumors by Oral Administration of MNNG Combined
with Various Kinds of Surfactant

| Group No. | Effective No. of rats | No. of tumors (%) | Glandular stomach | | | | Small intestine | |
| | | | Adenocarcinoma | | Sarcoma with adeno- carcinoma | | Carcinoma | Sarcoma |
			Well-differ- entiated (%)	Undiffer- entiated (%)				
I	13	10 (77)	6 (46)	4 (31)	2		2	3
II	15	12 (80)	9 (60)	3 (20)	1		2	5
III	15	9 (60)	7 (47)	2 (13)	2		0	1
IV	10	4 (40)	2 (20)	2 (20)	1		0	1
V	13	8 (62)	8 (62)	0 (0)	0		0	1

Ultrathin sections were cut on an LKB microtome with glass knives, and stained with uranyl acetate and lead citrate, and examined with a Hitachi HU-12 electron microscope. Thin sections were stained with Toluidin Blue, and other thin sections removed from Epon were stained with periodic acid-Schiff and Alcian Blue for light-microscopic studies.

The incidence of tumors of the glandular stomach and other sites in the body is summarized in Table I. As for the rate and time of the induced tumors, there were no differences between the experimental groups and the control. However, undifferentiated adenocarcinomas increased in the experimental groups.

Histological Criteria of Gastric Adenocarcinoma

The criteria used for adenocarcinoma of the glandular stomach included one of the following histological appearances: (1) atypical glands consisting of cells or nuclei with irregularity in size and shape or loss of glandular arrangement, invading the submucosa, the muscle layer or the serosa, (2) lymphatic or blood vascular invasion of tumor cells, or (3) presence of metastasis. Diagnostic criteria of undifferentiated adenocarcinoma were based on the absence of glandular structure of the tumor cells.

Microscopically, adenocarcinoma of the glandular stomach was divided into two histological types; well-differentiated and undifferentiated. The combined types showed an overlapping in histological patterns, i.e., anaplastic elements mixed with tubular pattern, but we classified such cases as undifferentiated adenocarcinomas in this paper.

Adenocarcinoma of the Glandular Stomach

In every group, the incidence of adenocarcinomas in the glandular stomach was 40–80%. Adenocarcinomas of the glandular stomach were found in 10 of 13 effective animals in Group I, in 12 of 15 in Group II, in 9 of 15 in Group III, in 4 of 10 in Group IV, and in 8 of 13 in Group V. Most of the tumors were located in the pyloric region and the antrum along the lesser curvature. The tumors formed polypoid nodules or ulcerative umbilicated nodules with elevated borders.

They were greyish white, and the size of the tumors varied from miliary nodules to a size large enough to occupy the lumina of the glandular stomach. Some of them infiltrated widely into the stomach wall and invaded the serosa in many cases, grossly showing nodules on the serosa. In a few cases in the experimental groups, the tumors adhered to the omentum and the liver.

Undifferentiated adenocarcinomas were observed in 4 of 10 adenocarcinomas in Group I, in 3 of 12 in Group II, in 2 of 9 in Group III, and in 2 of 4 in Group IV. There were no undifferentiated adenocarcinomas in Group V. In one case of Group I, anaplastic tumor cells infiltrated the omentum and the capsule of the liver, forming masses on the peritoneal surfaces. In another case of Group I, tumor cells invaded the neighboring organs, such as the omentum and the pancreas. Lymphatic invasion was sometimes observed in the submucosa and the serosa (Photos 4 and 7). Metastases in the intestinal lymph nodes were found in one case of Group I (Photo 8). Undifferentiated adenocarcinoma cells invaded the smaller nerve trunks in the omentum.

Histological Findings of Gastric Adenocarcinoma

The predominant features of the well-differentiated type consisted of typical glandular structure. The proliferating glands showing tubular, papillary, or cystic pattern, often exhibited cellular or structural atypism. In some cases the tumor tissues had a well-differentiated glandular pattern. The histological feature of the tumor indicated clearly low malignancy and in such cases, it was often difficult to distinguish them from adenomatous hyperplasia. However, these atypical glands invaded the muscle layer and the serosa. Neither direct spread to the neighboring organs nor metastasis was found. In a few cases cartilage formation in the stroma of the tumor tissues was observed.

Undifferentiated types were characterized by loss of glandular arrangement. The anaplastic tumor cells showed polymorphism, increased basophilia of the cytoplasm, and hyperchromatism of the nucleus (Photos 5 and 6). In several cases, there were many signet-ring cells which could easily be demonstrated with mucicarmine or periodic acid-Schiff stain. Two types of mucoid adenocarcinoma were observed. One was composed of signet-ring cells (Photo 3) and the other, of anaplastic glandular cells floating in pools of copious mucin (Photos 1 and 2). In a few cases, the scirrhous types with abundant fibrous stroma were found (Photo 3). These tumor cells frequently infiltrated into the muscle layer and the serosa (Photo 6).

Spread of Undifferentiated Adenocarcinoma

The spread of adenocarcinoma of the glandular stomach is summarized in Table II. In a few cases there was lymphatic invasion, direct spread to the neighboring organs, and metastasis in lymph nodes. These cases revealed histologically undifferentiated adenocarcinomas in the primary site.

Lymphatic invasion was found in 2 cases in Group I, 1 in Group II, 2 in Group III, and 1 in Group IV. Metastases to the intestinal lymph nodes were

TABLE II. Spread of Adenocarcinoma of the Glandular Stomach

Group No.	Total No. of adenocarcinoma	Lymphatic invasion	Metastases in lymph nodes	Direct spread	
I	10	2	1	2	Pancreas 1 Liver and omentum 1
II	12	1	0	0	
III	9	2	0	0	
IV	4	1	0	0	
V	8	0	0	0	

observed in 1 case in Group I. The direct spread was found in 2 cases in Group I, one to the omentum and the capsule of the liver as well, and the other to the pancreas. Neither lymphatic invasion nor metastasis was found in the control group.

Ultrastructural Findings of Undifferentiated Adenocarcinoma

Electron-microscopic examination revealed two types of signet-ring cells in undifferentiated adenocarcinomas. The cytoplasm of one type was closely packed with mucin, which stained strongly with periodic acid-Schiff and Alcian Blue in the thin section after the removal of Epon. The nucleus was compressed to one side of the cytoplasm. Electronmicroscopically, the cancer cell contained pale, large, and mutually fused mucin granules as in goblet cells (Photo 9). Only a few poorly developed microvilli were present (Photo 10) and these had fine filamentous coats. In the other type, cystic or vacuolar structures were found in Golgi area of the cells in the plastic sections. These structures varied in size up to 10.0 μm in diameter. Internal substances of the microcyst were demonstrated with a varying degree by periodic acid-Schiff staining. The microcyst often compressed the nucleus to one side. Under the electron microscope, the internal surface of the intracellular microcyst showed well-developed microvilli (0.2 to 0.5 μm long) closely arranged (Photos 11 and 12). These microvilli contained filamentous cores which were dispersed into the cytoplasm. Inside the microcyst, there were amorphous mucoid substances intermixed with a few of the myelin-like components, while outside were many filaments but no mucin granules.

DISCUSSION

Tween 60 and Nonipol are hydrophilic nonionic surfactants, and alkylbenzenesulfonate is hydrophilic and anionic. Alkylbenzenesulfonate has two types; one is called a hard type, which has an alkyl group of branched structure, and the other is a soft type with a straight alkyl chain. These surfactants possess powerful surface activities, namely, penetrating property in acid medium. Ekwall et al. (5) reported the ability of Tweens to enhance the penetration of a carcinogen, 3,4-benzopyrene, into the mucosa of the glandular stomach in mice and cats. Wissler et al. (29) and Mori et al. (15) indicated that dietary Tween 20 increased iron absorption from the intestinal tract in the hamster. Jones *et al.* (*10*) reported that in conditions of serious malnutrition secondary to such disturbances as celiac disease, sprue, chronic inflammatory diseases of the jejunum or the ileum, and anastomotic operations of the upper gastrointestinal tract, the absorption of dietary fats from the intestinal tract increased by adding Tween 80 to the diet. They also said that it was possible to influence the absorption of substances other than fat. Setälä *et al.* (*19–21*), Della *et al.* (*3*), and Dammert (*2*) reported that Tween 60 promoted induction of skin tumors in mice. However, there has never been a report that these surfactants themselves induce cancer (*13*).

Recently, we reported (*27, 28*) that undifferentiated adenocarcinoma of the glandular stomach was induced when 4-nitroquinoline 1-oxide combined with alkylbenzenesulfonate was administered to rats by esophageal intubation, although alkylbenzenesulfonate had no evidence of carcinogenicity (*26*). Sugimura *et al.* (*23–25*) found that MNNG produced well-differentiated adenocarcinoma of the glandular stomach in most cases in rats (*7*).

In the present experiment, induction of adenocarcinoma of the glandular stomach was observed frequently in every group. The remarkable results obtained were many cases of undifferentiated adenocarcinoma as well as well-differentiated one in the experimental groups. The undifferentiated adenocarcinomas were composed of anaplastic cells with increased basophilia in the cytoplasm, or contained mucin-like signet-ring cells. We also obtained two cases of mucoid adenocarcinoma with abundant extracellular mucin. In another case, a scirrhous part with abundant collagenous stroma was present. In regard to the behavior of the tumors, direct spread occurred to the omentum, liver, and pancreas. In these cases lymphatic invasion and metastases in the lymph nodes were found. Although the control group revealed well-differentiated adenocarcinomas in many cases, neither lymphatic invasion nor metastasis was found (Table II).

According to electron-microscopic observations of human gastric cancer (*11, 14, 16, 17*), mucin-containing cells and intracellular microcyst cells show signet-ring appearance. In this investigation, there were two types of signet-ring cells in undifferentiated adenocarcinomas. The mucin granules of one type were pale, large, and mutually fused, and similar to those of the goblet cells in the intestinal epithelium. This type is exactly identical with mucin-containing cells found in human gastric cancer. The other type had a cystic or vacuolar structure in the cytoplasm. The surface of the microcyst was stained with periodic acid-Schiff, and the microvilli covering it had filamentous cores. The microcyst was not the same as the intracellular canaliculus which was found in normal parietal cells. Kondo *et al.* (*11*) examined 23 cases of human gastric cancer by electron microscope and stated that the intracellular microcyst was found in undifferentiated adenocarcinoma cells. The cystic structure was very similar to that of experimental gastric cancer.

In conclusion, it is obvious that the four experimental groups exhibited prominent carcinogenesis as compared with the control group. This fact could be due to the surfactants used as a vehicle for MNNG. By virtue of the strong penetrating property of the surfactants, MNNG could invade the protective mucous barrier (*1, 8, 9*) of the stomach and directly contact with the gastric mucosa. Surfactants might facilitate penetration of the carcinogen into target cells of gastric mucosa. Consequently, in both aspects of the light- and electron-microscopic characteristics and the behavior, the undifferentiated adenocarcinoma of the experimental gastric cancer resembles those of human gastric cancer.

REFERENCES

1. Barrett, M. K. Avenues of approach to the gastric-cancer problem. *J. Natl. Cancer Inst.*, **7**, 127–157 (1946).
2. Dammert, K. Zur Histologie der chemischen Hautcarcinogenese im Licht der Zweiphasenhypothese Untersucht an Mäusen. *Acta Pathol. Scand.*, **124** (Suppl.), 1–139 (1957).
3. Della, G. P., Shubik, P., Dammert, K., and Terracini, B. Role of polyoxyethylene sorbitan monostearate in skin carcinogenesis in mice. *J. Natl. Cancer Inst.*, **25**, 607–625 (1960).
4. Druckrey, H., Preusmann, R., Ivankovik, S., So, B. T., Schmidt, C. H., and Bücheler, J. Zur Erzeugung subcutaner Sarkome an Ratten. Carcinogene Wirkung von Hydrazodicarbon-saüre-bis-(methyl-nitrosamid), N-Nitroso-N-*n*-butylharnstoff, N-Methyl-N-nitroso-nitroguanidin und N-Nitroso-imidazolidon. *Z. Krebsforsch.*, **68**, 87–102 (1966).
5. Ekwall, P., Ermala, P., Setälä, K., and Sjöblom, L. Gastric absorption of 3,4-benzpyrene. II. The significance of the solvent for the penetration of 3,4-benzpyrene into the stomach wall. *Cancer Res.*, **11**, 758–763 (1951).
6. Fishbein, L., Flamm, W. G., and Falk, H. L. Environmental effects on biological systems. *In* "Chemical Mutagens," ed. by D. H. K. Lee, E. W. Hewson, and D. Okun, Academic Press, New York/London, pp. 169–170 (1970).
7. Fujimura, S., Kogure, K., Sugimura, T., and Takayama, S. The effect of limited administration of N-methyl-N'-nitro-N-nitrosoguanidine on the induction of stomach cancer in rats. *Cancer Res.*, **30**, 842–848 (1970).
8. Hollander, F. Gastric mucus secretion in relation to cancer of the stomach. *Acta Unio Int. Contra Cancrum*, **17**, 307–312 (1961).
9. Ivy, A. C. Gastric physiology in relation to gastric cancer. *J. Natl. Cancer Inst.*, **5**, 313–337 (1945).
10. Jones, C. M., Culver, P. J., Drummery, G. D., and Ryan, A. E. Modification of fat absorption in the digestive tract by the use of an emulsifying agent. *Ann. Intern. Med.*, **29**, 1–10 (1948).
11. Kondo, K., Tamura, H., and Taniguchi, H. Intracellular microcyst in gastric cancer cells. *J. Electron Microsc.*, **19**, 41–49 (1970).
12. Mandel, J. D. and Greenberg, J. A new chemical mutagen for bacteria, 1-methyl-3-nitro-1-nitrosoguanidine. *Biochem. Biophys. Res. Commun.*, **3**, 575–584 (1960).
13. Merenmies, L. Zum Mechanismus der Hauttumorbildung bei Mäusen. *Acta Pathol. Microbiol. Scand.*, **130** (Suppl.), 1–107 (1959).
14. Ming, S. C., Goldman, H., and Freiman, D. G. Intestinal metaplasia and histogenesis of carcinoma in human stomach. *Cancer*, **20**, 1418–1429 (1967).
15. Mori, H. D., Barker, P. A., Juras, D. S., and Wissler, R. W. Study of the mechanism of increased iron absorption in hamsters fed Tween 20. *Lab. Invest.*, **6**, 421–446 (1957).
16. Onoe, T. Electron microscopic studies of human carcinoma. *J. Electron Microsc.*, **11**, 70–84 (1962).

17. Sasano, N., Nakamura, K., Arai, M., and Akazaki, K. Ultrastructural cell patterns in human gastric carcinoma compared with non-neoplastic gastric mucosa—Histogenetic analysis of carcinoma by mucin histochemistry. *J. Natl. Cancer Inst.*, **43**, 783–802 (1969).

18. Schoental, R. Carcinogenic activity of N-methyl-N-nitroso-N'-nitroguanidine. *Nature*, **209**, 726–727 (1966).

19. Setälä, H. Tumor promoting and co-carcinogenic effects of some non-ionic lipophilic-hydrophilic (surface active) agents. An experimental study on skin tumors in mice. *Acta Pathol. Microbiol. Scand.*, **115** (Suppl.), 1–93 (1956).

20. Setälä, K. Experimental chemical carcinogenesis and the influence of solvents. *Nature*, **174**, 873–875 (1954).

21. Setälä, K., Setälä, H., and Holsti, P. A new and physicochemically well-defined group of tumor-promoting (co-carcinogenic) agents for mouse skin. *Science*, **120**, 1075–1076 (1954).

22. Sugimura, T., Nagao, M., and Okada, Y. Carcinogenic action of N-methyl-N'-nitro-N-nitrosoguanidine. *Nature*, **210**, 962–963 (1966).

23. Sugimura, T. and Fujimura, S. Tumour production in glandular stomach of rat by N-methyl-N'-nitro-N-nitrosoguanidine. *Nature*, **216**, 943–944 (1967).

24. Sugimura, T., Fujimura, S., and Baba, T. Tumor production in the glandular stomach and alimentary tract of the rat by N-methyl-N'-nitro-N-nitrosoguanidine. *Cancer Res.*, **30**, 455–465 (1970).

25. Sugimura, T., Fujimura, S., Kogure, K., Baba, T., Saito, T., Nagao, M., Hosoi, H., Shimosato, Y., and Yokoshima, T. Production of adenocarcinomas in glandular stomach of experimental animals by N-methyl-N'-nitro-N-nitrosoguanidine. *GANN Monograph*, **8**, 157–196 (1969).

26. Swisher, R. D. Surfactant effects on humans and other mammals. *In* "Scientific and Technical Report, No. 4," The Soap and Detergent Assoc. of the U.S. (1966).

27. Takahashi, M. Effect of alkylbenzenesulfonate as a vehicle for 4-nitroquinoline 1-oxide on gastric carcinogenesis in rats. *Gann*, **61**, 27–33 (1970).

28. Takahashi, M. and Sato, H. Effect of 4-nitroquinoline 1-oxide with alkylbenzenesulfonate on gastric carcinogenesis in rats. *GANN Monograph*, **8**, 241–261 (1969).

29. Wissler, R. W., Bethard, W. F., Barker, P., and Mori, H. D. Effects of polyoxyethylene sorbitan monolaurate (Tween 20) upon gastrointestinal iron absorption in hamsters. *Proc. Soc. Exp. Biol. Med.*, **86**, 170–177 (1954).

EXPLANATION OF PHOTOS

PHOTO 1.   A mucoid adenocarcinoma with tumor cells floating in pools of copious mucin (No. N-41, Group II).

PHOTO 2.   Higher magnification of the area in the same tumor (No. N-41, Group II).

PHOTO 3.   Many signet-ring cells with abundant proliferation of fibrous stroma (No. N-41, Group II).

PHOTO 4.   Intralymphatic tumor cells in the muscle layer (No. N-41, Group II).

PHOTO 5.   Undifferentiated adenocarcinoma. Some of the cells are signet-ring shaped, and others are over-distended with mucin (No. T-13, Group I).

PHOTO 6.   Isolated tumor cells infiltrating the muscle layer (No. T-13, Group I).

PHOTO 7.   Lymphatic invasion of tumor cells in the serosa (No. T-13, Group I).

PHOTO 8.   Metastasis in the regional lymph node. The arrow indicates anaplastic tumor cells occupying the subcapsular sinus (No. T-13, Group I).

PHOTO 9.   Ultrastructural appearance of an undifferentiated adenocarcinoma cell. The mucin granules are large, pale, and closely packed. ×18,000.

PHOTO 10.   Another part of Photo 9. The cancer cells form an incomplete glandular arrangement. ×14,000.

PHOTO 11.   Ultrastructure of an intracellular microcyst cell showing a cystic structure in the cytoplasm. The cyst compresses the nucleus. ×15,000.

PHOTO 12.   The same type as Photo 11. The microvilli with filamentous cores are well developed and closely arranged. Amorphous mucoid substances are present in the microcyst. ×25,000.

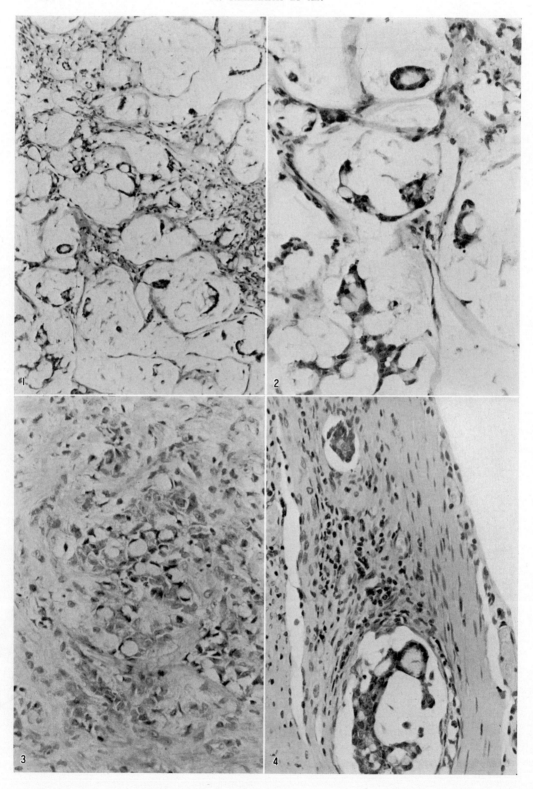

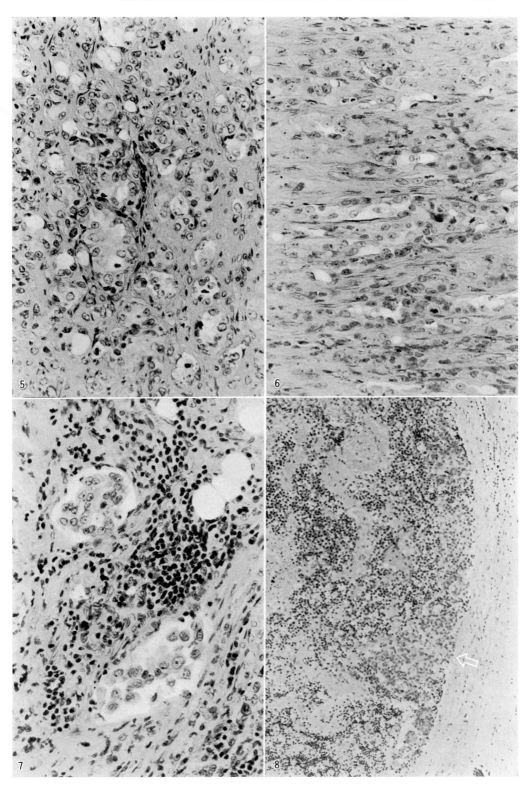

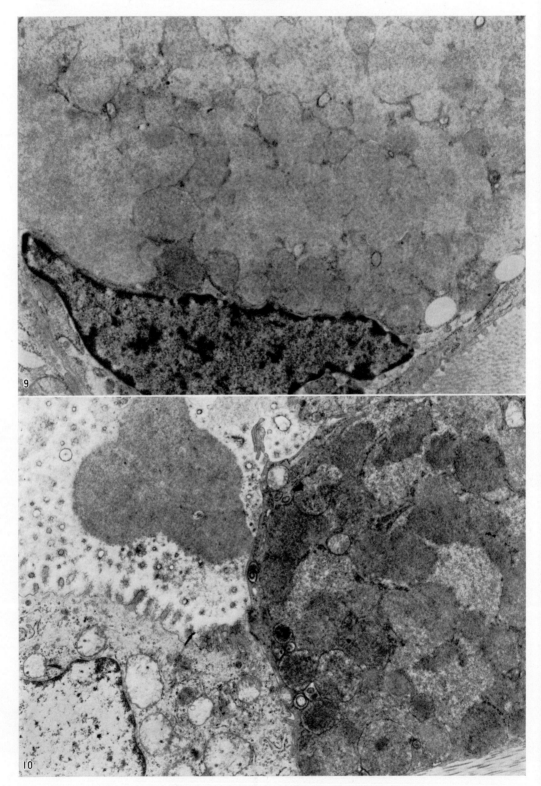

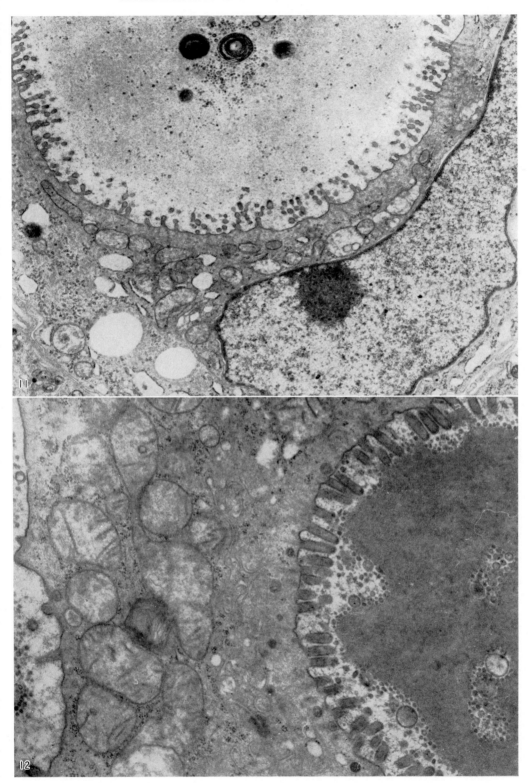

GANN Monograph on Cancer Research 17, 269–281 (1975)

MORPHOGENESIS OF DUODENAL ADENOCARCINOMAS INDUCED BY N-ETHYL-N'-NITRO-N-NITROSO-GUANIDINE IN MICE AND RATS[*1]

Mutsushi Matsuyama,[*2] Takaaki Nakamura,[*3] Harumi Suzuki,[*2] and Takeo Nagayo[*2]

*Laboratory of Pathology, Aichi Cancer Center Research Institute,[*2] and Second Department of Pathology, Nagoya City University[*3]*

Adenocarcinomas of the duodenum can be induced by continuous, oral administration of a concentrated solution of N-ethyl-N'-nitro-N-nitrosoguanidine (ENNG), in high incidence in mice and rats. Correlative examinations on stereomicroscopic and microscopic features of early morphological changes in ENNG carcinogenesis in duodenum revealed that neoplastic cells originated from proliferating zones of the crypts and penetrated into the lamina propria of the villi, forming intravillous lesions. The intravillous lesions subsequently encroached upwards and laterally, forming crater-form lesions visible with a stereomicroscope. The lesions then invaded the serosa and developed into macroscopic lesions. A quantitative account of the sequential development from the microscopic intravillous lesions to the macroscopic lesions through the stereomicroscopic crater-form lesions was obtained from an analysis of the lesions in the mice given ENNG for shorter (4 weeks) and longer (8 and 12 weeks) periods. Submicroscopically, cells constituting these three types of the lesion were almost identical, showing that these lesions represented various phases of the sequential development of neoplastic lesions. No erosion, ulcer, or benign tumor anteceded these lesions. It was considered from these morphological features that ENNG carcinogenesis in the duodenum occurred in one step.

In man approximately 3% of gastrointestinal carcinomas occur in the small intestine. Of these small-intestinal carcinomas, 45% originate in the duodenum (5). In a study on carcinomas of the duodenum, Jefferson, in 1916, stated "Considering the shortness of the duodenum, it is evident that inch for inch it is more liable to cancer than the rest of the small intestine." In animals spontaneous carcinoma of the duodenum occurs infrequently (12) and, when it occurs, it is difficult to differentiate it from ampullar carcinoma originating from the common bile duct and the pancreatic ducts. It has, therefore, been desired to have an experimental model system of unquestionable duodenal carcinoma to

[*1] The original studies cited from our laboratory were supported by Grants from the Ministry of Health and Welfare, Japan (Cancer Subsidies 1970-1, 1971-22, and 1972-20).

[*2] Kanokoden 81-1159, Chikusa-ku, Nagoya 464, Japan (松山睦司, 鈴木春見, 長与健夫).

[*3] Kawasumi-cho 1, Mizuho-ku, Nagoya 467, Japan (中村隆昭).

analyse the cause(s) of induction and developmental features of duodenal carcinomas in man.

Feeding and parenteral injection of many synthetic and natural chemical substances have induced intestinal carcinomas in mice, rats, and hamsters (reviewed in Refs. *2, 12, 20, 26*). However, the large majority of the induced carcinomas originated from the colon and ileum. Druckrey *et al.* (*4*) induced duodenal tumors with 1,2-dimethylhydrazine (DMH) in 7 out of 13 rats by subcutaneous injection and in 3 of 13 by intraperitoneal injection. The results were confirmed by Pozharisski, inducing duodenal tumors in 51% (*20*). The principal sites of DMH carcinogenesis were the colorectal segment. With propylnitrosourea carcinomas in various parts of the digestive tract were also induced by Druckrey (*2*). The incidence of duodenal carcinomas was 25%. Similar results, with a higher incidence of leukemias, were obtained by Ogiu *et al.* (*18*).

In the present article, the results of a series of three studies are described: (1) the induction of duodenal adenocarcinomas by N-ethyl-N'-nitro-N-nitrosoguanidine (ENNG), (2) the early morphological changes, and (3) ultrastructure of the early lesions.

Duodenal Adenocarcinomas Induced by N-Methyl-N'-nitro-N-nitrosoguanidine (MNNG) and ENNG

Stimulated by the success of induction of gastric adenocarcinomas in rats by Sugimura and his associates (*27*), we tested MNNG for its carcinogenicity in mice. In mice, however, MNNG given daily in the drinking water as a dilute solution of 50 mg/liter induced no gastric carcinoma, but resulted in induction of several duodenal adenocarcinomas (*14*). A more concentrated solution (200 mg/liter) was used in another laboratory, and induced no gastric tumors in mice (*11*). These results show that mouse stomach is refractory to MNNG.

Since the carcinogenic effect apparently is modified by the alkyl group (*2*), the ethyl homolog of MNNG, ENNG, was tested in the hope of inducing adenocarcinomas of the gastrointestinal tract in mice. In the first experiment a low dose of ENNG, as a solution of 50 mg/liter, was given to CBA/H-T6 mice for 10 months (*16*). Tumors of the duodenum were observed macroscopically in 19 (44%) of 43 treated mice, including 4 mice with hemangioendothelial sarcomas, after 10–18 months. Many tumors were single; 14 bulged from the serosa and formed a large elevation of the mucosa with a central crater, obstructing the lumen. Histologically, these 14 were adenocarcinomas, and 10 invaded the pancreas. A few other well-differentiated adenocarcinomas blocked the opening of the ampulla of Vater and were associated with pedunculated cysts growing from the serosa. Squamous cell carcinomas of the esophagus in 11 mice and adenomatous polyps and an adenocarcinoma of the glandular stomach in 3 mice were also induced.

In the second experiment higher doses of ENNG and also of MNNG, as solutions of 500 mg/liter, were given to several strains of mice for 5 months (*17*). The lower doses of both carcinogens were also given to other mice of the same strains for comparison. Duodenal adenocarcinomas were induced at higher rates

TABLE I. Carcinomas in Duodenum, Esophagus, and Forestomach in Mice of
Various Strains Given ENNG and MNNG[a]

Treatment (mg/liter, months)	Strain	Effective No. of mice[b]/ initial No. of mice	No. of mice with carcinomas in		
			Duodenum (%)	Esophagus (%)	Forestomach (%)
ENNG (500, 5)	CBA/H-T6	94/105	68 (72)	10 (11)	32 (37)
	CBA/H	52/60	31 (60)	5 (10)	33 (63)
	C3H/He	68/80	53 (78)	14 (21)	38 (56)
	C57B1/6	69/78	54 (78)	1 (1)	4 (6)
	dd/I	28/32	15 (54)	12 (43)	15 (54)
MNNG (500, 5)	CBA/H-T6	16/20	6 (38)	0 (0)	0 (0)
	C3H/He	21/27	6 (29)	1 (5)	8 (38)
	dd/I	34/40	8 (24)	2 (6)	4 (12)
ENNG (50, 10)	CBA/H-T6	212/297	13 (6)	58 (27)	9 (4)
	CBA/H	32/43	0 (0)	7 (22)	0 (0)
	C3H/He	85/134	0 (0)	18 (21)	2 (2)
	C57B1/6	38/45	11 (29)	5 (13)	2 (5)
MNNG (50, 10)	CBA/H-T6	70/93	4 (6)	8 (11)	4 (6)
	CBA/H	71/91	2 (3)	5 (7)	0 (0)
	C3H/He	41/55	0 (0)	4 (10)	0 (0)
Water[c] (—, —)	CBA/H-T6	38/45	0 (0)	0 (0)	0 (0)

[a] Carcinomas were diagnosed macroscopically and microscopically.   [b] Number of surviving mice when the first tumor was found in the group.   [c] Mice were killed 18 months after birth.

(54–78%) within shorter periods (3–7 months) in those strains of mice given the higher dose of ENNG, as compared to those on the low dose (Table I). The higher dose of MNNG also induced more duodenal carcinomas than the lower dose. There was no significant difference among the strains, except in the group given the lower dosage of ENNG. On the high dose, most of the adenocarcinomas were multiple, larger with deeper craters, and more invasive. More forestomach carcinomas and fewer esophageal carcinomas and hemangioendothelial sarcomas developed when the higher doses of the carcinogens were used. Druckrey reported that in order to induce intestinal cancer by the oral route, DMH had to be given at a dosage high enough to surpass the activation capacity of the relevant enzymes of the liver which were damaged by the hepatotoxicity of DMH (2).

As shown in Table I, ENNG gave rise to more carcinomas of the duodenum compared to MNNG, at both doses. The results were similar in the case of carcinomas of the esophagus and forestomach. Thus, these results established that ENNG was more effective than MNNG, when continuous doses of these compounds were given orally to mice. This may be due to a higher stability of ENNG than MNNG in neutral and acidic conditions (9). A difference in the affinity of the esophagus, forestomach, and duodenum to the two carcinogens may have a role in carcinogenesis. Conversely, ENNG induced fewer gastro-intestinal tumors than MNNG in rats and mice, when intragastric intubation or intraperitoneal injection was used by Schoental and Bensted (23). The dis-crepancy between our results and those of Schoental and Bensted may be due mainly to the difference in the route of administration and total amounts of the carcinogens.

A concentrated solution of ENNG (500 mg/liter), given continuously to Wistar rats for 5 months, induced duodenal adenocarcinomas in 59 of 62 treated rats (Nakamura and Matsuyama, unpublished). In rats the carcinomas were more frequently multiple and involved the upper part of the jejunum (Photo 1). Only 4 gastric adenocarcinomas were induced. In the exeperiment by Kogure *et al.* (*10*), Tween 60 solutions of ENNG (55 or 91 mg/liter) were given to rats, and carcinomas were induced in equal numbers in the glandular stomach and duodenum. This may be due to the smaller dose, since it was revealed by the experiments with MNNG and N-methyl-N-nitro-N'-acetylurea that the specific induction of gastric carcinomas could be obtained most effectively by using a low dosage for a limited period (*3, 8*). The accelerated impregnation of ENNG into the gastric mucosa by Tween 60 may have a role, as assumed by Takahashi *et al.* (*28*). It is, however, noteworthy that Kawachi *et al.* (*9*) also induced equal number of gastric and duodenal carcinomas in hamsters by ENNG (91 mg/liter) without Tween 60.

Early Morphological Changes in ENNG Carcinogenesis in the Duodenum

We have succeeded in inducing adenocarcinomas of the duodenum in about 70% of mice given ENNG (*17*). This result made it possible to analyze early sequential events in ENNG carcinogenesis (*13*), by taking advantage of the regularly situated, three-dimensional structures, the villi, of the duodenum. The small intestine contains villi and crypts supported by mesenchymal cells. The villi are the longest and the ratio of crypts to villi is the highest in the duodenum (*7*), denoting that the villi protrude more prominently from the base than in other segments of the small intestine. These features of the duodenum make it possible to visualize extremely small lesions occurring in the mucosa.

CBA/H-T6 mice were given ENNG continuously, dissolved in drinking water at a concentration of 500 mg/liter for 4, 8, or 12 weeks. They were then given plain water without ENNG for 8 weeks. The mice were killed, the duodenum was removed, opened, and placed on a filter paper. The organs were fixed and photographed through a stereomicroscope. They were embedded and cut serially for histological examinations.

There were two types of initial morphological changes in the development of lesions; enlargement of a single villus (A type, Photo 2) and fusion of several villi (B type, Photo 3) were seen 12 weeks after start of the administration of ENNG. In A type, single, atypical glands occupied the whole lamina propria of the villi as blind cysts without transitional communication with the covering epithelium. In B type, several atypical glands were situated, with several capillaries, in the lamina propria of the fused villi. The atypical glands in both types of lesions consisted of basophilically stained cells with a large number of mitotic figures. The nuclei were large and located at different levels in the cytoplasm.

With increased duration of the treatment, the cells of the intravillous lesions proliferated upwards and laterally, developing more complicated shapes of glands, and eroded the surface of the villi (crater-form lesion, Photo 4). The latter increased in size and developed into macroscopic lesions, invading through thickened muscle layers (Photo 5) and into the pancreas. The sequence of events is summarized in Fig. 1. Histologically, the cells of the macroscopic lesions were almost identical to those of the intravillous lesions.

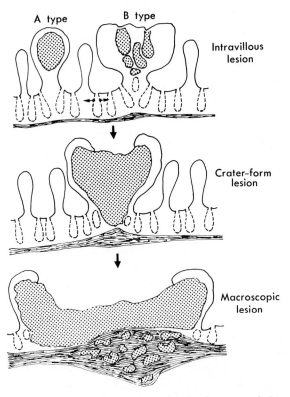

FIG. 1.   Schematic diagram of the sequential development of three types of lesions induced by ENNG in CBA/H-T6 mice

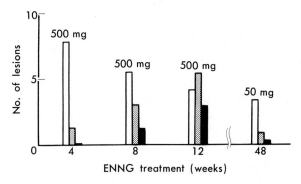

FIG. 2.   Dose response in the number of intravillous, crater-form, and macroscopic lesions in CBA/H-T6 mice given ENNG

The number per mouse is shown. □ intravillous lesion; ▨ crater-form lesion; ■ macroscopic lesion.

Counting and analysis of the number of the lesions revealed that the number of the intravillous lesions decreased and the number of the crater-form and macroscopic lesions increased, with the advancement of treatment period (Fig. 2). The mice given the dilute solution of ENNG (50 mg/liter) for 48 weeks had about half the number of intravillous and crater-form lesions, but 2 times the number of macroscopic lesions, as compared to the mice given the concentrated solution for 4 weeks. These facts suggest that the intravillous lesions actually developed into the crater-form and further into macroscopic lesions.

Wistar rats, which were given the concentrated solution of ENNG for 20 weeks, also had the three types of the lesion simultaneously. Other mice of the CBA/H-T6 strain, given the concentrated solution of ENNG for 1, 3, 7, or 28 days, showed neither erosion nor ulcer in the duodenum.

Systematic examination of serial sections of the intravillous lesions revealed that the surface cells of the villi and crypts, situated deep in the lamina propria, were normal; transitions from normal to abnormal were not observed. These findings suggest that neoplastic changes occurred in the middle proliferating zones of the crypts, penetrating directly into the lamina propria of the villi. Theoretically neoplastic cell(s) can penetrate the lamina propria in two directions; into the root of a villus or between the crypts, developing A or B type lesions, respectively (Fig. 1). In the latter case, penetrating neoplastic cells proliferated, forming glands and rose the base, and produced fused villi. A mechanism in which the neoplastic glands in both types of the lesions are drawn toward the luminal space of the duodenum can be assumed, since a few normal crypts situated in the stalks of the fused villi occupy a higher level than other crypts (Photo 3b).

Rogers et al. (21) reported that carcinomas in the colon induced by DMH originated from abnormal mucosal glands which lay over or localized within the lymphoid follicles. We also found that these mucosal glands were distorted in shape and strained basophilically, but all the intravillous lesions originated from the middle proliferating zones of the crypts, apart from the lymphoid follicles in the duodenum (Photo 4b). Schauer et al. (22) and Springer et al. (25) also assumed that intestinal tumors, induced by DMH, originated from the crypts. The induction of carcinoma in situ in the rat intestinal tract has been described by Spjut and Noall (24). However, the intravillous lesions, which sometimes consisted of a single gland, were probably the result of penetration into the lamina propria from the crypts. Therefore, we are unable to adopt the concept of "carcinoma in situ" for the intravillous lesions.

Rats fed bracken fern (Pteridium aquilinum) or N,N'-fluorenylenebisacetamide (FAA) developed mainly multiple adenomatous polyps and adenocarcinomas of the ileum (6, 15, 19, 29). In the duodena of the mice given ENNG, we never found adenomatous polyps. There is thus a correlation among the macroscopic form of the tumors, the segment involved, and the carcinogen used. We assume that the difference in the macroscopic forms of the tumors induced depends on the potency for malignant transformation of the carcinogen. ENNG may have a stronger potency for transformation of epithelial cells of the small intestine than bracken fern and FAA. Adenomatous polyps of man have generally been regarded as a precursor of carcinoma. However, Spjut and Noall (24) thought that the experimental data could not substantiate the hypothesis of conversion of polyps to carcinomas. It is clear from our results that adenocarcinomas initially develop from the normal appearing crypts in the duodenum.

Ultrastructure of Early Lesions in ENNG Carcinogenesis in Mouse Duodenum

Twenty-one lesions in various stages of development in the duodenum of 11 mice, which were given a concentrated solution of ENNG (500 mg/liter) for 20 weeks and maintained by plain water for further 4–8 weeks, were examined submicroscopically (Matsuyama, Nakamura, and Suzuki, unpublished). The duodenum was opened and placed in a petri dish containing a fixative, and lesions were selected under a stereomicroscope, removing non-involved areas. Careful correlative references were made between microscopic and submicroscopic features, using colored micrographs taken from semithin sections stained with Basic Fuchsin and Methylene Blue, such as Photo 6, to obtain correct boundaries of the lesions with normal covering epithelium of the villi and with crypts.

The ultrastructural features of the cells of the lesions were much like those of the proliferating cells of the normal crypts, but sharply differed from those of the surface absorptive cells of the villi (*1*). At the luminal surface the microvilli always appeared shorter and sparser than the normal (Photos 7, 8, and 9). The shape and distribution of the adhesive apparatus were variable. Polysomes were generally numerous and in many of the cells they were closely packed in the cytoplasm (Photos 8 and 9). Nuclear variation in size and shape was apparent and nucleoli were more prominent. Goblet cells and Paneth cells were not observed. These features were consistent among the intravillous (Photo 8), crater-form (Photo 7), and macroscopic lesions (Photo 9). The absorptive cells adjoining the larger lesions, crater-form or macroscopic, showed extremely complicated interdigitations of the cytoplasmic membranes (Photo 7). These submicroscopic features suggest that the lesions originated from the middle part of the crypts. An enzyme histochemical study also supports the results of the submicroscopical study, showing a similarity between the cells of the lesions and normal crypts (Matsuyama, Ito, Yamada, Nakamura, and Nagayo, unpublished).

Acknowledgments

We wish to thank Dr. H. Kishimoto of the Second Department of Pathology, Nagoya City University, and Dr. K. Kojima and Dr. M. Hoshino of the Aichi Cancer Center Research Institute, for their encouragement, Dr. E. D. Murphy of the Jackson Laboratory, for reviewing the manuscript, and Miss F. Kotani, Miss K. Sugiyama, and Mrs. K. Mizukoshi for their painstaking assistance.

REFERENCES

1. Bergener, M. Die Feinstruktur des Dünndarmepithels während der Physiologischen Milchresorption beim jungen Goldhamster. *Z. Zellforsch.*, **57**, 428–474 (1962).
2. Druckrey, H. Organospecific carcinogenesis in the digestive tract. *In* "Topics in

Chemical Carcinogenesis," ed. by W. Nakahara, S. Takayama, T. Sugimura, and S. Odashima, University of Tokyo Press, Tokyo, pp. 73–101 (1972).

3. Druckrey, H., Ivankovic, S., and Preussmann, R. Selektive Erzeugung von Carcinomen des Drüsenmagens bei Ratten durch orale Gabe von N-Methyl-N-nitroso-N'-acetylharnstoff (AcMNH). *Z. Krebsforsch.*, **75**, 23–33 (1970).

4. Druckrey, H., Preussmann, R., Matzkies, F., and Ivankovic, S. Selektive Erzeugung von Darmkrebs bei Ratten durch 1,2-Dimethyl-hydrazin. *Naturwissenschaften*, **54**, 285–286 (1967).

5. Eger, S. A. Primary malignant disease of the duodenum. *Arch. Surg.*, **27**, 1087–1108 (1933).

6. Evans, I. A. and Mason, J. Carcinogenic activity of bracken. *Nature*, **208**, 913–914 (1965).

7. Fujii, R. Quantitation of the number of villi and crypts in the intestine of rodent animals. *Experientia*, **28**, 1209–1210 (1972).

8. Fujimura, S., Kogure, K., Sugimura, T., and Takayama, S. The effect of limited administration of N-methyl-N'-nitro-N-nitrosoguanidine on the induction of stomach cancer in rats. *Cancer Res.*, **30**, 842–848 (1970).

9. Kawachi, T., Kogure, K., Tanaka, N., Tokunaga, A., Fujimura, S., Sugimura, T., Kuwabara, N., and Takayama, S. Induction of tumors in the stomach and duodenum of hamsters by N-ethyl-N'-nitro-N-nitrosoguanidine. *Z. Krebsforsch.*, **81**, 29–36 (1974).

10. Kogure, K., Kawachi, T., Tanaka, N., Kuwabara, N., Takayama, S., and Sugimura, T. Experimental stomach cancer in rats induced by N-methyl-N'-nitro-N-nitrosoguanidine and Tween 60. *Proc. Japan. Cancer Assoc., 30th Annu. Meet.*, 31 (1971) (in Japanese).

11. Kubo, T. Experimental approach to the promoting factors for gastric carcinogenesis. *Proc. Japan. Cancer Assoc., 28th Annu. Meet.*, 82 (1969) (in Japanese).

12. Lingeman, C. H. and Garner, F. M. Comparative study of intestinal adenocarcinomas of animals and man. *J. Natl. Cancer Inst.*, **48**, 325–346 (1972).

13. Matsuyama, M. and Nakamura, T. Early morphological changes in carcinogenesis by N-ethyl-N'-nitro-N-nitrosoguanidine in mouse duodenum. *Proc. Japan. Cancer Assoc., 32nd Annu. Meet.*, 140 (1973) (in Japanese).

14. Matsuyama, M., Suzuki, H., and Nakamura, T. Leiomyosarcomas induced by oral administration of N-methyl-N'-nitro-N-nitrosoguanidine in gastric cysts grafted in subcutaneous tissue of mice. *Gann*, **61**, 523–527 (1970).

15. Morris, H. P., Wagner, B. P., Ray, F. E., Snell, K. C., and Stewart, H. L. Comparative study of cancer and other lesions of rats fed N,N'-2,7-fluorenylenebis-acetamide or N-2-fluorenylacetamide. *Natl. Cancer Inst. Monogr.*, **5**, 1–53 (1961).

16. Nakamura, T., Matsuyama, M., and Kishimoto, H. Tumors of the esophagus and duodenum induced in mice by oral administration of N-ethyl-N'-nitro-N-nitrosoguanidine. *J. Natl. Cancer Inst.*, **52**, 519–522 (1974).

17. Nakamura, T., Matsuyama, M., and Kishimoto, H. Carcinomas of forestomach and duodenum in mouse induced by high concentrated solution of N-ethyl-N'-nitro-N-nitrosoguanidine. *Proc. Japan. Cancer Assoc., 32nd Annu. Meet.*, 140 (1973) (in Japanese).

18. Ogiu, T., Odashima, S., and Nakadate, M. Experimental leukemias in Donryu rats with 1-*n*-propyl-1-nitrosourea (PNU). *Proc. Japan. Cancer Assoc., 32nd Annu. Meet.*, 145 (1973) (in Japanese).

19. Pamukcu, A. M. and Price, J. M. Induction of intestinal and urinary bladder

cancer in rats by feeding bracken fern (*Pteris aquilina*). *J. Natl. Cancer Inst.*, **43**, 275–281 (1969).

20. Pozharisski, K. M. Tumours of the intestines. *In* "Pathology of Tumours in Laboratory Animals," ed. by V. S. Turusov, International Agency for Research on Cancer, Lyon, Vol. 1, Part 1, pp. 119–140 (1973).

21. Rogers, A. E., Herndon, B. J., and Newberne, P. M. Induction by dimethylhydrazine of intestinal carcinoma in normal rats and rats fed high or low levels of vitamin A. *Cancer Res.*, **33**, 1003–1009 (1973).

22. Schauer, A., Völlnagel, Th., and Wildanger, F. Cancerisierung des Rattendarmes durch 1,2-Dimethylhydrazin. *Z. Ges. Exp. Med.*, **150**, 87–93 (1969).

23. Schoental, R. and Bensted, J. P. M. Gastro-intestinal tumours in rats and mice following various routes of administration of N-methyl-N-nitroso-N'-nitroguanidine and N-ethyl-N-nitroso-N'-nitroguanidine. *Brit. J. Cancer*, **23**, 757–764 (1969).

24. Spjut, H. J. and Noall, M. W. Experimental induction of tumors of the large bowel of rats. A review of the experience with 3,2'-dimethyl-4-aminobiphenyl. *Cancer*, **28**, 29–37 (1971).

25. Springer, P., Springer, J., and Oehlert, W. Die Vorstufen des 1,2-dimethylhydrazin-induzierten Dick- und Dünndarmcarcinoms der Ratte. *Z. Krebsforsch.*, **74**, 236–240 (1970).

26. Stewart, H. L. Site variation of alimentary tract cancer in man and experimental animals as indicators of disease etiology. Proc. 9th Int. Cancer Congr., Springer-Verlag, Berlin, pp. 15–49 (1967).

27. Sugimura, T., Fujimura, S., and Baba, T. Tumor production in the glandular stomach and alimentary tract of the rat by N-methyl-N'-nitro-N-nitrosoguanidine. *Cancer Res.*, **30**, 455–465 (1970).

28. Takahashi, M., Fukushima, S., and Sato, H. Carcinogenic effect of N-methyl-N'-nitro-N-nitrosoguanidine with various kinds of surfactant in the glandular stomach of rats. *Gann*, **64**, 211–218 (1973).

29. Yamada, S., Ito, M., and Nagayo, T. Histological and autoradiographical studies on intestinal tumors of rat induced by oral administration of N,N'-2,7-fluorenylenebisacetamide. *Gann*, **62**, 471–478 (1971).

EXPLANATION OF PHOTOS

PHOTO 1. Papillomatosis in forestomach and several adenocarcinomas in duodenum and upper part of jejunum of a Wistar rat given a concentrated solution of ENNG (500 mg/liter) for 20 weeks.

PHOTOS 2–4. Stereomicrographs (a) and micrographs (b) of duodenal lesions in CBA/H-T6 mice given ENNG (500 mg/liter) for 4–8 weeks. 2: swollen single villi (arrow). 3: fused abnormal villi (arrow). 4: crater-form lesions. L, lymphoid follicle.

PHOTO 5. Macroscopic lesions (arrows in (a)) infiltrating the serosa (b) of a CBA/H-T6 mouse given ENNG for 8 weeks.

PHOTOS 6 and 7. Part of a crater-form lesion of a CBA/H-T6 mouse given ENNG for 20 weeks. Neoplastic glands (N) contact the normal covering epithelium (V) in back-to-back fashion. C, crypts; M, muscle layer.

PHOTO 8. Part of a neoplastic gland of an intravillous lesion in a CBA/H-T6 mouse given ENNG for 20 weeks.

PHOTO 9. Cells of a neoplastic gland infiltrating in the muscle layer in CBA/H-T6 mouse given ENNG for 20 weeks.

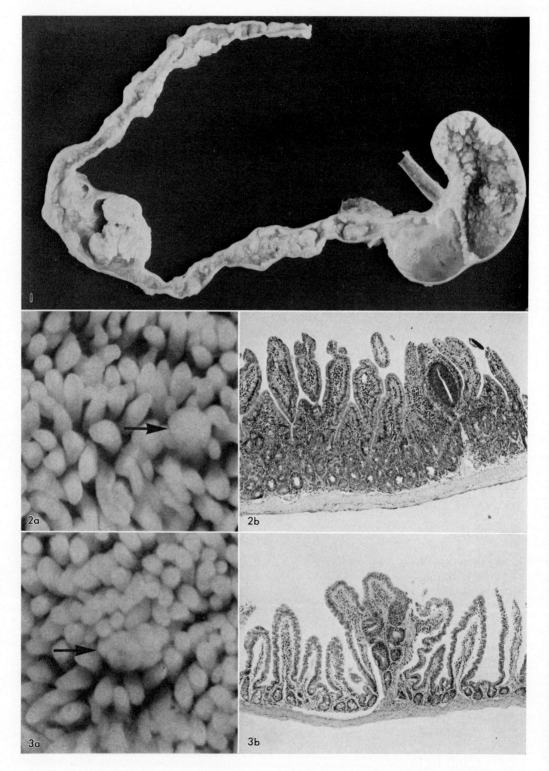

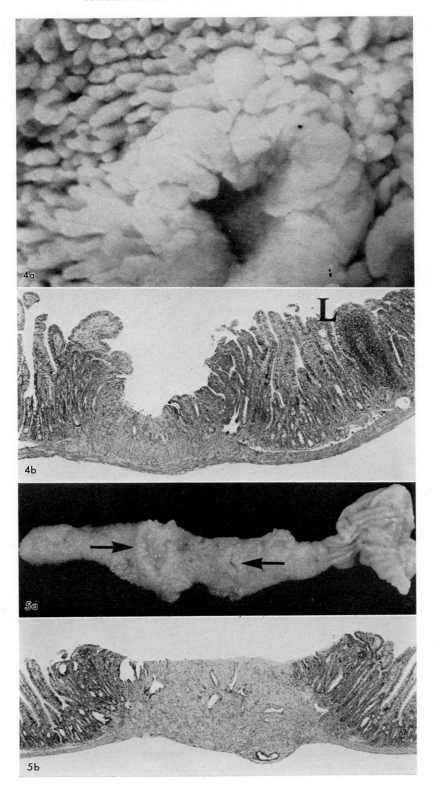

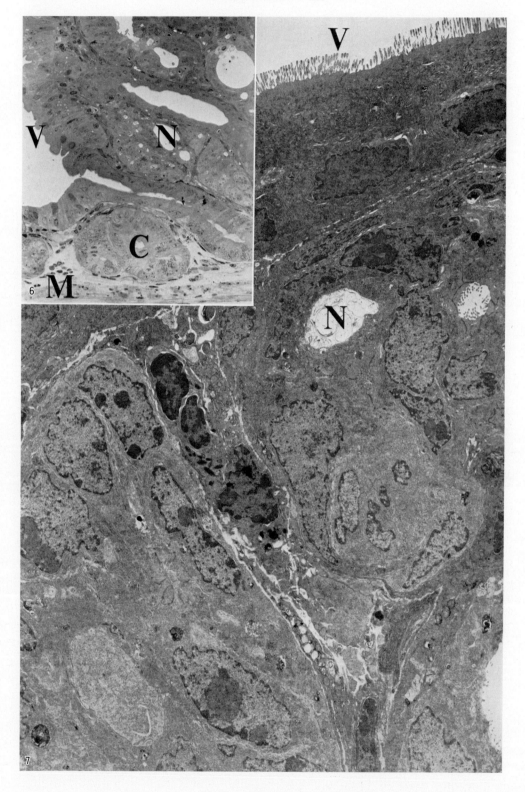

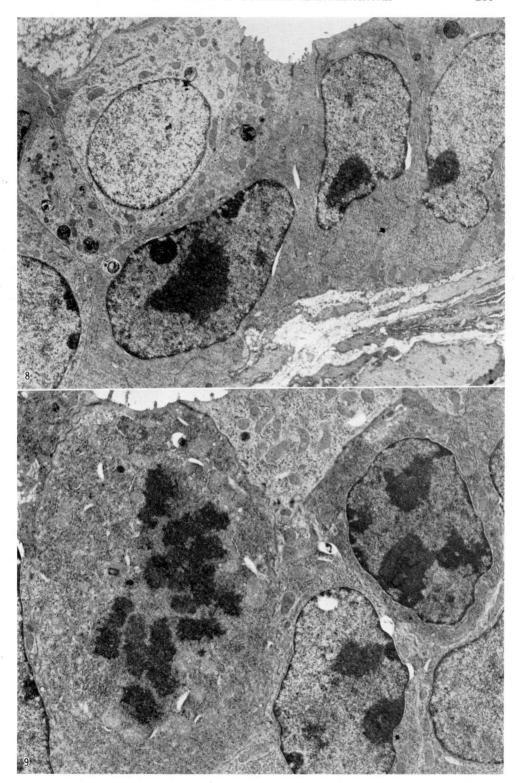

GANN Monograph on Cancer Research 17, 283–299 (1975)

AN ANTIGEN COMMON TO PRENEOPLASTIC HEPATOCYTE POPULATIONS AND TO LIVER CANCER INDUCED BY N-2-FLUORENYL-ACETAMIDE, ETHIONINE, OR OTHER HEPATOCARCINOGENS[*1]

Kiwamu OKITA and Emmanuel FARBER

Fels Research Institute and Departments of Pathology and Biochemistry, Temple University School of Medicine[*2]

A new common antigen, preneoplastic (PN) antigen, has been found in rats in both early and late hyperplastic nodules induced by N-2-fluorenylacetamide (2-FAA) or ethionine and in primary hepatocellular carcinomas induced by 2-FAA, ethionine, 3′-methyl-4-dimethylaminoazobenzene, dimethylnitrosamine, or diethylnitrosamine. This antigen so far has not been found in normal mature liver, fetal liver, amniotic fluid, adult normal serum, serum from rats with hyperplastic nodules or primary hepatomas, or in a variety of normal tissues. Immunofluorescent staining shows it to be present only in hepatocytes in hyperplastic nodules or in primary hepatomas. The PN antigen seems not to be related to rat group-specific (gs) 1-antigen or gs 3-antigen. However, further in-depth studies are needed before a positive or negative relationship to an RNA virus can be established. The possible relationship of the new PN antigen to an interruption in differentiation or remodeling of liver parenchyma is pointed out. In addition, the possible use of such an antigen in the study of human cirrhosis and cancer, and in carcinogenesis in other organs is briefly discussed.

Developments over the past several years have clearly shown that chemical carcinogenesis in liver, as in skin and in many other organs, is divisible into a rapid initial period, initiation, and a subsequent much longer period of evolution or development (*18, 20*). With most carcinogens, prolonged exposure over a period of 8 to 10 weeks is usually necessary to obtain a high incidence of liver cancer. However, if exposure to the carcinogen is given following partial hepatectomy, a single dose of dimethylnitrosamine (DMN) will induce a reasonably high incidence of hepatocellular carcinoma (*11, 12*). DMN is rapidly metabolized (*44*) so that under such circumstances the carcinogen is administered essentially

---

[*1] The research of the authors included in this brief review was supported in part by research grants from the National Institutes of Health (CA-12218, CA-10439, and AM-14882) and American Cancer Society (BC-7N and PRP-39), and by a contract (NOl-CP-33262) with the National Cancer Institute.

[*2] Philadelphia, Pennsylvania 19140, U.S.A. (沖田　極).

as a "pulse" lasting at most 24 to 48 hr. This special role of partial hepatectomy in the genesis of liver cancer is also seen with single doses of 7,12-dimethyl-benzanthracene (DMBA) (45, 49), urethan (9, 31, 40, 41), and β-propiolactone (10), and with dietary 2'-methyl-4-dimethylaminoazobenzene (2'-Me-DAB) (59).

The process of initiation is most easily viewed as consisting of the induction of many new "permanent" cell changes, akin to mutations, a few of which are the initial progenitors for the cancer that ultimately evolves from this new population. The relatively long period of development appears to consist of the progressive selection of new cell populations that have an increasing probability of developing and evolving into a population of malignant neoplastic cells (18–20, 23). Thus, processes akin to both somatic mutation and altered differentiation are considered to be involved in carcinogenesis.

From the present vantage point, one can observe three major areas in carcinogenesis, the elucidation of which are basic to an understanding of the pathogenesis of cancer in cellular and molecular terms. These are (a) the essential nature of the process of initiation, with clarification of the most important and critical target molecules and organelles in susceptible cells, (b) the identification of the number and nature of the cell population(s) that are the products of the initiation process and that appear to be sequential precursors for malignant neoplasia, and (c) the manner in which the various properties acquired at various stages in its life history during the development of cancer contribute to its malignant behavior (19). This formulation of liver carcinogenesis (17–20), which is very similar in outline to that proposed by Foulds for carcinogenesis generally (23), has as one of its essential attributes the more or less "independent progression of character" (23). Thus, any individual malignant neoplasm behaves at any moment in its life history in a manner which reflects the many and varied properties it has acquired progressively and seriatim since it began to evolve from initiated target cells.

In this presentation, we shall focus almost exclusively on (b) above. We shall review briefly the current knowledge concerning precursor populations for hepatocellular carcinoma and to present some new data that indicate the presence of a highly reproducible "positive" marker for preneoplastic liver cells. In addition, new data concerning the basis for nodular proliferation and a possible role of arrested differentiation in this phase of carcinogenesis will be included.

Preneoplastic Liver Cell Populations

Since the original discovery of an experimental model of liver carcinogenesis with o-aminoazotoluene (4-amino-2',3-dimethylazobenzene) by Sasaki and Yoshida (52), focal proliferative areas of liver cells, "hyperplastic nodules," have received major attention as ultimate precursors of cancer (16, 18–20). An apparently similar type of hyperplastic lesion has been suggested as a precursor for liver cancer in human cirrhosis (8, 27, 56). Parenthetically, the term "adenoma" appears periodically in the literature on liver carcinogenesis. We believe that its use offers nothing positive to our conceptual armanentarium today and only seems to confuse the picture at this time. Therefore, we prefer to use descriptive (*e.g.*, "hyperplastic," "proliferative," *etc.*) rather than interpretive nomenclature.

There are at least two types of "hyperplastic nodules"—an early, seemingly reversible (see below) nodule and a later more irreversible one (*17, 18, 21, 50, 57*). Although these new liver cell populations have been studied to some degree from the point of view of biochemical, biological, and morphological properties, as recently reviewed in detail (*18*), major critical issues concerning their role and meaning in carcinogenesis remain. These include (a) their role, either obligatory or facultative, as precursors for liver cancer, and (b) their characterization, both from a biological and a molecular point of view. Assuming them to be precursors, how do they differ from normal hepatocytes in their molecular and cellular characteristics and what mechanistic role do any of these differences play in the cellular evolution to malignant neoplasia? The second (b) must remain of necessity largely speculative until the means for a much more penetrating scientific analysis is developed.

The first issue, their role as precursor, has been receiving increasing attention and there is now growing evidence in support of the hypothesis that the hyperplastic nodule is a major progenitor for liver cancer. The evidence consists of the following (*18*): (a) virtually every hepatic carcinogen induces many changes in common in the liver including focal and nodular hyperplastic lesions of hepatocytes, (b) other compounds, often just as toxic (*e.g.*, α-naphthylisothiocyanate (ANIT), lithocholic acid), even though they induce many functional and structural changes in hepatocytes and ductular cells, do not give rise to hyperplastic nodules in the rat and do not lead to liver cancer, (c) there is a large body of observational experience in human disease, correlating nodular hyperplasia and liver cancer, (d) with one carcinogen, N-2-fluorenylacetamide (2-FAA), a bound form of carcinogen is found in glycogen in the hyperplastic nodule and in the ultimate cancer but not in the liver surrounding the nodules or the cancer (*15*), (e) areas of hyperbasophilia and histologic and cytologic atypia, indistinguishable from unequivocal hepatocellular carcinoma, can be seen arising in the interior of nodules without any evidence of cancer elsewhere (*14, 17*), and (f) α-fetoprotein (AFP), an important marker for hepatocellular carcinoma, has been found to be localized exclusively in hyperplastic nodules during liver carcinogenesis induced by 2-FAA (46a) and not in ductular cells or in the liver parenchyma surrounding nodules or cancer. Unfortunately, this first "positive" marker for preneoplastic cell populations, AFP, varies greatly in its occurrence in nodules and in liver cancer. Only a minority of nodules stain positively for AFP.

The most convincing evidence, in our opinion, is the presence of a new highly reproducible antigen, tentatively called preneoplastic (PN) antigen which appears in the earliest nodule population, which persists only in this focal population throughout carcinogenesis, and which is also present in primary hepatocellular carcinoma. Although the study of this new "positive" marker for new preneoplastic cell populations in liver carcinogenesis is still early, we would like to present the highlights to date and some of the possible implications for our understanding of the pathogenesis of liver cancer.

A Common PN Antigen

This study only became possible with the development of a reproducible method to obtain large nodules in sufficient quantity (*14*). Of necessity, all the

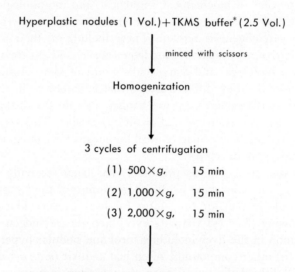

Fig. 1. Schematic outline of preparation of crude PN antigen from hyperplastic nodule tissue
* 0.05 M Tris-0.024 M KCl-0.005 M MgCl$_2$-0.25 M sucrose buffer.

TABLE I. Subcellular Distribution of PN Antigen
in Hyperplastic Nodule Tissue

	PN antigen[a]
Crude fraction	╫
Mitochondrial fraction	—
PMS[b]	╫
Cytosol (soluble supernatant)	+
Microsome preparation[c]	╫

[a] Semi-quantitative analysis by means of single radial immunodiffusion. [b] Post-mitochondrial supernatant. [c] Contains plasma membrane as well as endoplasmic reticulum.

TABLE II. Immunization Schedule in Rabbits

No. of injections (weekly)	Volume of antigen (ml)	Protein[a] (mg)	Adjuvant (ml)
1	2	36	2
2	1	18	1
3	1	18	1
↓	↓	↓	↓
Booster	1	18	0

[a] In this and all other experiments, protein was measured by the method of Layne (*42*).

TABLE III. Absorption of Antiserum against Crude PN Antigen from Hyperplastic Nodules with Crude Antigens from Normal Livers[a]

Absorption ratio (volume)	Normal liver protein added (mg/ml of antiserum)	Precipitation lines following reaction with antigen preparations from	
Antiserum : normal liver		Normal liver	Nodules
Absorption condition			
1 : 2	40	0	1[b]
1 : 1	20	0	1
2 : 1	10	0	1
3 : 1	6.6	2	3
4 : 1	5	5[c]	6[c]

[a] Aliquots of antisera were incubated at 37° for 2 hr with varying amounts of crude extract of normal liver prepared in similar manner to the crude antigens from hyperplastic nodules. The antigen-antibody precipitates were removed by centrifugation at 10,000 rpm for 10 min. Each supernatant was tested with Ouchterlony's double diffusion method for detection of the specific antibody against the hyperplastic liver nodules. [b] Very weak line. [c] This is the minimum number.

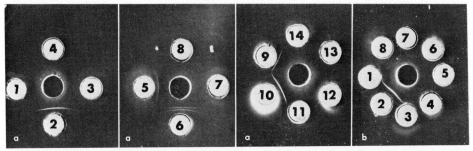

PHOTO 1. Demonstration of PN antigen which is specifically related to hyperplastic nodules and hepatomas, using Ouchterlony's double diffusion method

(a) A single precipitation line was seen between the wells containing antigen preparation from hyperplastic nodules or from hepatomas and the center well. Two lines were observed if the antigen preparation from hyperplastic nodules was left overnight at room temperature. This finding may indicate the instability of PN antigen or exogenous contamination. Center well: rabbit anti-hyperplastic nodule antiserum which was extensively absorbed with pooled normal rat liver. The remaining wells contained crude preparations from a variety of sources as follows: 1, pooled normal rat livers; 2, hyperplastic nodules induced by 2-FAA (fresh material); 3, pooled fetal rat liver (17-day-old); 4, amniotic fluid; 5, hepatoma induced by 2-FAA; 6, hyperplastic nodules induced by 2-FAA (old material); 7, regenerating rat liver 3 days after partial hepatectomy; 8, pooled sera from the rats with hyperplastic liver nodules; 9, hepatoma induced by ethionine; 10, hepatoma induced by DMN; 11, carcinoma of Zymbal's gland in the ear duct induced by 2-FAA; 12, spleen from a rat with myelogenous leukemia induced by 2-FAA; 13, clear cell carcinoma of the kidney induced by DMN; 14, Novikoff hepatoma.

(b) Rabbit anti-hyperplastic nodule antiserum absorbed with normal rat liver did not cross-react with tissue preparations from several organs from normal rats. Center well: same as (a). 1, liver; 2, hyperplastic nodules induced by 2-FAA; 3, brain; 4, heart; 5, lung; 6, kidney; 7, spleen; 8, gastrointestinal tract.

early screening studies have been done with fairly crude extract of hype:plastic nodules prepared by a modification of the method of Gajdusek (24). However, the essential validity of these results remains, as more purified antigen preparations are used.

The preparation of the crude microsomal fraction is outlined in Fig. 1. Preliminary assays indicate that the PN antigen is probably "microsomal" in distribution (Table I). Antisera to the crude antigenic preparations were induced in rabbits, as outlined in Table II. The antibody was titrated at weekly intervals by Ouchterlony's double diffusion method (47). When the antiserum titer was positive at dilutions greater than 1:32, a booster injection was given intramuscularly and the rabbits were bled 1 week later.

The antiserum was absorbed with a crude preparation from normal rat liver, made in a manner similar to that for the crude antigen from hyperplastic nodules. The supernatants after absorption were tested by the double diffusion method for the detection of antibody against hyperplastic liver nodules (Table III). A highly reproducible antibody to one or more components in the hyperplastic nodule was found in all antisera prepared against nodule tissue. An apparently identical precipitation line was found when antigen preparations from hyperplastic nodules or from primary hepatomas were used (Photo 1a). Thus the presumed preneoplastic and the neoplastic cell populations contain some antigenic component or components not apparently present in normal liver.

Specificity of the PN Antigen

The agarose gel reaction pattern obtained with antisera absorbed with normal liver indicated that the single precipitation line detectable following reaction with crude extract from hyperplastic nodules did not cross-react with extracts from normal liver, or from normal kidney, spleen, heart, lung, gastrointestinal tract or brain (Photo 1b). Also, normal rat serum proteins were negative. Absorption of the antiserum with preparations from either hyperplastic nodules or primary hepatomas each induced by 2-FAA or ethionine abolished the reaction with either antigen preparation interchangeably.

Immunoelectrophoresis as described by Scheidegger (54) performed with the soluble antigenic material of hyperplastic nodules against absorbed antiserum demonstrated a single precipitation line in the β-region. Moreover, the specificity of absorbed antiserum was examined by more sensitive methods such as microcomplement fixation as described by Levine and Van Vunakis (43) and by immunofluorescence. As shown in Fig. 2, absorbed antiserum specifically reacted to hyperplastic liver nodules and hepatoma induced by 2-FAA. The finding of about 30% fixed complement in the reaction between normal liver and the antiserum is probably due to the incomplete absorption of antiserum with normal liver. Beale (7) pointed out the possibility that such antigen-antibody reactions in complement fixation using liver components with serum γ-globulin-like substances. However, this possibility has been made less likely by the isolation of the antigenic activity in purified subcellular fractions washed free of any soluble "γ-globulin-like" protein (51). This complication will hopefully be

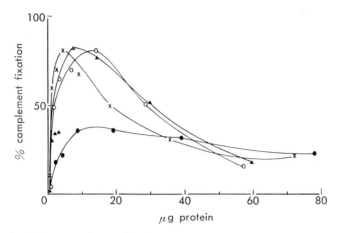

FIG. 2.   Micro-complement fixation

   Antibody titer of absorbed rabbit anti-hyperplastic nodule antiserum with
normal livers was previously examined according to the method of Levine and
Van Vunakis, and from this result the specific antiserum, diluted 1 : 800, was
used in this test. This result indicates the presence of a common antigen (PN
antigen) to hyperplastic nodules and hepatoma at various concentrations of
the antigen. × hyperplastic nodules in early stage during hepatocarcinogenesis
by 2-FAA; ○ in late stage; ▲ hepatoma induced by 2-FAA; ● pooled normal
rat livers.

obviated after purification of PN antigen from the hyperplastic liver nodules.

   In view of the increasing realization that neoplasms of diverse types produce
antigens characteristic of fetal tissue that were somehow "turned off" or "turned
down" during fetal or postnatal development and maturation (*e.g.*, Ref. *1, 25,
58*), and in view of the intimate association between AFP and liver cancer (*e.g.*,
Ref. *1, 35–37, 60*), it is very important to establish whether the PN antigen is a
fetal protein.

   Firstly, repeated attempts to show any identity or antigenic relationship of
AFP to PN antigen were uniformly negative. Also, whole fetuses (10- or 12-
day-old), fetal liver (14-, 16-, 18-, or 20-day-old), newborn livers, and amniotic
fluid (10-, 12-, 14-, 16-, 18-, or 20-day-old) were examined for PN antigen
activity. An insufficient amount of tissue from fetuses younger than 10 days has
been examined to date because of the small amount available. Crude extracts
comparable to those for liver, nodules, and cancer were used. PN antigen was
never detected in any of the tissues examined. Also, immunofluorescent study
of sections with specific antiserum failed to demonstrate any PN antigen in fetal
liver (Photo 5). However, it should be emphasized that the PN antigen could
still be a fetal antigen that appears only transitorily during development in the
liver or elsewhere.

   A variety of livers under various experimental conditions and some neoplasms
of other tissues were examined for the presence of PN antigen (Table IV).
Crude tissue preparations were made as described previously for hyperplastic
nodules. The whole liver or where appropriate the localized lesions in liver or

TABLE IV. Possible Presence of PN Antigen in Various Hepatic Lesions
and Non-hepatic Neoplasms

Lesions	Treatment	No. of rats tested	Positive PN antigen
Acute liver damage	CCl$_4$[a]	3	0/3
	DMN[b]	3	0/3
	ANIT[c]	3	0/3
Hyperplastic nodules			
Early stages[d]	2-FAA	46	46/46
Late stages[e]	,,	25	25/25
Early stages	Ethionine	24	24/24
Late stages	,,	11	11/11
Primary hepatomas	2-FAA	15	15/15
	Ethionine	8	8/8
	3'-Me-DAB	4	4/4
	DMN	5	5/5
	DEN	4	4/4
Transplanted hepatomas			
Novikoff	DAB	4	0/4
Morris 9618	2-Fluorenyldiacetamide	1	1/1
Morris 5123-C	,,	1	0/1
Morris 3924-A	,,	5	0/5
Sidransky	Ethionine	6	6/6
Other organ tumors			
Ear duct	2-FAA	2	0/2
Kidney	DMN or DEN	5	0/5
Leukemia[f]	2-FAA	3	0/3
Regenerating liver	Partial hepatectomy[g]	5	0/5
Normal liver		15	0/15

[a] 5 ml/kg in an equal volume of mineral oil by stomach tube—killed after 3 days.   [b] 30 mg/kg by intraperitoneal injection—killed after 3 days.   [c] 50 mg/kg in oil by stomach tube—killed after 24 hr.   [d] Whole liver was used.   [e] Hyperplastic nodules separated from liver were used.   [f] Spleen was used.   [g] Livers which were removed 3 days after partial hepatectomy.

elsewhere were used. As is evident from Table IV, PN antigen was present in every liver containing hyperplastic nodules or in every nodule examined induced by either 2-FAA or ethionine. In addition, the PN antigen was uniformly present in every primary hepatoma, whether induced by 2-FAA, ethionine, 3'-methyl-4-dimethylaminoazobenzene (3'-Me-DAB), DMN, or diethylnitrosamine (DEN). In contrast, it is only present in some transplantable hepatomas and not in others (Table IV). Although all animals with hyperplastic nodules and primary hepatomas showed the presence of PN antigen, the sera of these animals were uniformly negative. Thus, it appears that this antigen is not secreted under these conditions. However, the possibility of the antigen in the serum being complexed with antibody has yet to be explored.

The PN antigen could not be found at the current level of detection in livers of animals treated acutely with CCl$_4$, DMN, or ANIT, in regenerating liver, or in 3 types of neoplasms other than liver cancer—carcinoma of Zymbal's gland in the ear duct induced by 2-FAA, in renal carcinomas induced by DMN or DEN, or in leukemia induced by 2-FAA.

The absence of PN antigen in livers or sera of animals given CCl_4, ANIT, or DMN, or in some transplantable hepatomas is presumptive evidence in favor of the probability that the PN antigen is different from fetal α-2-glycoprotein, which Grabar *et al.* (*26*) have found in the sera of animals with a variety of acute and chronic toxic and neoplastic lesions.

Time of Appearance of PN Antigen during Carcinogenesis

If the PN antigen is truly closely related to preneoplastic cell populations, it should appear during carcinogenesis at or before the first appearance of recognizable hyperplastic nodules. This has been examined so far during carcinogenesis induced by 2-FAA. As seen in Table V, PN antigen appeared in 2 of 5 animals on the 2-FAA regimen for 2 weeks and in every animal thereafter at all time intervals up to 13 weeks. Very small hyperplastic nodules could usually be seen at 3 weeks and nodules of increasing size were always seen thereafter. Thus, the pattern of appearance of PN antigen is consistent with its being associated with new focal liver cell populations during carcinogenesis.

TABLE V. Relationship between Appearance of Hyperplastic Nodules and of PN Antigen during Liver Carcinogenesis Induced by 2-FAA

Time (weeks)	No. of rats	Hyperplastic nodules	PN antigen[a]
Before treatment	5	—	0/5
1	5	—	0/5
2	5	—	2/5
3	5	— ~ +	5/5
4	5	+	5/5
5	4	+	4/4
7	4	++	4/4
8	4	++	4/4
9	4	++	4/4
11	5	++	5/5
13	4	+++	4/4

[a] Whole liver and not isolated nodular or non-nodular tissue were used in the preparation of crude PN antigen in this experiment. The antigen was tested by the Ouchterlony double diffusion method using anti-hyperplastic nodule antiserum.

Localization of PN Antigen by Immunofluorescence

Localization of PN antigen in tissue section by immunofluorescence was accomplished using the indirect method. All tissues were fixed in 95% ethanol and then were embedded in paraffin by the method of Sainte-Marie (*53*). Microtome sections, 4 μm thick, were deparaffinized in xylene, and washed with precooled phosphate-buffered saline (PBS). After washing, rabbit anti-hyperplastic-

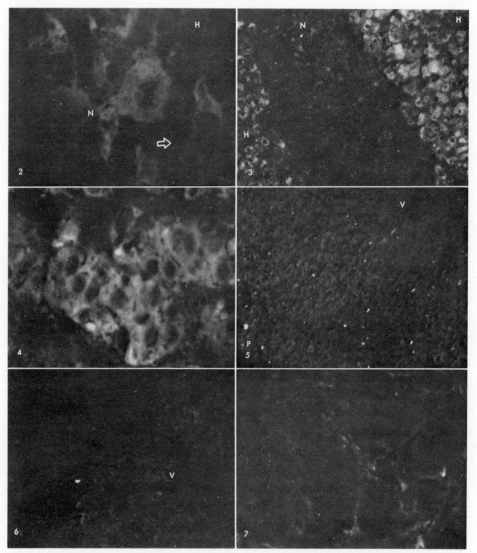

PHOTO 2.   Hyperplastic nodules in early stage during 2-FAA hepatocarcino-genesis
The bright fluorescence was observed mainly in the cytoplasm of hyper-plastic nodules as the fine granules. However, the specific fluorescence was also seen as a linear staining of what appeared to be the cell membrane (arrow). Note the absence of fluorescence in the non-nodular area. ×1,600. N, non-nodular area; H, hyperplastic nodule.

PHOTO 3.   Hyperplastic nodules in late stage during 2-FAA hepatocarcino-genesis
The specific fluorescence was observed only in the cytoplasm of hyperplastic nodules. ×400. N, non-nodular area; H, hyperplastic nodules.

PHOTO 4.   Hepatoma induced by 2-FAA
The specific fluorescence was observed in the cytoplasm. ×1,600.

PHOTO 5.   Normal rat liver
No fluorescence was observed. ×400. V, central vein; P, portal vein.

PHOTO 6.   Fetal rat liver
No fluorescence was seen. ×400. V: central vein.

PHOTO 7.   Cholangioma induced by 2-FAA
No fluorescence was seen. ×800.

liver nodule antiserum, repeatedly absorbed with normal liver, was added and the sections incubated at 37° for 30 min. After incubation, excess antiserum was washed out with PBS. To the sections were added fluorescent isothiocyanate (FITC)-labeled IgG from goat anti-rabbit IgG antiserum prepared by the method of Kawamura (34) and incubated at room temperature for 2 hr. The sections were then extensively washed with PBS and mounted in buffered glycerol. Stained sections were examined with a fluorescence microscope with UV exciter filters and barrier filters. Control sections were incubated with either pre-immune rabbit serum or rabbit anti-hyperplastic-liver nodule antiserum absorbed with hyperplastic liver nodules.

Intensive positive staining was observed in all early or later hyperplastic liver nodules (Photos 2 and 3) and primary hepatomas (Photo 4). Normal rat livers, fetal livers, or cholangioma did not show any specific fluorescence (Photos 5–7). In the stained cells, specific fluorescence was observed regularly in the cytoplasm as fine granules. Nuclei were uniformly negative. In some instances, fluorescence was also seen as a linear staining of what appeared to be the cell membrane. However, this was variable. These observations with fluorescent staining are consistent so far with the results of the early attempts to determine the intracellular localization of the PN antigen with simple differential centrifugation (Table I).

Possible Significance and Implications of PN Antigen

From the data summarized above, it appears that the focal liver cell populations called hyperplastic nodules uniformly contain an apparently new antigen in their endoplasmic reticulum and possibly also in the plasma membrane that is present uniformly in primary hepatomas as well. This new antigen appears very early during liver carcinogenesis and seems to persist throughout the carcinogenic process in the hepatocytes of hyperplastic nodules and in the neoplastic hepatocytes in all primary hepatomas. No evidence for the appearance of PN antigen in the surrounding non-hyperplastic or non-neoplastic liver parenchyma could be found. Thus, the PN antigen offers the strongest evidence for a unifying link between the hyperplastic cell populations at all time intervals from the very earliest to liver cancer.

The analysis of preneoplastic or premalignant cell populations for new antigens has been neglected generally probably because of the general unavailability of sufficient amounts of uniform tissue. Two systems, the papillomas in the skin and the hyperplastic nodules in the breast, have been studied from this point of view in Prehn's laboratory (38, 39, 55). In both instances, with chemical carcinogens, hyperplastic premalignant mammary gland lesions (55), and skin papillomas (38, 39) show neoantigenicity which persisted essentially unchanged through years of transplantation and was still present in the malignant neoplasms that subsequently developed. However, the antigens studied were apparently unique for each lesion and were not common to all of the similar lesions in one organ. Thus, no common antigen, analogous to the PN antigen in preneoplastic liver, has been found so far.

In regard to liver neoplasms, there are several reports of a marked decrease or loss of liver antigens in hepatomas (2, 22, 30, 46, 61). Also, an important study by Weiler (62) showed the loss of specific liver antigens in focal islands of liver cells, considered to be a presumptive preneoplastic population. We have found a similar loss of liver antigens early during liver carcinogenesis, within 2 weeks of beginning a 2-FAA feeding regimen (Okita and Farber, unpublished results).

In addition, new antigens have also been found in a variety of hepatomas (1, 3, 5, 6, 13, 28–30, see review by Baldwin (4)). Some of these seem to be unique for each hepatoma or for each group of hepatomas induced by a single carcinogen while others are probably fetal in type, including, of course, AFP. However, no single common antigen for primary hepatomas, other than AFP, has been reported. Thus, the PN antigen appears to be a new marker for hepatocellular carcinomas as well as for its precursor cells.

The nature and significance of the new PN antigen is both interesting and provocative. Any truly definitive establishment of the nature and significance of PN antigen must await its complete purification and definitive localization in the cell. Such studies are now in progress. However, it is still possible, even at this early stage in its history, to raise some legitimate questions concerning origin and meaning.

Is the PN antigen an altered protein pre-existing in the original liver? One trivial possibility could be as follows: a normal multi-unit protein may have an alteration or deficiency in one or more of its subunits, thus generating new antigenic sites now available. An attempt to study this was done by incubating crude extracts of hyperplastic nodules with similar extracts from normal liver at 37° for 2 hr. As controls, each type of extract was incubated separately under the same conditions. All preparations containing extracts from hyperplastic nodules gave equally strong reactions with antiserum to hyperplastic nodules and the presence of extracts from normal liver did not exert any observable influence. Also, since it is well established that some hepatic carcinogens induce new antigenic components in liver or serum with each carcinogen as a specific hapten (reviewed by Baldwin (4)), it is possible that the PN antigen is of such a nature. However, there are several compelling arguments that rule out this possibility; (a) nodules induced by 2-FAA or ethionine and primary hepatomas induced by 2-FAA, ethionine, 3'-Me-DAB, DMN, or DEN all have the same apparent PN antigen, and (b) two hepatomas, a Morris hepatoma 9618 induced by 2-fluorenyldiacetamide and the Sidransky hepatoma induced by ethionine, each have the PN antigen, even though these have been transplanted for many years. Thus, a relationship of PN antigen to a specific carcinogen-protein product is ruled out.

A much more plausible hypothesis is that the PN antigen is a viral antigen that has been encouraged to become active by treatment with the carcinogen and/or by the appearance of a new cell population that is much more favorable to the virus than is the original liver cell population. This hypothesis could easily explain the appearance of a common antigen in that sequence of cell populations related to the evolution of liver cancer. Obviously, it would be of the greatest importance to our understanding of carcinogenesis if liver cancer, so closely associated with chemical carcinogens, could be shown to be associated, *in vivo*, with a virus. Although viruses are now being found in some cultures of hepatomas *in vitro* (*e.g.*, Ref. *64*), their role in hepatocarcinogenesis is not evident.

One approach to this problem is to determine whether the PN antigen has any observable relationship to two viral group-specific (gs) antigens—gs-1 antigen, present only in rats and gs-3 antigen, common to RNA viruses of several species (*e.g.*, Ref. *32, 33*).

PN antigen has been examined for gs-1 antigen by Dr. Hatanaka and was found to be negative (personal communication). Rat anti-gs-3 antigen, supplied by Dr. Girardi of the Wistar Institute, was found not to react with PN antigen. These negative results, although important, do not rule out completely any relationship between PN antigen and a rat RNA virus. Obviously, further studies with varied approaches must be used to explore this potentially important aspect of the problem.

Another attractive hypothesis is that the PN antigen is a protein that is made or "turned on" in response to an interruption in differentiation that is associated with both hyperplastic nodules and primary hepatocellular carcinoma. It is now becoming evident that the hyperplastic nodule remains a discrete separate nodule because of a failure in remodeling, differentiation, or maturation of its parenchyma (*21*). It is now well known that hepatocytes in areas of regeneration of liver often show what appears to be immature architectural arrangements— *e.g.*, two-cell thick plates and tubularization (*48*). The hyperplastic nodules show a similar pattern. Normally, the hepatocytes then undergo remodeling to the mature adult arrangement of one-cell thick plate. The early hyperplastic nodule, the so-called reversible one, remains immature as long as the carcinogen is administered. However, on removing the carcinogen, the early nodules undergo remodeling and maturation to normal-looking liver and thus seem to "regress." The later nodules do not show this differentiation on removal of the carcinogen or do so only very slowly and thus are irreversible and can act as a precursor population for further evolution to liver cancer. The appearance of PN antigen might be related to this interruption in differentiation or maturation, since preliminary data show that it disappears from the nodule hepatocyte when the nodule is remodeled.

Thus, it is possible that the new PN antigen may not be a marker for the neoplastic growth but for the disturbance in differentiation that so regularly accompanies this type of relatively uncontrolled cell proliferation.

Regardless of its essential nature, the PN antigen opens new avenues for the study of liver carcinogenesis both in animals and in humans. Hopefully, a similar antigen may be found in the human. This would allow a more definitive identification of preneoplastic lesions and might well allow a better understanding between cirrhosis and liver cancer.

These new observations in liver also raise the distinct possibility that analogous antigens might be found in preneoplastic lesions in other organs and tissue. Such a realization could offer new possibilities in both the understanding and diagnosis of early lesions related to cancer.

In addition, the discovery of a *general* property of preneoplastic and neoplastic cell populations induced by several chemically different carcinogens offers a needed perspective in the study of carcinogenesis. Many biochemical and immunological studies over the past 25 years, designed to uncover unifying molecular or cellular properties of neoplastic cell populations, point on the whole to a contrary conclusion—the uniqueness of individual neoplasms rather than to their similarities (*e.g.*, see Refs. *4, 19*, and *63*). Even though an origin of many neoplasms from single cells by cellular evolution is highly probable, one cannot help being impressed by the many superficial similarities in the biological properties of various carcinogenic processes. The observation of a common antigenic marker for the many cell populations associated with one carcinogenic process raises again the prospect of discovering other common unifying markers in the development of cancer and of ultimately utilizing such markers in either the prevention or cure of cancer.

REFERENCES

1. Abelev. G. I. Alpha-fetoprotein in ontogenesis and its association with malignant tumors. *Adv. Cancer Res.*, **14**, 295–358 (1971).
2. Abelev, G. I. Antigenic structure of chemically induced hepatomas. *Prog. Exp. Tumor Res.*, **7**, 104–157 (1965).
3. Baldwin, R. W. Abnormal cell antigen in aminoazo dye-induced rat liver tumours. *Brit. J. Cancer*, **19**, 894–902 (1965).
4. Baldwin, R. W. Immunological aspects of chemical carcinogenesis. *Adv. Cancer Res.*, **18**, 1–75 (1974).
5. Baldwin, R. W. and Barker, C. R. Antigenic composition of transplanted rat hepatomas originally induced by 4-dimethyl-aminoazobenzene, *Brit. J. Cancer*, **21**, 338–345 (1967).
6. Baldwin, R. W. and Glaves, D. Solubilization of tumor specific antigen from plasma membrane of an aminoazo dye-induced rat hepatoma. *Clin. Exp. Immunol.*, **11**, 51–56 (1972).
7. Beale, G. H. The nature of the complement-fixing antigen in normal human liver extracts. *J. Lab. Clin. Med.*, **67**, 67–75 (1963).
8. Berman, C. Primary carcinoma of the liver. *Adv. Cancer Res.*, **5**, 55–96 (1958).
9. Chernozemski, I. N. and Warwick, G. P. Liver regeneration and induction of hepatomas in B6 Af$_1$ mice by urethan. *Cancer Res.*, **30**, 2685–2690 (1970).
10. Chernozemski, I. N. and Warwick G. P. Production of hepatomas in suckling mice after single application of β-propiolactone. *J. Natl. Cancer Inst.*, **45**, 709–717 (1970).
11. Craddock, V. M. Liver carcinomas induced in rats by single administration of dimethylnitrosamine after partial hepatectomy. *J. Natl. Cancer Inst.*, **47**, 899–905 (1971).
12. Craddock, V. M. Induction of liver tumours in rats by a single treatment with nitroso compounds given after partial hepatectomy. *Nature*, **245**, 386–388 (1973).
13. Deckers, C. and Deckers-Passau, L. Specific tumor antigens in rat hepatomas and leukosarcoma. *UICC Monogr.*, **2**, 34–41 (1966).
14. Epstein, S. M., Ito, N., Markow, L., and Farber, E. Cellular analysis of liver carcinogenesis: The induction of large hyperplastic nodules in the liver with 2-fluorenylacetamide or ethionine and some aspects of their morphology and glycogen metabolism. *Cancer Res.*, **27**, 1702–1711 (1967).

15. Epstein, S. M., McNary, J., Bartus, B., and Farber, E. Chemical carcinogenesis: Persistence of bound forms of 2-fluorenylacetamide. *Science*, **162**, 907–908 (1968).

16. Farber, E. Similarities in the sequence of early histological changes induced in the liver of the rat by ethionine, 2-acetylaminofluorene and 3'-methyl-4-dimethylaminoazobenzene. *Cancer Res.*, **16**, 142–148 (1956).

17. Farber, E. Ethionine carcinogenesis. *Adv. Cancer Res.*, **7**, 383–474 (1963).

18. Farber, E. Hyperplastic liver nodules. *Methods Cancer Res.*, **7**, 345–375 (1973).

19. Farber, E. Carcinogenesis—cellular evolution as a unifying thread: Presidential address. *Cancer Res.*, **33**, 2537–2550 (1973).

20. Farber, E., Sarma, D. S. R., Rajalakshmi, S., and Shinozuka, H. Liver carcinogenesis: A unifying hypothesis. *In* "Principles of Liver Disease," ed. by F. F. Becker, Marcel Dekker, New York, in press.

21. Farber, E. and Parker, S. Unpublished.

22. Fisher, E. and Weiler, E. Die histologische Darstellung der leberspezifischen Antigens und dessen Schwund in Hepatoma mit Hilfe fluoresceinmarkierten Anticomplements. *Z. Krebsforsch.*, **64**, 441–447 (1962).

23. Foulds, L. "Neoplastic Development," Academic Press, London, Vol. 1 (1969).

24. Gajdusek, D. C. An "autoimmune" reaction against human tissue antigens in certain acute and chronic diseases. *Arch. Intern. Med.*, **101**, 9–29 (1958).

25. Gold, P. and Freedman, S. O. Specific carcinoembryonic antigens in the human digestive system. *J. Exp. Med.*, **122**, 467–481 (1965).

26. Grabar, P., Stanislawski-Birencwajg, M., Iosgold, S., and Uriel, J. Immunochemical and enzymatic studies on chemically induced rat liver tumors. *UICC Monogr.*, **2**, 20–31 (1966).

27. Higginson, J. and Svoboda, D. J. Primary carcinoma of the liver as a pathologist's problem. *Pathol. Annu.*, **5**, 61–89 (1970).

28. Hirai, H., Taga, H., Isaka, H., Satoh, H., and Warabioka, K. The specificity of antigenic protein of rat ascites hepatoma cells. *Gann*, **54**, 177–183 (1963).

29. Hirai, H. Specific antigenic proteins of rat ascites hepatoma. *UICC Monogr.*, **2**, 42–66 (1966).

30. Hiramoto, R., Gurand, J., Bernecky, J., and Pressman, D. Immunochemical differences among N-2-fluorenylacetamide-induced rat hepatomas. *Cancer Res.*, **23**, 109–111 (1963).

31. Hollander, C. F. and Bentvelzen, P. Enhancement of urethan induction of hepatomas in mice by prior partial hepatectomy. *J. Natl. Cancer Inst.*, **41**, 1303–1306 (1968).

32. Huebner, R. J. and Todaro, G. J. Oncogenesis of RNA tumor viruses as determinants of cancer. *Proc. Natl. Acad. Sci. U.S.*, **64**, 1087–1094 (1969).

33. Huebner, R. J., Sarma, P. S., Kelloff, G. J., Gilden, R. V., Meier, H., Myers, D. D., and Peters, R. L. Immunological tolerance to RNA tumor virus genome expressions: Significance of tolerance and prenatal expressions in embryogenesis and tumorigenesis. *Ann. N.Y. Acad. Sci.*, **181**, 246–271 (1971).

34. Kawamura, A. "Fluorescent Antibody Techniques and Their Applications," University of Tokyo Press, Tokyo, and University Park Press, Baltimore/Manchester (1969).

35. Kitagawa, T., Yokochi, T., and Sugano, H. α-Fetoprotein and hepatocarcinogenesis in rats fed 3'-methyl-4-(dimethylamino)azobenzene or N-2-fluorenylacetamide. *Int. J. Cancer*, **10**, 368–381 (1972).

36. Kroes, R., Williams, G. M., and Weisburger, J. H. Early appearence of serum

α-fetoprotein during hepatocarcinogenesis as a function of age of rats and extent of treatment with 3'-methyl-4-dimethylaminoazobenzene. *Cancer Res.*, **32**, 1526–1532 (1972).

37. Kroes, R., Williams, G. M., and Weisburger, J. H. Early appearance of serum α-fetoprotein as a function of dosage of various hepatocarcinogens. *Cancer Res.*, **33**, 613–617 (1973).

38. Lappé, M. A. Evidence for the antigenicity of papilloma induced by 3-methyl-cholanthrene. *J. Natl. Cancer Inst.*, **40**, 823–846 (1968).

39. Lappé, M. A. Tumor specific transplantation antigens: Possible origin in pre-malignant lesions. *Nature*, **223**, 82–84 (1969).

40. Lane, M., Liebelt, A., Calvert, J., and Liebelt, R. A. Effect of partial hepatectomy on tumor incidence in BALB/c mice treated with urethan. *Fed. Proc.*, **26**, 625 (1967).

41. Lane, M., Liebelt, A., Calvert, J., and Liebelt, R. A. Effect of partial hepatectomy on tumor incidence in BALB/c mice treated with urethan. *Cancer Res.*, **30**, 1812–1816 (1970).

42. Layne, E. Spectrophotometric and turbidimetric methods for measuring proteins. *Methods Enzymol.*, **3**, 447–454 (1957).

43. Levine, L. and Van Vunakis, H. Micromplement fixatoin. *Methods Enzymol.*, **11**, 928–936 (1967).

44. Magee, P. N. and Barnes, J. M. Carcinogenic nitroso compounds. *Adv. Cancer Res.*, **10**, 163–256 (1967).

45. Marquardt, H., Steinberg, S. S., and Philips, F. S. Dimethylbenz(a)anthracene and hepatic neoplasia in regenerating rat liver. *Chem.-Biol. Interact.*, **2**, 401–403 (1971).

46. Nairn, R. C., Richmond, H. G., and Fothagill, J. E. Immunological differences between normal and malignant cells. *Brit. Med. J.*, **2**, 1335–1340 (1960).

46a. Okita, K., Gruenstein, M., Klaiber, M., and Farber, E. Localization of alpha-fetoprotein by immunofluorescence in hyperplastic nodules during hepatocarcino-genesis induced by 2-acetylaminofluorence. *Cancer Res.*, **34**, 2758–2763 (1974).

47. Ouchterlony, O. Antigen-antibody reaction in gels. *Acta Pathol. Microbiol. Scand.*, **26**, 507–515 (1949).

48. Phillips, M. J. and Steiner, J. W. Electron microscopy of cirrhotic nodules. Tubu-larization of the parenchyma by biliary hepatocytes. *Lab. Invest.*, **15**, 801–817 (1966).

49. Pound, A. W. Carcinogenesis and cell proliferation. *N. Z. Med. J.*, **67**, 88–99 (1968).

50. Reuber, M. D. Development of preneoplastic and neoplastic lesions of the liver in male rats given 0.025 percent of N-2-fluorenylacetamide. *J. Natl. Cancer Inst.*, **34**, 697–723 (1965).

51. Roitt, I. M., Ling, N. R., Doniach, D., and Conchman, K. G. The cytoplasmic auto-antigen of the human thyroid. I. Immunological and biochemical charac-teristics. *Immunology*, **7**, 375–393 (1964).

52. Sasaki, T. and Yoshida, T. Experimentelle Erzeugung des Lebercarcinoms durch Fütterung mit o-Amidoazotoluol. *Arch. Pathol. Anat. Physiol.*, **295**, 175–200 (1935).

53. Sainte-Marie, G. A paraffin embedding technique for studies employing im-munofluorescence. *J. Histochem. Cytochem.*, **10**, 250–256 (1962).

54. Scheidegger, J. J. Une micro-méthode de l'immunoélectrophorése. *Int. Arch. Allergy*, **7**, 103–110 (1955).

55. Slemmer, G. Host response of premalignant mammary tissues. *Natl. Cancer Inst. Monogr.*, **35**, 57–71 (1972).

56. Steiner, P. E. Carcinoma of the liver in the United States. *Acta Unio Int. Contra Cancrum*, **13**, 628–645 (1947).

57. Teebor, G. W. and Becker, F. F. Regression and persistence of hyperplastic nodules induced by N-2-fluorenylacetamide and their relationship to hepatocarcinogenesis. *Cancer Res.*, **31**, 1–3 (1971).

58. von Kleist, S. and Burtin, P. Isolation of fetal antigen from human colonic tumors. *Cancer Res.*, **29**, 1961–1964 (1966).

59. Warwick, G. P. Covalent binding of metabolites of tritiated 2-methyl-4-dimethylaminoazobenzene to rat liver nucleic acids and proteins and the carcinogenicity of the unlabelled compound in partially hepatectomized rats. *Eur. J. Cancer*, **3**, 227–233 (1967).

60. Watabe, H. Early appearance of embryonic α-globulin in rat serum under carcinogenesis with 4-dimethylaminoazobenzene. *Cancer Res.*, **31**, 1192–1194 (1971).

61. Weiler, E. Loss of specific cell antigen in relation to cancer. *Ciba Found. Symp. on Carcinogenesis—Mechanisms of Action*, 165–175 (1958).

62. Weiler, E. Die Änderung der serologischen Spezifität von Leberzellen der Ratte während der Carcinogenese durch *p*-Dimethylaminoazobenzol. *Z. Naturforsch.*, **116**, 31–38 (1956).

63. Weinhouse, S. Glycolysis, respiration and anomalous gene expression in experimental hepatomas—G. H. A. Clowes Memorial Lecture. *Cancer Res.*, **32**, 2007–2016 (1972).

64. Weinstein, I. B., Gebert, R., Stadler, U. C., Orenstein, J. M., and Axel, R. Type C virus from cell cultures of chemically induced rat hepatomas. *Science*, **178**, 1098–1100 (1972).

GANN Monograph on Cancer Research 17, 301–342 (1975)

EVOLUTION OF HYPERPLASIA, HYPERPLASTIC NODULES, AND CARCINOMAS OF THE LIVER INDUCED IN RATS BY N-2-FLUORENYL-DIACETAMIDE[*1]

Melvin Dwaine REUBER[*2]

National Cancer Institute[*3]

Hyperplastic cells are dependent upon the continued feeding of the chemical stimulus. If the chemical is discontinued early, hyperplasia will not progress to hyperplastic nodules. If the chemical is continued, however, hyperplasia will begin to appear as nodules of hyperplasia. Only few areas ever progress to nodules, whereas most develop degenerative changes in the cytoplasm.

Hyperplastic nodules have reached the stage when they are no longer dependent upon continued exposure to the chemical. If the chemical is discontinued, these nodules will continue to progress and become carcinomas only in the host liver. Hyperplastic nodules must be distinguished from cirrhotic nodules by their gross appearance and histology.

Carcinomas less than 5 mm are less likely to metastasize, *i.e.*, spread and grow in organs other than the liver, than are carcinomas greater than 5 mm. Small carcinomas, as with hyperplastic nodules, will invariably progress in the host liver to become larger carcinomas. They will survive and grow in the liver of another animal as a small carcinoma, but probably will not reach a larger size.

Large carcinomas are capable of metastasizing and are also able to kill the host animal. They grow on transplantation in the same or other animals of the same inbred strain in the liver, spleen, lungs, muscle, subcutaneous tissues, or peritoneum.

There is an excellent correlation between the histological pattern of carcinomas, *i.e.*, well-differentiated *vs.* poorly or undifferentiated, and their biological behavior, as shown in the host and on transplantation to isologous animals.

Hyperplasia is the forerunner of carcinoma of the liver in the experimental animal (*1–3*) and has been postulated to precede carcinoma in human beings. In animals fed a carcinogen, the transformation from hyperplasia to neoplasia takes place gradually. The evidence for this is based on the development of both hyperplasia and neoplasia from the same cells in the same organ, the finding that

---

[*1] Chemical Abstracts' nomenclature: N,N-diacetyl-2-fluorenamine or N,N-diacetyl-2-aminofluorene. Also in the literature as 2-diacetylaminofluorene and 2-diacetamidofluorene.

[*2] Present address: 11014 Swansfield Road, Columbia, Maryland 21044, U.S.A.

[*3] Bethesda, Maryland 21044, U.S.A.

hyperplasia appears before the development of carcinoma, the apparent occurrence of histological transformation of hyperplastic tissue into a carcinomatous growth, and the lack of similar hyperplastic or neoplastic changes in notable numbers in other cells or organs.

N-2-Fluorenyldiacetamide (FdiAA) has provided a useful model for the study of preneoplastic and neoplastic lesions of the liver in rats (*1, 2*). The lesions develop slowly over a period of months and can be followed from hyperplastic areas to hyperplastic nodules to small hepatocellular carcinomas and later large well-developed hepatocellular carcinomas often with metastases. Cirrhosis develops along with the hyperplastic lesions. The experiment utilizes a relatively low dose of FdiAA, 0.025%, added to a semi-synthetic diet with a good source of protein (*2*). For the best regimen the carcinogen-containing diet is given for 4-week periods with rest periods on the basal diet so that animals can recover

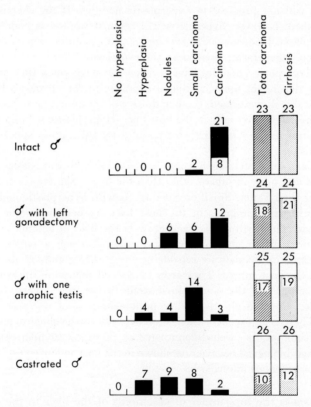

FIG. 1. Intact male rats, male rats with left gonadectomy, male rats with one atrophic testis, and castrated male rats ingesting 0.025% FdiAA for a total of 16 weeks

Only the most advanced lesion in a given animal is indicated. Cirrhosis is included in last bar to allow comparison with carcinomas. Number above each black bar is the total number of animals developing such lesions. Under "carcinomas" white area designates number of animals with metastases. "Total carcinomas" and "cirrhosis" show number of animals in group as well as number with those lesions. These designations apply to all the figures using this classification.

from toxic effects and weight loss, until a total of 16 weeks of FdiAA has been administered. Animals are placed on the basal diet or laboratory pellets for the remainder of the experiment. This allows the hyperplastic areas and nodules to progress to carcinomas, and the cirrhosis to regress or decrease in severity. Most carcinomas are large and 100% over 1.0 cm in size can be transplanted in isologous hosts, *i.e.*, inbred rats of the same strain (*9–11*).

The development of hyperplastic and neoplastic lesions of the liver is dependent upon the presence of the testes, or more specifically of endogenous testosterone in male rats, or exogenous testosterone administered to female rats. The incidence of carcinomas and the number of rats with large carcinomas, multiple carcinomas, and metastases is highest in intact rats. The incidence and size not only decrease in the animals with one or both testes removed, but the decrease is directly related to the bulk and weight of the testis or testes in rats. The incidence is lowest in rats with both testes removed (Fig. 1) (*7*). Thyroidectomy also decreases the development of carcinomas of the liver in male rats and this decrease is probably related to atrophy of the testes (*5, 6*). Extensive studies concerning the role of hormones in hepatic carcinogenesis have been carried out with this model (*2, 4–8*).

The liver of the rat is particularly useful for the study of preneoplastic hyperplasia and neoplasia induced by carcinogens. Laparotomy can be carried out, the liver examined for gross lesions, and biopsies of lesions taken for histological study or transplantation (*9–11*). The criteria for malignancy are based upon morphology and/or growth when transplanted to another animal of the same strain.

Animals can be injected with materials that are taken up by normal parenchymal cells or Kupffer cells, or chemicals that damage normal cells. Rose Bengal dye or India ink can be injected intravenously prior to killing of animals (*3*). Normal liver is stained bright pink by Rose Bengal, whereas lesions stain either lighter pink or remain untinted. India ink is taken up by and detects the presence of functioning Kupffer cells in normal liver or in the lesions.

The findings in the livers of animal were classified (*2, 3, 9*) and tabulated as follows:

1) No hyperplasia. This also included animals with diffuse increase in size of cells in the periportal areas.

2) Hyperplasia. These were in animals with livers containing multiple small foci or larger areas of hyperplasia distinct from the surrounding liver and often showing somewhat different architectural arrangement from the normal lobule. Degenerating areas of hyperplasia were those in which the cells showed hydropic or fatty change of the cytoplasm.

3) Hyperplastic nodules. These were in animals in which the hyperplasia had progressed to the formation of clearly defined nodules of parenchymal cells with distinct compression of surrounding parenchyma. The architecture in these nodules varied from well-organized adult cords to a disorderly pattern of growth, at times with atypicality of cells. Focal malignant change was often seen in hyperplastic nodules.

4) Small hepatocellular carcinomas. These represented the earliest and smallest lesions that could be morphologically accepted as malignant; yet by definition, they were limited to lesions no more than 5 mm in greatest diameter.

5) Well-developed (large) hepatocellular carcinomas. These were malignant tumors of parenchymal cells which were well-differentiated, poorly differentiated, or undifferentiated growths larger than 5 mm in diameter. Occasionally there were cholangiomatous areas in the hepatocellular carcinomas.

6) Metastases. Invasion of portal or hepatic veins was frequent, and in some animals multiple emboli or metastases were seen in the lungs. In some animals there were omental and peritoneal implants or invasion of adjacent organs.

7) Cirrhosis. Simultaneously there was often proliferation of small bile ducts and accompanying fibroblastic activity progressing to apparent isolation of hepatic cells and lobules.

Hyperplastic and Neoplastic Lesions of the Liver

1. Areas of hyperplasia

Grossly the earliest change was the finely granular surface of the liver which gradually became coarsely granular (Photo 1). Microscopically the earliest change was diffuse periportal hyperplasia and proliferation of small bile ducts (Photos 2 and 3). Fairly discrete foci of hyperplasia that could not be recognized grossly developed in the periportal zone (Photo 4).

Foci of hyperplasia increased in size and became areas of hyperplasia, measuring 1 to 3 or 4 mm in diameter. Areas of hyperplasia could be seen on gross examination (Photos 1 and 9). The cytoplasm of the cells was usually somewhat eosinophilic (Photos 5 and 6), sometimes basophilic or only faintly colored (Photo 8). The cytoplasm of hyperplastic cells rarely contained glycogen (Photo 25). Kupffer cells were increased in number.

Areas of hyperplasia in some parts of the liver expanded to constrict and compress the adjacent liver cords, at first focally (Photo 10) and later on all margins, and formed hyperplastic nodules. Hyperplastic cells that did not continue to grow developed hydropic or fatty change within the cytoplasm (Photos 11 and 12).

2. Nodules of hyperplasia

Nodules of hyperplasia could be recognized grossly as discrete nodules, which were tan or colored similar to the adjacent liver, and measured 4 to 6 mm (Photo 13). A prominent vessel could often be seen over the surface of the nodule. Histologically, the cells in the nodules were identical to those in areas of hyperplasia, and at first were arranged in cords and sheets (Photos 14, 15, and 18). As a nodule increased in size the cytoplasm became more eosinophilic staining. Increased number of Kupffer cells lined the vascular sinusoids.

Areas and nodules of hyperplasia collided and appeared to form one lesion grossly (Photos 9 and 24), however, the individual lesions could be detected on microscopic examination (Photo 17).

Later the hyperplastic parenchymal cells were atypical and then underwent malignant change in focal areas (Fig. 8). This change was characterized by the formation of double cords with prominent sinusoids and was often located in the center, but also could be seen in the periphery (Photos 19 to 22). The cytoplasm of the cells became more darkly eosinophilic. Hyperplastic cells in nodules gradually became malignant and developed into small carcinomas.

3. Small hepatocellular carcinomas

Small carcinomas were liver-colored or tan and showed, especially at laparatomy, a similar prominent vessel with small ramifications over the surface as did the hyperplastic nodules (Photo 16). There were variations in the cytologic characteristics of small carcinomas just as there were in nodules of hyperplasia. Because their histological pattern resembled that of larger hepatocellular carcinomas (Photo 23), they were considered to be analogous to "carcinoma *in situ.*"

Small carcinomas continued to increase in size and became large well-developed carcinomas (Photo 44).

4. Well-developed hepatocellular carcinomas

Large hepatocellular carcinomas measured more than 5 mm in diameter. They could be separated into 3 types on the basis of their histological pattern, transplantability, and biological behavior (9–11). The poorly differentiated and undifferentiated carcinomas made up a small percentage, with the predominant carcinoma being well-differentiated. From biopsy specimens, growth on transplantation, and findings at autopsy, the pattern of a particular carcinoma did not change with time.

1) *Well-differentiated hepatocellular carcinomas* were soft and tan, brown, or liver-colored, and were sometimes stained with bile. They were nodular, had several prominent vessels with branches over the surface, and sometimes reached 4.5 to 5.0 cm in diameter but were more often 3.5 cm (Photo 28).

Histologically, well-differentiated carcinomas retained many of the characteristics of normal parenchymal cells. These characteristics were the formation or cords, two to several layers in thickness, with canaliculi, and prominent sinusoids with lining cells. The cytoplasm was usually darkly eosinophilic, but sometimes was basophilic; and was either decreased or increased in amount. The nuclei were vesicular with prominent nucleoli. Double nucleated cells or mitotic figures were usually absent (Photos 29, 30, 33, 34, and 36). Formation of cords with canaliculi was often the most helpful indication of well-differentiated carcinomas (Photo 33). Adjacent to these there often were strands of connective tissue with macrophages containing lipofuchsin, ceroid, and/or lipid (Photo 43).

The cells of some well-differentiated carcinomas had bile pigment in the cytoplasm and bile casts in canaliculi (Photo 41). Glycogen was rarely present within the cytoplasm of well-differentiated carcinomas (Photo 42).

2) *Poorly differentiated hepatocellular carcinomas* were firm, gray or white, coarsely lobulated, and fairly well demarcated from the adjacent liver parenchyma and reached 6.0 cm in size (Photo 45). These carcinomas had the characteristics of anaplasia, but retained a resemblance in some parts to hepatic cells. The cells varied in size and shape, grew in sheets, and sometimes grew in cords many cells in thickness (Photos 46 and 48). Nuclei were vesicular with prominent

nucleoli. The cytoplasm was usually basophilic, but was occasionally darkly eosinophilic. Abnormal mitotic figures were present. Focally cells attempted to form canaliculi (Photo 48) and even rarely secreted bile pigment (Photo 47).

Poorly differentiated carcinomas were occasionally made up of cells that varied greatly in size and shape (Photo 50). The vesicular nuclei were large with large nucleoli and the cytoplasm was darkly eosinophilic (Photo 51).

3) *Undifferentiated carcinomas* were firm, gray or white, involved much of the liver, and invaded the adjacent liver (Photo 54). Centrally there was extensive necrosis. Undifferentiated carcinomas grew in sheets. They were more anaplastic than poorly differentiated carcinomas and had greater variation in size and shape of nuclei and cells. The cytoplasm was usually basophilic but sometimes was eosinophilic. Abnormal mitoses were frequent. Nucleoli were prominent and often there were more than one (Photos 55, 56, 59, and 60).

5. *Well-developed cholangiocellular carcinomas*

Grossly cholangiocellular carcinomas were hard and white, often contained mucus, and measured 3 to 5 cm in size (Photo 65). These carcinomas retained many of the characteristics of bile duct cells, *i.e.*, columnar cells with lightly basophilic cytoplasm and oval nuclei. Well-differentiated cholangiocellular carcinomas formed ducts sometimes containing mucin in the cytoplasm or lumens; the cytoplasm was lightly basophilic; there was a "desmoplastic" background of fibrous connective tissue; nuclei were oval with inconspicuous nucleoli (Photos 63, 64, 67, and 68).

Hepatocellular cholangiocarcinomas resembled hepatocellular carcinomas grossly, but microscopically they contained areas of varying size that formed a cholangiomatous pattern (Photo 62).

6. *Degenerative changes in hyperplastic lesions*

Microscopically, in a few areas of hyperplasia, the cytoplasm was clear or foamy after 20 weeks, and in most areas of hyperplasia, such cells were present terminally (Photos 11 and 12). No glycogen was demonstrable, and the foamy cells contained fat. By contrast with areas of hyperplasia the cells in nodules of hyperplasia did not undergo diffuse hydropic or fatty change.

7. *Degenerative changes in carcinomas*

Degenerative changes were most marked in the large tumors, and they were present more often in the poorly differentiated than in the well-differentiated tumors. The signs of degeneration consisted of hyaline inclusions or lipid vacuoles in the cytoplasm, necrotic cells, and areas of recent or old hemorrhage. The well-differentiated tumors occasionally had macrophages containing lipid, iron, and ceroid within strands of connective tissue (Photo 43).

8. *Metastases*

Well-differentiated carcinomas metastasized to the lungs in one-third to one-half of the animals, and also occasionally to portahepatic lymph nodes. The peritoneum and organs adjacent to the liver were not involved. These carcinomas also did not metastasize to other parts of the same lobe or to other lobes of the liver. There was a direct correlation between the size of the primary carcinoma, venous invasion, and presence and size of metastases in the lungs. Microscopic emboli or tiny metastases were not observed until the primary carcinoma was approximately 3 cm in diameter. The metastases were about the same size and were scattered diffusely throughout the lungs (Photo 35).

Poorly differentiated and undifferentiated carcinomas metastasized in all of the animals. The sites of the metastases and local extension were related to the size of the primary carcinoma and its location in the liver. Metastases were observed in the lungs when the primary carcinoma was 1 cm in size. The metastatic growths varied more and reached larger sizes than did those of the well-differentiated carcinomas (Photo 58). With larger carcinomas emboli were seen in many sinusoids, veins, and portal lymphatics within the liver. The carcinomas invaded the stomach, spleen, diaphragm, mesentery, or abdominal muscles, and metastasized to portahepatic and retroperitoneal lymph nodes (Photo 57). Tumor grew out into the portal vein and inferior vena cava (Photo 61). Occasionally, there was reddish or brownish blood in the peritoneum of animals with poorly differentiated carcinomas apparently from the rupture of a dilated vessel over the surface of the carcinoma (Photo 40).

Cholangiocellular carcinomas metastasized to the lungs and/or portahepatic lymph nodes. The metastases to the lungs varied not only in size, but also in involvement of the different lobes of the lungs (Photo 66).

The histological pattern of the metastases was identical to that of the primary carcinoma (Photos 52 and 53). Degenerative changes were noted in the center of metastatic growths that measured 3 mm or larger. Metastases did not occur from primary tumors with bile pigment; however, metastases in the lungs of well-differentiated transplantable Reuber hepatocellular carcinoma-35 contained bile pigment following irradiation of the primary transplant (M. D. Reuber, unpublished data) or after administration of large doses of testosterone propionate (12) (Photo 38). Metastasis to the lungs of one well-differentiated hepatocellular carcinoma containing glycogen has been observed (Photo 37).

A comparison of the well-differentiated and poorly differentiated metastatic carcinomas is given in Table III (p. 309).

Transplantation Studies

1. Hyperplastic lesions

Areas of hyperplasia will not survive on transplantation to any site in an isologous host. Nodules of hyperplasia will survive and even increase in size only following intrahepatic transplantation to isologous hosts. Nodules reached a larger size in the liver of male than of female host rats. The cells eventually develop degenerative cytoplasmic changes identical to those seen in the primary hyperplastic lesions that do not progress to carcinomas. Since hyperplastic lesions involve much of the liver, they cannot be transplanted from one lobe into another lobe of the same liver.

2. Small hepatocellular carcinomas

The fate of small hepatocellular carcinomas following transplantation depends upon the degree of differentiation. Those with well-differentiated cells progress to well-differentiated carcinomas only in the liver in which they developed. When transplanted to the liver of isologous hosts they grew only as small hepatocellular carcinomas and never reached a large or well-developed size. These small carcinomas grew better in the liver of male than of female animals.

Small carcinomas with poorly differentiated cells, when transplanted to the spleen, muscle, and subcutaneous tissue, grew both autologously and isologously. Since they were uncommon in this experiment small poorly differentiated carcinomas were not transplanted intrahepatically to isologous hosts. In the spleen they never reached a large size; however, in the subcutaneous tissue or in muscle they were several centimeters in diameter, a finding comparable to that of well-developed carcinomas.

3. Well-developed carcinomas of the liver

Carcinomas 1.0 cm or larger in size can be easily transplanted to liver, lungs, spleen, peritoneum, muscle, or subcutaneous tissues. Once a tumor transplant was palpable it increased in size or remained the same size but never decreased in size or regressed.

The biological behavior of transplanted carcinomas was closely related to the morphological pattern. Undifferentiated carcinomas grew rapidly; well-differentiated carcinomas grew slowly; whereas the growth of poorly differentiated carcinomas was intermediate.

The transplantable carcinomas grossly and microscopically resembled the primary carcinomas in early generation transplants (Photos 30, 32, and 49), however, in later generation transplants the morphology and growth rates of well-differentiated carcinomas resembled those of poorly differentiated carcinomas.

Bile pigment was observed more often in transplanted well-differentiated hepatocellular carcinomas than in the primary carcinomas (Photos 30 and 31). Such pigment was usually seen adjacent to strands of fibrous connective tissue with macrophages containing ceroid, lipid, or bile in their cytoplasm (Photo 43). It is felt that the cells in well-differentiated carcinoma transplants are unable to secrete bile into the circulation.

Appearance and Growth of Hyperplastic and Neoplastic Lesions

The earliest change noted microscopically consisted of diffuse periportal hyperplasia. Fairly discrete foci of hyperplasia that could not be recognized grossly were observed later in the same zone. All lobes of the liver were equally involved at this stage.

Foci of hyperplasia increased in size and occupied larger areas. Hyperplastic areas appeared first in the left and caudate lobes, and later in the median and right lobes of the liver. Hyperplastic areas gradually increased in size, with the increase in size occurring first in the left lobe and later in other lobes. They were easily seen grossly, involved most of the liver, and were sometimes confluent.

Areas of hyperplasia in the periportal region expanded to compress and constrict the adjacent liver cords with the formation of hyperplastic nodules. The compression began formally along the margin of a hyperplastic area and continued until the liver around the whole circumference was compressed. Nodules were found first in the left lobe of the liver, as were the earlier hyperplastic lesions. Nodules in some parts of the liver sometimes collided.

The cells in nodules of hyperplasia became malignant and were then small hepatocellular carcinomas and, as they increased in size, large well-developed carcinomas. Small and large carcinomas of the liver appeared first in the periportal region in the left lobe of the liver as did areas and nodules of hyperplasia. The left lobe was the site of the largest number of carcinomas. The number of carcinomas per liver gradually increased from 1 to about 4 or 5. Carcinomas grew progressively until the death of the host.

TABLE I. Comparison of Rates of Development of Carcinomas, Metastases, and Cirrhosis of the Liver and of Metastases after Feeding of FdiAA for 12 or 16 Weeks and Killed at Various Time Intervals

Time killed (wk)	Incidence (%)		Aver. size (cm)		Aver. No. per liver		Metastases (%)		Cirrhosis (%)	
	12	16	12	16	12	16	12	16	12	16
26	0	90	—	0.5	0	1	0	0	—	100
36	50	85	1.2	1.0	1	1.5	8	33	33	44
48	50	93	1.5	1.5	1.5	2	7	50	50	71
60	75	92	1.5	2.5	1.5	3	8	38	75	100
68	80	100	1.5	3.0	1.5	4	10	43	70	100
84	100	—	2.7	—	2	—	0	—	71	—

TABLE II. Comparison of Well-differentiated and Poorly Differentiated Primary Carcinomas in Animals Fed FdiAA for 16 Weeks

Items	Well-differentiated	Poorly differentiated
Largest size	4.5 cm	6.0 cm
Adjacent liver	Compression	Invasion
Total per liver	1–5	1
Solitary tumor	Left lobe	Right lobe
Growth per 6 wk	0.5–1.0 cm	1.5–2.0 cm
Death of animals	68 wk	40 wk

TABLE III. Comparison of Well-differentiated and Poorly Differentiated Metastatic Carcinomas

Items		Well-differentiated	Poorly differentiated
Lungs	Microscopic	3.0 cm	1.0 cm
	Gross	4.0 cm	2.0 cm
Peritoneum		—	6.0 cm
Number of animals		33–50%	100%
Carcinogen		16 wk	12 or 16 wk

The biological behavior of carcinomas was related to their histological pattern. A comparison of well- and poorly differentiated carcinomas and their metastases is given in Tables I, II, and III.

1. Response of hyperplastic and neoplastic lesions to Rose Bengal

Areas of hyperplasia, which at first stained pink following the injection of Rose Bengal dye, later remained untinted (Photo 24). The number of unstained areas gradually increased until only an occasional area was pink. The first areas to remain untinted were observed first in the left lobe of the liver and later in the other lobes.

Approximately one-fourth of hyperplastic nodules were light to dark pink following the injection of Rose Bengal dye; the remainings were not tinted by the dye. Approximately one-fourth of the well-differentiated tumors mostly in rats given 12 weeks of carcinogen stained pink after the injection of Rose Bengal dye. The 6 tumors with bile were among the group with this characteristic. All poorly differentiated or undifferentiated carcinomas remained untinted by the injection of Rose Bengal dye.

2. Phagocytosis of India ink

Some Kupffer cells in foci, areas and nodules of hyperplasia were functional,

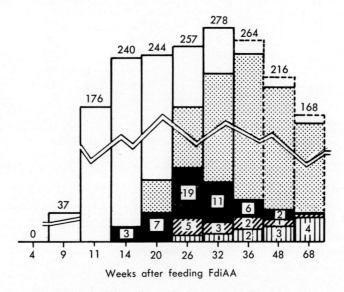

Fig. 2. Average number of lesions per liver after feeding 0.025% FdiAA for a total of 16 weeks

Hyperplastic and neoplastic lesions were counted after the injection of Rose Bengal dye. As the number of hyperplastic nodules and small carcinomas decreases, the number of large carcinomas increases. The number of carcinomas is smaller than the number of hyperplastic nodules because nodules collide and form one large carcinoma. The development of lesions after 12 weeks of feeding was similar except that there were fewer nodules and carcinomas and the animals survived for an average of 84 weeks. ☐ areas; ■ nodules; ◪ small hepatomas; ▥ large hepatomas; ▨ degenerating areas.

as revealed by phagocytosis of India ink after its injection just before the animals
were killed (Photo 7). In contrast to the areas and nodules of hyperplasia in which
India ink was phagocytized, the sinusoidal lining cells in small hepatocellular
carcinomas failed to pick up India ink. Functioning Kupffer cells also could not
be detected in well-developed carcinomas. A similar finding for the gradual loss
of functioning Kupffer cells in hyperplastic hepatic lesions has also been described
with loss of ability to phagocytize iron (*13*).

3. Fate of hyperplastic lesions

Nodules with differing cytological characteristics were sometimes adjacent
to one another. As they increased in size, they sometimes collided and, except
for differing cytologial characteristics, they resembled a single nodule. By con-

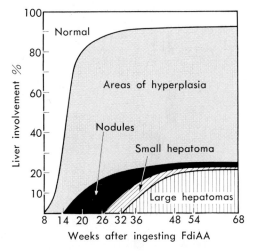

Fig. 3.   Percentage of liver involvement by hyperplasia and carcinomas
The development of areas of hyperplasia, nodules of hyperplasia, small
carcinomas, and large carcinoma in rats ingesting 0.025% FdiAA for a total
of 16 weeks is shown by the percentage of liver involvement.

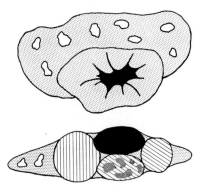

Fig. 4.   Collison of lesions in the liver
Externally the lesion appears to be a solitary tumor (above). On the cut
surface this tumor is made up of four separate lesions (below). □ areas of
hyperplasia; ■ nodules of hyperplasia; ◨ small hepatoma; ▥ well-developed
hepatoma.

312   M. D. REUBER

trast with areas of hyperplasia, the cells in nodules of hyperplasia usually did
not undergo degenerative changes but rather either persisted as nodules or
apparently progressed to formation of carcinomas.

It seemed to take nodules of hyperplasia with well-differentiated cells
about 6 weeks to develop atypical cells and 6 more weeks to become small hepatocellular carcinomas. Those nodules present when the carcinogen was with-
drawn, as demonstrated by laparotomy and biopsy, appeared to become carcinomas
if the animal survived long enough; however, nodules developing later were more
apt to remain as nodules and less apt to become carcinomas. As the number
of nodules per liver decreased with time, the number of carcinomas increased.

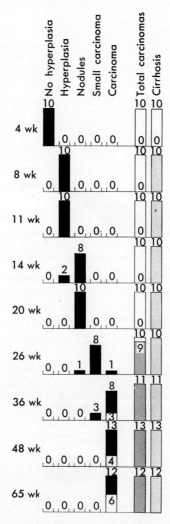

FIG. 5. Development of preneoplastic and neoplastic lesions in male rats
ingesting 0.025% FdiAA in the diet for a total of 16 weeks, after which time
the carcinogen was discontinued

Note the development of lesions from hyperplastic areas to hyperplastic
nodules, and small and large carcinomas with time.

It is apparent from the large number of hyperplastic areas that only a small number develop into hyperplastic nodules and that the remaining cells undergo degenerative cytoplasmic changes.

Small carcinomas were rarely found terminally and there were no degenerative changes of the cytoplasm to indicate regression. It appeared that every small carcinoma would become a larger hepatocellular carcinoma if the animal were to live long enough. Well-developed carcinomas, which compressed the adjacent liver cells or were surrounded by thick strands of fibrous connective tissue, sometimes appeared lobulated. Often the histologic pattern varied somewhat from one lobulation to another, which represents the collision of nodules of hyperplasia or smaller carcinomas (Figs. 2 and 4).

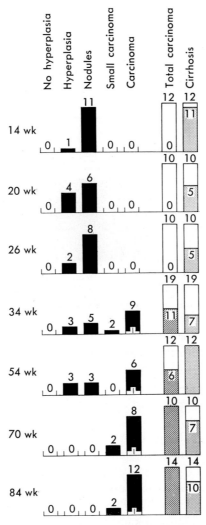

FIG. 6. Development of preneoplastic and neoplastic lesions in male rats ingesting 0.025% FdiAA in the diet for a total of 12 weeks, after which time the carcinogen was discontinued

The development of hyperplasia and carcinomas progresses at a slower rate.

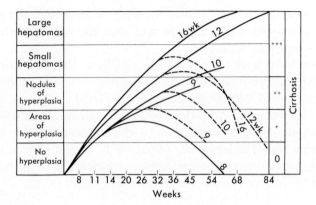

Fig. 7. Development of hyperplastic and neoplastic lesions of the liver after feeding of FdiAA for varying lengths of time

Hyperplastic and neoplastic lesions shown by solid line and the degree of cirrhosis shown by broken lines, have been graded from 1 to 3 plus. Length of time the carcinogenic diet was fed is given on each solid and broken line. Survival time in weeks is on the lower margin. —— tumors; - - - - cirrhosis.

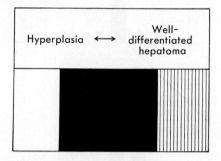

Fig. 8. Mixture of hyperplastic and malignant cells

During the transition stage there are both hyperplastic cells and malignant cells (shown in black) present in the same lesion.

4. Relationship of tumors to cirrhosis of the liver

Simultaneously with the parenchymal cell hyperplasia, there was proliferation of small bile ducts and fibroblastic activity that progressed to isolation of hepatic cells and lobules (cirrhotic nodules) (Photos 2 and 3). There were often bands of connective tissue, particularly in animals fed carcinogen for longer periods of time.

Proliferation of small bile ducts appeared first in the left and caudate lobes of the liver and later in the remaining lobes, as did the parenchymal cell hyperplasia. Both developed together as long as the carcinogen was fed. However, areas and nodules of hyperplasia continued to grow and involved much of the liver, whereas the cirrhosis regressed and became focalized after the carcinogen feeding was discontinued (Fig. 7). Although the incidence of cirrhosis increased (Figs. 5 and 6), the degree of cirrhosis decreased. Some degree of cirrhosis was usually present in livers with carcinomas.

5. *Cirrhotic nodules versus hyperplastic nodules*

Cirrhotic nodules differed from hyperplastic nodules in that they always stained pink after intravenous injection of Rose Bengal dye, did not have a prominent vessel over the surface, and were completely surrounded by proliferating bile ducts or fibroblasts.

The cells in hyperplastic nodules also fail to take up iron (*13*), and resist the toxic effects of carbon tetrachloride or dimethylnitrosamine (Photo 26) (E. Farber, personal communication). The cells in hyperplastic nodules also contain more radioactive carcinogen than do the cells in adjacent parenchyma or cirrhotic nodules (H. Dyer and M. D. Reuber, unpublished data).

6. *Length of carcinogen administration and the development of hepatic lesions*

If the carcinogen-containing diet was discontinued after 8 weeks of feeding, the hyperplastic foci and areas disappeared within 65 weeks. After 9 or 10 weeks of carcinogen feeding, the areas of hyperplasia became nodules of hyperplasia or small hepatocellular carcinomas after many subsequent weeks on the noncarcinogenic diet (Fig. 7). The hyperplastic nodules and small hepatocellular carcinomas were located in the left or caudate lobes, the same lobes in which areas of hyperplasia first appeared. Apparently an area of hyperplasia was no longer capable of disappearing after it lost the ability to stain pink with Rose Bengal dye.

There were fewer hyperplastic nodules and carcinomas, and less severe cirrhosis in rats fed carcinogen for 10 or 12 weeks than in those fed carcinogen for 16 weeks. There were a larger number of hyperplastic nodules, small carcinomas, and more advanced cirrhosis in rats fed carcinogen for 20 weeks (*3*). In both the 12- and 20-week groups, the nodules of hyperplasia were more difficult to distinguish from the carcinomas histologically, and they grew more slowly than in animals fed the carcinogen for 16 weeks.

The cells were so well formed in the well-differentiated hepatocellular carcinomas that they were difficult to distinguish from hyperplastic nodules and even from normal liver in the 12-week group. The well-differentiated carcinomas also failed to metastasize and took a longer time to kill the animals, *i.e.*, rats lived for 76 to 115 weeks (average, 84). Only 50% were transplantable isologously (*9*). Massive hemorrhage into a tumor occurred only in well-differentiated carcinomas in animals fed carcinogen for 12 weeks (Photo 39).

The poorly differentiated hepatocellular carcinomas did not depend on the duration of feeding the carcinogen; in rats fed carcinogen for 12 or 16 weeks, the metastatic growths were associated with a primary tumor 1.0 cm in diameter and the animals died in 38 to 45 weeks.

The differences between primary carcinomas after 12 or 16 weeks of feeding the carcinogen are summarized in Tables I and II.

DISCUSSION

The carcinogen fed in the diet induced hyperplasia of liver cells. This hyperplastic hepatic tissue then behaved in one of several ways. The cells usually underwent degenerative changes or disappeared, but some of them also progressed to a more advanced stage of hyperplasia. Only a small number of hyperplastic areas ever became hyperplastic nodules and carcinomas. Progression of the hyperplastic areas was dependent upon the carcinogenic chemical. The longer the carcinogen was fed, the greater the number of hyperplastic areas that progressed.

In contrast to hyperplastic areas, the nodules of hyperplasia were of less frequent occurrence but of greater importance. They were relatively few. These nodules either remained as nodules or progressed to carcinomas and did not disappear or undergo diffuse degenerative changes. Hyperplastic nodules continued to grow even though the carcinogenic stimulus was discontinued. The longer the feeding period of the carcinogen (up to 16 weeks), the faster the nodules grew.

Small carcinomas, like hyperplastic nodules, were no longer dependent upon the carcinogen, but continued to increase in size and became large well-developed carcinomas. Even after the development of small carcinomas, other factors were involved. Time, size, and degree of differentiation were important, as indicated by metastases, transplantability, and the growth rate.

The feeding of carcinogen for 16 weeks and then killing the rats after 65 weeks offered an advantageous model of study because all the animals developed carcinomas terminally and most of the nodules in any one liver had become well-developed carcinomas, so that the problem of differentiation between hyperplasia and carcinoma was minimal. It was convenient to follow the changes preceding the appearance of well-differentiated carcinoma, since the hyperplastic and neoplastic changes took place over a long period of time. The various stages of the poorly differentiated or undifferentiated carcinomas could not be followed readily because of the rapid growth of the tumors and because they were few in number.

Generally, the histologic pattern of the carcinoma was determined from the earliest hyperplastic stage, which then continued to increase in size until a carcinoma was formed. The histologic pattern varied slightly within one carcinoma because of the collision at an early stage of nodules of hyperplasia or small carcinomas (see Photo 17 and Fig. 4). After the development of a carcinoma, the histological pattern did not change.

The relationship of the histological pattern, amount of carcinogen ingested, and the biological behavior of the primary hepatocellular carcinoma in the host animal is identical to those for the transplants. Primary well-differentiated carcinomas metastasized, grew more rapidly, and killed the host more readily in animals fed carcinogen for 16 weeks than in those fed carcinogen for 12 weeks. The poorly differentiated and undifferentiated carcinomas grew most rapidly and metastasized and killed the host sooner.

Cirrhosis appeared at the same time as areas of parenchymal cell hyperplasia and progressed during the period of feeding the carcinogen.

After withdrawal of the carcinogen, the same hyperplastic lesions continued to progress, whereas the cirrhotic changes regressed or decreased in severity and at death were often minimal and focal. The cirrhosis was more severe in animals fed for 16 weeks than for shorter periods of time. Since the carcinomas in animals ingesting the carcinogen for 16 weeks were more malignant than those in animals fed for shorter periods, it seems that the carcinomas developing in livers with more cirrhosis were the most malignant.

If the carcinogen is fed for too long a period of time (longer than 16 weeks), then the animals die from toxic effects such as cirrhosis of the liver. Such animals will have hyperplastic lesions and early carcinomas, but will not develop large as many well-developed carcinomas with metastases.

In the progress of neoplasia, there is a gradual transition from the state of dependency toward one of autonomy. Study of the lesions grossly and microscopically provides general information of predictive value in assessment of the probable relative degree of dependency or autonomy of the lesions as shown by the subsequent biologic behavior in the host or on transplantation. Study of lesions in experimental animals aids in their interpretation in human beings.

REFERENCES

1. Firminger, H. I. Histopathology of carcinogenesis and tumors of the liver in rats. *J. Natl. Cancer Inst.*, **15** (Suppl.), 1427–1442 (1955).

2. Firminger, H. I. and Reuber, M. D. Influence of adrenocortical, androgenic, and anabolic hormones on the development of carcinoma and cirrhosis of the liver in A×C rats fed N-2-fluorenyldiacetamide. *J. Natl. Cancer Inst.*, **27**, 559–595 (1961).

3. Reuber, M. D. Development of preneoplastic and neoplastic lesions of the liver in male rats ingesting 0.025 percent N-2-fluorenyldiacetamide. *J. Natl. Cancer Inst.*, **34**, 697–724 (1965).

4. Reuber, M. D. and Firminger, H. I. Effect of progesterone and diethylstilbestrol on hepatic carcinogenesis and cirrhosis in A×C rats fed N-2-fluorenyldiacetamide. *J. Natl. Cancer Inst.*, **29**, 933–943 (1962).

5. Reuber, M. D. The thyroid gland and N-2-fluorenyldiacetamide carcinogenesis and cirrhosis of the liver in Wistar male rats. *J. Natl. Cancer Inst.*, **35**, 959–966 (1965).

6. Reuber, M. D. Importance of thyroid hormone and testosterone in the induction of carcinomas, and cirrhosis of the liver in female Wistar rats ingesting N-2-fluorenyldiacetamide. *J. Natl. Cancer Inst.*, **36**, 775–781 (1966).

7. Reuber, M. D. Importance of testosterone in the induction of hyperplastic nodules, carcinomas, and cirrhosis of the liver in A×C strain male rats ingesting 0.025 percent N-2-fluorenyldiacetamide. *J. Natl. Cancer Inst.*, **53**, 883–886 (1974).

8. Reuber, M. D. Influence of hormones on N-2-fluorenyldiacetamide induced hyperplastic hepatic nodules in rats. *J. Natl. Cancer Inst.*, **43**, 445–452 (1969).

9. Reuber, M. D. and Firminger, H. I. Morphologic and biologic correlation of lesions obtained in hepatic carcinogenesis in A×C rats given 0.025 percent N-2-fluorenyldiacetamide. *J. Natl. Cancer Inst.*, **31**, 1407–1429 (1963).

10. Reuber, M. D. and Odashima, S. Further studies on the transplantation of lesions in hepatic carcinogenesis in rats given 0.025 percent 2-(diaceto-amido)-fluorene. *Gann*, **58**, 513–520 (1967).

11. Reuber, M. D. Histopathology of transplantable hepatic carcinomas induced by chemical carcinogens in rats. *GANN Monograph*, **1**, 43–54 (1966).

12. Reuber, M. D. Influence of sex and hormones on transplantable hepatocellular carcinoma in the rat. *Pathol. Microbiol.*, in press (1975).

13. Williams, G. M. and Yamamoto, R. S. Absence of stainable iron from preneoplastic and neoplastic lesions in rat liver with 8-hydroxyquinolone-induced siderosis. *J. Natl. Cancer Inst.*, **44**, 685–692 (1974).

EXPLANATION OF PHOTOS

Histological sections are stained with Hematoxylin and Eosin unless otherwise indicated.

PHOTO 1.   Areas of hyperplasia. Early areas of hyperplasia in liver from rat that was previously injected with Rose Bengal dye. Areas of hyperplasia are white, fairly well demarcated from adjacent liver and measure 1 to 3 mm in diameter compared to remainder of liver that was pink in color. The surface of the liver is finely granular, which is indicative of proliferation of small bile ducts.

PHOTO 2.   Cirrhosis of the liver. Proliferation of small bile ducts or spindle-shaped cells with isolation of hepatic parenchymal cells and lobules of varying sizes. ×54.

PHOTO 3.   Cirrhosis of the liver. ×170.

PHOTO 4.   Focus of hyperplasia. Cells have increased lighter eosinophilic cytoplasm and often double nuclei. Cells are not clearly demarcated from adjacent parenchymal cells. This lesion cannot be recognized grossly. ×210.

PHOTO 5.   Area of hyperplasia. Cells are similar to those in focus of hyperplasia, but are increased in size, the number of cells is larger and the junction with the surrounding hepatic cells is well demarcated. There are double nucleated cells and occasional mitotic figures. ×150.

PHOTO 6.   Area of hyperplasia. ×320.

PHOTO 7.   Hyperplastic hepatic parenchymal cells. Some Kupffer cells in an area of hyperplasia have phagocytized India ink in the cytoplasm. Glycogen is absent. Periodic acid-Schiff stain. ×380.

PHOTO 8.   Hyperplastic hepatic parenchymal cells. Cytological appearance of cells in hyperplastic area. Cells are large with vesicular nuclei, prominent nucleoli, and palely eosinophilic cytoplasm. There are occasional double nucleated cells. ×340.

PHOTO 9.   Areas of hyperplasia and early nodules of hyperplasia in liver from rat that was previously injected with Rose Bengal dye. Some white areas with early compression of adjacent liver tissue measure up to 5 mm in diameter. Remaining liver stained pink in color. Areas are colliding and appearing as larger areas.

PHOTO 10.   Area of hyperplasia. There is early compression and constriction of surrounding parenchymal cells. This is a later stage of an area of hyperplasia similar to that in Photo 5. ×100.

PHOTO 11.   Area of hyperplasia with degenerative change. Cytoplasm contains water or lipid many weeks after the carcinogen was discontinued. ×95.

PHOTO 12.   Area of hyperplasia with degenerative change. Hydropic change involving the cytoplasm of hyperplastic cells. ×430.

PHOTO 13.   Nodules of hyperplasia in liver from rat previously injected with Rose Bengal. The largest nodule located on the lower right has a blood vessel over its surface and appears white beside the adjacent pink tissue. Other nodules do not have a vessel over their surface, are colored pink, and are part of the cirrhosis seen here, rather than being hyperplastic nodules.

PHOTO 14.   Nodule of hyperplasia. The cells in this early nodule of hyperplasia are similar to those in areas of hyperplasia but they are increased in number. The cytoplasm is eosinophilic and the sinusoids are more conspicuous and some cells are atypical. There are more double nucleated cells and mitotic figures. There is focal early compression of adjacent parenchymal cells. ×120.

PHOTO 15.   Nodule of hyperplasia. Cells in this nodule are smaller, have less cytoplasm and the cytoplasm is basophilic as compared to those in Photo 14. Adjacent hepatic cells are compressed and constricted. Sinusoids are prominent in lower right corner. ×120.

PHOTO 16. Small hepatocellular carcinoma. A small well-demarcated carcinoma, with blood vessels on the surface, protrudes from the surface of a cirrhotic liver at the bottom (left). A hyperplastic nodule with its own blood supply is seen at the right of the small carcinoma. This animal was not injected with Rose Bengal dye and the nodule and small carcinoma appear the same color as the adjacent liver. The only way a hyperplastic nodule in this liver can be distinguished from a cirrhotic nodule is by the blood vessel on the surface or by histologic examination.

PHOTO 17. Colliding areas and nodules of hyperplasia. This lesion appeared as one separate lesion grossly, however, on microscope examination there are several areas and early small hyperplastic nodules. ×80.

PHOTO 18. Cytology of cells in hyperplastic nodule. Cells are large with eosinophilic cytoplasm and are similar to cells with lightly eosinophilic cytoplasm in an area of hyperplasia. Nuclei are larger and cytoplasm more eosinophilic. ×340.

PHOTO 19. Nodule of hyperplasia with atypical cells. Cells are forming cords and sinusoids are prominent focally. Cells (on the left) are atypical and resemble those in a small carcinoma. Nuclei have conspicuous nucleoli and the cytoplasm is decreased. There is increased compression of adjacent parenchymal tissue. ×100.

PHOTO 20. Nodule of hyperplasia with focal hepatocellular carcinoma. Hyperplastic cells are present in the center. Well-differentiated carcinoma cells are seen forming cords and canaliculi focally, particularly on the left side of the nodule. ×100.

PHOTO 21. Nodule of hyperplasia with focal hepatocellular carcinoma. Well-differentiated carcinoma can be seen on the right side of the nodule. The sinusoids are greatly increased in size. ×87.

PHOTO 22. Nodule of hyperplasia with focal hepatocellular carcinoma. There is poorly differentiated carcinoma, particularly on the left side of this nodule. Note the large vessel supplying this nodule. ×95.

PHOTO 23. Small poorly differentiated hepatocellular carcinoma. This carcinoma has large cells of varying sizes and shapes, with eosinophilic cytoplasm and large nuclei and nucleoli. Most of the cells are malignant, however few cells still resemble hyperplastic cells. ×108.

PHOTO 24. Lesions in a liver from a rat that was previously injected with Rose Bengal dye. A, colliding areas of hyperplasia; N, hyperplastic nodule; C, carcinoma. Some areas of hyperplasia failed to stain the same pink color as the adjacent liver.

PHOTO 25. Nodule of hyperplasia. The cytoplasm does not contain stainable glycogen. Periodic acid-Schiff stain. ×140.

PHOTO 26. Nodule of hyperplasia. This nodule was taken from a rat that had ingested DMN and later was injected with carbon tetrachloride. The hyperplastic cells were resistant to the toxic effects when compared to the adjacent parenchymal cells with coagulation necrosis. There is focal malignant change with formation of double cell cords and prominent sinusoids on the right. × 90. (Courtesy of Dr. E. Farber, Fels Research Institute and Temple University School of Medicine)

PHOTO 27. Nodule of hyperplasia. This nodule was taken from a rat that had hydroxyquinoline and ferrous gluconate in the diet. Hyperplastic or Kupffer cells in the nodule fail to take up the iron, whereas cells adjacent to the nodule take up iron. Perls' stain. ×40. (Courtesy of Dr. G. Williams, Temple University School of Medicine)

PHOTO 28. Well-differentiated hepatocellular carcinoma. This carcinoma is liver-colored and is well-differentiated histologically. This carcinoma is the primary from which Reuber hepatocellular carcinoma-35 was started. In addition to the carcinoma there is mild cirrhosis of the liver and small cysts.

PHOTO 29. Well-differentiated hepatocellular carcinoma. Carcinoma cells resemble hepatic parenchymal cells with large round nuclei, prominent nucleoli, and abundant eosinophilic cytoplasm. They form canaliculi in some parts. ×210. Such carcinomas arise from nodules of hyperplasia with the pattern illustrated in Photos 20 and 21.

PHOTO 30. Transplantable Reuber hepatocellular carcinoma-35. Carcinoma cells are well-differentiated and are the same as those is the primary carcinoma. They resemble hepatic parenchymal cells and form canaliculi. ×415.

Photo 31.   Bile in Reuber hepatocellular carcinoma-35. Canalicular structures between adjacent carcinoma cells contain bile casts. ×415. This was the first time bile was observed in a hepatic carcinoma in experimental animals.

Photo 32.   Transplantable Reuber hepatocellular carcinoma-35. Carcinoma transplant resembling liver tissue is partitioned by wide bands of darkly green bile-stained connective tissue. Bile-stained parts of tumor tissue are adjacent to connective tissue. There are cysts containing bile-stained fluid.

Photo 33.   Well-differentiated hepatocellular carcinoma. Cytoplasm is darkly eosinophilic and cells are growing in cords several layers thick. Nuclei are vesicular and nucleoli prominent. There are occasional canaliculi. Lining cells are present. ×340.

Photo 34.   Well-differentiated hepatocellular carcinoma. The prominent dilated sinusoids shown here are often seen in well-differentiated hepatocellular carcinomas. ×290.

Photo 35.   Well-differentiated hepatocellular carcinoma metastatic to lungs. There are multiple small growths of carcinoma scattered throughout the lung parenchyma, a typical finding with metastases of well-differentiated hepatocellular in rats.

Photo 36.   Well-differentiated hepatocellular carcinoma. Cells are growing in cords several layers wide with lining cells. Fibrous connective tissue is present at the lower right side. ×260.

Photo 37.   Well-differentiated hepatocellular carcinoma metastatic to lung. The cells of this metastatic carcinoma contain glycogen. Periodic acid-Schiff stain. ×160.

Photo 38.   Well-differentiated hepatocellular carcinoma, metastatic to lung. There is a small bile cast in a canaliculus in this carcinoma metastatis seen on the right. Lung is present on the left. ×390. This metastasis was from a castrated female rat with subcutaneous Reuber hepatocellular carcinoma-35 that had received testosterone (12).

Photo 39.   Hemorrhage into hepatocellular carcinoma. The external and cut surfaces show a large part of the carcinoma replaced by clotted blood.

Photo 40.   Large hepatocellular carcinoma. This dilated aneurysm-like blood vessel on the surface of this primary carcinoma of the liver is one source of bleeding into the peritoneum, which is commonly found at necropsy as a cause of death.

Photo 41.   Bile in well-differentiated hepatocellular carcinoma. Bile pigment is within the cytoplasm and a bile cast is in the canaliculus. ×680.

Photo 42.   Glycogen in well-differentiated hepatocellular carcinoma. The glycogen within the cytoplasm of some of the cells of this carcinoma stains darkly with periodic acid-Schiff stain. ×380.

Photo 43.   Well-differentiated hepatocellular carcinoma. Strands of fibrous connective tissue with macrophages containing ceroid pigment from Reuber hepatocellular carcinoma. Such parts of carcinoma can contain lipid and bile pigment as well, and can also be seen in primary hepatic carcinomas. Periodic acid-Schiff stain. ×293. Ceroid also stains with Oil Red-O on frozen or paraffin sections.

Photo 44.   Hepatocellular carcinomas of the liver. The carcinoma of the liver in the left lobe of the liver (on the right) is larger than the carcinoma of the liver in the median lobe (on the left) and are intermediate in size between small and large well-developed carcinomas. The carcinoma in the median lobes appears to be better differentiated than that of the left lobe. Cirrhosis of the liver has almost regressed.

Photo 45.   Poorly differentiated hepatocellular carcinoma. This carcinoma is firm and white, and is fairly well demarcated at the margins. There is mild cirrhosis of the liver.

Photo 46.   Poorly differentiated hepatocellular carcinoma. Cells are small with basophilic cytoplasm and vesicular nuclei with nucleoli. Cells grow in sheets, but sometimes have the appearance of growing in broad cords. The cells sometimes form structures resembling canaliculi. Lining cells may be present or absent. This carcinoma arises from a nodule of hyperplasia like the one illustrated in Photo 15. ×290.

Photo 47.   Bile pigment in poorly differentiated hepatocellular carcinoma. Bile pigment is present in a space resembling a poorly formed canaliculus. ×680.

Photo 48.   Poorly differentiated transplantable hepatocellular carcinoma. The cells are growing in sheets and are forming canaliculi focally and resemble the primary. ×290.

Photo 49.   Transplantable poorly differentiated hepatocellular carcinoma. This carcinoma
growing on subcutaneous transplantation is firm and white and resembles the primary.

Photo 50.   Poorly differentiated hepatocellular carcinoma. The cells in this 7-mm carcinoma
are large with much darkly eosinophilic cytoplasm and vesicular nuclei. There are some double
nucleated hyperplastic cells mixed in with the malignant cells. This carcinoma arose in a
small carcinoma similar to that illustrated in Photo 23. ×108.

Photo 51.   Poorly differentiated hepatocellular carcinoma. The cells are growing in sheets.
There is also cirrhosis of the liver shown by the strands of fibrous connective tissue. The
various parts separated by connective tissue arose as separate carcinomas from separate
hyperplastic areas and nodules. ×208.

Photo 52.   Metastases of well-differentiated hepatocellular carcinoma to lung. There are
multiple small growths of carcinoma. The histologic characteristics are those of a well-differentiated carcinoma. ×72.

Photo 53.   Metastases of poorly differentiated hepatocellular carcinoma to lung. The cells in
this carcinoma have the characteristics of a poorly differentiated primary carcinoma of the
liver. ×210.

Photo 54.   Undifferentiated carcinoma of the liver. This carcinoma is firm and white, and
infiltrates the adjacent hepatic tissue. It is capable of metastasing to other parts of the same
lobe of the liver. There is moderate cirrhosis of the liver.

Photo 55.   Undifferentiated carcinoma of the liver. Cells grow in solid sheets. The cell outlines
are indistinct, the nucleus and nucleolus make up much of the cell and the scanty cytoplasm
is darkly basophilic. ×290.

Photo 56.   Undifferentiated carcinoma of the liver. Cells are growing in sheets. The nuclei of
the cells in this carcinoma are often oval. There is decreased basophilic cytoplasm. ×290.

Photo 57.   Invasive undifferentiated carcinoma of the liver. This carcinoma has extended into
the intestine and is growing in the omentum.

Photo 58.   Metastases of undifferentiated carcinoma to lung. The metastatic growths vary in
size and shape and are present in all lobes of the lung. Poorly differentiated hepatocellular
carcinoma to the lung has a similar appearance.

Photo 59.   Undifferentiated carcinoma of the liver. The cells of this carcinoma grow in sheets.
Nuclei vary in shape and the cytoplasm is basophilic. There is loss of cohesiveness. ×180.

Photo 60.   Undifferentiated carcinoma of the liver. The cells of this carcinoma are anaplastic.
The nuclei and cells vary in size and shape, and hyperchromasia. Cytoplasm is eosinophilic,
but can be basophilic. This carcinoma cannot be recognized as primary in liver without
gross identification. ×190.

Photo 61.   Undifferentiated carcinoma. There is invasion of the diaphragm on the upper left
and middle and growth into hepatic vein and inferior vena cava. Cirrhosis of the liver is
present on the upper right.

Photo 62.   Cholangio-hepatocellular carcinoma. Columnar cells with oval basilar hyperchro-
matic neuclei and eosinophilic cytoplasm forming duct-like structure in upper center. Elsewhere cells are arranged in sheets or cords and have vesicular central nuclei, nucleoli, and
less dense eosinophilic cytoplasm, and form occasional canaliculi. ×475.

Photo 63.   Cholangiocellular carcinoma. Columnar cells with pseudostratified oval basal nuclei
and light amphophilic cytoplasm forming ducts. Tumor contains moderate amount of
fibrous desmoplastic stroma. ×190.

Photo 64.   Cholangiocellular carcinoma. The cells contain mucus in the cytoplasm. Periodic
acid-Schiff stain. ×350.

Photo 65.   Cholangiocellular carcinoma. This carcinoma is hard and white, and protrudes from
the under surface of the left lobe of the liver. Remaining liver is cirrhotic.

PHOTO 66. Cholangiocellular carcinoma metastatic to lungs. The metastatic growths vary in size and are characteristic of cholangiocellular carcinoma. The metastasis in the left lobe is much larger than the others. Compare the metastases in this photo with those of well-differentiated hepatocellular carcinoma in Photo 35 and undifferentiated carcinoma in Photo 58.

PHOTO 67. Well-differentiated cholangiocellular carcinoma. The cells form ducts with pseudo-stratified oval nuclei located at the base. Cytoplasm varies from lightly basophilic to lightly eosinophilic. The stroma is made up of dense fibrous connective tissue. ×210.

PHOTO 68. Mucus in well-differentiated cholangiocellular carcinoma. Dark staining mucus is present at the apical surface of the ducts. Periodic acid-Schiff stain. ×290.

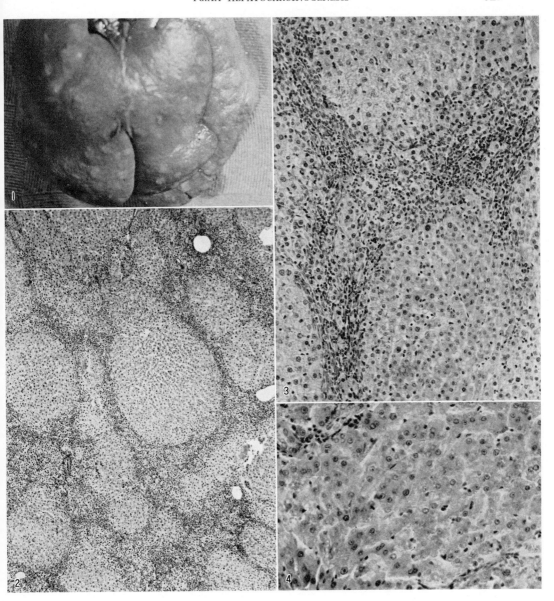

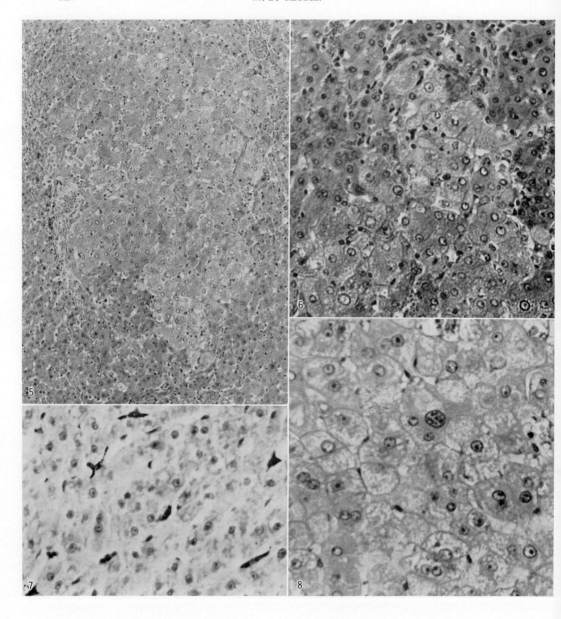

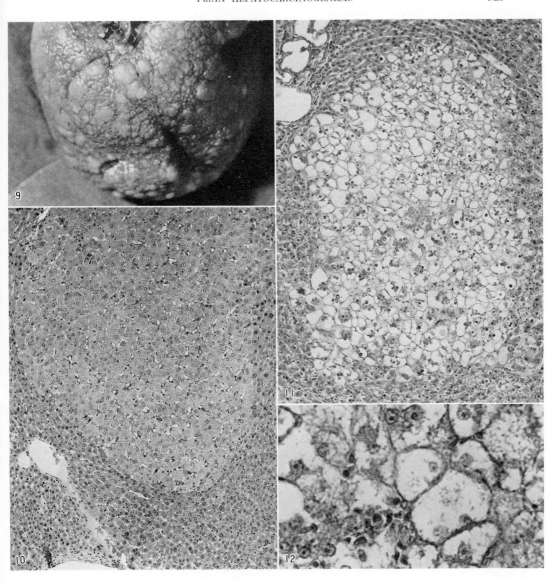

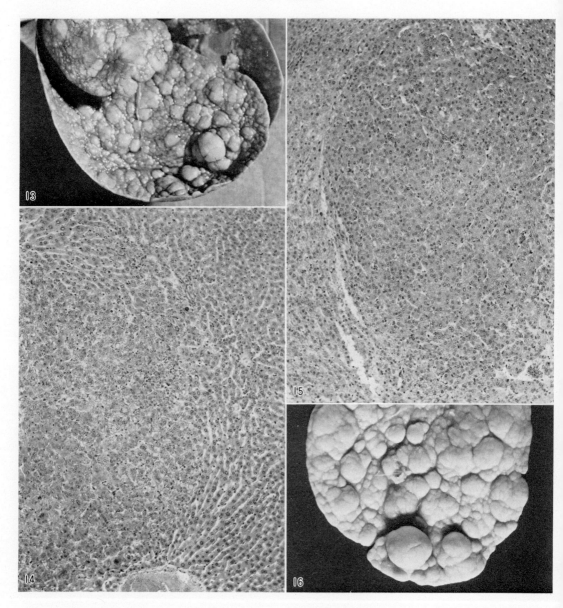

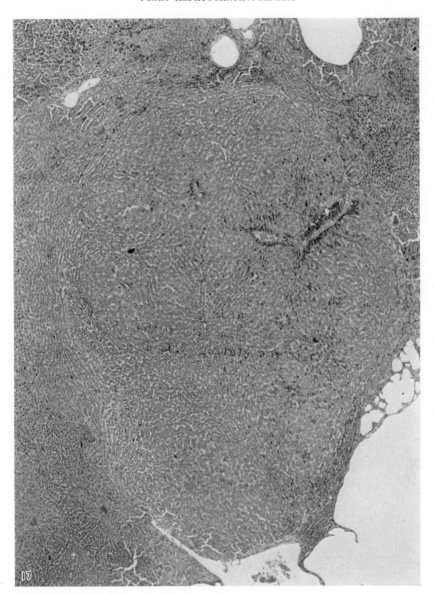

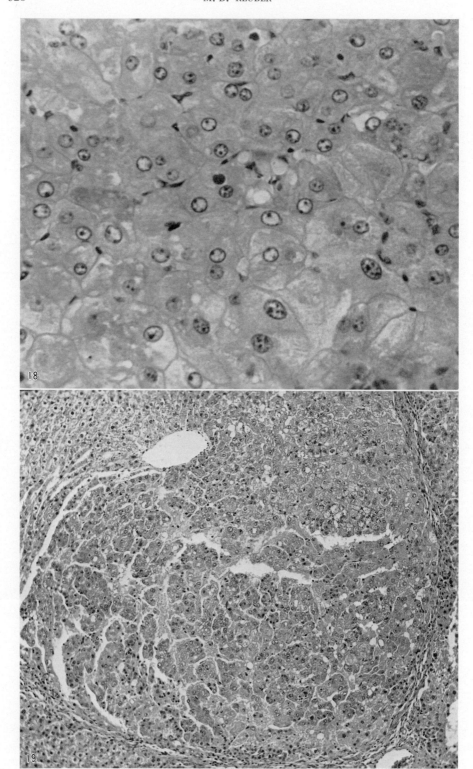

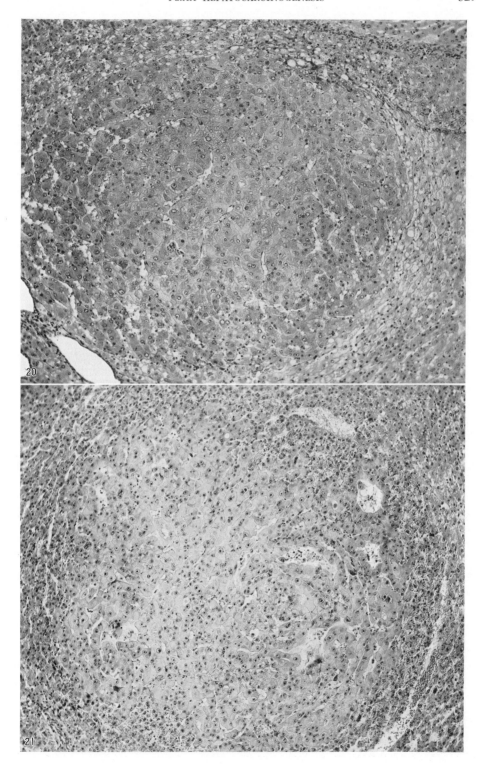

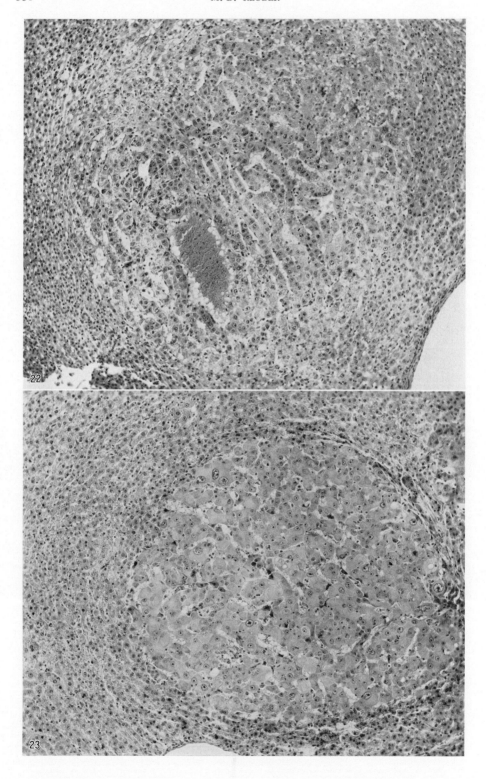

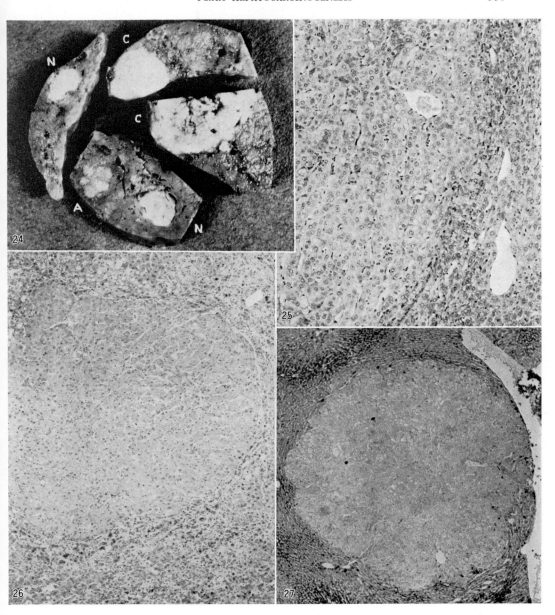

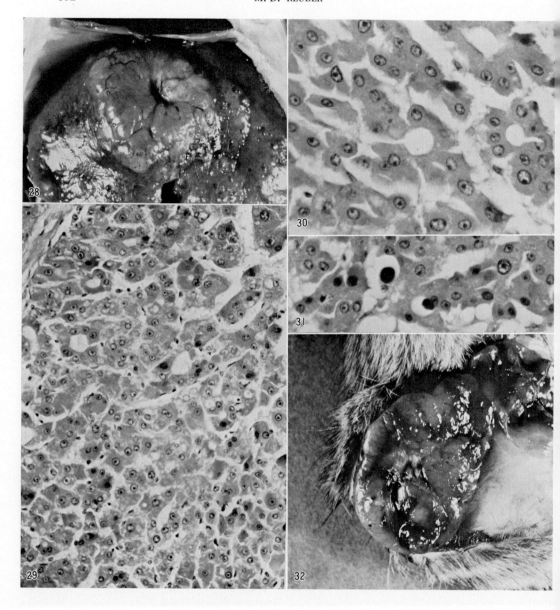

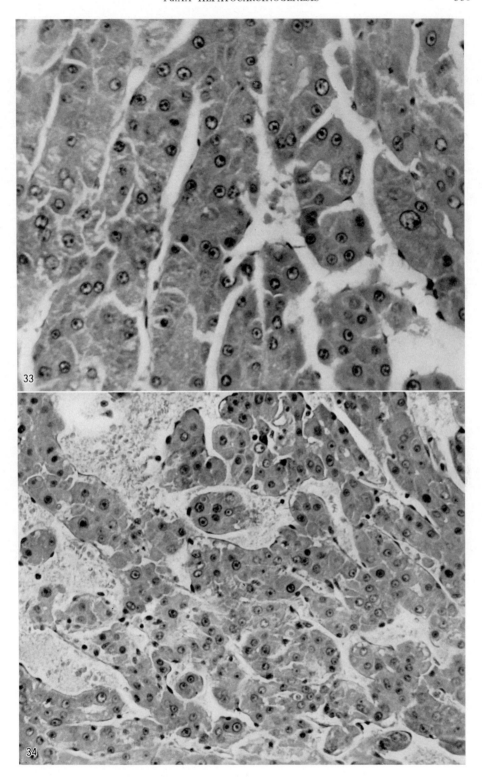

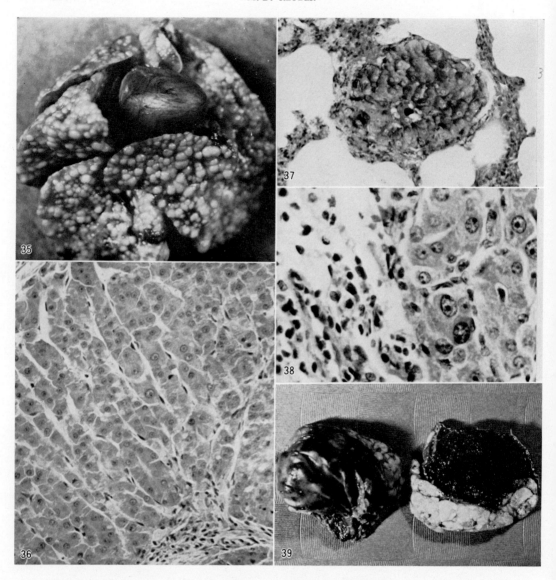

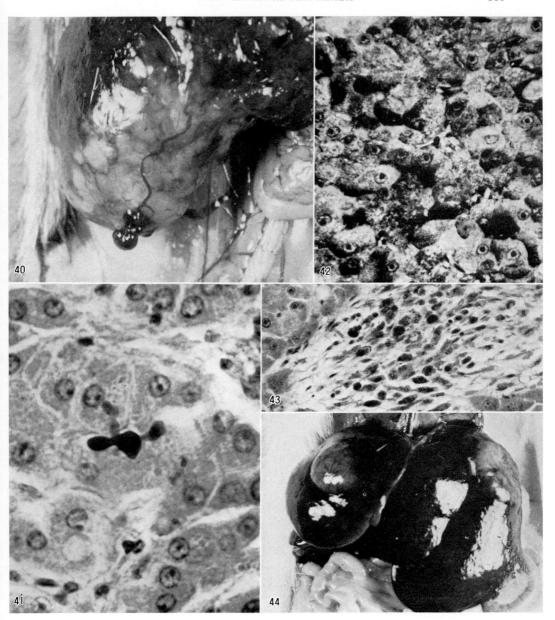

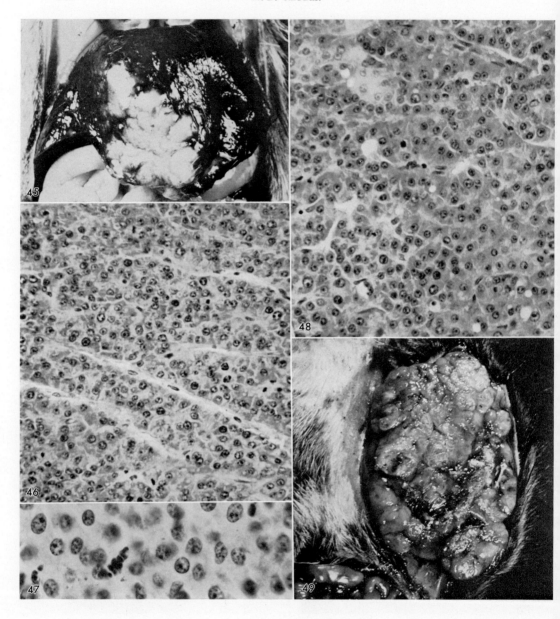

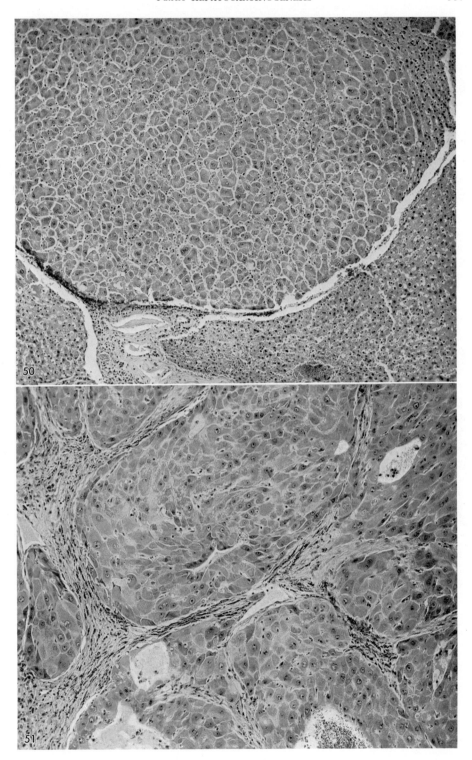

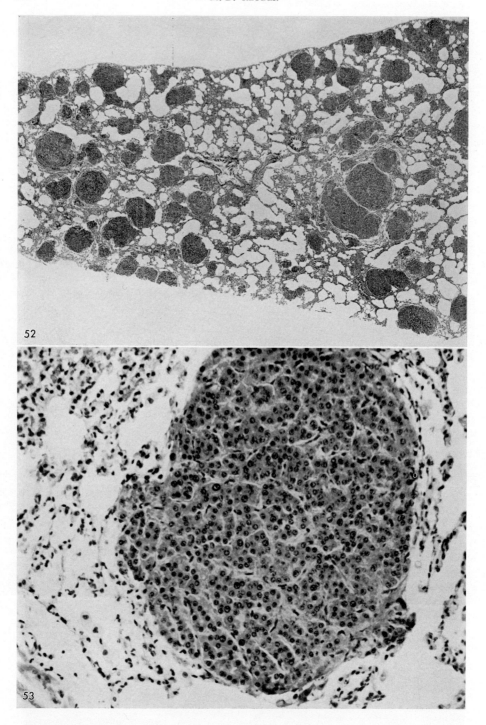

52

53

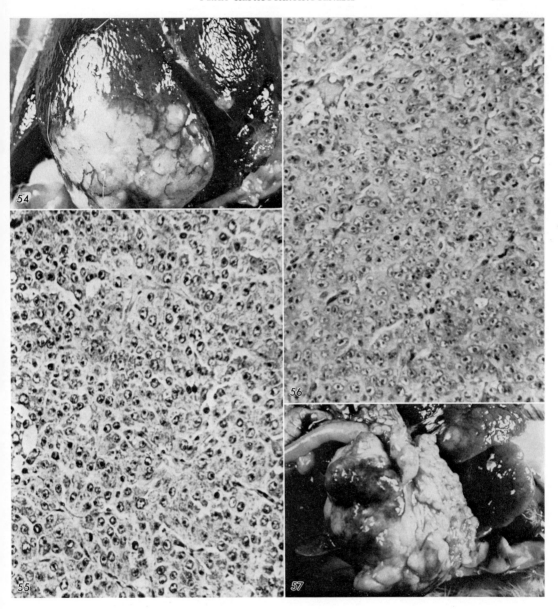

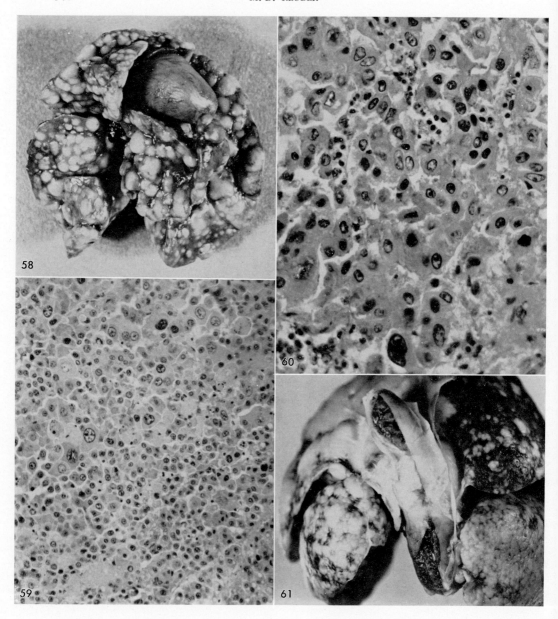

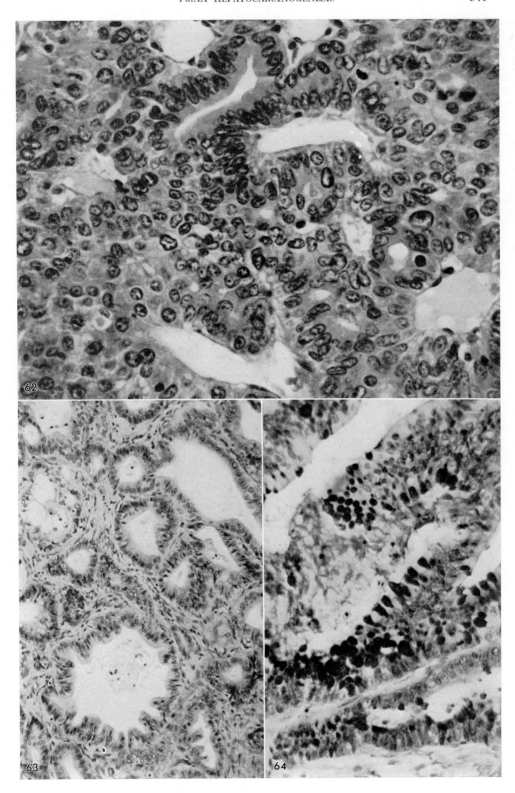

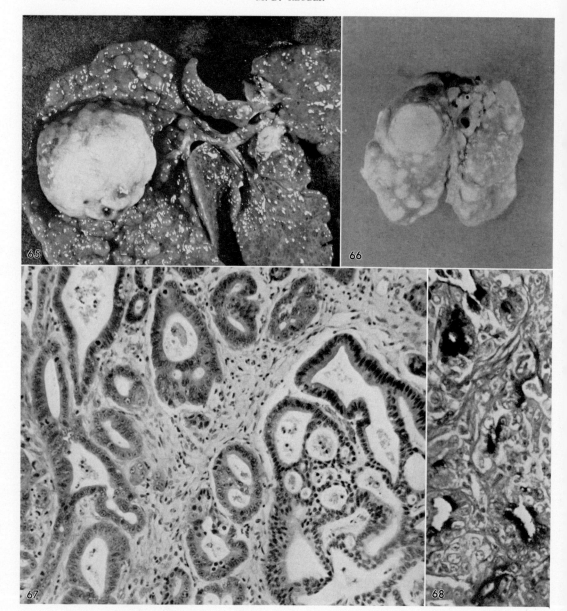

GANN Monograph on Cancer Research 17, 343–354 (1975)

HISTOLOGICAL AND CYTOLOGICAL STUDIES ON HEPATOCARCINOGENESIS IN RATS BY ADMINISTRATION OF DIETHYLNITROSAMINE

Shozo Takayama,[*1] Masahito-Hitachi,[*1] and Kiyomi Yamada[*2]

*Department of Experimental Pathology and Laboratory of Director, Cancer Institute,[*1] and Department of Cytogenetics, Medical Research Institute, Tokyo Medical and Dental University[*2]*

Administration of 50 ppm of diethylnitrosamine (DEN) in drinking water to male Donryu rats for 3 weeks resulted in the formation of liver tumors after a long latent period. Histologically, the so-called area of hyperplasia was produced in the liver after the end of DEN administration, nodular hyperplasia after 14 weeks, and then liver tumors developed.

Chromosomal analysis carried out in parallel with histological examination showed that the cells with abnormal chromosome constitution appeared in rats sacrificed at a later period and this was paralleled with morphological changes. Appearance of polyploid cells increased after stopping of DEN administration. A large part of the dividing cells in liver cell carcinomas induced by DEN was characterized by chromosomally abnormal cells of the diploid range.

Yoshida, in his book "Carcinogenesis" (*23*), wrote that oral administration of the so-called *o*-aminoazotoluene (4-amino-2′,3-dimethylazobenzene) (OAT) in rats results in appearance of mitosis in liver cells near the central vein, later in the periphery of the lobule, and continued feeding of OAT for one month resulted in the proliferation of liver cells in the periphery. Yoshida stated that the most important finding in the experimental hepatocarcinogenesis by OAT was a simple and unilateral proliferation of liver cells and this proliferation progressed finally to the formation of a tumor nodule. In other words, Yoshida considers that this proliferation of liver cells is the only essential change and other lesions, even if found rarely, are accessory finding and have no significance in cancerization.

It is known that liver tumors are readily induced in rats by continuous administration of diethylnitrosamine (DEN) for 5 months (*21*). However, the fact that tumors are observed after 5 months does not necessarily mean that cancerization of individual cells requires a long period of treatment. It seems likely that cancerization of cells actually occurs much earlier. It would be valuable, therefore, to determine the time at which some indicator of cancerization of cells could first be observed after administration of DEN.

[*1] Kami-Ikebukuro 1-37-1, Toshima-ku, Tokyo 170, Japan (高山昭三, 常陸宮正仁親王).
[*2] Yushima 1-5-45, Bunkyo-ku, Tokyo 113, Japan (山田清美).

The present paper reports studies on cytogenetic and morphological changes associated with the development of liver tumors in rats receiving DEN in their drinking water.

According to Opie (16) and Orr (17), who reported the hepatocarcinogenesis in rats by oral administration of 4-dimethylaminoazobenzene (DAB), degeneration of liver cells begins soon after the administration is started, followed by their regeneration, and cell proliferation to nodule formation progresses finally to liver tumor. Similar histological observations have been reported for experiments with carcinogens other than azo dyes. For our experiments, chemical compounds which show nonspecific toxicity to liver cells were not appropriate even if they have a strong carcinogenicity. Therefore, a number of carcinogens were selected and administered to rats in various doses to find the conditions for inducing simple proliferation of liver cells. Finally, administration of drinking water containing 50 ppm of DEN was selected. DEN is characterized by (1) having the action to induce proliferation of liver cells by the administration of a small dose, (2) being able to form only liver cell carcinoma in various experimental animals (21), and (3) comparatively low toxicity (9).

Production of Rat Liver Tumors by Administration of Water Containing 50 ppm of DEN

Oral administration of water containing 100 ppm DEN in rats over a long period can induce liver tumor reliably but, from preliminary experiments, water containing 50 ppm of DEN was found to be more appropriate in obtaining mitosis without marked degeneration of liver cells, and 50 ppm of DEN was used for subsequent experiments.

The animals used were male Donryu rats (Nihon Rat Co., Tokyo) and DEN administration was started at 8 weeks of age. Rats were housed individually in a plastic cage and given commercial diet CE-2 (CLEA Japan Inc., Tokyo).

In order to determine the carcinogenicity of water containing 50 ppm of DEN against rat liver, this water was given as drinking water for 2, 3, and 4 weeks. The rats were then given ordinary drinking water and observed for a maximum of 76 weeks. The rats were examined by abdominal palpation once a week and those in which tumor nodules were palpated were killed for histological examination.

The first liver tumor was found in one of the rats killed during the 34th week from a group given water with 50 ppm of DEN for 2 weeks. A total of 24 rats were killed up to 78 weeks and liver cell carcinoma was found in 3 of these rats. In a group given water with 50 ppm of DEN for 3 weeks, a liver tumor was found in a rat killed in the 31st week of experiment. A total of 32 rats were examined during 59 weeks of experiment and 14 cases of liver cell carcinoma were found. In a group given water with 50 ppm of DEN for 4 weeks, the first liver tumor was found in a rat killed in the 16th week of experiment. A total of 20 rats were autopsied during 44 weeks of the experiment and liver cell carcinoma was histologically diagnosed in 9 rats.

The above results provide a basis for the assumption that potential cancer cells and/or definitely cancerized cells originate in 2 weeks or less after the administration of DEN. The foregoing experiment has shown that administration of DEN for 2 or 3 weeks produces liver tumor after a long latent period. The next experiment was carried out to see when potential cancer cells and/or some indicator of cancerization of cells would be observed after discontinuation of the carcinogen.

The animals used were male Donryu rats, 8 weeks of age. The animals were given water containing 50 ppm of DEN for 3 weeks and then ordinary drinking water, and killed periodically for histological and cytogenetic examinations.

Morphologically diffuse periportal hyperplasia was seen in the liver immediately after administration of DEN water for 3 weeks. In some zones, the cytoplasm was lightly eosinophilic, often with double nuclei, and not clearly demarcated from adjacent parenchymal cells, the so-called area of hyperplasia. This area of hyperplasia grew rapidly in the animals given further DEN water and began to replace major part of the liver. If DEN water was given only for 3 weeks and then changed to ordinary drinking water, areas of hyperplasia decreased markedly 4 weeks after stopping of DEN water.

The areas of hyperplasia formed by the administration of drinking water containing DEN occurred in two types, one with an acidophilic cytoplasm and the other with basophilic cytoplasm. In some cases, the two types were intermingled. Mitotic figures were seen in the periphery of the area of hyperplasia.

In the animals given DEN drinking water for 3 weeks and then ordinary water, nodular hyperplasia was observed in the liver 14 weeks after discontinuation of the carcinogen. These lesions were seen first in the left lobe of the liver, and then dispersed over the whole lobe in a later period. The size of this lesion was 4–8 mm in diameter and appeared white. Histologically, the cells in these nodules were identical to those in the area of hyperplasia, were arranged in cords and sheets, and mitotic figures were also seen. Later, the parenchymal cells showed atypism, formed 2-cell cords, and expanded by compressing the adjacent liver cell cords.

Initial Changes in Rat Liver after Administration of Various Hepatocarcinogens

According to Farber (5) and Kitagawa (12), continuous administration of a diet containing 0.06% of 3'-methyl-4-dimethylaminoazobenzene (3'-Me-DAB) to rats results in the proliferation of oval cells and small liver cells in the periphery of the liver lobe from about the 2nd week. Areas of hyperplasia appear in about the 6th week and the liver is soon replaced by this lesion. This proliferation of oval cells becomes very active.

Continuous administration of a diet containing 0.03% of N-2-fluorenyl-acetamide (2-FAA) results in a slight proliferation of oval cells in the periportal area during the 3rd to 6th week. If the feeding of the carcinogen is continued, areas of hyperplasia appear in the periportal area, and the major part of the liver is replaced by this lesion in 12 weeks (12, 18).

Administration of drinking water containing 100 ppm of DEN to rats results in scattered cell necrosis or centrolobular focal necrosis of liver cells in the initial stage but not the formation of cellular proliferation in the periportal area as was seen after feeding of 3'-Me-DAB or 2-FAA (*11, 12*). The area of hyperplasia appeared when this feeding was continued for 4 weeks.

Thus, the area of hyperplasia is formed by various liver carcinogens. This area of hyperplasia increases by compressing the adjacent parenchymal cells and grows to nodules of hyperplasia or nodular hyperplasia. The fact that this nodular hyperplasia is a likely precursor of liver cell carcinoma has been reported by many workers experimenting by the administration of 2-FAA (*3, 11, 18*), ethionine (*4–6*), various kinds of azo dye (*2*), aflatoxin-B$_1$ (*15*), and DEN (*12*).

Enzymic Deviation in Area of Hyperplasia and Nodular Hyperplasia

Histochemical studies on enzymic deviation in proliferative cells, area of hyperplasia, and nodular hyperplasia have been reported by many workers (*7, 10, 12, 19, 20, 22*), and most of their results were similar to enzymic feature shown by liver cell carcinoma.

Scherer and others (*19*) made histochemical examination of the area of hyperplasia and nodular hyperplasia formed by DEN administration, and observed a marked deficiency in adenosine triphosphatase, glucose-6-phosphatase, and β-glucuronidase in these lesions, naming this phenomenon "enzyme-deficient island" or "island." Since the "island" induced by DEN showed entirely the same histochemical pattern as liver cell carcinoma formed by DEN administration, this "island" was considered to be an irreversible lesion and they suggested

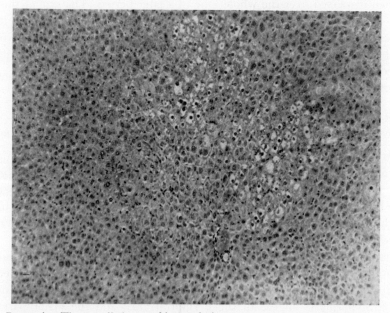

PHOTO 1.   The so-called area of hyperplasia

The cytoplasm is lightly eosinophilic, often double nuclei are present. Mitotic figures are present in the periphery of the lesion. Hematoxylin-Eosin stain.

×270

the presence of a cell which had the capacity to become liver cell carcinoma in these "island cells."

From these bibliographic evidences and from our experiments, it became certain that a characteristic lesion appears in rat liver after administration of DEN water and the lesion progresses to liver tumor. Consequently, this hepato-carcinogenic process was further studied by making chromosome analysis of the rat liver after administration of DEN water (Photo 1).

Chromosome Changes in Rat Liver Cells after Administration of DEN

Owing to technical difficulties, there have been few reports on chromosomal changes in the liver during chemical carcinogenesis (8, 13, 14). Grover (8) ex-amined chromosomal abnormality in liver cells after continuous subcutaneous injection of DEN (10 mg/kg body weight) in rats, found changes in chromosomal pattern from the 3rd day, and a similar pattern was seen even on the 48th day. He also found the same change in the malignant nodule found in rat liver induced by DEN.

Male Donryu rats, 8 weeks of age, were given drinking water containing 50 ppm of DEN freely for 3, 4, and 5 weeks, and changes in chromosomes were examined immediately after the end of DEN administration. Chromosomal changes in the liver were also followed for 20 weeks in the animals given drinking water with 50 ppm of DEN for 3 weeks and ordinary water without the carcinogen for subsequent period, and aminals killed every 4 weeks.

Cytological Preparations for Chromosome Analysis

To arrest mitosis, rats were injected intraperitoneally with 0.1 mg/100 g body weight of colchicine 3 hr before being sacrificed. The piece of liver tissue to be analyzed was minced with fine scissors, and the cells were suspended by pipet-ting in 20 ml of Hanks' balanced salt solution in a test tube. The suspension was allowed to stand for a few minutes to allow relatively large pieces of tissue to sediment and then approximately 15 ml of the upper part of the suspension was centrifuged at 1,000 rpm for 5 min. The cells that sedimented were re-suspended in a hypotonic solution (0.9% sodium citrate) and allowed to stand for 20 min at room temperature. The suspension was recentrifuged and then the cells were fixed with a fixative of methanol-acetic acid mixture (3:1). After three changes of the fixative, at intervals of 30 min, the cells were suspended in a small volume of the fixative. A few drops of the suspension were placed on a clean cold slide glass and quickly dried by the aid of the flame of a gas burner. Then the preparations were stained with Giemsa solution and mounted.

Classification of Chromosomes

The 42 chromosomes of normal male rats of the Donryu strain were arranged according to the proposed numbering system reported by animal chromosome study group (1). In Donryu rats, 5 pairs of autosomes (Nos. 1, 2, 11, 12, and 13) and Y chromosome can be identified by their morphological characteristics. In the present study, chromosome Nos. 11, 12, and Y could be identified in some metaphase cells in good quality preparations, but usually this was not possible. Therefore, in this study the normal 42 chromosomes were tentatively classified into 6 groups; No. 1, No. 2, Nos. 3–12, No. 13, Nos. 14–18, and Nos. 19–20. Sex chromosomes were included in the Nos. 3–12 group.

Periodical Changes in Chromosomes until Formation of Liver Tumor

In the liver of rats immediately after ingestion of DEN drinking water for 3, 4, and 5 weeks, cells in the diploid range were 95.2, 95.2, and 86.7%, respectively, and those in the polyploid range were 4.8, 4.8, and 13.3%, respectively.

TABLE I.   Percentage Distribution of Cells by Ploidy

Ploidy	Experimental group[a]							
	3	4	5	3–4	3–8	3–12	3–20	Control
2n[b]	95.2 (73.4)	95.2	86.7	76.4 (73.9)	79.5 (82.1)	82.5 (75.2)	91.0	100 (82.0)
3n	0.2 (3.0)	0	4.2	7.3 (1.0)	6.2 (1.0)	7.0 (0.9)	1.8	0 (0.7)
4n	4.6 (23.6)	4.6	8.9	14.8 (22.2)	14.3 (16.9)	10.1 (23.9)	7.0	0 (17.3)
6n–8n	0 (0)	0.2	0.2	1.5 (2.9)	0 (0)	0.4 (0)	0.2	0 (0)
No. of cells analyzed	500 (203)	500	503	330 (207)	161 (207)	286 (206)	442	251 (306)
No. of rats used	10 (2)	12	14	4 (2)	4 (2)	4 (2)	4	4 (2)

[a] No. of weeks treated–No. of weeks after treatment.   Values in parentheses indicate ploidy rates of liver cells after partial hepatectomy.   [b] Ranges of chromosome numbers: 2n (38–52), 3n (53–73), 4n (74–94), 6n–8n (116–178).

TABLE II.   Results of Analyses of

Exp. group[a]	Distribution of chromosome												
	38	39	40	41	42	43	44	45	46	47	48	49	50
Control					13								
3 wk	1	2	3	10	156	1							
4 wk				9	98								
5 wk		2	1	10	89	1							
3–4 wk				2	9	1				2	1		
3–8 wk			1	2	7	1	1						
3–12 wk			1	3	13			1		2			
3–20 wk		2	5	5	14	6	3	1		1			

[a] No. of weeks treated–No. of weeks after treatment.   [b] Karyotypes lacking only one or two as artifacts during the preparation.

Near-triploid and tetraploid cells appeared in the animals given the DEN water for a long period of time.

When the DEN drinking water was discontinued after 3 weeks, the appearance of near-triploid and tetraploid cells was 22.2% four weeks after cessation, 20.5% eight weeks after, and decreased to 8.8% after 20 weeks (Table I). Exact analysis of the number of chromosomes and karyotype was made with metaphase cells of good quality. As shown in Table II, majority of the cells contained 42 chromosomes in any of the groups immediately after cessation of the DEN administration but in 194 cells in which karyotype analysis was made, chromosome abnormality was found in 10 of them. In the control untreated rats, chromosome number was all in the diploid range and abnormal cells did not appear.

Chromosome Analysis of Primary Liver Tumors Induced by DEN

In the animals given DEN drinking water for 3 weeks and subsequently water not containing the carcinogen, liver tumors were produced 28 weeks after stopping of DEN administration. Tumor size, histological diagnosis, and cytogenetic characteristics of liver tumors in 12 animals are listed in Table III. Of these 12 liver tumors 8 were diagnosed histologically as carcinomas (Nos. 1 to 8), 3 as adenomas (Nos. 9 to 11), and one was intermediate between an adenoma and a carcinoma.

The results of ploidy analysis in these 12 tumors are summarized in Table IV. In the 8 carcinomas, the chromosomes of most cells were in the diploid range. In 3 of the 4 adenomas, the mode of chromosome number was in the diploid range, while in one (No. 9), 63.3% of the cells were in the tetraploid range.

As shown in Table V, the chromosome number in tumor cells was distributed mostly in the diploid range of 38 to 48, the majority of them being around 42. In a few of the tumors, however, a few cells had a chromosome number in the triploid and tetraploid range.

Chromosome Numbers and Karyotypes

numbers						No. of cells analyzed	Karyotype analysis	
51–55	56–60	61–65	66–70	71–75	76–80		Normal cell	Abnormal cell[b]
						13	5	0
	1					174	98	4
						107	51	2
						103	35	4
1	4	7	6	7	2	42	4	1
2		3	2	3		22	2	0
	5	4	6	2	1	38	4	0
				1		38	7	2

chromosomes from the normal complement were excluded, because such cells might be produced

TABLE III. Size, Histological Diagnosis, and Cytogenetic Characteristics of Liver Tumors

Tumor No.	Weeks after DEN treatment	No. of animals	Tumor nodule diameter (mm)	Histological diagnosis	Percentage of cells with 42 chromosomes	Mitotic index	Mean
1	28	3	4–5, 4–5, 10–10	Hepatocellular carcinoma	26.5	0.38%	
2	32	1	4–5	,,	34.8	0.33	
3	38	1	4–5	,,	50.9	0.57	0.42%
4	40	1	10–10	,,	18.0	0.41	
					32.6		
5	40	1	20–20	,,	24.3	0.23	
6	41	1	15–15	,,	9.0	0.33	
7	44	1	12–15	,,	37.5	0.56	0.33
8	49	1	25–40	,,	6.9	0.20	
					19.4		
9	28	1	4–5	Adenoma	19.1	0.35	
10	30	2	7–8, 9–12	,,	8.0	0.37	
11	34	1	7–10	,,	9.4	0.43	0.35
12	38	1	8–10	Adenoma (intermediate tumor)	33.2	0.25	
					17.4		

TABLE IV. Percentage Distribution of Liver Tumor Cells by Ploidy

Ploidy	Tumor No.[a]											
	1	2	3	4	5	6	7	8	9	10	11	12
2n[b]	74.6	98.8	95.5	93.4	72.8	85.7	98.0	97.0	31.9	95.9	89.6	63.3
3n	1.5	0.4	5.7	1.0	0	2.4	0	0	3.0	0	0.5	5.7
4n	21.4	0.4	3.2	6.6	24.8	13.3	2.0	3.0	63.3	4.5	9.9	26.2
6n–8n	2.5	0.4	0.3	0	0	0.5	0	0	1.8	0	0	4.8
No. of cells analyzed	201	242	309	229	206	196	203	203	166	202	203	210

[a] Nos. 1–8 were hepatocellular carcinoma and Nos. 9–12 were adenoma. [b] Ranges of chromosome numbers: 2n (38–52), 3n (53–73), 4n (74–94), 6n–8n (116–178).

TABLE V. Chromosome Numbers and

Tumor No.	Distribution of chromosome												
	38	39	40	41	42	43	44	45	46	47	48	49	50
1	1	1	4	5	11	6	3						
2	6	6	6	12	49	55	4		1				
3	1	2	1	4	16			1	2	1	2		
4	1	3	3	4	5	1	3	1	3	1	1		
5			1	4	5	5							
6	3	4	6	3	2	1							
7	2	1	4	9	13	1	1	1		2			
8	1		4	2	2	3	3	10	3				
9				2	3								
10		3	4	3	1	1							
11	3	1	2	3	2	3	2		2				1
12				1	11								

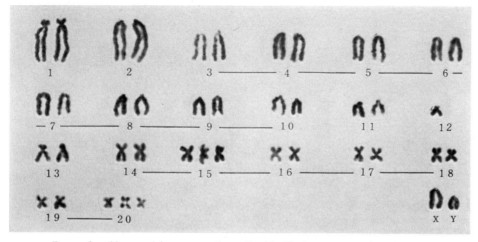

PHOTO 2. Abnormal karyotype of a cell with 43 chromosomes from a small nodule of hepatocellular carcinoma (No. 2), showing monosomy in No. 12 and trisomy in Nos. 14–18 and 19–20

Karyotype analysis revealed that the cells with chromosome number other than 42 were characterized by monosomy and/or trisomy of many chromosomes and by structurally abnormal chromosomes which are called marker chromosomes (Photos 2 and 3).

Percentages of Cells with 42 Chromosomes and the Mitotic Frequency

The percentages of cells with 42 chromosomes among the total dividing cells and mitotic frequencies were analyzed in hepatocellular carcinomas in relation to the size of the tumor nodules, and these results are given in Table III. The percentages of cells with 42 chromosomes tended to decrease with increase

Karyotypes of Liver Tumor Cells

numbers							No. of cells analyzed	Cells with marker chromosomes	Karyotype analysis by photography	
51–55	56–60	61–65	66–70	71–75	76–80	81–90			Normal	Abnormal
			1	1		1	34	1	6	7
1		1	1			1	143	3	14	26
1	1						32	0	3	1
							26	1	0	0
			1	5	5	12	38	0	1	8
1			1	2	1	1	25	18	1	0
							34	1	8	1
							28	6	0	7
						3	8	2	1	0
					1		13	0	0	0
	1	1			2		23	2	0	0
		2			10	10	34	17	7	3

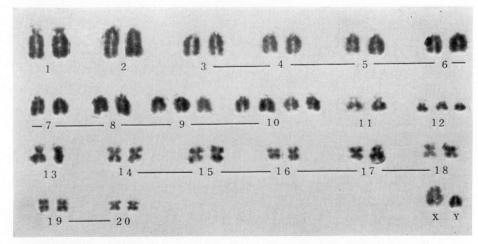

PHOTO 3.   Abnormal karyotype of a cell with 46 chromosomes from a small
nodule of hepatocellular carcinoma (No. 8), having 4 extra chromosomes

in the size of tumor nodules. To test the validity of this observation, the tumors
were grouped according to size into one group of less than 10 mm diameter
(Nos. 1–4), and another of over 10 mm diameter (Nos. 5–8). The mean percentages
of cells with 42 chromosomes were $32.6 \pm 12.1\%$ in the latter group, but the
difference between these values was not statistically significant ($t=1.52$, $d.f.=7$,
$0.1 < P < 0.2$). The mean mitotic frequency in the former group was higher than
that of the latter group.

The relationship between the mitotic frequencies and the percentages of
cells with 42 chromosomes at intervals after DEN treatment is shown in Fig. 1.
The mean mitotic frequency was higher in rats sacrificed after DEN treatment,

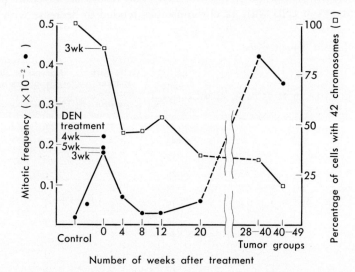

FIG. 1.   Relationship between mitotic frequencies and percentages of total
dividing cells with 42 chromosomes at intervals after DEN treatment and in
tumors

while the percentage of cells with 42 chromosomes seemed to decrease gradually with increase in the period after treatment.

CONCLUSIONS

Administration of 50 ppm of DEN in drinking water for 2 or 3 weeks resulted in the production of liver tumor after a long latent period. This fact indicates that either cancerized cells were formed during the 2 or 3 weeks of carcinogen administration or potential cancer cells were produced within a short period after administration of DEN.

In order to obtain more detailed information on the early stages of tumor development, DEN drinking water was given to rats for 3 weeks, the animals were killed periodically, and morphological and cytogenetic examinations were made on the liver. Histologically, the so-called area of hyperplasia was produced in the liver after the end of DEN administration, nodular hyperplasia after 14 weeks, and liver tumors were formed after about 30 weeks.

Chromosomal analysis carried out in parallel with this histological examination showed that the cells with abnormal chromosome constitution appeared in rats sacrificed at a later period and this was in parallel with morphological changes. Appearance of polyploid cells increased 4, 8, and 12 weeks after stopping of DEN administration but tended to decrease after 20 weeks. A large part of the dividing cells in liver cell carcinomas induced by DEN was characterized by chromosomally abnormal cells of the diploid range.

However, the study has demonstrated that cytogenetic changes occur in liver cells during and after DEN administration. As a working hypothesis it may be postulated that these changes are relevant to the subsequent development of tumors.

Acknowledgments

We are grateful to the late Professor Tomizo Yoshida, the former Director of the Cancer Institute, Dr. Haruo Sugano, the present Director of the Cancer Institute, and Professor Takashi Fujii, Consultant of the Cancer Institute, for their valuable discussion and encouragement.

This investigation was supported by grants from the Ministry of Education (801062-1973) and the Society for the Promotion of Cancer Research (1973), Japan.

REFERENCES

1. Committee for a Standardized Karyotype of *Rattus norvegicus*. Standard karyotype of the Norway rat, *Rattus norvegicus*. *Cytogenet. Cell Genet.*, **12**, 199–205 (1973).
2. Daoust, R. and Calamai, R. Hyperbasophilic foci as sites of transformation in hepatic parenchyma. *Cancer Res.*, **31**, 1290–1296 (1971).
3. Epstein, S., Ito, N., Merkow, L., and Farber, E. Cellular analysis of liver carcinogenesis: The induction of large hyperplastic nodules in the liver with 2-fluorenylacetamide or ethionine and some aspects of their morphology and glycogen metabolism. *Cancer Res.*, **27**, 1702–1711 (1967).
4. Faber, E. Hyperplastic liver nodules. *Methods Cancer Res.*, **7**, 345–375 (1973).

5. Faber, E. Similarities in the sequence of early histological changes induced in the liver of rats by ethionine, 2-acetylaminofluorene, and 3'-methyl-4-dimethylamino-azobenzene. *Cancer Res.*, **16**, 142–148 (1956).

6. Farber, E. Ethionine carcinogenesis. *Adv. Cancer Res.*, **7**, 383–474 (1963).

7. Friedrich-Freksa, H., Gössner, W., and Börner, P. Histochemische Untersuchungen der Cancerogenese in der Rattenleber nach Dauergaben von Diäthylnitrosamin. *Z. Krebsforsch.*, **72**, 226–239 (1969).

8. Grover, S. and Fischer, P. Cytogenetic studies in Sprague-Dawley rats during the administration of a carcinogenic nitroso compound—diethylnitrosamine. *Eur. J. Cancer*, **7**, 77–82 (1971).

9. Heath, D. F. The decomposition and toxicity of dialkylnitrosamines in rats. *Biochem. J.*, **85**, 72–91 (1962).

10. Kitagawa, T. Histochemical analysis of hyperplastic lesions and hepatomas of the liver of rats fed 2-fluorenylacetamide. *Gann*, **62**, 207–216 (1971).

11. Kitagawa, T., Yokochi, T., and Sugano, H. α-Fetoprotein and hepatocarcinogenesis in rats fed 3'-methyl-4-dimethylaminoazobenzene or N-2-fluorenylacetamide. *Int. J. Cancer*, **10**, 368–381 (1972).

12. Kitagawa, T. and Sugano, H. Timetable for hepatocarcinogenesis in rat. *In* "Analytic and Experimental Epidemiology of Cancer," ed. by W. Nakahara, T. Hirayama, K. Nishioka, and H. Sugano, University of Tokyo Press, Tokyo, p. 91 (1973).

13. Masahito-Hitachi. Chromosome changes in rat liver cells after administration of diethylnitrosamine. *Proc. Japan. Cancer Assoc., 30th Annu. Meet.*, 3 (1971) (in Japanese).

14. Masahito-Hitachi, Yamada, K., and Takayama, S. Chromosome changes in rat liver cells induced by diethylnitrosamine. *J. Natl. Cancer Inst.*, unpublished.

15. Newberne, P. M. and Wogan, G. N. Sequential morphologic changes in aflatoxin B₁ carcinogenesis in the rat. *Cancer Res.*, **28**, 770–781 (1968).

16. Opie, E. L. The pathogenesis of tumors of the liver produced by butter yellow. *J. Exp. Med.*, **80**, 231–246 (1944).

17. Orr, J. W. The histology of the rat's liver during the course of carcinogenesis by butter yellow (*p*-dimethylaminoazobenzene). *J. Pathol. Bacteriol.*, **50**, 393–408 (1940).

18. Reuber, M. D. Development of preneoplastic and neoplastic lesions of the liver in male rats given 0.025% N-2-fluorenyldiacetamide. *J. Natl. Cancer Inst.*, **34**, 697–724 (1965).

19. Scherer, E., Hoffmann, M., Emmelot, P., and Freidrich-Freksa, M. Quantitative study on foci of altered liver cells induced in the rat by a single dose of diethylnitrosamine and partial hepatectomy. *J. Natl. Cancer Inst.*, **49**, 93–106 (1972).

20. Schmitz-Moormann, P., Gedigk, P., and Dharamadhach, A. Histologische und histochemische Frühveränderungen bei der experimentellen Erzeugung von Lebercarcinomen durch Diäthylnitrosamin. *Z. Krebsforsch.*, **77**, 9–16 (1972).

21. Thomas, G. Zur Morphologie der durch Diäthylnitrosamin erzeugten Leberveranderungen und Tumoren bei der Ratte. *Z. Krebsforsch.*, **64**, 224–233 (1961).

22. Wachstein, M. and Meisel, E. Enzyme histochemistry of ethionine-induced liver cirrhosis and hepatoma. *J. Histochem. Cytochem.*, **7**, 189–201 (1959).

23. Yoshida, T. "Gan no Hassei (Carcinogenesis)," Nippon Ishoshuppan, Tokyo, p. 99 (1944) (in Japanese).

GANN Monograph on Cancer Research 17, 355–365 (1975)

MORPHOLOGICAL ASPECTS OF EXPERIMENTAL RENAL TUMOURS

W. H. Butler

*MRC Toxicology Unit, Medical Research Council Laboratories**

In untreated rats adenomas and adenocarcinomas have been reported. Similar epithelial tumours may be induced by a variety of chemical agents. Spontaneous mesenchymal tumours are very rare but may be readily induced by the nitrosamines. The mesenchymal tumours are histologically very pleomorphic but the predominant cell type is a spindle cell. In many areas the tumour appears as a fibrosarcoma but both smooth and striated muscle are a very common feature. All tumours have a conspicuous vascular bed. At an ultrastructural level the neoplastic cells form rudimentary vascular structures suggesting a designation of angiosarcoma. The histogenesis of this lesion has been studied from the first day after treatment. An early acute lesion is seen in the cortical fibroblasts and afferent arteries. At 2 days mitoses are found in fibroblast-like cells and by 7 days in endothelial cells within the renal cortex. Ultrastructurally abnormal capillary endothelial cells are present at 7 days as well as an acute inflammatory reaction. The inflammatory reaction subsides by 4 weeks, leaving a few abnormal spindle cells usually associated with the glomeruli. By 8 weeks there is an increase of plasma cells and lymphocytes associated with the hypercellular foci. However, by 12 weeks the hypercellular foci, when found, are composed of rapidly proliferating spindle and endothelial cells which take the form of the final tumour. The development of the epithelial tumour has received less attention. The adenocarcinomas appear to develop from the proximal tubules at which site necrotic damage is present one day after treatment with nitrosamines. However, it has not been possible to study the development of this lesion in detail as the system used produced a much lower incidence of the adenocarcinoma as compared with the mesenchymal angiosarcoma.

Renal tumours are found in untreated rats and mice, and may be induced by a wide range of compounds. In untreated rats the common tumour seen is an epithelial adenoma or adenocarcinoma. Similar epithelial tumours may be induced by lead salts (*23*), nitrosamines (*6, 14*), and aflatoxin (*2, 3*). Mesenchymal tumours are rare in untreated rats but may be readily induced by the nitrosamines (*6, 14, 21*) and cycasin or its aglycone methylazoxymethanol (*13*) and virus (*19*). There is some confusion over the identity of these neoplasms which have

---

* Woodmansterne Road, Carshalton, Surrey, U.K.

been referred to as nephroblastomas, embryonal nephroma, Wilms' tumour, anaplastic tumour or carcinoma, fibrosarcoma, interstitial tumour, stromal nephroma, or mesenchymal tumour. This neoplasm and its development will be described in detail later and should be distinguished from the nephroblastoma. Nephroblastoma has been induced by parental administration of dimethyl-benzanthracene (12). This tumour is histologically distinct from the mesenchymal tumours induced by the nitrosamines and there is little evidence of a mesenchymal origin. The nephroblastoma possibly represents an undifferentiated carcinoma.

Epithelial Tumours

The nitrosamines and the closely related nitrosamides have been used extensively in the study of renal carcinogenesis. This group of compounds produces both epithelial and mesenchymal neoplasms which have been studied at the light-microscopic and the ultrastructural level. The epithelial tumours have been termed adenomas or adenocarcinomas but a rigid classification which distinguishes between the two types of epithelial lesions is difficult. The epithelial tumours are usually multiple, well-circumscribed lesions compressing the surrounding structures. These tumours seldom give metastases. In such cases diagnosis of carcinoma rests upon the presence of local invasion. Histologically the tumours consist of cells arranged in columns, lobules, or cords and are frequently eosinophilic (Photo 1). Other tumours may have a basophilic staining reaction or consist of clear cells (Photo 2). The clear cell carcinoma is very similar in appearance to the hypernephroma or Grawitz tumour as described in man. However, such terms should not be used. In some instances tumours consist of tubules surrounded by a scant fibrous framework. In the large tumours, areas of haemorrhage and necrosis (Photo 3) are invariably found. Variable numbers of mitoses are present in all epithelial neoplasms. In the small spontaneous lesions where there is little necrosis and haemorrhage, and no evidence of invasion, mitoses may be rare, while in the undifferentiated invasive carcinomas mitoses are abundant.

There have been several reports of the ultrastructural characteristics of induced adenomas and adenocarcinomas (6, 11, 15). The tumour cells vary considerably in size and within a single lesion show a wide range of cytoplasmic differentiation. In many cells cytoplasmic organelles are sparse while in others there are abundant mitochondria and a well-developed pattern of cytoplasmic membranes (Photo 4). The acini are bound by a thickened basement membrane. In all published reports the most characteristic feature of this neoplasm is the synthesis of large areas of brush border lying between the tumour cells (Photo 5). Foci of this microvillus brush border are seen in abnormal locations occurring as deep intracellular invaginations. Similar findings have been reported in clear cell and granular cell carcinomas in man (16–18).

It has been recognized that renal adenomas and adenocarcinomas arise within the renal cortex. Magee and Barnes (14) described the first stage of development as the appearance of tubules lined by irregular epithelium which forms papilliary projections into the lumen. We have studied the sequence of epithelial changes following dimethylnitrosamine (DMN) administration (7) and found occasional proliferative tubules within 6 weeks of a single dose of the compound (Photo 6). These lesions were similar to those reported by Magee and Barnes (14) and invariably involve tubules located near glomeruli. These lesions were studied at an ultrastructural level and were shown to possess many of the features of the fully developed neoplasm and in particular the abnormal clumps of basement membrane and foci of microvilli. Apart from the abnormal brush border both the small proliferating tubules and the final tumours contained peroxiscmes which are organelles characteristically found in the proximal tubules of a normal kidney (1). The ultrastructural characteristics of the early lesions and their position within the renal cortex would identify the site of development of the tumours as the first segment of the proximal tubule.

Mesenchymal Tumours

The demonstration that administration of a single dose of DMN to a protein-depleted rat would lead to the induction of 100% incidence of mesenchymal tumours provides an excellent experimental system for studying the histogenesis of these tumours (21). The final neoplasm, which invariably invades surrounding tissue and may give distant metastases, displays a wide spectrum of cell and tissue types within each individual tumour (4, 13, 14, 20, 22). The predominant cell type is the spindle cell which is seen at the invading edge of the lesion, where it infiltrates the surrounding normal renal tubules (Photo 7). In other areas the spindle cells form sheets of fibrosarcoma characterised by a herring-bone or storiform pattern (Photo 8). In the central areas, particularly in large tumours, the lesion is less cellular with bundles of collagen and areas of myxoid degeneration (Photo 9). In most of the tumours studied at either a light or electron-microscopical level smooth muscle is present and in some instances striated muscle (Photo 10) and rhabdomyoblasts. A characteristic finding in all the tumours studied was an abundant vascular bed. In many cases the development of abnormal vascular structures appears to form an integral part of the neoplastic tissues, and resemble capillary or cavernous haemangiomas and haemangiopericytomas (Photo 11).

When the tumours were studied at an ultrastructural level the vascular nature of the lesion became more apparent (8). In all areas of the neoplasm the spindle cells appeared to be forming vascular spaces (Photo 12). It was possible to demonstrate red cells within the rudimentary lumens of the capillary haemangiomas (Photo 13). As commented on above, muscle fibres were a consistent feature of these tumours and at an ultrastructural level these fibres demonstrated the features of vascular, rather than visceral smooth muscle.

In the literature, confusion as to the nature of these neoplasms has arisen as a result of the presence of epithelial structures within the neoplasm. At the invading edge of the neoplasm the spindle cells can be seen surrounding renal tubules and within the depths of the tumour residual glomeruli are present. In a response to the invading neoplasm the tubular epithelium may become hyperplastic but there is no evidence that it is neoplastic or has a structure similar to that seen in the adenocarcinomas described above. In some instances the primitive mesenchymal cells invaginate pre-existing tubules giving rise to the appearance of a primitive glomerulus (Photo 14). This, however, should not be considered to be evidence of multipotential differentiation. On analysis of the developed neoplasm at a light and ultrastructural level it is apparent that this neoplasm is a mesenchymal tumour of vascular origin and should be designated an angiosarcoma.

The sequence of events following a single dose of DMN and the conditions which lead to the induction of 100% incidence of these angiosarcomas has been studied by Hard and Butler (5, 9). These studies trace the origin of this apparent heterogeneous tumour from 24 hr to a time when the full characteristics of the tumour are evident. The initial lesion in interstitial space adjacent to the glomerular hilus was demonstrated at 24 hr after treatment with DMN. At this time there was evidence of acute damage of the afferent artery and the surrounding pericytes and fibroblasts. The interstitial cells immediately adjacent to the hilus contained abundant anastomosing channels of rough endoplasmic reticulum and were often found next to free red cells. By 2 days, within this area, mitosis was present in the fibroblast-like cells. This cell division and an inflammatory reaction of mononuclear phagocytes and lymphocytes constitute the hypercellular foci which can be seen between 3 to 4 days reaching a maximum between 7 and 14 days. During this time mitosis can be identified both in cortical fibroblasts and capillary endothelium. In 7 days within these hypercellular foci a few capillary endothelium cells were greatly increased in size with abundant cytoplasmic organelles (Photo 15). Their nuclei were often irregular. These atypical endothelial cells appeared to extend beyond the vessel walls into the interstitial space. Between 7 and 14 days the interstitial infiltration with lymphocytes and macrophages extended throughout the cortex and was probably associated with the epithelial necrosis also induced by the DMN. This initial lymphocytic and macrophage reaction which reached its peak between 7 and 14 days slowly subsided, so that by between 3 and 4 weeks the hypercellular foci consisted only of lymphocytes. Although at this stage the lymphocytes were the predominant cell form seen, a few large cells with many of the characteristics of fibroblasts remained. These cells with unusual mitochondria, large nuclei, and hypertrophied nucleoli, often appeared to encircle tubules. A few cells identified as smooth muscle cells were also present. These hypercellular foci were found in the vicinity of many glomeruli. By 8 weeks there was an increase in the number of plasma cells present and the hypercellular foci became more apparent. Within these lesions there were the abnormal fibroblast-like cells, bizarre capillaries, lymphocytes, plasma cells, and macrophages (Photo 16). This apparent immunological response to the abnormal cells appears in many cases to be successful in removing the abnormal cell type as the number of foci within a kidney is greatly reduced. However, by 12 weeks there is a sudden reduction in the immunological cells within the persisting foci which now assume the form of aggregations of cells morphologically similar to the abnormal cells seen as early as 1 week. There is rapid proliferation of these cells so that by 16 weeks macroscopic neoplasms are present which display the characteristic spectrum

of vascular differentiation observed in the final tumour. In no stage of the development of these neoplasms is there evidence of development from multiple
cell types.

DISCUSSION

There can be little doubt that the proliferating lesion seen at 12 weeks is
identical to that of the macroscopic tumour seen later. The nature of the enlarged
bizarre cells seen prior to 12 weeks have not been conclusively demonstrated but
it would appear that these represent neoplastic cells which are derived from the
interstitial cells, either fibroblasts or pericytes, in the vicinity of the damaged
afferent artery.

In the study of renal carcinogenesis induced by nitrosamines we have an
excellent system for investigating the mechanisms of carcinogenesis. Within
this organ there is a specific site from which the neoplasm develops, that is, the
glomerular hilus and specifically the interstitial fibroblasts or pericytes around
the afferent artery. These cells react to a single dose of carcinogen and in the
right dietary conditions result in 100% incidence of sarcoma. It would appear
from these studies that there is rapid induction of neoplasia without evidence
of a multiple stage phenomenon. It is of interest that at 7 days it is possible to
culture transformed cells from the renal cortex of treated animals (10) and that
there is no evidence of a "pre-neoplastic lesion" or evidence of "tumour progression." A further interesting feature of this system is the intense immunological response to the foci of abnormal cells occurring between about 8 and 12
weeks. This immunological surveillance appears to be partially successful in
that following this it is difficult to find such hypercellular foci. In the rats receiving 60 mg/kg DMN where all the animals developed sarcoma, it was always
possible to find foci after the cessation of the immunological response. But when
the dose was reduced to 30 mg/kg most animals showed the changes in the
region of the glomerular hilus in the acute phases but only 30% of the animals
had persistent chronic lesions developing into macroscopic neoplasms. Such
studies demonstrate the importance and relevance of morphological studies in
experimental carcinogenesis.

REFERENCES

1. Beard, M. E. and Novikoff, A. B. Distribution of peroxisomes (microbodies) in
    the nephron of the rat. A cytochemical study. *J. Cell Biol.*, **42**, 501–518 (1969).
2. Butler, W. H., Greenblatt, M., and Lijinsky, W. Carcinogenesis in rats by
    aflatoxins B_1, G_1, and B_2. *Cancer Res.*, **29**, 2206–2211 (1969).
3. Epstein, S. M., Bartus, B., and Farber, E. Renal epithelial neoplasm induced in
    male Wistar rats by oral aflatoxin B_1. *Cancer Res.*, **29**, 1045–1050 (1969).
4. Hard, G. C. and Butler, W. H. Cellular analysis of renal neoplasia: Induction of
    renal tumors in dietary-conditioned rats by dimethylnitrosamine, with a reappraisal
    of morphological characteristics. *Cancer Res.*, **30**, 2796–2805 (1970).
5. Hard, G. C. and Butler, W. H. Cellular analysis of renal neoplasia: Light micro-
    scope study of the development of interstitial lesions induced in the rat kidney by

a single carcinogenic dose of dimethylnitrosamine. *Cancer Res.*, **30**, 2806–2815 (1970).

6. Hard, G. C. and Butler, W. H. Ultrastructural aspects of renal adenocarcinoma induced in the rat by dimethylnitrosamine. *Cancer Res.*, **31**, 366–372 (1971).

7. Hard, G. C. and Butler, W. H. Morphogenesis of epithelial neoplasms induced in the rat kidney by dimethylnitrosamine. *Cancer Res.*, **31**, 1496–1505 (1971).

8. Hard, G. C. and Butler, W. H. Ultrastructural analysis of renal mesenchymal tumor induced in the rat by dimethylnitrosamine. *Cancer Res.*, **31**, 348–365 (1971).

9. Hard, G. C. and Butler, W. H. Ultrastructural study of the development of inter-stitial lesions leading to mesenchymal neoplasia induced in the rat renal cortex by dimethylnitrosamine. *Cancer Res.*, **31**, 337–347 (1971).

10. Hard, G. C., Borland, R., and Butler, W. H. Altered morphology and behaviour of kidney fibroblasts *in vitro*, following *in vivo* treatment of rats with a carcinogenic dose of dimethylnitrosamine. *Experientia*, **27**, 1208–1209 (1971).

11. Jasmin, G. and Cha, J. W. Renal adenomas induced in rats by dimethylnitrosamine. An electron microscope study. *Arch. Pathol.*, **87**, 267–278 (1969).

12. Jasmin, G. and Riopelle, J. L. Nephroblastomas induced in ovariectomized rats by dimethylbenzanthracene. *Cancer Res.*, **30**, 321–326 (1970).

13. Laqueur, G. L. and Matsumoto, H. Neoplasm in female Fischer rats following intraperitoneal injection of methylazoxymethanol. *J. Natl. Cancer Inst.*, **37**, 217–232 (1966).

14. Magee, P. N. and Barnes, J. M. Induction of kidney tumours in the rat with dimethylnitrosamine (N-nitroso-dimethylamine). *J. Pathol. Bacteriol.*, **84**, 19–31 (1962).

15. Merkow, L. P., Epstein, S. M., Slifkin, M., and Pardo, M. The ultrastructure of renal neoplasms induced by aflatoxin B_1. *Cancer Res.*, **33**, 1608–1614 (1973).

16. Oberling, C., Rivière, M., and Haguenau, F. Ultrastructure des epithéliomas à cellules claires du rein (Hypernéphromas on tumeurs de Grawitz) et son implication pour l'histogénèse de ces tumeurs. *Bull. Assoc. Franc. Étude Cancer*, **46**, 356–381 (1959).

17. Oberling, C., Rivière, M., and Haguenau, F. Ultrastructure of the clear cells in renal carcinomas and its importance for the demonstration of their renal origin. *Nature*, **186**, 402–403 (1960).

18. Okada, K., Yokoyama, M., Tokue, A., and Takayasu, H. Ultrastructure of renal cell carcinoma. *Urologia (Treviso)*, **36**, 11–19 (1969).

19. Prechtel, K. and Zobl, H. Sarkobildung durch Polyoma-virus im der Niere von Ratten. *Verh. Dtsch. Ges. Pathol.*, **51**, 354–356 (1967).

20. Riopelle, J. L. and Jasmin, G. Nature, classification and nomenclature of kidney tumours induced in the rat by dimethylnitrosamine. *J. Natl. Cancer Inst.*, **42**, 643–662 (1969).

21. Swann, P. F. and McLean, A. E. M. The effect of diet on the toxic and carcinogenic action of dimethylnitrosamine. *Biochem. J.*, **107**, 14–15 (1968).

22. Thomas, C. and Schmahl, D. Zur Morphologie der Nierentumoren bei der Ratte. *Z. Krebsforsch.*, **66**, 125–137 (1964).

23. Zollinger, H. U. Durch chronische Bleivergiftung erzeugte Nierenadenome und Carcinome bei Ratten und ihre Beziehungen zu den entsprechenden Neubildungen des Menschen. *Arch. Pathol. Anat. Physiol.*, **323**, 694–710 (1953).

EXPLANATION OF PHOTOS

PHOTO 1.   Cortical adenoma from a rat showing regular columns and acini of epithelial cells. There is no haemorrhage or necrosis. Hematoxylin-Eosin stain (H-E). ×160.

PHOTO 2.   Clear cell adenocarcinoma from a rat showing irregular acini and sheets of cells. H-E. ×160.

PHOTO 3.   Cortical adenocarcinoma from a rat showing irregular sheets of cells and extensive haemorrhage and necrosis. H-E. ×160.

PHOTO 4.   Electron micrograph of a cortical adenocarcinoma showing a cell with cytomembranes and other organelles and adjacent cells with sparse cytoplasmic organelles. The acinus is limited by a basement membrane. ×10,000. (From Ref. 6)

PHOTO 5.   Electron micrograph of a cortical adenocarcinoma showing a focus of microvilli between two epithelial cells. ×13,000. (From Ref. 6)

PHOTO 6.   Early proliferative focus of epithelial cells within the renal cortex. H-E. ×160.

PHOTO 7.   Edge of a cortical angiosarcoma showing infiltration of tubules by spindle cells. H-E. ×300.

PHOTO 8.   Area of a cortical angiosarcoma showing the storiform pattern of a fibrosarcoma. H-E. ×160.

PHOTO 9.   Central area of a cortical angiosarcoma showing dense collagen and myxoid degeneration surrounding a pre-existing glomerulus and tubules. H-E. ×160.

PHOTO 10.   Area of striated muscle in a cortical angiosarcoma. P.T.A.H. stain. ×350.

PHOTO 11.   Area of a cortical angiosarcoma showing multiple vascular spaces similar to a haemangiopericytoma. H-E. ×160.

PHOTO 12.   Electron micrograph of a spindle cell from a cortical angiosarcoma showing a small cleft-like space with the cytoplasm (↑). ×4,250.

PHOTO 13.   Electron micrograph of a cortical angiosarcoma showing abnormal vascular channels in a degenerative stroma. ×1,500.

PHOTO 14.   Area of a cortical angiosarcoma showing invagination of spindle cells into a dilated tubule giving rise to the appearance of a primitive glomerulus. H-E. ×160.

PHOTO 15.   Electron micrograph of an abnormal fibroblast-like cell with a 7 day after treatment with DMN periglomerular hypercellular focus. ×10,000. (From Ref. 9)

PHOTO 16.   Electron micrograph of a cortical hypercellular 8 weeks after treatment with DMN showing collections of plasma cells (P) and lymphocytes (L). ×3,500. (From Ref. 9)

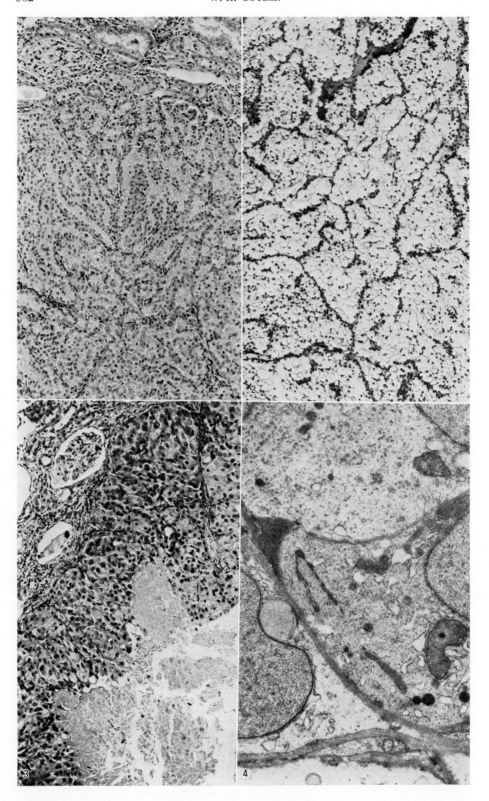

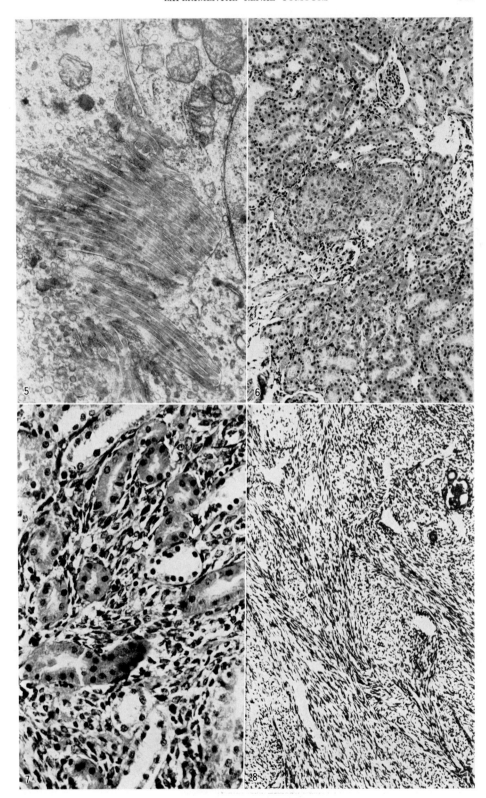

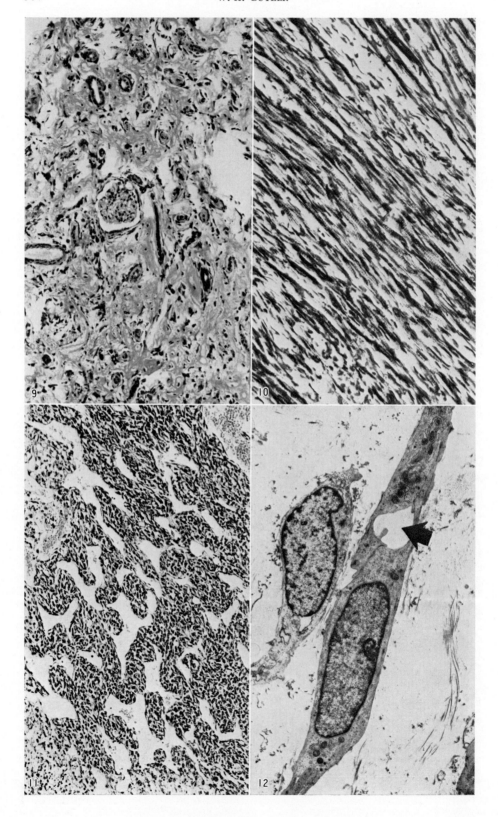

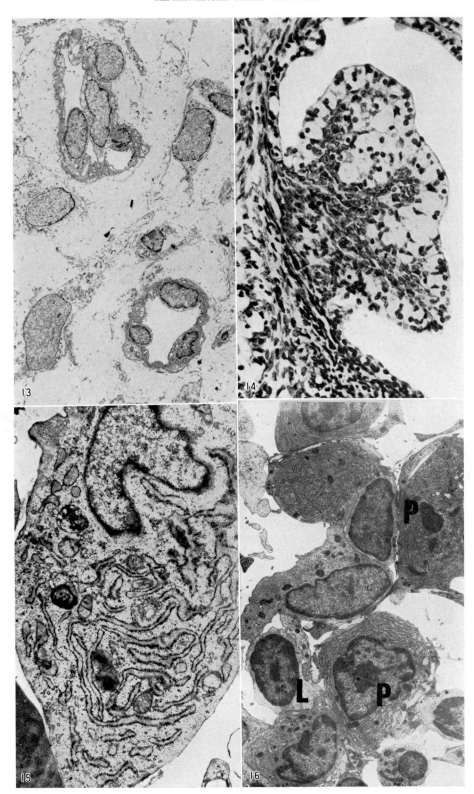

GANN Monograph on Cancer Research 17, 367–381 (1975)

EXPERIMENTAL URINARY BLADDER TUMORS INDUCED BY N-BUTYL-N-(4-HYDROXYBUTYL)-NITROSAMINE[*1]

Nobuyuki Ito,[*2] Masayuki Arai, Seiichi Sugihara, Kazuya Hirao, Sachio Makiura, Kinuko Matayoshi, and Ayumi Denda

Department of Oncological Pathology, Cancer Center Institute, Nara Medical University[*3]

The specificities of the morphological, histological, and histochemical changes induced in the urinary bladder by N-butyl-N-(4-hydroxybutyl)nitrosamine (BBN) were investigated in various animals. Results showed that this carcinogen is very useful in studies on urinary bladder carcinogenesis. Several factors, such as age, sex, strain, and species differences in animals, on urinary bladder carcinogenesis induced by BBN were analysed. Clear relationships were found between the concentration of this carcinogen and its period of administration and the development of urinary bladder cancer.

The effects of various chemicals on development of bladder tumors in rats induced by BBN were studied.

There are many reports on the carcinogenic effect of various compounds on the urinary bladder in experimental animals (*4, 34*). Recently, several nitroso compounds were found to have carcinogenic effects on the urinary bladder of rats (*8, 17, 25, 35, 36*). Druckrey *et al.* (*9*) first reported the selective carcinogenic activity of N-butyl-N-(4-hydroxybutyl)nitrosamine (BBN) on the urinary bladder of rats and, since then, there have been many reports on the histology, histogenesis, and ultrastructure of urinary bladder tumors induced in rats, mice, and dogs by this carcinogen (*1, 2, 18–23, 26, 27, 33*).

The present paper surveys biological aspects of the urinary bladder tumors in experimental animals induced by BBN, including histological, histochemical, and electron-microscopic analyses of data obtained in our laboratory.

Pathology of Urinary Bladder Tumors

1. Gross findings

When rats and mice are treated with BBN the outer wall of the urinary bladder becomes thickened, usually with vascular dilatation of the wall, while

[*1] This work was supported in part by Grants-in-Aid for Scientific Research from the Ministry of Education of Japan (No. 92338, 1971, No. 90319, 1972, and No. 801062, 1973), by a grant from Tokyo Biochemical Research Foundation, and by a grant from the Experimental Pathological Research Association (1972 and 1973). These grants are gratefully acknowledged.

[*2] Present address: The 1st Department of Pathology, Nagoya City University Medical School, Kawasumi, Mizuho-cho, Mizuho-ku, Nagoya 467, Japan.

[*3] Shijo-cho 840, Kashihara, Nara 634, Japan (伊東信行, 荒井昌之, 杉原誠一, 平尾和也, 牧浦幸男, 又吉絹子, 伝田阿由美).

the inside shows papillomatous and hemorrhagic changes due to development of neoplasms (Photo 1).

In most mice and in some rats, urinary bladder tumors showed infiltrative growth into the bladder wall. Metastatic lesions in the mesenteric or para-aortic lymph nodes were seen. Non-papillomatous areas frequently showed focal hyperplastic patches.

2. Light microscopy

For histopathological studies, the urethra was ligated and 0.5 ml of 10% buffered formaldehyde solution was injected into the bladder. Then, tissues were fixed and stained with Hematoxylin and Eosin, van Gieson's stain, or Mallory's stain.

The normal distended urinary bladder of rats, mice, hamsters, and guinea pigs has a mucosal epithelium, which is 2 to 4 cells thick (Photo 2). On treatment with a carcinogen the epithelium increases diffusely to a thickness of 5 to 8 cells. The following three kinds of focal changes of the bladder epithelium were found in experimental animals treated with BBN; hyperplasia (Photo 3), papilloma (Photo 4), and transitional cell carcinoma (Photo 5), including squamous metaplasia (Photo 6). These histological changes resemble those induced in the urinary bladder of animals by other chemicals (3, 11, 13–15, 31, 32).

3. Histochemistry

After treatment of animals with BBN, the urinary bladder was frozen, cut into sections of 10 μm width, and incubated at room temperature in Gomori's acid and in suitable media to test the activities of alkaline phosphatase, succinate dehydrogenase, monoamine oxidase, glucose-6-phosphatase, and β-glucuronidase (18).

Histochemical findings on urinary bladder tumorigenesis in rats induced by BBN are summarized in Table I. Hyperplastic lesions showed low activities of several enzymes, especially alkaline phosphatase. However, the activities of succinate dehydrogenase and β-glucuronidase were increased. Papillomatous and cancerous tissue usually gave strong positive reactions for monoamine oxidase and β-glucuronidase.

TABLE I. Histochemical Activities of Urinary Bladder Epithelium in Rats after Treatment with BBN

	Normal	Hyperplasia	Papilloma	Cancer
Alkaline phosphatase	+	± ~ +	± ~ +	− ~ +
Acid phosphatase	+	+ ~ ⧺	± ~ ⧺	± ~ ⧺
β-Glucuronidase	+	± ~ ⧺	± ~ ⧻	+ ~ ⧻
Succinate dehydrogenase	+	+ ~ ⧺	+ ~ ⧺	± ~ ⧺
Monoamine oxidase	±	± ~ +	+ ~ ⧺	+ ~ ⧻
Glucose-6-phosphatase	⧺	± ~ +	± ~ +	± ~ +
Periodic acid-Schiff reaction	−	±	±	±

− none; ± trace; + weak; ⧺ moderate; ⧻ marked.

4. Scanning electron microscopy

Rat bladders were injected with 2.5% glutaraldehyde in 0.1 M phosphate buffer (pH 7.2) at 4°. After 30 min, the bladders were cut open and rinsed. Then the tissue was put into liquid CO_2 in a critical-point drying apparatus. The resulting dry specimens were lightly coated with carbon and then with gold-palladium, and examined in a Hitachi Model HHS-2R scanning electron microscope, operated at 20 kV.

In a normal bladder, large polygonal cells were seen arranged fairly regularly, with slightly upturned edges along their margins of contact (Photo 7). In animals after treatment with BBN for 12 weeks, elevated, hyperplastic cells were clearly seen arranged irregularly and their surface was uneven with numerous microvilli (Photo 8). Papillomatous areas showed papillary proliferation, resembling a cauliflower (Photo 9). The surface of tumor areas was irregular with numerous, short tubular microvilli of uniform diameter, some of which arose from flat excrescences of the surface (Photos 10 and 11).

5. Transmission electron microscopy

After treatment of rats with BBN the bladder tissue was fixed in buffered glutaraldehyde and osmium tetroxide, and embedded in epoxide resin. The preparations were mounted on Formvar-coated copper specimen grids and double stained, first with aqueous uranyl acetate and then with lead citrate. Sections were examined with a Hitachi HU-12 electron microscope.

Normal bladder cells were clear with numerous fusiform vesicles and free ribosomes. Their nuclear margin was smooth (Photo 12). Hyperplastic areas consisted of both dark and clear cells with few fusiform vesicles, and enlarged nuclei and nucleoli. The cytoplasm of dark hyperplastic cells contained many free ribosomes. Both dark and clear hyperplastic cells contained many tonofibrils (Photo 13). Papillomatous and cancerous cells had many microvilli and these cells also had either dark or clear cytoplasm. The cytoplasm of cancer cells usually contained tonofilaments of various sizes, but no fusiform vesicles were seen. The cytoplasm of dark tumor cells occasionally showed invaginated canaliculi with many microvilli. The nuclei were oval or round, like those of normal bladder cells, and nucleolar hypertrophy was marked (Photos 14 and 15).

Factors Affecting Development of Bladder Tumors

1. Age, sex, strain, and species differences

The effects of sex and age on carcinogenesis were studied in rats. Male and female Wistar strain rats of 4, 8, 12, and 24 weeks old were given water containing 0.01% BBN for 20 weeks and then water without the carcinogen for 20 weeks.

Histological findings in these animals are summarized in Table II. The incidence of cancer of the bladder was higher in older rats than in younger ones. The development of squamous metaplasia in cancerous areas also tended to increase with increasing age of the rats. No significant sex difference was observed in the incidence of urinary bladder cancer.

Strain differences in carcinogenesis were studied using Wistar, ACI, BDIX,

TABLE II. Effect of Age on the Incidence of Urinary Bladder Tumors in Male
and Female Rats Treated with BBN[a]

Initial age (weeks)	Sex	Effective No. of rats	Changes in urinary bladder (%)			With squamous metaplasia	With invasion
			Hyperplasia	Papilloma	Cancer		
4	M	6	6 (100.0)	6 (100.0)	5 (83.3)	0 —	0 —
	F	11	11 (100.0)	11 (100.0)	7 (63.6)	1 (9.1)	1 (9.1)
8	M	13	13 (100.0)	13 (100.0)	10 (76.9)	2 (15.4)	3 (23.1)
	F	9	9 (100.0)	8 (88.9)	7 (77.8)	4 (44.4)	0 —
12	M	11	11 (100.0)	11 (100.0)	9 (81.8)	5 (45.5)	2 (18.2)
	F	13	13 (100.0)	13 (100.0)	12 (92.3)	7 (53.8)	5 (38.5)
24	M	10	10 (100.0)	10 (100.0)	10 (100.0)	6 (60.0)	3 (30.0)
	F	8	8 (100.0)	8 (100.0)	8 (100.0)	5 (62.5)	2 (25.0)

[a] 0.01% BBN for 20 weeks and then water for 20 weeks.

TABLE III. Strain Difference in the Incidence of Urinary Bladder Tumors
in Male Rats Treated with 0.05% BBN for 8 Weeks[a]

Strain	No. of rats	Changes in urinary bladder (%)			Changes in kidney
		Hyperplasia	Papilloma	Cancer	
ACI/NC	6	6 (100.0)	6 (100.0)	6 (100.0)	0
Wistar	14	14 (100.0)	13 (92.3)	12 (85.7)	1[b]
BDIX/N	10	10 (100.0)	9 (90.0)	5 (50.0)	0
Sprague-Dawley	10	10 (100.0)	6 (60.0)	4 (40.0)	1[c]
Lewis	9	9 (100.0)	3 (33.3)	0 —	0

[a] Examined after 40 weeks.   [b] Transitional cell carcinoma in the renal pelvis.   [c] Nephroblastoma in the renal cortex.

TABLE IV. β-Glucuronidase Activities in Homogenates of Liver, Kidney,
and Urinary Bladder of Various Strains of Rats

Strain	No. of rats	Specific activity of β-glucuronidase[a]		
		Bladder	Liver	Kidney
ACI/NC	3	23.73±0.50	78.57± 3.32	27.33±7.02
Wistar	3	21.48±1.77	115.44±13.75	30.40±2.74
BDIX/N	3	24.83±1.94	73.03± 3.97	24.17±1.63
Sprague-Dawley	3	20.93±2.18	166.60±33.69	30.47±2.76
Lewis	3	21.03±3.70	215.53±11.65	45.50±3.71

[a] Values are mean±SD. 1 unit: μmoles of phenolphthalein broken down/hr/mg protein.

Sprague-Dawley, and Lewis strain rats. The incidence of bladder cancer was
highest in the ACI strain followed in that order by the Wistar, BDIX, Sprague-
Dawley, and Lewis strains (Table III). These different strains also showed difference in the activity of β-glucuronidase in the liver, kidney, and bladder (Table
IV), and the difference in the activities in the liver and urinary bladder was not
related to the difference in the incidence of bladder cancer.

Species differences in carcinogenesis were studied using male golden Syrian hamsters, guinea pigs, dd mice, and Wistar rats. No cancer developed in the urinary bladder of guinea pigs or hamsters, though a very low incidence of hyperplasia of the bladder epithelium was observed. This result showed that male dd mice also developed cancer of the urinary bladder on treatment with this carcinogen and that invasive growth of cancer cells into the bladder walls, like that seen in rats, was especially marked in mice.

2. Concentration and period of administration of carcinogen

Relationship between the concentration and period of administration of BBN and the incidence of cancer was examined in male rats, 7 to 8 weeks old. Rats were given water containing 0.1, 0.05, 0.01, 0.005, or 0.001% carcinogen for 2 to 40 weeks and all were killed for histological observation 40 weeks after the start of the experiments.

TABLE V. Incidence of Urinary Bladder Changes in Male Rats Treated with BBN for Various Periods at Various Concentrations

Administration of BBN		No. of rats	Changes in urinary bladder (%)		
Period (weeks)	Concentration (%)		Hyperplasia	Papilloma	Cancer
2	0.1	10	9 (90.0)	4 (40.0)	0 —
	0.05	18	12 (66.7)	3 (33.3)	0 —
	0.01	13	3 (23.1)	0 —	0 —
	0.005	14	0 —	0 —	0 —
4	0.1	12	12 (100.0)	11 (91.7)	4 (33.3)
	0.05	11	11 (100.0)	8 (72.7)	2 (18.2)
	0.01	14	6 (42.9)	1 (7.1)	0 —
	0.005	15	1 (6.7)	1 (6.7)	0 —
6	0.1	13	13 (100.0)	10 (76.9)	7 (53.8)
	0.05	17	16 (94.1)	15 (88.2)	11 (64.7)
	0.01	14	7 (50.0)	5 (35.7)	1 (7.1)
	0.005	13	5 (38.5)	0 —	0 —
8	0.1	12	12 (100.0)	12 (100.0)	11 (91.7)
	0.05	10	10 (100.0)	9 (90.0)	9 (90.0)
	0.01	15	10 (66.7)	2 (13.3)	0 —
	0.005	11	5 (45.5)	2 (18.2)	0 —
12	0.05	9	9 (100.0)	9 (100.0)	9 (100.0)
	0.01	11	8 (72.7)	4 (36.4)	2 (18.2)
	0.005	13	7 (53.8)	3 (23.1)	2 (15.4)
20	0.01	7	7 (100.0)	7 (100.0)	7 (100.0)
	0.005	8	8 (100.0)	5 (62.5)	2 (25.0)
	0.001	9	0 —	0 —	0 —
40	0.01	10	10 (100.0)	10 (100.0)	10 (100.0)
	0.005	6	6 (100.0)	6 (100.0)	3 (50.0)
	0.001	6	0 —	0 —	0 —
Control		7	0 —	0 —	0 —

Histological findings in the urinary bladders of rats which received various concentrations of BBN in the drinking water for different periods are summarized in Table V. Clear relationship was seen between the concentration and period of administration of carcinogen and changes in the urinary bladder. For the development of urinary bladder cancer in rats, the minimum dose of BBN in the drinking water was 0.005%, while the maximum non-carcinogenic dose was 0.001%. The minimum period required for induction of urinary bladder cancer on administration of 0.1% carcinogen solution to rats was 4 weeks.

3. Effect of other chemicals

The influence of nephrotoxic and hepatotoxic chemicals on induction of urinary bladder cancer by BBN was examined. Rats were treated with 4-chloro-acetanilide (4CA) or N-(3,5-dichlorophenyl)succinimide (NDPS), as nephrotoxic chemicals, or with 1-naphthylisothiocyanate (ANI) or dimethylnitrosamine (DMN) as hepatotoxic chemicals (23) before administration of BBN. The changes seen in the urinary bladder epithelium of these rats are summarized in Table VI. These results showed that induction of urinary bladder cancer by BBN was inhibited by 4CA or ANI. But, pretreatment with DMN increased the incidence of papillomas and cancers of the urinary bladder.

TABLE VI. Effect of Pretreatment with Various Hepatotoxic or Nephrotoxic Chemicals on the Induction of Urinary Bladder Tumors in Rats by BBN

Treatment with chemical (weeks)[a]		No. of rats	Changes of urinary bladder (%)		
Pretreatment	BBN		Hyperplasia	Papilloma	Cancer
None	(8)	13	13 (100.0)	7 (53.8)	5 (38.5)
4CA (8)	(8)	18	17 (94.4)	11 (61.1)	2 (11.1)
4CA (8)	—	11	0 —	0 —	0 —
NDPS (8)	(8)	13	12 (92.3)	8 (61.5)	6 (46.2)
NDPS (8)	—	10	0 —	0 —	0 —
ANI (8)	(8)	25	14 (56.0)	5 (20.0)	1 (4.0)
ANI (8)	—	12	0 —	0 —	0 —
DMN (4)	(8)	15	14 (93.3)	11 (73.3)	8 (53.3)
DMN (4)	—	14	0 —	0 —	0 —

[a] BBN: 0.025% BBN in drinking water. 4CA: 0.25% 4CA in diet. NDPS: 0.5% NDPS in diet. ANI: 0.06% ANI in diet. DMN: 0.01% DMN in diet. Rats were killed 12 weeks after the period of administration of BBN.

4. Administration with another carcinogen

The effect of another urinary bladder carcinogen, N-2-fluorenylacetamide (2-FAA) (11, 24, 28–30), on the carcinogenic effect of BBN was studied in rats. Animals were given drinking water containing 0.001% BBN and/or fed on basal diet containing 0.005% 2-FAA or 1.5% DL-tryptophan (Trp) for 40 weeks. The experimental groups and findings in the urinary bladder of these rats are summarized in Table VII.

TABLE VII. Effect of Administration of 2-FAA or DL-Tryptophan with
BBN for 40 Weeks on Urinary Bladder Carcinogenesis in Rats

Treatment[a]	No. of rats	Changes of urinary bladder (%)			Liver cancer
		Hyperplasia	Papilloma	Cancer	
BBN	10	0 —	0 —	0 —	0
BBN+2-FAA	11	9 (81.8)	6 (54.5)	1 (9.1)	1
BBN+2-FAA+Trp	14	13 (92.9)	9 (64.3)	1 (7.1)	0
BBN+Trp	14	2 (14.3)	0 —	0 —	0
2-FAA	13	0 —	0 —	0 —	1
2-FAA+Trp	13	5 (38.5)	0 —	0 —	0
Trp	15	0 —	0 —	0 —	0
Control	6	0 —	0 —	0 —	0

[a] BBN: 0.001% BBN in drinking water. 2-FAA: 0.005% 2-FAA in diet. Trp: 1.5% DL-tryptophan in diet.

No changes were found in the urinary bladder epithelium of rats which had received 0.001% BBN or 0.005% 2-FAA only for 40 weeks. However, about 82% of those which received both BBN and 2-FAA for 40 weeks developed hyperplasia and of these animals about 55% developed papillomas while only 9% developed cancer. Groups treated with both carcinogens plus Trp showed similar urinary bladder changes to rats treated with both carcinogens only. However, induction of hyperplasia of the urinary bladder epithelium by BBN or 2-FAA was slightly increased by administration of Trp. No remarkable changes were seen in rats treated with Trp alone for 40 weeks. The results showed that a combination of BBN and 2-FAA had a greater tumorigenic effect in rats than either compound alone.

DISCUSSION

Recent results have shown that several nitroso compounds have a carcinogenic action on the urinary bladder of experimental animals (8, 17, 25, 35, 36). Results have shown that BBN has a selective carcinogenic effect on the urinary bladder of rats and mice when given orally but not when given subcutaneously.

Previously we found that this chemical has a carcinogenic action not only on the urinary bladder but also on the renal pelvis and the ureter when the latter is ligated (18, 21). The tumors that developed in these three organs of the urinary system were transitional cell carcinomas or papillomas. This shows that transitional cells are more sensitive to BBN than renal parenchymal tissue or tubular epithelium of other organs.

Histological, histochemical, and electron-microscopic findings on urinary bladder tumors in rats and mice induced by BBN were very similar to findings on tumors induced by other chemical carcinogens (3–4, 5–7, 10–12, 28, 31, 37). Most chemicals which induce bladder cancer also induce cancer of the liver and other organs. However, oral administration of the two carcinogens, BBN and N-[4-(5-nitro-2-furyl)-2-thiazolyl]formamide induced a high incidence of papillomatous cancers of the bladder epithelium in rats and mice within a short period, without causing changes in other organs.

Scanning electron microscopy of urinary bladder tumors in rats induced by BBN showed marked changes in areas of hyperplastic lesions. Previous studies have suggested that focal hyperplasia of the bladder epithelium is a pre-cancerous lesion (*18, 20, 32*). Thus, superficial changes of the bladder epithelium induced by many chemicals at a rather early stage may be important for progress of urinary bladder tumorigenesis. Analytical studies on urinary bladder tumorigenesis by scanning electron microscopy may be useful in studies on early changes of the urinary bladder surface.

Our results showed a species difference in bladder tumorigenesis of BBN, and clear relationship between the incidence of urinary bladder tumors and the concentration and period of administration of the carcinogen in rats. These results in rats should be useful in studies on the clinical or fundamental chemotherapy of bladder cancer. Pretreatment with 4CA or ANI was found to inhibit the induction of urinary bladder cancer by BBN. These results suggest that some kidney or liver injury may have an important effect on the development of urinary bladder cancer in man.

When the two carcinogens, BBN and 2-FAA, were administered together, their carcinogenic action on the urinary bladder was synergistic. Moreover, Trp promoted their action in producing urinary bladder tumors in rats. In these studies, non-carcinogenic doses of both BBN and 2-FAA were used. Previously, Okajima *et al.* (*25*) reported the synergistic effect of Trp and BBN or N-dibutyl-nitrosamine, and Dunning *et al.* (*11*) showed that Trp increased the incidence of urinary bladder tumors in rats induced by 2-FAA. These results suggest that the carcinogenic effect of BBN and 2-FAA on the urinary bladder of rats is related to some intrinsic factors. The metabolism of BBN and related compounds have been studied by Hashimoto *et al.* (*16*). Progress in these studies should be of great value in solving the many biological, pathological, and histological problems related to urinary bladder tumorigenesis in animals treated with BBN. Moreover, further studies on the synergistic or antagonistic effects on this carcinogen of many chemicals, including both those with known and unknown carcinogenic actions, should be valuable in providing means of protecting man from bladder cancer.

REFERENCES

1. Akagi, G., Akagi, A., Kimura, M., and Otsuka, H. Comparison of bladder tumors induced in rats and mice with N-butyl-N-(4-hydroxybutyl)nitrosamine. *Gann*, **64**, 331–336 (1973).
2. Bertram, J. and Craig, A. W. Specific induction of bladder cancer in mice by butyl-(4-hydroxybutyl)nitrosamine and the effects of hormonal modifications on the sex difference in response. *Eur. J. Cancer*, **8**, 587–594 (1972).
3. Bryan, G. T., Brown, R. R., and Price, J. M. Incidence of mouse bladder tumors following implantation of paraffin pellets containing certain tryptophan metabolites. *Cancer Res.*, **24**, 582–585 (1964).

4. Clayson, D. B. and Cooper, E. H. Cancer of the urinary tract. *Adv. Cancer Res.*, **13**, 271–381 (1970).

5. Cohen, S. M., Headley, D. B., and Bryan, G. T. The effect of adult thymectomy and adult splenectomy on the production of leukemia and stomach neoplasms in mice by N-[4-(5-nitro-2-furyl)-2-thiazolyl]acetamide. *Cancer Res.*, **33**, 637–640 (1973).

6. Cohen, S. M., Lower, G. M., Ertürk, E., Jr., and Bryan, G. T. Comparative carcinogenicity in Swiss mice of N-[4-(5-nitro-2-furyl)-2-thiazolyl]acetamide and structurally related 5-nitrofurans and 4-nitrobenzenes. *Cancer Res.*, **33**, 1593–1597 (1973).

7. Croft, W. A. and Bryan, G. T. Production of urinary bladder carcinomas in male hamsters by N-[4-(5-nitro-2-furyl)-2-thiazolyl]formamide, N-[4-(5-nitro-2-furyl)-2-thiazolyl]acetamide, or formic acid 2-[4-(5-nitro-2-furyl)-2-thiazolyl]hydrazine. *J. Natl. Cancer Inst.*, **51**, 941–949 (1973).

8. Denlinger, R. H., Swenberg, J. A., Koestner, A., and Wechsler, W. Differential effect of immunosuppression on the induction of nervous system and bladder tumors by N-methyl-N-nitrosourea. *J. Natl. Cancer Inst.*, **50**, 87–93 (1973).

9. Druckrey, H., Preussmann, R., Ivankovic, S., and Schmidt, C. H. Selektive erzeugung von Blasenkrebs an Ratten durch Dibutyl- und N-butyl-N-butanol(4)-nitrosamin. *Z. Krebsforsch.*, **66**, 280–290 (1964).

10. Dukes, C. E. "Tumors of the Bladder," E. & S. Livingstone, Edinburgh, p. 105 (1959).

11. Dunning, W. F., Curtis, M. R., and Maun, M. E. The effect of added dietary tryptophan on the occurrence of 2-acetylaminofluorene-induced liver and bladder cancer in rats. *Cancer Res.*, **10**, 454–459 (1950).

12. Engelbart, K., Brunk, R., and Schütz, E. Über die Entwicklung von Harnblasencarcinom bei Ratte und Hund unter der Verfütterung von 1,2-Dihydro-2-(5'-nitrofuryl)-4-hydroxychinazolin-3-oxid. *Z. Krebsforsch. Klin. Onkol.*, **79**, 165–175 (1973).

13. Ertürk, E., Cohen, S. M., and Bryan, G. T. Urinary bladder carcinogenicity of N-[4-(5-nitro-2-furyl)-2-thiazolyl]formamide in female Swiss mice. *Cancer Res.*, **30**, 1309–1311 (1970).

14. Ertürk, E., Cohen, S. M., Price, J. M., and Bryan, G. T. Pathogenesis, histology, and transplantability of urinary bladder carcinomas induced in albino rats by oral administration of N-[4-(5-nitro-2-furyl)-2-thiazolyl]formamide. *Cancer Res.*, **29**, 2219–2228 (1969).

15. Ertürk, E., Price, J. M., Morris, J. E., Cohen, S. M., Leith, R. S., von Esch, A. M., and Crovetti, A. J. The production of carcinoma of the urinary bladder in rats by feeding N-[4-(5-nitro-2-furyl)-2-thiazolyl]formamide. *Cancer Res.*, **27**, 1998–2002 (1967).

16. Hashimoto, Y., Suzuki, E., and Okada, M. Induction of urinary bladder tumors in ACI/N rats by butyl (3-carboxypropyl)nitrosoamine, a major urinary metabolite of butyl(4-hydroxybutyl)nitrosoamine. *Gann*, **63**, 637–638 (1972).

17. Hicks, R. M. and Wakefield, J. St. J. Rapid induction of bladder cancer in rats with N-methyl-N-nitrosourea. I. Histology. *Chem.-Biol. Interact.*, **5**, 139–152 (1972).

18. Ito, N. Experimental studies on tumors of the urinary system of rats induced by chemical carcinogens. *Acta Pathol. Japon*, **23**, 87–109 (1973).

19. Ito, N., Hiasa, Y., Tamai, A., Okajima, E., and Kitamura, H. Histogenesis of

urinary bladder tumors induced by N-butyl-N-(4-hydroxybutyl)nitrosamine in rats. *Gann*, **60**, 401–410 (1969).

20. Ito, N., Hiasa, Y., Toyoshima, K., Okajima, E., Kamamoto, Y., Makiura, S., Yokota, Y., Sugihara, S., and Matayoshi, K. Rat bladder tumors induced by N-butyl-N-(4-hydroxybutyl)nitrosamine. *In* "Topics in Chemical Carcinogenesis," ed. by W. Nakahara, S. Takayama, T. Sugimura, and S. Odashima, University of Tokyo Press, Tokyo, pp. 175–197 (1972).

21. Ito, N., Makiura, S., Yokota, Y., Kamamoto, Y., Hiasa, Y., and Sugihara, S. Effect of unilateral ureter ligation on development of tumors in the urinary system of rats treated with N-butyl-N-(4-hydroxybutyl)nitrosamine. *Gann*, **62**, 359–365 (1971).

22. Ito, N., Matayoshi, K., Arai, M., Yoshioka, Y., Kamamoto, Y., Makiura, S., and Sugihara, S. Effect of various factors on induction of urinary bladder tumors in animals by N-butyl-N-(4-hydroxybutyl)nitrosamine. *Gann*, **64**, 151–159 (1973).

23. Ito, N., Matayoshi, K., Matsumura, K., Denda, A., Kani, T., Arai, M., and Makiura, S. Effects of various carcinogenic and non-carcinogenic substances on development of bladder tumors in rats induced by N-butyl-N-(4-hydroxybutyl)-nitrosamine. *Gann*, **65**, 123–130 (1974).

24. Melicow, M. M., Uson, A. C., and Prise, T. D. Bladder tumor induction in rats fed 2-acetaminofluorene (2-FAA) and a pyridoxine deficient diet. *J. Urol.*, **91**, 520–529 (1964).

25. Okajima, E., Hiramatsu, T., Motomiya, Y., Iriya, K., Ijuin, M., and Ito, N. Effect of DL-tryptophan on tumorigenesis in the bladder and liver of rats treated with N-nitrosodibutylamine. *Gann*, **62**, 163–169 (1971).

26. Okajima, E., Hiramatsu, T., Motomiya, Y., Iriya, K., Ijuin, M., Kondo, T., Hirao, Y., Matsushima, S., Ikuma, S., Yamada, K., and Sugihara, S. Development of urinary bladder tumors in dogs induced by N-nitrosodibutylamine (DBN) and N-butyl-N-(4-hydroxybutyl)nitrosamine (BBN) (2nd report). *Proc. Japan. Cancer Assoc., 32nd Annu. Meet.*, 134 (1973) (in Japanese).

27. Okajima, E., Hiramatsu, T., Motomiya, Y., Kondo, T., and Hirao, Y. Effects of foreign bodies on development of urinary bladder tumors in rats treated with N-butyl-N-(4-hydroxybutyl)nitrosamine. *Urol. Res.*, **1**, in press (1973).

28. Oyasu, R., Kitajima, T., Hopp, M. L., and Sumie, H. Enhancement of urinary bladder tumorigenesis in hamsters by coadministration of 2-acetylaminofluorene and indole. *Cancer Res.*, **32**, 2027–2033 (1972).

29. Oyasu, R., Kitajima, T., Hopp, M. L., and Sumie, H. Induction of bladder cancer in hamsters by repeated intratracheal administrations of 2-acetylaminofluorene. *J. Natl. Cancer Inst.*, **50**, 503–506 (1973).

30. Oyasu, R., Miller, D. A., McDonald, J. H., and Hass, G. M. Neoplasma of rat urinary bladder and liver. Rats fed 2-acetylaminofluorene and indole. *Arch. Pathol.*, **75**, 184–190 (1963).

31. Scott, W. W. and Boyd, H. L. A study of the cacinogenic effect of beta-naphthylamine on normal and substituted isolated sigmoid loop bladder of dogs. *J. Urol.*, **70**, 914–925 (1953).

32. Tiltman, A. J. and Friedell, G. H. The histogenesis of experimental bladder cancer. *Invest. Urol.*, **9**, 218–226 (1971).

33. Toyoshima, K., Ito, N., Hiasa, Y., Makiura, S., and Kamamoto, Y. Tissue culture of urinary bladder tumor induced in a rat by N-butyl-N-(4-hydroxybutyl)nitrosamine: Establishment of cell line, Nara bladder tumor. II. *J. Natl. Cancer Inst.*, **47**, 979–986 (1971).

34. Veenema, R. J., Fingerhut, B., and Lattimer, J. K. Experimental studies on the biological potential of bladder tumors. *J. Urol.*, **93**, 202–211 (1965).
35. Wakefield, J. St. J. and Hicks, R. M. Bladder cancer and N-methyl-N-nitrosourea. II. Sub-cellular changes associated with a single noncarcinogenic dose of MNU. *Chem.-Biol. Interact.*, **7**, 165–179 (1973).
36. Weisburger, J. H., Hadidian, Z., Fredrickson, T. N., and Weisburger, E. K. "A Symposium, Bladder Cancer, 45," Esculpius Publ. Co., Birmingham (1966).
37. Yalciner, S. and Friedell, G. H. Cilia in the epithelium of the urinary bladder during experimental carcinogenesis. *J. Natl. Cancer Inst.*, **51**, 501–505 (1973).

EXPLANATION OF PHOTOS

PHOTO 1. Cut surface of rat urinary bladder tumor induced by BBN. The bladder cavity is filled with the tumor mass.

PHOTO 2. Normal bladder epithelium of 1 to 3 cell thickness. Hematoxylin-Eosin stain (H-E). ×200.

PHOTO 3. Focal hyperplastic area of the urinary bladder of a rat induced by BBN. Nuclear irregularities and growth of stromal tissue are rare. H-E. ×200.

PHOTO 4. Papillomatous lesion of the urinary bladder in a rat induced by BBN. H-E. ×200.

PHOTO 5. Area of transitional cell carcinoma in the urinary bladder of a rat induced by BBN, showing nuclear irregularities and mitotic figures, and slight growth of stromal tissue. H-E. ×100.

PHOTO 6. Squamous metaplasia in an area of transitional cell carcinoma of the urinary bladder of a rat induced by BBN. Clear cancer pearls are seen. H-E. ×200.

PHOTO 7. Appearance of normal rat urinary bladder epithelium by scanning electron microscopy, showing the polygonal arrangement of the surface cells. H-E. ×1,500.

PHOTO 8. Scanning electron-microscopic appearance of a hyperplastic lesion of the urinary bladder of a rat induced by BBN. Hyperplastic cells are elevated and many enlarged, irregular shaped cells are seen. ×1,500.

PHOTO 9. Appearance of a papillomatous tumor by scanning electron microscopy, showing the irregular surface. ×170.

PHOTO 10. Appearance of an area of papillomatous tumor by scanning electron microscopy. The surface of tumor cells is irregular with numerous short microvilli. ×3,000.

PHOTO 11. Scanning electron-microscopic appearance of papillomatous tumor cells. Microvilli of uniform diameter are seen. ×10,000.

PHOTO 12. Transmission electron-microscopic appearance of epithelial cells in the urinary bladder of a rat, showing numerous fusiform vesicles and free ribosomes. ×25,000.

PHOTO 13. Transmission electron-microscopic appearance of a hyperplastic lesion of the urinary bladder of a rat induced by BBN. Both clear and dark cells are seen. Fusiform vesicles are reduced in number but no nuclear changes are seen. ×14,000.

PHOTO 14. Transmission electron-microscopic appearance of a transitional cell carcinoma in a rat induced by BBN. Both dark and clear tumor cells contain many free ribosomes and tonofibrils. Dark cells frequently show intracellular invagination of clear cells. ×16,000.

PHOTO 15. Transmission electron-microscopic appearance of the surface of a cell in a transitional cell carcinoma with many small microvilli. The nucleus and nucleolus are enlarged and irregular. The number of free ribosomes is markedly increased. ×20,000.

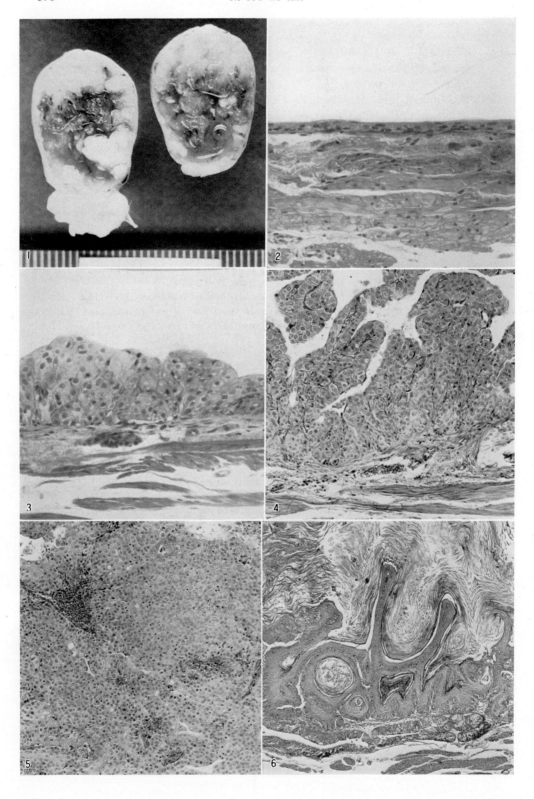

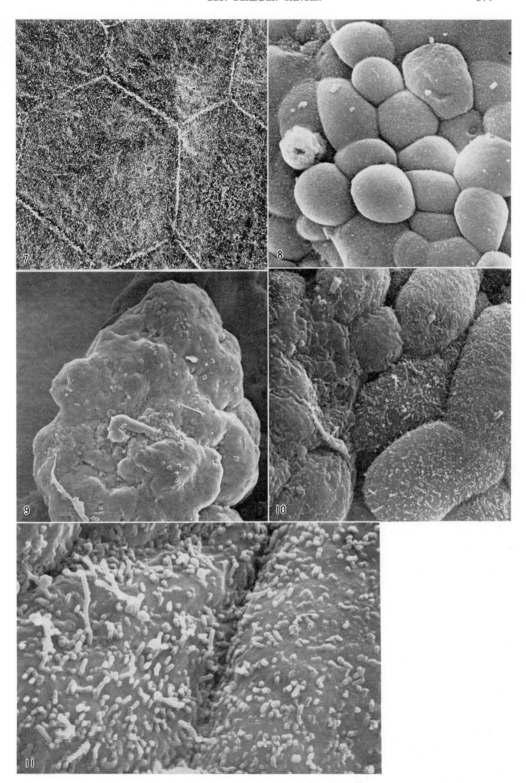

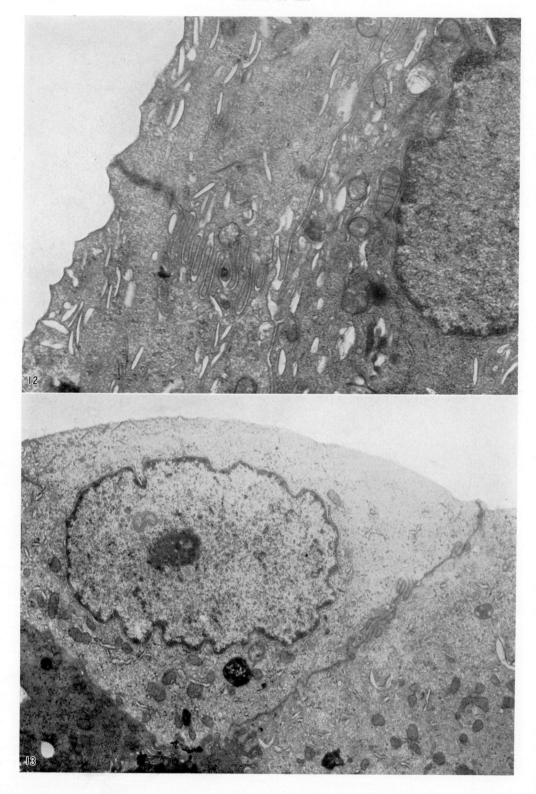

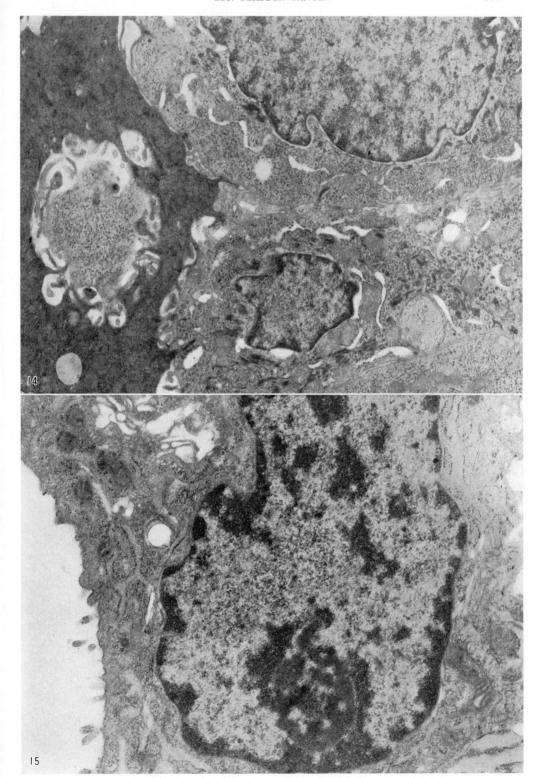

GANN Monograph on Cancer Research 17, 383–392 (1975)

CARCINOGENESIS BY CHEMICALS IMPLANTED INTO THE BLADDER: AN EVALUATION

J. W. Jull[†]

*Cancer Research Centre, University of British Columbia**

The technique of bladder implantation is reviewed and the following new data presented:

Paraffin wax pellets, made in two different laboratories and implanted into the bladder lumen of mice, induced 0 and 10.6% of carcinomas, respectively, after 40–50 weeks. The incidences of carcinomas observed after 70–80 weeks with the same lots of pellets were 33.3 and 26.8%. There was 53.8% of carcinomas in mice implanted with the second lot of wax pellets and killed between 100 and 110 weeks. Wax pellets incorporating 1-phenylazo-2-naphthol induced significantly higher incidences of bladder carcinomas at 40–50 weeks, 70–80 weeks, and 100–110 weeks than did the wax alone. The incidences of carcinomas in bladders exposed to 2-acetamidofluorene, 1-hydroxy-2-acetamidofluorene, 3-hydroxy-2-acetamidofluorene, or N-hydroxy-2-acetamidofluorene contained in paraffin wax pellets were greater than found with the wax alone, but did not differ between the various chemicals.

It is concluded that cancer of the bladder can be induced in mice and rats by the presence of a foreign body only. The tumours so induced are malignant, but their incidence cannot be used as a measure of carcinogenic activity in the conventional sense.

The technique of testing chemicals for carcinogenic activity by incorporating them into a paraffin wax vehicle and implanting the resulting mixture as pellets into the bladders of mice, was introduced in 1951 (*14*). The end point of the assay was taken as the percentage of carcinomas of the bladder which arose within a fixed time, usually 40 weeks, after implantation (*2, 3, 7*). A comprehensive bibliography and summary of the results obtained in various centres, using this technique, has recently been compiled (*8*).

The method was designed so that small quantities of compounds could be brought into contact with the bladder epithelium for protracted periods whilst the organ was functioning under approximately normal physiological conditions. It was considered that any substance so applied to the bladder would be subject only to the action of the urine before coming into contact with the bladder epithelium; thus metabolic changes in chemical structure subsequent to feeding or injection would be obviated. The paramount advantage envisaged was that only small quantities of substances to be tested would be required.

---

† Deceased on October 2, 1974.

* Vancouver 8, Canada.

The end point for assays by the bladder implantation technique has always been based on the assessment of proliferative changes in the bladder epithelium by the examination of histological sections (4). It was demonstrated that provided the bladders were moderately distended with fixative postmortem, and provided that the sections examined included those areas which were macroscopically abnormal, then exhaustive sectioning through the remainder of the bladder did not reveal more advanced hyperplastic or neoplastic lesions than those originally presented. It was also found that a number of pathologists, experienced in examining animal tissues, did not vary to any great extent in their classification of the same sections under the headings of hyperplasia, benign tumour, or carcinoma. Extensive later experience has not refuted these basic findings.

For the purpose of assay of suspected carcinogens the proliferative lesions induced by implanted pellets in mouse bladders have been classified as hyperplasia, adenoma, or papilloma and varying stages of carcinoma from I in which there was invasion of the sub-epithelial tissues, II in which there was invasion of the underlying muscle, and III in which complete penetration of the bladder wall by cancer cells had occurred. Distant metastasis from such bladder tumours is reported in one case in the present communication, but there is no previous record of this happening.

The fact that the changes observed histologically in implanted bladders represent a graded series of changes from simple downgrowth to infiltrating carcinoma, has been emphasised by Roe (18). In experiments terminated at fixed times, therefore, there has been an element of uncertainty as to the ultimate fate of early hyperplastic lesions. It would be expected that if early hyperplastic lesions eventually give rise to neoplasia and carcinoma, then there would be an increase in the incidence of carcinomas with time of exposure to bladder pellets, even those containing no added carcinogen. The fact that all "inert" substances used in bladder implantation have induced some incidence of carcinomas (8) has made this aspect of the problem more urgent.

Another facet of the results of bladder implantation studies which requires explanation is that in some instances the method demonstrates carcinogenic activity in substances for which there is no other supporting biological data.

The experiments reported in the next section were designed to clarify these aspects of the results reported so far.

New Experimental Data

The objective was to determine over an extended period the course of the early proliferative changes seen after the implantation of paraffin wax pellets into mouse bladders, and to compare the relative activities of 2-acetamidofluorene and its metabolites in inducing epithelial neoplasia of the bladder, when incorporated into such pellets.

1. Experimental design

A stock of paraffin wax was obtained from the same supplier as that used by the Leeds group (British Drug Houses, Ltd.). The plain wax pellets were used

TABLE I. Incidence of Hyperplasia and Neoplasia in Mice with Bladder Pellets of Various Compositions

Group No.	Source of wax vehicle	Chemical	Length of exp. (weeks)	Total No. mice	Hyperplasia No.	Hyperplasia %	Adenoma No.	Adenoma %	Carcinoma I No.	Carcinoma II No.	Carcinoma III No.	Carcinoma Total %	Total hyperplasia and neoplasia (%)
1a	Vancouver	—	40–50	36	4	11.1	2	5.6	0	0	0	0	16.7
1b		—	70–80	27	6	22.2	3	11.1	5	3	1	33.3	66.6
2a	Vancouver	N-Hydroxy-2-acetamido-fluorene	40–50	11	1	9.1	2	18.2	1	0	0	9.1	36.4
2b			70–80	20	3	15.0	3	15.0	6	4	0	50.0	80.0
3a	Vancouver	1-Hydroxy-2-acetamido-fluorene	60–70	46	11	23.9	10	21.7	8	2	0	21.7	67.3
3b			70–80	23	4	17.4	3	13.0	10	4	0	60.9	91.3
4a	Vancouver	3-Hydroxy-2-acetamido-fluorene	60–70	21	2	9.5	4	19.0	7	0	0	33.3	61.8
4b			70–80	26	3	11.5	5	19.2	9	4	2	57.7	88.4
5a	Vancouver	2-Acetamidofluorene	60–70	22	2	9.1	1	4.5	6	2	0	36.4	50.0
5b		”	70–80	39	4	10.3	8	20.5	12	4	1	43.6	74.4
6a	Leeds	—	40–50	66	31	47.0	15	22.7	6	1	0	10.6	80.3
6b		—	70–80	56	17	30.4	13	23.2	11	4	0	26.8	80.4
6c		—	100–110	39	6	15.4	5	12.8	17	4[a]	0	53.8	82.0
7a	Leeds	1-Phenylazo-2-naphthol	40–50	60	14	23.3	10	16.7	14	6	0	33.3	73.3
7b		—	70–80	36	4	11.1	3	8.3	12	10	0	61.1	80.5
7c		—	100–110	26	0	0	2	7.7	3	12	8	88.5	96.2

[a] One with multiple liver metastases.

alone in control experiments, and 2-acetamidofluorene or its derivatives, N-hydroxyacetamidofluorene, 1-hydroxyacetamidofluorene, or 3-hydroxyacetamido-fluorene was incorporated into pellets of this wax at a concentration of 12.5% as previously described (2). For purposes of comparison similar wax pellets, as used in bladder implantation studies in Leeds, were used in some experiments. A known potent carcinogen by the bladder implantation method, 1-phenylazo-2-naphthol, incorporated into Leeds wax, was also used to give a high incidence of bladder tumours for the study of the emergence of the more advanced lesions. It was planned to terminate groups of mice carrying pellets of wax, with or without added chemicals, at different times after implantation, to see in what manner the hyperplastic changes progressed with time. In fact, groups of mice were killed during 40–50, 60–70, 70–80, and 80–100 weeks.

Pellets were implanted into the bladders of female $B6AF_1/J$ (Jackson Laboratory) mice by the modified method (1) of Jull (14), except that in most cases relaxation of the plain muscle of the bladder was achieved by topical application of a drop of 1% atropine sulphate in saline. Surgical trauma was much reduced thereby. The mice were killed at the times shown in Table I and their bladders processed for microscopical examination as described by Bonser and Jull (4). Those showing hyperplasia were assigned to one of the degrees of proliferative change described below. Where more than one type of proliferative change was present, the mouse was included only in the most advanced class. In some cases other tissues, suspected of containing metastases, were examined histologically. Classification of proliferative changes of the bladder epithelium was done according to the criteria illustrated by Bonser and Jull (4).

The following classifications were adopted depending on the extent of the lesion.

Hyperplasia: when downgrowth was limited to a few nests of cells.

Adenoma or papilloma: when downgrowths of epithelium formed a small nodule not considered to be malignant.

Carcinoma Grade I: tumours more advanced than adenomas and considered to be malignant, but not invading the underlying muscle of the bladder wall.

Grade II: those in which invasion of muscle could be demonstrated.

Grade III: those in which the tumour had completely penetrated the bladder wall.

Metastasis to a distant site was observed only once, in the liver of a mouse which was killed 110 weeks after implantation (Table I).

2. Results

The incidences of hyperplasia and tumours observed are shown in Table I. In group 1a, using pellets made in Vancouver, and group 6a, using paraffin pellets made in Leeds, the incidences of carcinomas of the bladder in mice killed between 40 and 50 weeks were 0 and 10.6%, respectively. These incidences would have been accepted as within the normal range of control groups of mice in previous work. It should be noted, however, that the incidences of hyperplasia and papilloma in mice implanted with Leeds wax were much greater than those in mice exposed to the wax used in Vancouver, although the specification and supplier were the same. Between 70 and 80 weeks the incidence of neoplasia rose sharply in mice exposed to either type of wax pellet. The carcinoma incidences in the Vancouver and Leeds wax groups were 33.3 and 26.8%, respectively, which is a significant increase compared to 40 to 50 weeks ($P<0.01$ and $P<0.05$) and is comparable to the differences observed between control groups and those exposed to chemicals accepted as carcinogenic as a result of the bladder implantation test. Mice implanted with Leeds wax and observed for 100 to 110 weeks showed a further significant rise in carcinoma incidence ($P< 0.01$).

Mice with bladder carcinoma were not included in the "hyperplasia" or "adenoma" columns, even though they invariably showed one of these conditions as well. The total number of mice showing some degree of hyperplastic change, from minimal to very advanced (carcinoma) in groups (6a, b, and c) implanted with the wax vehicle only, over the three time periods studied were, therefore, 80.3, 80.4, and 82.0%, respectively. It must be concluded that increases in the incidences of carcinoma took place, with time, in bladders which were already hyperplastic, suggesting that there is a continuity of change from initial hyperplasia to advanced carcinoma. The unique observation (group 6c) of an instance in which there were liver metastases from a bladder tumour illustrates that this ultimate criterion of malignant change can be achieved. These data reinforce the subjective impression gained from the microscopical examination of thousands of bladders in different stages of hyperplasia from many experiments, that the ultimate malignant nature of the epithelial changes is a progressive development from the initial hyperplastic downgrowths which can be detected at a very early stage.

The incidence of carcinomas in group 7a at 40–50 weeks with pellets containing 1-phenylazo-2-naphthol was significantly higher than the control incidence with wax only (group 6a, $P<0.01$). This conforms to previous findings (8) that this compound is a potent bladder carcinogen when implanted into the lumen of the bladder in pellet form. Similarly, the incidences of tumours at 70–80 weeks and at 100–110 weeks, with 1-phenylazo-2-naphthol, were significantly higher than the controls at the corresponding time periods. Despite the differences in carcinoma incidence which can be demonstrated between the chemical-containing pellets of group 7 and the plain vehicle of group 6, however, the total number of mice in group 7a, b, and c, which showed hyperplasia at different times (73.3, 80.5, and 96.2%) were not different from the percentages of mice in groups with plain wax (6a, b, and c), which had hyperplasia or more advanced lesions. An unprejudiced assessment of the results in these two groups suggests, therefore, that the changes induced by the pellets containing the added chemical were qualitatively similar to those induced by the plain wax pellets, but proceeded at a faster rate in the presence of the chemical.

3. Conclusions from these experiments

The basic concepts implicit in the development of bladder implantation as a routine assay for the detection of carcinogenic activity have been concisely expressed by Clayson and Cooper (8), who suggest that the chemical is required to bring about conversion of normal epithelial cells to latent tumour cells, and the presence of the pellet provides the proliferative stimulus which causes development of the latent tumour cells to overt neoplasia.

An alternative concept which arises from the new results presented above is that tumorigenesis in implanted mouse bladders occurs as a result of protracted stimulation of proliferation, which can be provided by the pellet alone over a sufficient period, but is significantly accentuated by the addition of irritative or toxic substances to the vehicle. It seems reasonable to postulate that when implanted in a solid vehicle in the bladder lumen, added chemicals achieve a more intimate association with the epithelium over a more protracted period than can be achieved by systemic administration. Arguments against the idea that the wax vehicle or other foreign objects such as glass beads implanted in the bladder have low amounts of a carcinogenic initiator have been presented by Clayson et al. (9). The fact that 0.05 or 0.5% of methylcholanthrene in paraffin wax pellets did not cause a significant increase in the incidence of carcinomas above that seen with the control wax alone indicates that even relatively high amounts of a carcinogen of unquestionable potency in the pellet vehicle does not enhance its tumourigenicity.

The experiments of groups 2, 3, 4, and 5 failed in their primary objective, which was to demonstrate differences in carcinogenic potency between 2-acetamidofluorene and its metabolites when applied locally to the bladder epithelium. There was no difference in the incidence of carcinomas present between 60 and 70 weeks whether the compound in the pellet was 1-hydroxyacetamidofluorene, 3-hydroxyacetamidofluorene, or the parent amine. At 70–80 weeks the incidences of carcinoma with these three compounds and with N-hydroxyacetamidofluorene were virtually the same. No conclusions can be drawn from the small number of mice observed between 40 and 50 weeks with the latter compound, but the limited observations do not suggest potent local carcinogenic activity. These results of bladder implantation are in sharp contrast to the extensive evidence that the tumourigenic activity of 2-acetamidofluorene is expressed through an N-hydroxy metabolite (15). There is no other evidence than that presented here that either 1-hydroxy- or 3-hydroxyacetamidofluorene has local tumourigenic activity.

Significance of Bladder Implantation Results

The validity and utility of results obtained by bladder implantation, in testing compounds for carcinogenic activity, have been favourably assessed by Clayson et al. (7), Bryan (5), and by Clayson and Cooper (8). Doubts have been expressed, however, by Irving et al. (13) and more recently by Price (17).

The new results described above constitute an additional major paradox which must be explained. A ready solution could be that the strain of mice used (B6AF$_1$) have unusually high concentrations of an endogenous urinary metabolite, which with the additional stimulus of a foreign body in the bladder lumen precipitates a high incidence of epithelial hyperplasia and tumours. The experiments of Bryan and Springberge (6) lend weight to this possibility. They showed that the subcutaneous (s.c.) injection of 1 mg of xanthurenic acid 8-methyl ether three times weekly induced carcinomas in 30% of 38 mice which had bladder implants of cholesterol pellets, but induced no lesions in the bladders of mice which did not have pellets. In their experiments cholesterol pellets alone in the bladder gave rise to carcinomas in 8% of 294 mice. $B6AF_1$ mice are genetically standardised and commercially available in large numbers, so that it would be possible to investigate in them the role of a strain-variable, carcinogenic, urinary factor.

It seems equally likely, however, that the development of bladder tumours and hyperplasia in the experiments presented above is a consequence of protracted stimulation by the pellet. Where the incidence of neoplasia is increased by the addition of chemicals to the pellet, it seems simplest to suppose that the action of the chemical is to increase the effective stimulation of hyperplasia in the bladder epithelium. The ability of substances, for which there is no other evidence of carcinogenic activity, to increase the incidence of tumours induced by pellet implantation suggests that it is some general property of the compounds, such as toxicity, and not a specific cancer-initiating action which is responsible for this.

In view of the considerations referred to above, bladder implantation results alone cannot be accepted as assays of the carcinogenic activity of chemicals. An explanation must still be offered, however, for the undoubtable fact that pellet implantation into the bladder, with or without added chemicals, is followed in sufficient time by a high incidence of carcinoma. The histological findings of the present study leave no doubt that the lesions induced by this method are malignant. Wax pellets alone were markedly carcinogenic, underlining the lack of necessity for specific chemicals in the implanted body.

The idea that chemical carcinogenesis follows a pattern of initiation and promotion in tissues other than the skin is one which is often accepted as axiomatic. It seems, however, that a concept of carcinogenesis which postulates that cancer is the result of protracted hyperstimulation is perhaps more tenable. The question is whether a chemical interaction by the "carcinogenic agent" with a specific cellular constituent to form a "latent tumour cell," is in fact a necessary step in tumour induction. Alternative interpretations of a variety of forms of cancer induction, which offer plausible explanations for the involvement of chemicals in the initial stages, have been put forward in detail by Poel (16). The wider application of these ideas might resolve many of the difficulties in the interpretation of chemical carcinogenesis. In particular the role of the chemical in bladder implantation tumourigenesis might be regarded as simply the action of a non-specific toxin whose action is to destroy successive layers of cells, with which it comes into contact. A continuous loss of epithelial cells, due to the protracted presence of the chemical, would be expected to result in stimulation of cellular replication in the basal cells. The consequent chronic hyperplasia might be expected to increase the possibility of neoplasia.

Observations on Rats

Shortly after the initial experiments with bladder implants in mice, it was found in rats (*3*) that the implantation of wax pellets alone caused hyperplasia and papilloma formation in the bladders of all of 7 rats surviving more than 10 weeks and in 5 of 8 rats implanted with pellets of wax containing 2-amino-1-naphthol hydrochloride.

The photomicrographs and descriptions of the bladder lesions in these rats are suggestive of the changes which have been seen frequently in much larger numbers of mice implanted with pellets of various kinds, and which in mice are considered to be the immediate precursors of infiltrating carcinoma. Bonser *et al.* (*3*) in fact suggested that the presence of metaplasia and tumours in the bladders of the rats appeared to be related to the presence of a foreign body, rather than to the presence of a carcinogenic chemical.

The significant suggestion was also made (*3*) that the concretions present in the bladders of rats treated with estrogens (*11, 12*) might be the responsible agents for the occurrence of bladder carcinomas in animals so treated. In more recent work bladder cancers have been found in rats treated with high doses of cyclamate (*10*), but in all the treated rats the initial changes were extensive stone formation and calcification throughout the urinary tract. Bladder stones were present in all animals which had malignant epithelial tumours. In this experiment also the stones in the bladder could have been the precipitating agents for tumour formation.

CONCLUSIONS

The possibility that carcinoma of the bladder can be induced in experimental animals by the presence of only a foreign body in the bladder lumen without an additional chemical stimulus, is supported by the following evidence:

a)   Cancer induction in mouse bladders by the implantation of pellets made from a variety of otherwise innocuous substances.

b)   The evidence presented above that in the mouse bladder, cancer incidence increases progressively with the time of exposure to wax pellets alone, as well as with pellets containing incorporated chemicals.

c)   The demonstration that wax pellets alone induce advanced hyperplastic lesions in the bladders of rats.

d)   The presence of cancer in the bladders of rats containing concretions induced by estrogen administration.

e)   The presence of cancer in the bladders of rats containing concretions induced by cyclamate administration.

It does not seem justified, therefore, to use the incidence of bladder tumours induced in mice by pellets containing an added chemical as an index of the carcinogenic activity of that chemical in the conventional sense. It is established, however, that the tumours induced by bladder implantation frequently proceed to malignancy, and the histological interpretations which have been accepted appear to be valid.

The mechanisms involved in carcinogenesis by chemicals with this technique do not seem to be parallel to their mode of action in other systems.

Acknowledgments

I wish to thank Dr. D. B. Clayson for his cooperation in supplying the Leeds wax and 1-phenylazo-2-naphthol pellets, Dr. J. Miller for his gift of the 2-acetamido-fluorene and its metabolites, and Dr. T. Lloyd Fletcher who prepared the 1-hydroxy- and 3-hydroxy-2-acetamidofluorenes. This work was supported by the National Cancer Institute of Canada.

REFERENCES

1. Allen, M. J., Boyland, E., Dukes, C. E., Horning, E. S., and Watson, J. G. Cancer of the urinary bladder induced in mice with metabolites of aromatic amines and tryptophan. *Brit. J. Cancer*, **11**, 212–228 (1957).
2. Bonser, G. M., Bradshaw, L., Clayson, D. B., and Jull, J. W. A further study of the carcinogenic properties of orthohydroxyamines and related compounds by bladder implantation in the mouse. *Brit. J. Cancer*, **10**, 539–546 (1956).
3. Bonser, G. M., Clayson, D. B., Jull, J. W., and Pyrah, L. N. The induction of tumours of the bladder epithelium in rats by the implantation of paraffin wax pellets. *Brit. J. Cancer*, **7**, 456–459 (1953).
4. Bonser, G. M. and Jull, J. W. The histological changes in the mouse bladder following surgical implantation of paraffin wax pellets containing various chemicals. *J. Pathol. Bacteriol.*, **12**, 489–495 (1956).
5. Bryan, G. T. Pellet implantation studies of carcinogenic compounds. *J. Natl. Cancer Inst.*, **43**, 255–261 (1969).
6. Bryan, G. T. and Springberg, P. D. Role of the vehicle in the genesis of bladder carcinomas in mice by the pellet implantation technique. *Cancer Res.*, **26**, 105–109 (1966).
7. Clayson, D. B., Jull, J. W., and Bonser, G. M. The testing of orthohydroxyamines and related compounds by bladder implantation and a discussion of their structural requirements for carcinogenic activity. *Brit. J. Cancer*, **12**, 222–230 (1958).
8. Clayson, D. B. and Cooper, E. H. Cancer of the urinary tract. *Recent Adv. Cancer Res.*, **13**, 271–381 (1970).
9. Clayson, D. B., Pringle, J. A. S., Bonser, G. M., and Wood, M. The technique of bladder implantation: Further results and assessment. *Brit. J. Cancer*, **22**, 825–832 (1968).
10. Friedman, L., Richardson, H. L., Lethco, E. J., Wallace, W. C., and Sauro, F. M. Toxic response of rats to cyclamates in chow and semisynthetic diets. *J. Natl. Cancer Inst.*, **49**, 751–764 (1972).
11. Dunning, W. F., Curtis, M. R., and Segaloff, A. Strain differences in response to diethylstilbestrol and the induction of mammary gland and bladder cancer in the rat. *Cancer Res.*, **7**, 511–521 (1947).
12. Dunning, W. F., Curtis, M. R., and Segaloff, A. Strain differences in response to estrone and the induction of mammary gland, adrenal and bladder cancer in rats. *Cancer Res.*, **13**, 147–152 (1953).
13. Irving, C. C., Gutman, H. R., and Larson, D. M. Evaluation of the carcinogenicity of aminofluorenols by implantation into the bladder of the mouse. *Cancer Res.*, **23**, 1782–1791 (1963).

14. Jull, J. W. The induction of tumours of the bladder epithelium in mice by the direct application of a carcinogen. *Brit. J. Cancer*, **5**, 328–330 (1951).

15. Miller, J. A. Carcinogenesis by chemicals: An overview—G.H.A. Clowes Memorial Lecture. *Cancer*, **30**, 559–576 (1970).

16. Poel, W. E. The cause and nature of cancer. *Prog. Exp. Tumor Res.*, **5**, 53–84 (1964).

17. Price, J. M. Etiology of bladder cancer. *In* "Benign and Malignant Tumours of the Urinary Bladder," ed. by E. Maltry, Jr., Medical Examination Publ. Co., New York (1971).

18. Roe, F. J. C. An illustrated classification of the proliferative and neoplastic changes in mouse bladder epithelium in response to prolonged irritation. *Brit. J. Urol.*, **36**, 238–253 (1964).

GANN Monograph on Cancer Research 17, 393–403 (1975)

CHROMATID REARRANGEMENT AND CARCINOGENESIS[*1]

Taketoshi Sugiyama

Department of Pathology, Kobe University School of Medicine[*2]

The results obtained in the cytogenetic studies on aromatic hydrocarbon-induced rat leukemia with specific chromosomal abnormalities are reviewed. The chemicals induce non-random chromatid breakage in the late DNA-replicating heterochromatic regions. The chromosomal abnormalities in the leukemia are induced in relation to the heterochromatic regions. The essential underlying change has been suggested to be crossing-over of parent DNA strands in these regions. Based on these facts and on the relationship between chromatid breakage and carcinogenesis and between heterochromatin and nucleoli, a hypothesis is presented that cancer is a disease of gene dosage possibly with increased nucleolar cistrons brought by asymmetric crossing-over of the DNA strands in the specific chromosomal regions. The hypothesis explains various aspects of cancers induced by chemicals, viruses, and radiations as well.

A large body of informations has been obtained about the molecular interaction between chemical carcinogens and cellular macromolecules (*1*). Since the growth characteristic is usually altered in cancer cells, the essential change may be in the genes concerned with cell growth and reproduction. However, because of the complex genetic constitution of eukaryotic cells, the problems of carcinogen target remain to be resolved. On the other hand, recent cytogenetic studies have shown a significant relationship between the chromosome-damaging capacity of chemicals, viruses, and radiations and their carcinogenicity. Some investigators regard this as a common pathway to cancer cells (*25*), although no direct relationship between the acute effect and the genome change in cancer cells has been established.

Recent works on aromatic hydrocarbon-induced rat leukemia with specific chromosomal abnormalities reviewed below suggest that chromatid rearrangements play a role in carcinogenesis.

Chromosomal Abnormalities in Chemically Induced Rat Leukemia

In 1967, the present author reported the presence of highly consistent chromosomal abnormalities in primary erythroblastic leukemia induced in Long-

[*1] This work was supported by a Grant-in-Aid for Scientific Research from the Ministry of Education of Japan.

[*2] Kusunoki-cho 7-12, Ikuta-ku, Kobe 650, Japan (杉山武敏).

Evans (LE) rats by pulse injection of 7,12-dimethylbenz(a)anthracene (DMBA) (*32*). Almost half of the leukemias had trisomy of the largest telocentric chromosome (No. 2, according to the internationally proposed nomenclature for rat chromosome (*16*)), or C-1 (*32*) (Photo 1) in the predominant leukemia stemline or sidelines (*19, 20*). Partial duplication of No. 2 chromosome (Long No. 2, Long C-1) (Photo 2) was also found in some leukemias. They were also found

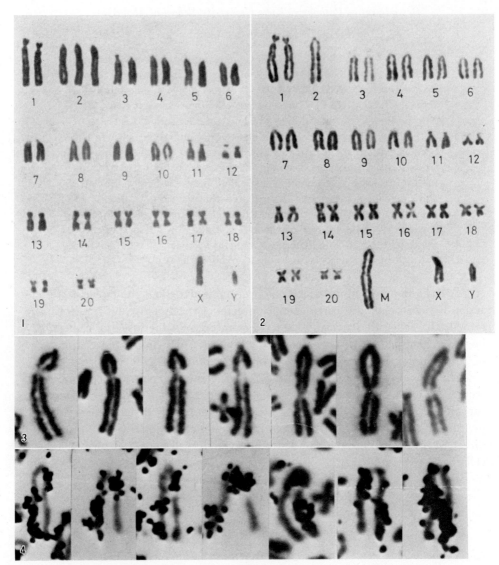

PHOTO 1.   No. 2 trisomy
PHOTO 2.   Long No. 2
PHOTO 3.   Chiasma and breaks localizing in two chromosomal regions of No. 2 chromosome
PHOTO 4.   Autoradiographically   demonstrated   chromatid   exchange   in   the specifically vulnerable regions of No. 2 chromosome
Some are accompanied with a break or a gap (see text and Ref. *35*).

TABLE I. Classification of Rat Leukemia According to the Predominant Stemline

	DMBA	6,8,12-TMBA	7,8,12-TMBA	Total
No. 2 trisomy	38 (2)[a]	0	27	65
Long No. 2	3	1	5	9
Other changes	16	0	13	29
Normal karyotype	70 (6)	1	84	155
Total	127 (8)	2	129	258

[a] Figure in parentheses indicates leukemias in Sprague-Dawley rats.

in leukemias induced by 6,8,12- and 7,8,12-trimethylbenz(a)anthracene (TMBA) (34). The leukemias in Sprague-Dawley (Table I) and Wistar rats (9) as well as in a different colony of LE rats (29) showed similar chromosomal changes. The same changes were also found in DMBA-induced rat fibrosarcoma (23) and N-butylnitrosourea (BNU)-induced rat leukemia in LE rats (Uenaka, Ueda, and Sugiyama, unpublished). Thus No. 2 abnormalities were shown to be rather a general change. Table I shows classification of 258 leukemias in LE rats induced by these three hydrocarbon carcinogens. Although No. 2 abnormalities appeared reproducibly, a considerable number of leukemias had normal karyotype. Therefore, the duplication of No. 2 chromatid itself is not a primary requisite for leukemic change. Some phenotypic differences between No. 2 trisomy and normal karyotype leukemia were demonstrated (33).

Detailed karyotype analysis showed 5 translocation types of No. 2 trisomy. They consisted of No. 2 chromosome fused with long arm of Nos. 1, 2, 9?, 12, and 13 at the centromeric or telomeric regions. Other chromosomal abnormalities in Table I represent various markers and aneuploidy involving Nos. 1, 3, 9?, 11, 13, and 19 chromosomes. They were also involved in additional changes of No. 2 trisomic cells (20, 34).

In summary, certain chromosomes were more frequently involved in chromosomal changes than the rest of chromosomes. Since they contained late-replicating DNA as a common property, the late-replicating DNA seemed to play a role in the origin of the above chromosomal abnormalities (35).

Chromatid Rearrangement as a Result of Carcinogen Action

Single intravenous pulse injection of lipid emulsion of DMBA given to 26-day-old male rats (50 mg/kg body weight) damages the chromosomes of the bone marrow cells (21). Aberrant metaphase cells rise within 3 hr, reach the maximum level at 18 hr, and decrease thereafter. The distribution of breaks and gaps among and within chromosomes is non-random and time-dependent; No. 2 chromosome is especially vulnerable to DMBA in the late S phase at least in 2 chromatid regions. Chiasma-like interactions between sister chromatids are observed in the same regions often associated with a break and a gap (Photo 3), suggesting a role in breakage formation. Therefore, the incidence of sister chro-

TABLE II. Incidence of Sister Chromatid Exchange Revealed by Autoradiography in the Bone Marrow Cells in Rats Treated with DMBA and in Control Animals (34)

	Control	DMBA	Difference
Cells with exchanges	23.7%	46.5%	$P<0.01$
Exchanges in No. 2	5.0	16.9	$P<0.001$
Exchanges in No. 1	5.8	6.3	—
Exchanges in No. 3	1.1	1.6	—
Exchanges in other chromosomes	0.08	0.33	$P<0.02$

TABLE III. Incidence of Chromatid Breakage in the Bone Marrow Cells after Treatment with ^{3}H-Thymidine and Non-labeled Thymidine

Time (hr)	Treatment		Aberrant metaphases (%)
0	None		1.8
6	^{3}H-Thymidine	75 μCi	4.5
	"	125	7.5
	"	250	8.5
	Thymidine[a]		1.8
15	^{3}H-Thymidine	125	10.0
	Thymidine[a]		1.8
24	^{3}H-Thymidine	125	12.5
	Thymidine[a]		1.8

[a] Non-labeled thymidine, equivalent amount to 125 μCi (specific activity of 3.0 mCi/μmole).

matid exchange (crossing-over) in the above regions before and after DMBA treatment was examined autoradiographically by Taylor's technique (39). Although some sister chromatid exchanges were induced in the absence of DMBA, the incidence was significantly higher after DMBA treatment (35) (Table II, Photo 4). Since ^{3}H-thymidine used for labeling chromatids induces chromatid breaks in a considerable frequency while cold thymidine did not (Table III), the present author considers that the sister chromatid exchanges in the control group may have been induced by radioactivity of thymidine. It is worth of note that other leukemogens such as TMBA, urethan, and BNU, induce sister chromatid exchange localizing in the same chromosomal regions (Sugiyama, unpublished).

On the other hand, the target regions for the chromatid exchange were shown to replicate DNA in the late S phase, therefore, heterochromatic (35). The vulnerability of the heterochromatic regions in plant and animal cells has long been recognized (8, 18). The involvement of heterochromatin in interchromosomal exchange has been indicated (4, 24). Quinacrine fluorescence analysis of two types of Long No. 2 chromatid revealed a partial chromatid duplication formed by the exchange at the vulnerable regions (Sugiyama, unpublished). Therefore, it is likely that carcinogenic chemicals rearrange chromatids and induce various chromosome abnormalities by acting on the heterochromatic regions.

Parallelism between Chromatid Rearrangement and Carcinogenesis

From the above findings, the present author supposes that chromatid rearrangement plays a role in carcinogenesis. This view is consistent with Nichols' view that single breaks with chemicals, viruses, and radiations are a common pathway to cancer (*25*). The bone marrow cells in a plethoric rat become sensitive to the chromosome-breaking action of DMBA by previous injection of sheep erythropoietin. The incidence of leukemia in the animals made anemic before each DMBA treatment is high and the incidence in the animals made plethoric is low (*36*). In other words, the hormone-induced enhancement of chromatid breaks is reflected by enhanced leukemogenesis. In another experiment, the chromosome-breaking capacity of various benz(a)anthracene derivatives parallels with their carcinogenicity (*37*) (Fig. 1). Both results support the view that chromatid rearrangement underlying breaks is related to carcinogenesis.

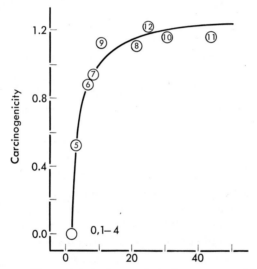

FIG. 1.   The relationship between the chromosome-breaking capacity and the carcinogenicity of various benz(a)anthracene (BA) derivatives (*37*)

Carcinogenicity: incidence of sarcomas (in %) following intramuscular injection of 5 mg of samples dissolved in sesame oil to mean latent period (days). Chromosome damage: aberrant metaphases (%) 12–24 hr after intravenous injection of 50 mg/kg body weight in lipid emulsion. 0, control; 1, BA; 2, 7,12-diethyl-BA; 3, 7-ethyl-BA; 4, 12-ethyl-BA; 5, 12-ethyl-7-methyl-BA; 6, 6,7,12-TMBA; 7, 3-methylcholanthrene; 8, 7-ethyl-12-methyl-BA; 9, 3,4-benzopyrene; 10, 6,8,12-TMBA; 11, DMBA; 12, 7,8,12-TMBA.

Cancer, a Disease of Nucleolar Gene Dosage?

The target DNA for carcinogens, heterochromatin, has been shown to be localized in several specific chromosomal regions such as centromere, telomere, and the nucleolar regions. It consists of reiterated base sequences different from

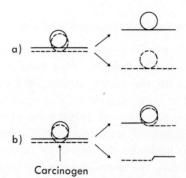

FIG. 2. (a) Symmetric division of the genes in normal mitosis, and (b) carcinogen-induced asymmetric division of the genes in the target region

the main nuclear DNA and therefore sediments as satellite DNA. Various roles in cell function are supposed. It protects vital areas such as nucleolar regions from mechanical stress and mutation, providing spacer DNA for nucleolar cistrons (6, 42).

From the above relationship between heterochromatin and nucleoli, the present author considers that the target regions contain nucleolar cistrons and that the chromatid rearrangement in these regions results in rearrangement of nucleolar cistrons. Asymmetric exchange between two nucleolar regions in the sister DNA strands or in different chromosomes produces two daughter cells with different amount of nucleolar cistrons rather than with a gene mutation. Although Revell (30) did not mention the nature of the target for exchange, his exchange hypothesis obviously implies the asymmetric nature of the exchange. As shown in Fig. 2, a DNA segment containing nucleolar cistrons, indicated by a loop, moves from one parent DNA strand to another after DMBA treatment. Consequently, after cell division, nucleolar cistrons become increased in one daughter cell at the expense in another. This could be a fairly possible mechanism of inducing gene unbalance in eukaryotic cells, since only certain genes are increased without a proportional gain of others. The exchange may take place between any two nucleolar regions present in different chromosomes but closely organized in an interphase nucleolus. Some exchange may form a marker chromosome through reciprocal translocation. No visible change results if the loop is small and the exchange occurs between sister chromatids. Aneuploidy, probably the result of nondisjunction and nucleolar persistence frequently observed after chemical treatment, may be brought by delayed separation of the affected regions. Markers and aneuploidy are induced *in vitro* 24–48 hr after carcinogen treatment during transformation process (2) and frequently observed in natural and induced cancers (28). Essential is not a chromosomal change but unequal division of nucleolar cistrons into 2 daughter cells.

The above hypothesis that cancer is a gene-dosage disease is based on the following additional facts and speculations. (1) In 1906, Boveri (3) proposed a chromosome-balance concept of malignant tumors. Yosida (41) proposed a similar concept on the progression of tumor cell stemlines. The drawback of Boveri's hypothesis, a fact that not all cancers have visible chromosomal abnormalities,

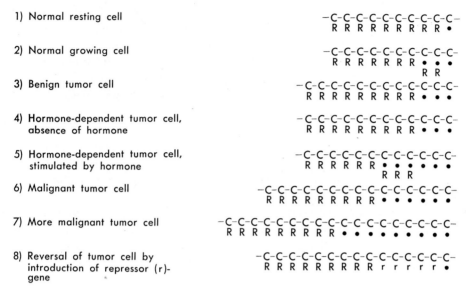

FIG. 3. A hypothetical scheme showing relationship between gene-dosage abnormality and nucleolar transcriptive activity in various growth states

C, nucleolar cistrons; R, repressor; ●, nucleolar cistrons being transcribed.

has been overcome in the present hypothesis. (2) There are various grades in malignancy of tumors, from normal to malignant and from malignant to highly malignant. Sudden or gradual change of malignancy is often observed in clinics as well as in experimental tumors. The alteration of malignancy is often accompanied by a chromosomal change and hard to explain by gene mutation theory. The present gene-dosage concept solves this problem (Fig. 3). Hormone dependency may be explained similarly; a hormone-dependent prostate cancer behaves as a normal tissue in the absence of a de-repressor of nucleolar cistrons, testosterone. It may become independent by additional gain of nucleolar cistrons. (3) Despite the extensive biochemical studies, no definite gene mutation has been detected in cancers. The only change found is a deviated metabolic flow similar to that of regenerating and embryonic tissues (*40*). Tumor cells can be reverted by the action of cyclic AMP and feeder layer factors (*14, 15*). Therefore the genes involved in cell differentiation are not defective in cancer cells. (4) The fact that cell fusion reverts the transformed cells (*12*) suggests that the excess genes in cancer cells can be rebalanced by introduction of repressor genes or chromosomes from outside as human rRNA cistrons are repressed by introduction of mouse chromosomes (*7*) (Fig. 3). (5) There is increasing evidence of chromosome rearrangement in cancer cells. The Philadelphia chromosome was recently shown to be a G22 chromosome of which the deleted part of the long arm was translocated to the long arm of a C9 chromosome (*31*). The cultured and biopsied cells from Burkitt lymphoma revealed a consistent presence of extra marker band in a D14 chromosome, an evidence of chromatid rearrangement in virus-induced tumors (*22*). (6) Most chemical carcinogens interact with DNA by alkylating guanine and other bases. Similar alteration of DNA bases occur after irradiation. Two repair mechanisms, excision and recombination, remove the altered bases. Recent studies on xeroderma pigmentosum suggest that the latter is the main mechanism involved in UV carcinogenesis (*38*). The recombination repair results in crossing-over of parent DNA strands as supposed in the present hypothesis. (7) The hypothesis regards carcinogenesis with chemicals, viruses, and radiation as a common process. The chromosome-breaking capacity of oncogenic viruses such as Rous, SV40, polyoma, and adenoviruses, has been indicated (*25*). Non-random distribution of virus-induced chromatid breaks in secondary constrictions with nucleolar heterochromatin has been indicated (*17*). In virus-infected cells, natural or reversely transcribed viral DNA are integrated into the host DNA. Various enzymes such as endonuclease, DNA polymerase, and ligase present in the viruses are involved in this process. Chromatid exchange may occur when two closely located parent DNA strands are individually integrated by viral DNA and misjoined. Since chromatid exchange is a 2-hit phenomenon (*30*), chemical carcinogens and ionizing radiations help this process by raising the chance of DNA strand scission (cocarcinogenesis). The chemically induced enhancement of virus-induced chromosome breakage (*27*) supports this view. (8) For cell transformation, cells must go through at least one mitotic phase, as well recognized in chemical, viral, and radiation carcinogenesis, probably because the gene-dosage abnormality is established during mitosis.

The present author assumes that the cells with large nucleoli with prominent RNA synthetic activity cannot differentiate and always tend to proliferate. Since the nucleolar predominance is inherited from a cell to the progeny cells, the clonal growth continues until the host becomes unable to supply nutrition. In this meaning, a cancer cell is a mutant cell *de novo* produced from a somatic cell by abnormal cell division and behaves wildly in a well-controlled cell society. The process is comparable to a mutant evolution in animal populations in which asymmetric crossing-over and chromatid rearrangement during meiosis in germ cells play an important role (*26*). The gene amplification in oocytes (*5*) is different from the above-suggested gene unbalance of cancer cells in that the former is a normal process carefully controlled.

Most chemical carcinogens induce mutation and malformation in variety of organisms. Obviously, the alteration of DNA bases leads to these phenomena. Some malformations are caused by aneuploidy in germ cells (see D18 trisomy syndrome), whereas others are induced by the action of chemicals, viruses, and radiations on developing embryos. From the evident association of aneuploidy and malformation in the former, it is possible that the gene-dosage problems such as aneuploidy and chromatid rearrangement are also involved in the latter cases. This may explain why certain neoplasms have their origin in tissue malformation.

Measurement of the amount of nucleolar cistrons (rDNA) in cancer cells has rarely been performed. Higashi *et al.* (*13*) measured the amount of rRNA hybridizable to the nuclear DNA from Ehrlich ascites tumor and normal liver cells and found no difference. However, some important problems seem to lie in evaluation of rDNA of the somatic tissues; since rDNA appears to replicate late in the S phase (*10, 11,* and Kano *et al.,* unpublished), the value for rDNA in tumors rich in the S-phase cells and the S-phase death must be considerably lower than that of the normal liver where the majority of the cells are in the G_1 phase and have a complete set of rDNA. Actually our measurement in growing embryos shows a considerably lower rDNA value than the normal liver in the rat. Careful determination of rDNA in various tumors is now in progress in our laboratory.

Acknowledgment

The author thanks late Dr. Tomizo Yoshida, and Dr. Kaneyoshi Akazaki and Dr. Yasuaki Nishizuka of Aichi Cancer Center Research Institute, and Professor Charles Huggins of University of Chicago for valuable suggestions, help, and encouragement.

Note Added in Proof

The present concept of carcinogenesis has been described in *Proc. Japan. Cancer Assoc., 29th and 31st Annu. Meet. (1970, 1972),* and in *Igaku-no-Ayumi (The Stride of Medicine),* **84,** 812–819 (1973). Another gene-dosage concept of cancer has been proposed by A. Gaudin (*J. Theor. Biol.,* **41,** 191–200 (1973)).

REFERENCES

1. Arcos, J. C. and Argus, M. P. Molecular geometry and carcinogenic activity of aromatic compounds. New perspectives. *Adv. Cancer Res.,* **11,** 305–504 (1968).
2. Benedict, W. F. Early changes in chromosomal number and structure after treatment of fetal hamster cultures with transforming doses of polycyclic hydrocarbons. *J. Natl. Cancer Inst.,* **49,** 585–590 (1972).
3. Boveri, T. "The Origin of Malignant Tumors, Jena (1914)," Williams & Wilkins, Baltimore (1929).
4. Brøgger, A. and Johansen, J. A model for the production of chromosome damage by Mitomycin C. *Chromosoma,* **38,** 95–104 (1972).
5. Brown, D. D. and David, I. B. Specific gene amplification in oocytes. *Science,* **160,** 272–280 (1968).
6. Brown, S. W. Heterochromatin. *Science,* **151,** 417–425 (1966).
7. Eliceiri, G. L. and Green, H. J. Ribosomal RNA synthesis in human-mouse hybrid cells. *J. Mol. Biol.,* **41,** 253–260 (1969).
8. Evans, H. J. and Bigger, T. R. L. Chromosome aberrations induced by ionizing radiations. *Int. Rev. Cytol.,* **13,** 221–322 (1962).
9. Fichidzhyan, V. S. and Pogoyants, E. E. Chromosomal characteristics of three transplantable leukemias of rats. *Vopr. Onkol.,* **9,** 47 (1963); *Fed. Proc.,* **23,** T1018–1020 (1964) (English translation).
10. Giacomoni, D. and Finkel, D. Time of duplication of ribosomal cistrons in a cell line of *Potorous tridactylis* (rat kangaroo). *J. Mol. Biol.,* **70,** 725–728 (1972).
11. Guttes, E. and Guttes, S. Replication of nucleolus-associated DNA during "G_2 phase" in *Physarum polycephalum. J. Cell Biol.,* **43,** 229–236 (1969).
12. Harris, H., Miller, O. J., Klein, G., Worst, P., and Tachibana, O. Suppression of malignancy by cell fusion. *Nature,* **223,** 363–368 (1969).
13. Higashi, K., Kuragano, T., Hanasaki, N., Matsuhisa, T., and Sakamoto, Y. Distribution of ribosomal cistrons in the nuclei of Ehrlich ascites tumor and hepatic cells from mice. *Cancer Res.,* **33,** 734–738 (1973).

14. Hsie, A. W. and Puck, T. T. Morphological transformation of Chinese hamster cells by dibutyryladenosine cyclic 3', 5'-monophosphate and testosterone. *Proc. Natl. Acad. Sci. U.S.*, **68**, 358–361 (1971).

15. Ichikawa, Y. Differentiation of leukemic myeloblasts. *GANN Monograph on Cancer Research*, **12**, 215–230 (1972).

16. International Committee for a Standardized Karyotype of *Rattus norvegicus*. Standard karyotype of the Norway rat, *Rattus norvegicus. Cytogenet. Cell Genet.*, **12**, 199–205 (1973).

17. Kato, R. Localization of "spontaneous" and Rous sarcoma virus-induced breakage in specific regions of the chromosomes of the Chinese hamster. *Hereditas*, **58**, 240–245 (1967).

18. Kihlman, B. A. "Actions of Chemicals on Dividing Cells," Prentice-Hall, Inc., Englewood Cliffs, N. J. (1966).

19. Kurita, Y., Sugiyama, T., and Nishizuka, Y. Cytogenetic studies on rat leukemia induced by pulse-doses of 7, 12-dimethylbenz(a)anthracene. *Cancer Res.*, **28**, 1738–1752 (1968).

20. Kurita, Y., Sugiyama, T., and Nishizuka, Y. Cytogenetic analysis of cell population in rat leukemia induced by pulse-doses of 7,12-dimethylbenz(a)anthracene. *Gann*, **60**, 529–535 (1969).

21. Kurita, Y., Sugiyama, T., and Nishizuka, Y. Chromosome aberration induced in rat bone marrow cells by 7,12-dimethylbenz(a)anthracene. *J. Natl. Cancer Inst.*, **43**, 635–641 (1969).

22. Manolov, G. and Manolova, Y. Marker band in one chromosome 14 from Burkitt lymphomas. *Nature*, **237**, 33–34 (1972).

23. Mitelman, F., Mark, J., Levan, G., and Levan, A. Tumor etiology and chromosome pattern. *Science*, **176**, 1340–1341 (1972).

24. Natarajan, A. T. and Ahnström, G. Heterochromatin and chromosome aberrations. *Chromosoma*, **28**, 48–61 (1969).

25. Nichols, W. W. Chromosome abnormalities and carcinogenesis. *In* "Handbook of Molecular Cytology," ed. by A. Lima-de-Faria, Elsevier, Amsterdam/London, pp. 732–750 (1969).

26. Ohno, S. "Evolution by Gene Duplication," Springer-Verlag, New York/Heidelberg/Berlin (1970).

27. O'Neill, F. J. and Rapp, F. Synergic effect of herpes simplex virus and cytosine arabinoside on human chromosomes. *J. Virol.*, **7**, 692–695 (1971).

28. Porter, I. H., Benedict, W. F., Brown, C. D., and Paul, B. Recent advances in molecular pathology: A review. Some aspects in chromosome changes in cancer. *Exp. Mol. Pathol.*, **11**, 340–367 (1969).

29. Rees, E. D., Majumdar, S. K., and Shuck, A. Changes in chromosomes of bone marrow cells after intravenous injections of 7,12–dimethylbenz(a)anthracene and related compounds. *Proc. Natl. Acad. Sci. U.S.*, **66**, 1228–1235 (1970).

30. Revell, S. H. A new hypothesis for "chromatid" exchanges. *In* "Radiobiology Symposium, Liége, 1954," ed. by Z. M. Bacq and P. Alexander, Butterworth Scientific Publ., London (1955).

31. Rowley, J. D. A new consistent chromosomal abnormality in chronic myelogenous leukemia identified by quinacrine fluorescence and Giemsa staining. *Nature*, **243**, 290–293 (1973).

32. Sugiyama, T., Kurita, Y., and Nishizuka, Y. Chromosomal abnormalities in rat leukemia induced by 7,12-dimethylbenz(a)anthracene. *Science*, **159**, 1058–1059 (1967).

33. Sugiyama, T., Kurita, Y., and Nishizuka, Y. Biologic studies on 7,12-dimethyl-benz(a)anthracene-induced rat leukemia with special reference to the specific chromosomal abnormalities. *Cancer Res.*, **29**, 1117–1124 (1969).

34. Sugiyama, T. and Brillantes, F. Cytogenetic studies of leukemia induced by 6, 8,12- and 7,8,12-trimethylbenz(a)anthracene. *J. Exp. Med.*, **131**, 331–341 (1970).

35. Sugiyama, T. Specific vulnerability of the largest telocentric chromosome of rat bone marrow cells to 7,12-dimethylbenz(a)anthracene. *J. Natl. Cancer Inst.*, **47**, 1267–1275 (1971).

36. Sugiyama, T. Role of erythropoietin in 7,12-dimethylbenz(a)anthracene induction of acute chromosome aberration and leukemia in the rat. *Proc. Natl. Acad. Sci. U.S.*, **68**, 2761–2764 (1971).

37. Sugiyama, T. Chromosomal aberrations and carcinogenesis by various benz(a)-anthracene derivatives. *Gann*, **64**, 637–639 (1973).

38. Takebe, H. The relationship between the repair defect and cancer in xeroderma pigmentosum. *Igaku-no-Ayumi* (*The Stride of Medicine*), **86**, 799–804 (1973) (in Japanese).

39. Taylor, J. H. Patterns and mechanisms of genetic recombination. *In* "Molecular Genetics. Part II," ed. by J. H. Taylor, Academic Press, New York/London (1967).

40. Weber, G. Hormonal control of metabolism in normal and cancer cells. *In* "Exploitable Molecular Mechanisms and Neoplasia," University of Texas M. D. Anderson Hospital and Tumor Institute of Houston, pp. 521–550 (1966).

41. Yosida, T. H. Relationship between chromosomal alteration and development of tumors *in vivo* and *in vitro*. *In* "Cancer Cells in Culture," ed. by H. Katsuta, University of Tokyo Press, Tokyo, pp. 171–194 (1968).

42. Yunis, J. J. and Yasmineh, W. G. Heterochromatin, satellite DNA, and cell function. *Science*, **174**, 1200–1209 (1971).

GANN Monograph on Cancer Research 17, 405–415 (1975)

LEUKEMIAS INDUCED BY 1-ALKYL-1-NITROSOUREAS IN DONRYU RATS[*1]

Shigeyoshi ODASHIMA,[*2] Toshiaki OGIU,[*2] Akihiko MAEKAWA,[*2]
and Masahiro NAKADATE[*3]

*Departments of Chemical Pathology[*2] and Synthetic Chemistry,[*3]
National Institute of Hygienic Sciences*

Leukemogenic activity of 1-ethyl-, 1-propyl-, and 1-butyl-1-nitrosoureas (ENU, PNU, and BNU) was studied in the female Donryu rat that received the chemical continuously in the drinking water. The incidence of leukemia was highest in ENU, lowest in PNU, and in-between in BNU. The average period until the leukemic rats were killed for autopsy was shortest in ENU, longest in PNU, and in-between in BNU. The major type of leukemias induced by ENU was erythroleukemia, that induced by BNU was myeloblastic leukemia, and that induced by PNU was myelocytic leukemia. There was thus a close relation of leukemogenic activity of chemicals, incidence of leukemia, average period until leukemic rats were killed for autopsy, and the types of leukemias induced.

Among various carcinogens, 7,12-dimethylbenz[a]anthracene (DMBA), its analogs, and 1-butyl-1-nitrosourea (BNU) have been employed as the most useful potent leukemogens in rats and mice. The former was first introduced by Huggins and Sugiyama (4), and induced stem cell leukemia associated with erythremia when it was injected intravenously, 1 to 5 times weekly, into the rat. Leukemogenic activity of the latter was first reported by Odashima (6, 7), and it induced myelogenous leukemias and erythroleukemia in Donryu rats when given continuously in the drinking water. Subsequently, the carcinogenic effects of BNU has been studied widely by several Japanese investigators (2, 3, 9, 10).

The present paper describes the results of comparative studies on leukemias induced by BNU, 1-ethyl- and 1-propyl-1-nitrosourea (ENU and PNU) in Donryu rats. Briefly, the leukemogenic activity was highest in ENU, followed by BNU and PNU. On the other hand, the type of leukemia induced by these 3 chemicals was different, as ENU induced erythroleukemia, BNU developed myeloblastic leukemia, and PNU produced myelocytic leukemia in the majority of cases.

[*1] This work was supported by Grant DRG-96At from the Damon Runyon Memorial Fund for Cancer Research, Inc., New York, U.S.A., Research Grant from the Princess Takamatsu Cancer Research Fund, Tokyo, and a Grant-in-Aid for Scientific Research from the Ministry of Education, Japan.
[*2],[*3] Kamiyoga 1-18-1, Setagaya-ku, Tokyo 158, Japan (小田嶋成和, 荻生俊昭, 前川昭彦, 中舘正弘).

Incidence of Leukemia and Other Tumors

1. Effect of ENU (Table I)

Female Donryu rats were randomly divided into 2 groups, consisting of 36 rats when they were 11 weeks old. Freshly prepared 400 or 100 ppm solution of ENU in distilled water was placed daily in a shielded glass bottle in each cage of Groups I and II, respectively. The ENU solution was given daily until the 7th week, and 5 days a week thereafter until the rat was killed for autopsy. The rat took the solution *ad libitum*.

In Goup I, 34 (97%) out of 35 rats that survived more than 10 weeks developed leukemia. Survival time of the leukemic rats was as short as 70–113 days (86±10 days). No extrahematopoietic tumors were detected in any of these 34 rats.

In Group II, 21 (58%) out of 36 rats died between the 16th and 25th experimental week. Leukemia developed in 18 (86%) of the 21 rats, and extrahematopoietic tumor was detected in the mammary gland of only one rat. The animal experiment of this group is still continuing.

TABLE I. Leukemia and Mammary Tumor Induced by ENU in Donryu Rats

Group	Conc. of ENU (ppm)	No. of rats with tumors (%)	Leukemia (%)	Mammary tumor (%)
I	400	34/35 (97)	34 (100)	0 (0)
II[a]	100	18/21 (86)	18 (100)	1 (6)
Total		52/56 (93)	52 (100)	1 (2)

[a] This animal experiment is still in progress.

2. Effect of PNU (Table II)

Female Donryu rats were randomly divided into 3 groups, consisting of 36 rats, when they were 11 weeks old. Similar to Experiment I, freshly prepared

TABLE II. Tumors in Various Organs and Leukemia Induced by PNU in Donryu Rats

Group	Conc. of PNU (ppm)	No. of rats with tumors (%)	Survival days (mean ±SD)	Leukemia (%)	Digestive tract (%)	Mammary glands (%)	Ear duct (%)	Thymus (%)	Others (%)
I	600	28/36 (78)	205±35	19 (68)	9 (32)	2 (7)	4 (14)	2 (7)	6[a] (21)
II	300	30/35 (86)	215±53	19 (63)	14 (47)	4 (13)	3 (10)	2 (7)	6[b] (20)
III	150	36/38 (95)	246±51	24 (67)	8 (22)	8 (22)	2 (6)	2 (6)	12[c] (33)
Total		94/109 (86)	224±54	62 (66)	31 (33)	14 (15)	9 (10)	6 (6)	24 (26)

SD: standard deviation. [a] Three in spleen, one each in liver, pancreas, and ovary. [b] Two in liver, one each in spleen, uterus, brain, and subcutis. [c] Two each in liver and kidney, one each in spleen, pancreas, uterus, brain, subcutis, adrenal gland, thyroid gland, and lung.

600, 300, and 150 ppm solution of PNU in distilled water was given 5 days a week continuously to Groups I, II, and III, respectively, until the rats were killed for autopsy.

There was no dose-effect relationship in the incidence of tumors in various organs among the 3 groups as shown in Table II. In these 3 groups, tumors were observed in 94 (86%) out of 108 rats. Among them, leukemia was found in the highest frequency, in 62 (66%) rats. Extrahematopoietic tumors were found mainly in the digestive tract, in 31 (33%) rats, followed by the mammary glands, ear duct, thymus, liver, and spleen. Incidence of tumors in other organs was very low as shown in Table II.

3. Effect of BNU (Table III)

Three groups of female Donryu rats, consisting of 32 rats, were given 15 ml/day/rat of 400, 200, and 100 ppm solution of BNU for 18, 24, and 46 weeks, respectively. Animals that died during the 19 experimental weeks were not included in the results because blood smears were not made during this period. However, most of these animals had hepatosplenomegaly.

As shown in Table III, leukemia developed in 42 (91%) out of 46 tumor rats. In general, the higher the concentration of BNU in the drinking water, the higher was the incidence of leukemia, and the rats that developed leukemia died early, and those that did not develop leukemia died of extrahematopoietic tumors in later stage of experimental period. The extrahematopoietic tumors were found in the esophagus, ear duct, mammary gland, and small intestine in 7, 6, 1, and 1 rat, respectively.

TABLE III. Tumors in Various Organs and Leukemia Induced by BNU in Donryu Rats

Group	Conc. of BNU (ppm)	No. of rats with tumor (%)	Leukemia (%)	Esophagus (%)	Ear duct (%)	Mammary gland (%)	Small intestine (%)
I	400	13/13 (100)	13 (100)	1 (8)	0 (0)	0 (0)	0 (0)
II	200	19/21 (90)	17 (90)	2 (10)	3 (16)	0 (0)	1 (5)
III	100	14/20 (70)	12 (86)	4 (28)	3 (21)	1 (7)	0 (0)
Total		46/54 (85)	42 (91)	7 (15)	6 (13)	1 (2)	1 (2)

Macroscopic Findings of Leukemic Rats

Anemia and diffuse enlargement of the liver, spleen, adrenal glands, and cisternal group of lymph nodes, due to the proliferation of leukemic cells, were commonly observed in leukemic rats (Photo 1). Bone marrow was usually anemic and slightly yellow. In the early stage of leukemic disease, tiny white spots were seen sporadically in the marrow of various bones. In some cases, the bone marrow and other organs with leukemic lesions were a characteristic greenish color resembling that in chloroma or chloroleukemia in human beings.

Classification of Leukemias

Leukemias were classified macroscopically into chloroleukemia and non-chloroleukemia. Animals with the former had greenish tumor nodules, hepatosplenomegaly, and anemia. Those with the latter had also hepatosplenomegaly and anemia, but tumor nodules were not greenish. These leukemias were classified cytologically into four types, myelocytic, myeloblastic, erythroblastic, and lymphoblastic leukemias, on the peripheral blood smears stained with the Wright-Giemsa solution.

1. Myelocytic leukemia

The cells were similar to normal promyelocytes. The cytoplasms contained azurophilic granules and stained blue to reddish purple. The nuclei were oval or kidney-shaped and the nuclear chromatin was somewhat coarser than that of a myeloblast. Nucleoli were still present (Photo 2). In a few cases, the cytoplasm was light blue to pinkish, and contained fine neutrophilic granules. In these cases, the nuclei were round, oval, or kidney-shaped, and the nuclear chromatin consisted of thick strands. There were a few nucleoli in the nucleus.

2. Myeloblastic leukemia

The cells were round and mononucleated. The cytoplasm stained moderately deep blue, often lighter in the perinuclear area, and exhibited no granules or a very few azurophilic granules. The nuclei were round or oval, and occupied about four-fifths of the cell body. The nuclear chromatin stained reddish purple, with fine strands and reticular formation. There were 2 to 4 nucleoli, generally sharply defined, with a well-marked chromatin border (Photo 3).

3. Erythroleukemia

The cells in the peripheral blood were quite similar to those in erythroblasts. The cytoplasm was usually found as a very narrow rim around the nuclei and stained deep blue to polychromatic hue. The size of these cells varied depending on the stage of maturation. The nucleus was generally round and the chromatin was thick and coarse. There were several darkly stained nucleoli in the tumor cells in immature stage (Photo 4). In some cases, a few tumor cells of myelocytic types coexisted in the peripheral blood.

4. Lymphoblastic leukemia

The tumor cells resembled lymphoblasts, and had no granules in the cytoplasm that stained blue at the periphery and lighter at the perinuclear area. The nucleus was round and large, and the nuclear chromatin was reticular. One or two nucleoli were found in the nucleus.

In addition to these four types, there was aleukemic leukemia in which leukemic lesions were found in organs, such as bone marrow, liver, spleen, or lymph nodes, although leukemic cells were not detected in the peripheral blood.

Incidence of Various Types of Leukemia in the Three Experiments

1. Leukemias induced by ENU

The 34 cases induced in the rat given 400 ppm ENU solution were erythroleukemia, and 18 leukemic rats induced by 100 ppm solution included 8 (44%) erythroleukemia, 5 (28%) myeloblastic leukemia, 2 (11%) myelocytic leukemia, 1 (6%) lymphoblastic leukemia, and 2 (11%) aleukemic leukemia.

2. Leukemias induced by PNU

There was no relation between the incidence of each type of leukemia and the dose of PNU given to the animals, as shown in Table IV. Among 62 leukemic rats, chloroleukemia and nonchloroleukemia were found in 23 (37%) and 39 (63%) rats, respectively. Cytologically, myelocytic, myeloblastic, erythro- and lymphoblastic leukemias were seen in 36 (58%), 14 (23%), 10 (16%), and 1 (2%) cases, respectively. In addition, there was one aleukemic leukemia in which leukemic invasion was seen in the liver and spleen.

TABLE IV. Cytological Types of Leukemia Induced by PNU in Donryu Rats

Group	Conc. of PNU (ppm)	No. of rats with leukemia (%)	Survival days (mean ±SD)	Myelo-cytic leukemia (%)	Myelo-blastic leukemia (%)	Erythro-leukemia (%)	Lympho-blastic leukemia (%)	Aleukemic leukemia (%)
I	600	19/36 (53)	190±34	11 (58)	4 (21)	3 (16)	0 (0)	1 (5)
II	300	19/45 (54)	207±50	11 (58)	4 (21)	3 (16)	1 (5)	0 (0)
III	150	24/38 (63)	232±48	14 (58)	6 (25)	4 (17)	0 (0)	0 (0)
Total		62/109 (57)	212±48	36 (58)	14 (23)	10 (16)	1 (2)	1 (2)

3. Leukemias induced by BNU

Among 42 leukemic rats, only one was myelocytic leukemia and the others were myeloblastic leukemia including a few cases of erythroleukemia.

Relation between Macroscopic and Microscopic Types of Leukemia

The relationship between the chloroleukemia, nonchloroleukemia, and various types of leukemia observed in Experiment II is given in Table V. Although myelocytic, myeloblastic, and erythroleukemias were found in equal

TABLE V. Chloroleukemias and Their Cell Types

Macro-scopic \ Micro-scopic	Myelo-cytic leukemia (%)	Myelo-blastic leukemia (%)	Erythro-leukemia (%)	Lympho-blastic leukemia (%)	Aleukemic leukemia (%)	Total
Chloroleukemia	21 (91)	2 (9)	0 (0)	0 (0)	0 (0)	23
Nonchloroleukemia	15 (38)	12 (31)	10 (26)	1 (3)	1 (3)	39
Total	36 (58)	14 (23)	10 (16)	1 (2)	1 (2)	62

frequency among 39 rats with nonchloroleukemia, myelocytic leukemia was found in as many as 21 (91%) among 23 rats with chloroleukemia.

Invasive Patterns of Leukemic Cells in the Liver

Invasive pattern of leukemic cells in the liver was microscopically divided into three types. The first type had a tendency to have invasive lesions in and around Glisson's capsule (Photo 5), and this was seen in the majority of myelocytic leukemia and in some of myeloblastic leukemia. In the second type, leukemic cells making small or large clusters of tumor cells invaded diffusely into sinusoids, and this was seen in the majority of cases with erythroleukemia (Photo 6). In the third type, although leukemic cells also invaded diffusely into sinusoids, they did not make clusters of aggregations with each other (Photo 7). A number of myeloblastic leukemia had widely and extensively distributed invasion of this type.

The weights of the body, liver, and spleen of leukemic rats in Experiment II are shown in Table VI. The liver weight was the heaviest in the rats with erythroleukemia, followed by myelocytic leukemia. On the other hand, the weight of the spleen was heavier in myelocytic leukemia and erythroleukemias than in myeloblastic leukemia.

TABLE VI. Average Survival Period and Average Weight of Body, Liver, and Spleen of Rats with Various Types of Leukemia

	Myelo-cytic leukemia	Myelo-blastic leukemia	Erythro-leukemia	Lympho-blastic leukemia	Aleukemic leukemia
No. of cases	36	14	10	1	1
Survival days	220 ±46[a]	208 ±49	197 ±47	137	187
Body weight (g)	172 ±28	182 ±28	173 ±17	139	96
Liver weight (g)	11.1± 3.1	10.4± 2.4	18.3± 7.5	12.4	3.8
Spleen weight (g)	2.7± 3.6	1.9± 1.3	2.2± 1.1	0.7	0.3

[a] Mean±SD.

DISCUSSION

It was clearly demonstrated through the present series of animal experiments that ENU, PNU, and BNU have a very potent leukemogenic activity on Donryu rats when given continuously in the drinking water. The incidence of leukemia was highest in ENU, lowest in PNU, and in-between in BNU. The average period until the leukemic rats were killed for autopsy was shortest in ENU, longest in PNU, and in-between in BNU. The major type of leukemias induced by ENU was erythroleukemia, that induced by BNU was myeloblastic leukemia, and that induced by PNU was myelocytic leukemia. There was thus a close relation in leukemogenic activity of chemicals, incidence of leukemia, average period until leukemic rats were killed for autopsy, and the types of leukemia induced.

It is generally accepted that 1-methyl-1-nitrosourea (MNU) does not produce leukemias in the rat. This was also confirmed in our experiment using the Donryu rat given MNU (8) or 3-acetyl-1-methyl-1-nitrosourea (5) continuously in the drinking water. On the other hand, our incomplete animal experiments, in which the Donryu rats were given 1-butyl-3-dimethyl-1-nitrosourea, 1,3-dibutyl-1-nitrosourea, or 1-amyl-1-nitrosourea continuously in the drinking water, have induced leukemias in some animals. Therefore, it is apparent that the number of carbons in the alkyl group in 1-position should be more than 2 for the induction of leukemias in the rat.

The results of our experiments as well as those of other Japanese investigators employing BNU showed that pulse doses of BNU, given intravenously, subcutaneously, or into the stomach by means of a stomach tube, resulted in a lower incidence of leukemias than continuous administration of BNU in the drinking water. Therefore, continuous action of BNU or its metabolites in very low concentration in the serum on bone marrow cells was most effective for their leukemogenic conversion. Similar effect was observed in ENU and continuous administration of this chemical in the drinking water caused the development of erythroleukemia in 100% in our experiment although Druckrey et al. (1) found leukemia in less than two-thirds of their animals that received pulse doses of ENU intravenously.

Lower doses of BNU resulted in extrahematopoietic tumors in some rats that did not have leukemia in the early part of the experimental period. PNU, which showed lower leukemogenic activity than ENU and BNU, induced extrahematopoietic tumors in many animals in the later part of the experimental period. Therefore, there seemed to be a minimum effective daily dose for development of leukemia in both BNU and PNU.

The authors consider ENU, PNU, and BNU as very useful leukemogens for studying experimental leukemia in the rat, especially in analyzing the target cell for various types of leukemia.

REFERENCES

1. Druckrey, H., Preussmann, R., Ivankovic, S., and Schmähle, D. Organotrope carcinogene Wirkungen bei 65 verschiedenen N-Nitroso-Verbeindungen an BD Ratten. *Z. Krebsforsch.*, **69**, 103–201 (1967).
2. Fukunishi, R., Terashi, S., and Kawaji, K. Tumors in rats by multiple oral administration of N-nitrosobutylurea. *Kagoshima Daigaku Igaku Zasshi* (*Med. J. Kagoshima Univ.*), **23**, 1039–1046 (1971).
3. Hosokawa, M., Gotohda, E., and Kobayashi, H. Leukemia and mammary tumor in the rats administered N-nitrosobutylurea. *Gann*, **62**, 557–559 (1971).
4. Huggins, C. B. and Sugiyama, T. Induction of leukemia in rat by pulse doses of 7, 12-dimethylbenz[a]anthracene. *Proc. Natl. Acad. Sci. U.S.*, **55**, 74–81 (1966).
5. Maekawa, A. Personal communication.
6. Odashima, S. Leukemogenesis of N-nitrosobutylurea in the rat. I. Effect of various concentrations in the drinking water to female Donryu rats. *Gann*, **61**, 245–253 (1970).

7. Odashima, S. Leukemogenic effects of N-butyl-N-nitrosourea in mice and rats. *GANN Monograph on Cancer Research*, **12**, 283–296 (1972).

8. Ogiu, T. Personal communication.

9. Takizawa, S. and Yamasaki, T. Role of ovarian hormones in mammary tumorigenesis by a continuous oral administration of N-nitrosobutylurea in Wistar/Furth rats. *Gann*, **62**, 485–493 (1971).

10. Yokoro, K., Imamura, N., Takizawa, S., Nishihara, H., and Nishihara, E. Leukemogenic and mammary tumorigenic effects of N-nitrosobutylurea in mice and rats. *Gann*, **61**, 287–289 (1970).

EXPLANATION OF PHOTOS

PHOTO 1.   Leukemic rat that was continuously administered 300 ppm PNU solution for 33 weeks. Diffuse swelling of the liver (10.35 g) and spleen (2.95 g) is seen. The leukemia was a myelocytic type and the white cell count was 242×10^3 at autopsy.

PHOTO 2.   Myelocytic leukemic cells in the peripheral blood of a rat that was continuously given 600 ppm PNU solution for 33 weeks. Abundant azurophilic granules were seen in the cytoplasms that stained blue to reddish purple.

PHOTO 3.   Myeloblastic leukemic cells in the peripheral blood of a rat that received continuously 300 ppm PNU solution for 24 weeks. The cytoplasms were stained moderately deep blue and exhibit none or a very few azurophilic granules.

PHOTO 4.   Erythroleukemic cells in the peripheral blood of a rat that was continuously given 150 ppm PNU solution for 24 weeks. The cytoplasms were seen as very narrow rims around the nuclei and stained deep blue to polychromatic hue.

PHOTO 5.   Leukemic lesions in the liver of a rat that received continuously 150 ppm PNU solution for 40 weeks. Leukemic cells invaded in and around Glisson's capsule. This pattern was seen in many cases of myelocytic and myeloblastic leukemia.

PHOTO 6.   Leukemic invasion in the liver of a rat that was continuously administered 150 ppm PNU solution for 42 weeks. Leukemic cells are growing making small or large clusters in sinusoids. This pattern was seen in half the cases of erythroleukemia.

PHOTO 7.   Leukemic infiltration in the liver of a rat that was continuously given 150 ppm PNU solution for 42 weeks. Leukemic cells distributed widely and extensively into acini of the liver. This pattern was seen in many cases of myeloblastic and erythroleukemia, and in a few cases of myelocytic leukemia.

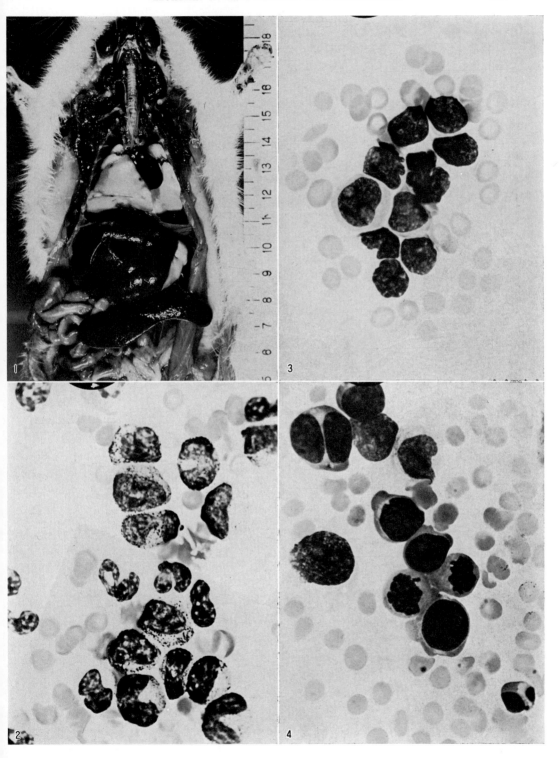

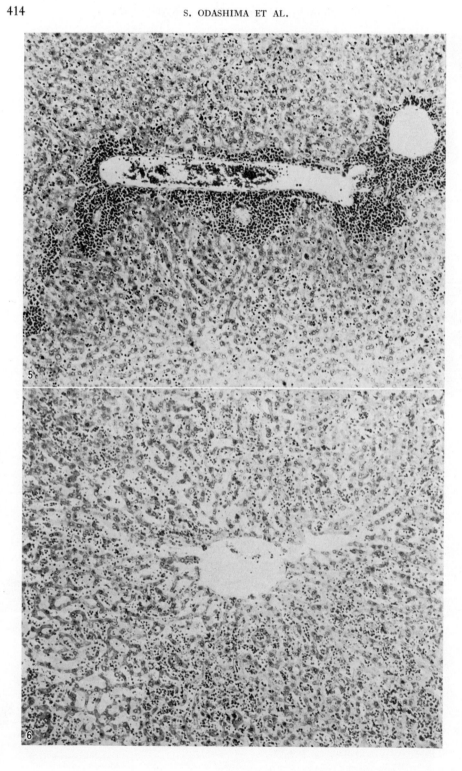

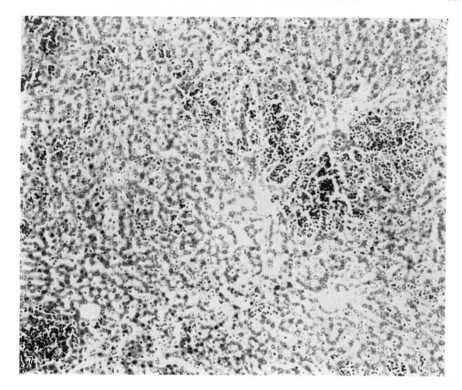

GANN Monograph on Cancer Research 17, 417–424 (1975)

A COMPARATIVE STUDY OF LEUKEMIA INDUCED BY N-NITROSOBUTYLUREA[*1] IN MICE AND RATS

Kenjiro Yokoro, Nobutaka Imamura, Yuzuru Kawamura, and Kenji Nagao

Department of Pathology, Research Institute for Nuclear Medicine and Biology, Hiroshima University[*2]

The continuous oral administration of N-nitrosobutylurea(NBU) resulted in a high yield of leukemia in both mice and rats. The type of leukemia induced in mice was invariably thymic lymphoma, the incidence of which was very high irrespective of the strain tested. In rats, on the other hand, a variety of leukemia types were encountered and the strain difference in the incidence and the type of leukemia was noted. Examinations for the possible role of leukemogenic virus as the etiological factor in NBU-induced leukemogenesis revealed that there may be active participation of the leukemogenic virus, probably of Gross type, as the causative agent in mice, but not in rats. However, the results of XC plaque assay for murine leukemia virus infectivity during the course of NBU- and N-nitrosoethylurea-induced leukemogenesis in mice did not necessarily support the principal role of the virus; there seemed no direct correlation between viral infectivity in various tissues and the target of leukemia. This may also imply the functional diversity of the morphologically indistinguishable type-C virus population.

Further studies are required to answer the question of whether there are truly different mechanisms for induction of leukemia in the two species of animals, or our present methods for viral detection are insufficiently sensitive to show that leukemia induction in the two species is basically alike.

The recent availability of such potent leukemogenic chemicals as certain aromatic polycyclic hydrocarbons and nitrosourea compounds enabled us to study the various aspects of the mechanism of leukemogenesis more in detail. The carcinogenic effect of N-nitrosobutylurea (NBU), one of the synthesized alkylnitrosourea compounds, was first demonstrated by Druckrey *et al.* in 1966 (*2*). They observed the development of sarcomas at the site of application in rats that received repeated subcutaneous injections of NBU dissolved in oil. Following this observation, the prominent leukemogenic effect of NBU in rats was first reported by Odashima in 1969 (*20*) and in mice by us in 1970 (*27*). Owing to its potent leukemogenicity and low toxicity, NBU became a popular tool for the study of leukemia in both rats and mice.

The present discussion is based mainly on recent experimental results ob-

---

[*1] Chemical Abstracts' nomenclature: N-butylnitrosourea (BNU).

[*2] Kasumi-cho 1-2-3, Hiroshima 734, Japan (横路謙次郎, 今村展隆, 河村　譲, 長尾健治).

tained in our laboratory. Our interest has been focused on the comparison of leukemogenic mechanisms in mice and rats elicited by NBU with special reference to the implication of a virus as an etiological agent in leukemia induction.

Induction of Leukemia in Mice by NBU

The prominent leukemogenic effect of NBU in mice was demonstrated by a high yield of thymic lymphomas with a short latent period in C57BL/Ka and ICR/JCL strains of mice following the continuous oral administration of NBU. The development of lymphomas was inhibited by the removal of the thymus prior to the administration of NBU, but the other type of leukemia with a longer latent period occurred in some of these thymectomized mice (29). These responses of mice to NBU bear striking similarity to those elicited by total body X irradiation (14), neonatal inoculation of the Gross virus (16), and are also similar to spontaneous lymphomas in AKR mice (18).

Search for the Implication of Leukemogenic Virus in NBU-induced Leukemia in Mice (9, 10, 28)

1. Cytotoxic effect of anti-Gross lymphoma serum on NBU-induced lymphoma cells

The etiological implication of the leukemogenic virus in radiation leukemogenesis in mice has been claimed by several investigators. Among them, it was reported by Kaplan that the radiation leukemia virus (RadLV), recovered from radiation-induced thymic lymphoma in C57BL/Ka mice, appears immunologically indistinguishable from the Gross virus which is considered to be the prototype of the murine leukemia virus (MuLV). Accordingly, the possible implication of the Gross virus in NBU leukemogenesis in C57BL/Ka mice was examined. Several cases of NBU-induced thymic lymphomas were incubated in vitro with antiserum against the Gross lymphoma-specific cell-surface antigen, and the cytotoxic index was estimated. It was revealed that many of NBU-induced lymphomas showed significantly higher cytotoxic indices as compared with those of normal thymocytes, some of which were almost comparable to those of the Gross virus-induced lymphomas. These results may indicate the etiological implication of a leukemogenic agent antigenically related to the Gross virus.

2. Cell-free transmission of NBU-induced mouse lymphomas

Cell-free transmissibility of NBU-induced mouse lymphomas was tested in both mice and rats. Several cell-free filtrates or supernatants were prepared from NBU-induced thymic lymphomas in C57BL/Ka mice, and were inoculated into syngeneic newborn mice or newborn Wistar/Furth(W/Fu) rats. One of the filtrates showed fairly high leukemogenicity, showing the development of either thymic or non-thymic lymphomas in 37% of inoculated mice with a mean latent period of 400 days. Another supernatant, derived from thymic lymphoma developed in a male C57BL/Ka mouse, showed remarkable leukemogenicity in a litter of W/Fu rats following the intrathymic inoculation within 24 hr after birth. Six of 7 inoculated rats developed either thymic lymphomas or reticulum cell neoplasm within 240 days. A potent leukemogenic virus was isolated from one of these cell-free transmitted thymic lymphomas by serial cell-free passage in newborn W/Fu rats, and the latent period of lymphoma development shortened to approximately 100 days with 100% incidence. In addition to the isolation of an agent eliciting thymic lymphomas in rats, another leukemogenic agent was recovered during the cell-free transmission experiment in rats. This agent is capable of inducing erythroblastic leukemia, resembling the Friend- or Rauscher-type lesion in both rats (W/Fu, ACI, and (W/Fu ×ACI)F$_1$) and mice (C57BL/Ka) with a short latent period. To the best of our knowledge, a leukemogenic agent capable of eliciting the Friend- or Rauscher-type lesion in rats has never been described.

3. Detection of cell-surface antigens of cell-free transmitted leukemias in rats by cytotoxicity test

The antigenicity of various types of cell-free transmitted rat leukemias was examined by cytotoxicity test with anti-Gross, anti-Rauscher, and anti-erythroblastic leukemia sera. Anti-Gross lymphoma serum showed a very high cytotoxic activity in every case of thymic lymphoma; the anti-Gross serum was also highly cytotoxic in cases of erythroblastic leukemia. A remarkable finding was that anti-erythroblastic leukemia serum reacted distinctly with erythroblastic leukemia cells even after the serum was absorbed with Gross virus-induced lymphoma cells. On the other hand, if anti-Rauscher serum was absorbed with Gross virus-induced lymphoma cells, it was no longer cytotoxic for erythroblastic leukemia cells. Cytotoxicity of anti-Gross lymphoma serum for reticulum cell neoplasm was less than that of thymic lymphoma but significantly higher than that of normal thymocytes. The effect of anti-erythroblastic leukemia serum on thymic lymphoma or reticulum cell neoplasm was not tested. From these findings, it is concluded that thymic lymphomas developing in cell-free passages carry at least the Gross lymphoma-specific cell-surface antigen, and erythroblastic leukemias carry both the erythroblastic leukemia virus-specific cell-surface antigen and the Gross antigen.

4. Virus neutralization test: cross-reactivity of the erythroblastic leukemia virus and the Gross virus

The immunological cross-reactivity of an agent, eliciting erythroblastic leukemia, with the Gross virus was demonstrated by the virus neutralization test. It was shown that leukemogenic activity of cell-free supernatant prepared from the erythroblastic leukemia tissue of ACI rats was completely lost after incubation *in vitro* with anti-Gross virus serum.

5. Electron-microscopic demonstration of virus particles

In order to visualize the erythroblastic leukemia agent, electron-microscopic observation was made of the leukemic tissues. As was expected, the presence of numerous mature type-C virus particles was invariably demonstrated in intercellular spaces of leukemic tissues of rats with cell-free transmitted erythro-blastic leukemia. The budding form of the virus was also observed on the surface of leukemia cells.

6. Quantitative assay for MuLV in leukemogenesis in mice induced by NBU and other nitrosourea compounds

A sensitive and quantitative method for detection of MuLV was recently devised by Rowe et al. (22). This method, XC plaque assay technique, is being applied in our laboratory to study the viral implication and pattern of organ distribution of the virus in chemical and radiation leukemogenesis in mice and rats in comparison with those in spontaneously developing leukemias or Gross virus-induced leukemia. The leukemogenicity of various nitrosourea compounds other than NBU, such as N-nitrosoethylurea (NEU), N-nitrosomethylurea (NMU), and N-nitrosopropylurea (NPU), was tested in the same manner as NBU in ICR/JCL mice. It was shown that these compounds possess a comparable or even stronger leukemogenicity than NBU(details will be reported elsewhere). The XC plaque assay was applied to leukemias induced by these compounds. Twenty-two out of 32 (68.7%) such leukemia cases showed a positive reaction for the presence of MuLV in varying titers.

In addition to the assay for established leukemia cases, the appearance and quantity of MuLV in various organs of NBU- or NEU-treated ICR/JCL mice are also being studied. The preliminary results revealed that MuLV activity could be detected from as early as the 12th day of continuous oral administration of chemicals in such tissues as uterus, spleen, and lymph nodes, but no activity was found in the thymus which is the primary target of the leukemia. The pattern of organ distribution of MuLV in these mice resembled that of spontaneously occurring lymphomas in AKR mice (23).

Induction of Leukemia in Rats by NBU, and Search for the Implication of Leukemogenic Virus

Following the pioneering work of Odashima (20) in inducing leukemia in Donryu rats by oral administration of NBU, we have reconfirmed his results using ACI and W/Fu rats (27). Approximately 90% of ACI rats of both sexes developed leukemia after a continuous oral administration of NBU. Majority of these cases were accompanied with prominent hepato-splenomegaly and the appearance of immature erythrogenic cells in the peripheral blood, and were cytologically diagnosed as erythroblastic leukemia. In W/Fu rats, however, a variety of leukemia types, including myeloid, erythroblastic, and undifferentiated cell types, were encountered, though the induction rate was lower and the latent period was longer than in ACI rats. Every type of leukemia, developing either in ACI or W/Fu rats, was invariably transplantable in the adult syngeneic recipients by inoculation of leukemic blood or cell suspension of leukemic tissue.

In an attempt to demonstrate the possible implication of leukemogenic virus in NBU-induced leukemogenesis in rats, the following studies were carried out but, in spite of our efforts, there has been no evidence supporting the viral implication in NBU-induced leukemogenesis in rats (9, 10, 28).

1) Virus particles were never demonstrated by electron-microscopic observations of leukemic tissues from primary or transplanted cases in ACI rats though the examined cases were limited only to erythroblastic leukemia.

2) In order to demonstrate the cell-free transmissibility, leukemic cell-free extracts were prepared from several cases of erythroblastic leukemia in ACI rats, and were inoculated into syngeneic newborn rats. No leukemia occurred in these recipients during an observation period of one year.

3) Anti-Gross lymphoma serum showed no detectable cytotoxic effect on the primary or transplanted leukemia cases in both ACI and W/Fu rats regardless of leukemic cell type.

4) Although the number of cases tested has been limited, none of the leukemia cases showed positive infectivity of MuLV by the XC plaque assay.

DISCUSSION

It is apparent from our present studies that NBU and related compounds are very useful tools in studying the mechanism of chemical leukemogenesis.

The isolation of the leukemogenic virus by Gross (4, 5) from spontaneous leukemia in AKR mice stimulated investigators to search for leukemogenic viruses from other sources and to consider whether there is a virus involved in the induction of leukemia in other mammals including man. This resulted in the isolation of a variety of new leukemogenic viruses from transplantable mouse tumors, in which these viruses existed as "the passenger virus" (21). Furthermore, the cell-free transmissibility of radiation-induced leukemias in mice was reported by several investigators, and they tended to take this as an evidence that radiation-induced leukemia in mice is viral in nature (6, 13, 17). Ito, in our laboratory, was also able to demonstrate the cell-free transmissibility of ^{90}Sr-induced leukemia in mice and speculated the etiological implication of a leukemogenic virus (12).

There have also been several reports dealing with the role of leukemogenic virus in chemical leukemogenesis in mice including our own studies presented here (7, 9–11, 26). All these observations led many of us to speculate that both physical and chemical agents may act merely as triggers for the activation of the latent leukemogenic virus preexisting in the host. On the other hand, it was assumed that natural transmission (vertical transmission) of leukemia in AKR mice is achieved by the exposure of germ cells to the leukemogenic virus during passage in the genital tracts of the parents (3). However, no concrete explanations either for the mechanism of "viral activation" or the origin of the virus has been given. The oncogene theory, proposed by Huebner and Todaro (8), is revolutionary and appears to be attractive in explaining the hitherto unsolved questions as to viral leukemogenesis apart from whether the theory is applicable to all vertebrates. But the experimental data for the foundation of the theory is based mainly on quantitation of the type-C virus *in vitro* and the appearance of virus-associated antigens; but the association of these data and leukemogenicity of the virus has not been critically evaluated. Recently, Aoki and Todaro (1) described the evidence that at least two closely related but nevertheless distinct type-C viruses are produced by cloned mouse embryo cells *in vitro*, suggesting the functional diversity of the morphologically similar viruses.

In our recent work, it was demonstrated in W/Fu rats inoculated with "rat-adapted Gross virus" at birth that the time of appearance and tissue distribution of the inoculated virus closely paralleled the clinical and pathological courses as revealed by the XC plaque assay. From these results we presume that "rat-adapted Gross virus" is composed mainly of the potent leukemogenic virus with little contamination of non-leukemogenic virus population. On the other hand, viral infectivity in tissues of mice during the course of NBU- or NEU-induced leukemogenesis was different from that in Gross virus-infected W/Fu rats, and showed no direct relation to the target tissue of leukemia; the distribution of viral activity was similar to that in AKR mice (*23*). These findings suggest that every type-C virus present in various tissues may not necessarily be involved in leukemogenesis. Here, we may need to reconsider the concept as to the leukemogenic mechanism in mice that the latent leukemogenic virus is activated by physical or chemical agent. This concept ignores the direct oncogenic potency of the agents interacting with cell components. Most known leukemogenic viruses in mice were isolated by chance under favorable conditions from various trans-plantable tumors, in which these viruses existed as a passenger virus without any causal relation to the tumor. It can be speculated in chemical or radiation leukemogenesis in mice that, here again, the propagation of the preexisting "leukemogenic passenger virus" in the host is favored by lowered immunological capability of the host and a large increment of target cell population after treatment, and finally by serial cell-free passage in immunologically inert newborn recipients. Thus, there is a possibility that the principal role of radiation or chemical agents as etiological factors in primary leukemogenesis has been relegated to a position of secondary importance by the fortuitous presence of the "thriving leukemogenic passenger virus" which has come to be regarded as the primary cause of leukemia in mice.

In recent years, there have been numerous reports dealing with the presence and production of type-C virus in the primary, transplanted, or *in vitro*-cultured tumor cells of rat origin (*15*). And some authors tend to assume that these type-C particles are the causative agents and the tumors are of viral origin. However, the biological activity of these particles present in rat tumors, and especially their oncogenicity, with one exception (*25*), have never been unequivocally demonstrated. Furthermore, a few reports have appeared describing the production of type-C particles in cultured cells which were derived from normal rat tissues (*19, 24*), suggesting the existence of indigenous viruses in rats with the morphology of type-C virus.

Finally, we see the intriguing difference between the two animal species, where virus seems to be effective in inducing leukemia in mice but not in rats. Is this difference qualitative or quantitative? Are there truly different mechanisms for inducing leukemia in the two animal species, or are our present methods for viral detection insufficiently sensitive to show that leukemia induction in the two species is really basically alike?

Acknowledgments

The authors express their thanks to Mr. T. Nishioka, Mr. K. Shitasue, Miss M. Sato, and Miss R. Ohkura for their excellent technical assistance. This work was supported by a Grant-in-Aid for Cancer Research from the Ministry of Education.

REFERENCES

1. Aoki, T. and Todaro, G. J. Antigenic properties of endogenous type-C viruses from spontaneously transformed clones of BALB/3T3. *Proc. Natl. Acad. Sci. U.S.*, **70**, 1598–1602 (1973).

2. Druckrey, H., Preussmann, R., Ivankovic, S., So, B. T., Schmidt, C. H., and Bucheler, J. Zur Erzeugung subcutaner Sarkome an Ratten. Carcinogene Wirkung von Hydrazodicarbonsäure-bismethylnitrosamid, N-Nitroso-N-*n*-butylharnstoff, N-Methyl-N-nitroso-N-nitrosoguanidin, und N-Nitroso-imidazolidon. *Z. Krebsforsch.*, **68**, 87–102 (1966).

3. Feldman, D. G. and Gross, L. Electron microscopic study of the distribution of the mouse leukemia virus (Gross) in genital organs of virus-injected C3Hf mice and Ak mice. *Cancer Res.*, **27**, 1513–1527 (1967).

4. Gross, L. "Spontaneous" leukemia developing in C3H mice following inoculation, in infancy, with Ak-leukemia extracts, or Ak-embryos. *Proc. Soc. Exp. Biol. Med.*, **76**, 27–32 (1951).

5. Gross, L. Development and serial cell-free passage of a highly potent strain of mouse leukemia virus. *Proc. Soc. Exp. Biol. Med.*, **94**, 767–771 (1957).

6. Gross, L. Serial cell-free passage of a radiation activated mouse leukemia agent. *Proc. Soc. Exp. Biol. Med.*, **100**, 102–105 (1959).

7. Haran-Ghera, N. A leukemogenic filtrable agent from chemically-induced lymphoid leukemia in C57BL mice. *Proc. Soc. Exp. Biol. Med.*, **124**, 697–699 (1967).

8. Huebner, R. J. and Todaro, G. J. Oncogenes of RNA tumor viruses as determinants of cancer. *Proc. Natl. Acad. Sci. U.S.*, **64**, 1087–1094 (1969).

9. Imamura, N. Evidence of viral implication in experimental leukemia induced by N-nitrosobutylurea in mice. *Gann*, **64**, 47–57 (1973).

10. Imamura, N. Murine erythroblastosis by a novel viral agent. *Gann*, **64**, 121–131 (1973).

11. Irino, S., Ota, Z., Sezaki, T., and Suzaki, K. Cell-free transmission of 20-methylcholanthrene-induced RF mouse leukemia and electron microscopic demonstration of virus particles in its leukemic tissue. *Gann*, **54**, 225–237 (1963).

12. Ito, T. Leukemogenic effect of radiostrontium(^{90}Sr) in mice: A comparative study of leukemogenicity of ^{90}Sr and X-rays. II. Transmissibility of the induced leukemias, alkaline phosphatase activity and cytogenetic changes of leukemic cells. *Nippon Ketsueki Gakkaishi* (*Acta Haematol. Japon.*), **33**, 432–448 (1970) (in Japanese).

13. Jenkins, V. K. and Upton, A. C. Cell-free transmission of radiogenic myeloid leukemia in the mouse. *Cancer Res.*, **23**, 1748–1755 (1963).

14. Kaplan, H. S. Influence of thymectomy, splenectomy and gonadectomy on incidence of radiation-induced lymphoid tumors in strain C57 black mice. *J. Natl. Cancer Inst.*, **11**, 83–90 (1950).

15. Kodama, T., Hosokawa, M., Gotohda, E., Sendo, F., and Kobayashi, H. Virus particles in rat leukemias induced by N-nitrosobutylurea. *Gann*, **63**, 261–263 (1972).

16. Levinthal, J. D., Buffett, R. F., and Furth, J. Prevention of viral lymphoid leukemia of mice by thymectomy. *Proc. Soc. Exp. Biol. Med.*, **100**, 610–614 (1959).
17. Lieberman, M. and Kaplan. H. S. Leukemogenic activity of filtrates from radiation-induced lymphoid tumors of mice. *Science*, **130**, 387–388 (1959).
18. McEndy, D. P., Boon, M. C., and Furth, J. On the role of thymus, spleen and gonads in the development of leukemia in a high-leukemia stock of mice. *Cancer Res.*, **4**, 377–383 (1944).
19. Oboshi, S., Miyamoto, K., Yanagihara, K., Seido, T., Yoshida, K., Inoue, J., Kuga, N., and Watanabe, S. Type-C virus in cultured cells derived from normal and tumor cells of a rat. *Gann*, **64**, 515–517 (1973).
20. Odashima, S. Development of leukemia in rats by oral administration of N-nitrosobutylurea in the drinking water. *Gann*, **60**, 237 (1969).
21. Rich, M. A. Virus-induced murine leukemia. *In* "Experimental Leukemia," ed. by M. A. Rich, North-Holland Publ. Co., Amsterdam, pp. 15–49 (1968).
22. Rowe, W. P., Pugh, W. E., and Hartley, J. W. Plaque assay techniques for murine leukemia viruses. *Virology*, **42**, 1136–1139 (1970).
23. Rowe, W. P. and Pincus, T. Quantitative studies of naturally occurring murine leukemia virus infection of AKR mice. *J. Exp. Med.*, **135**, 429–436 (1972).
24. Sarma, P. S., Dej Kunchorn, P., Vernon, M. L., Gilden, R. V., puꞓ Bergs, V. Wistar-Furth rat C type virus. Biologic and antigenic characterization. *Proc. Soc. Exp. Biol. Med.*, **142**, 461–465 (1973).
25. Svec, F. and Hlavay, E. Transmission of a filtrable agent from rat leukemia induced by X-ray irradiation and treatment with methylcholanthrene. *Acta Haematol.*, **26**, 252–260 (1960).
26. Toth, B. Development of malignant lymphomas by cell-free filtrates prepared from a chemically induced mouse lymphoma. *Proc. Soc. Exp. Biol. Med.*, **112**, 873–875 (1963).
27. Yokoro, K., Imamura, N., Takizawa, S., Nishihara, H., and Nishihara, E. Leukemogenic and mammary tumorigenic effects of N-nitrosobutylurea in mice and rats. *Gann*, 287–289 (1970).
28. Yokoro, K., Imamura, N., Kajihara, H., Nakano, M., and Takizawa, S. Association of virus in radiation and chemical leukemogenesis in rats and mice. *In* "Unifying Concepts of Leukemia," ed. by R. M. Dutcher and L. Chieco-Bianchi, S. Karger, Basel, pp. 603–616 (1973).
29. Yokoro, K., Takizawa, S., Kawamura, Y., Nakano, M., and Kawase, A. Multicarcinogenicity of N-nitrosobutylurea in mice and rats as demonstrated by host conditioning. *Gann*, **64**, 193–196 (1973).

GANN Monograph on Cancer Research 17, 425–438 (1975)

HISTOPATHOLOGY AND CELLULAR ORIGIN OF LEUKEMIAS INDUCED BY CHEMICAL CARCINOGENS IN THE MOUSE[*1]

Hayase Shisa, Yasuaki Nishizuka, Hiroshi Hiai,
and Yasue Matsudaira

*Laboratory of Experimental Pathology, Aichi Cancer
Center Research Institute*[*2]

Leukemias were induced in Swiss and C57BL mice, and in other inbred and hybrid mice by the administration of chemical carcinogens, 7,12-dimethylbenz[a]anthracene and N-butylnitrosourea, to neonates and adults. It was demonstrated that three types of leukemia, thymic lymphoblastic, θ-alloantigen-positive (T cell) leukemia, non-thymic, poorly differentiated lymphoblastic, θ-negative leukemia, and stem cell leukemia, can be distinguished by their histopathology. The frequency of each type may be correlated with host factors and in some instances with the method of leukemia induction. Histopathological observations on the thymus in preleukemic stages revealed that marked depletion of lymphocytes from the thymic cortex seems to be a pathognomonic and prerequisite change prior to the appearance of leukemia.

Studies with cell-surface markers of lymphocytes and of a chromosome marker in neoplastic cells appear to indicate the *in situ* occurrence of neoplastic cells in the depleted thymic cortex. However, no definite proof was obtained for the presence of bone marrow-derived cells (B cell) leukemia, in spite of the rather frequent appearance of a non-thymic type. It seems probable that B cells are sensitive to chemical leukemogens and form non-thymic leukemias. Stem cell leukemia may originate from more primitive cells in the bone marrow. The multiple origin of neoplastic cells in different hematopoietic tissues is also demonstrated by the chromosome analysis of leukemic cells.

Since the first report in 1959 by Pietra *et al.* (*14*) indicating that 7,12-dimethylbenz[a]anthracene (DMBA) is a very potent leukemogen, chemically induced leukemias in the mouse have been used as a tool for study of chemical carcinogenesis from various aspects. Recently, the strong leukemogenicity of N-butylnitrosourea (BNU) has been demonstrated (*11, 21*). The majority of mouse leukemias induced by chemical leukemogens show primary involvement of the

[*1] This work was supported in part by a Grant-in-Aid for Scientific Research from the Ministry of Education of Japan.
[*2] Kanokoden 81-1159, Tashiro-cho, Chikusa-ku, Nagoya 464, Japan (志佐　湍, 西塚泰章, 日合　弘, 松平康枝).

thymus, with or without subsequent dissemination to the spleen, lymph nodes, liver, and other organs (*14, 19*). It is also a distinct characteristic that leukemias affecting mostly the spleen and lymph nodes can be elicited in higher frequency when thymectomized mice or adult mice are exposed to the chemical (*10, 19*). This is in sharp contrast to Gross virus and X-ray induced leukemias which appear, as a rule, in only intact mice, and not in thymectomized mice (*cf.* Ref. *10*). In other words, chemically induced mouse leukemias may arise from both thymus and other lymphoid tissues and, therefore, are possibly separable into thymic and non-thymic types (*9, 19*). Both leukemias are essentially composed of lymphoblastic cells and should be distinguished from "lymphoma" of reticulum cell type according to Dunn's criteria (*3*). The mouse leukemias are different from chemically induced rat leukemias which are of myelogenous type in almost all strains and systems employed (*11, 20*).

This communication gives a survey of the histopathology of chemically induced mouse leukemias, with reference to preleukemic changes in thymic and other tissues, and of the cellular origins of thymic and non-thymic leukemias.

Histopathology and Target Cells in Chemical Leukemogenesis

The histogenesis of chemically induced leukemia has been studied mostly in Swiss mice that received, within 24 hr after birth, a single subcutaneous injection of DMBA in the form of a fat emulsion at a dose of 60 μg/mouse. Additional studies have also been made on Swiss mice with oral administration of BNU dissolved in the drinking water at a concentration of 0.04% for 60 days, starting at the age of 35 days. Swiss mice are very susceptible to chemical leukemogens and show a leukemia incidence of about 85% when given DMBA and of up to 100% when given BNU, with average latent periods of 107 days and 73 days, respectively (*9, 10*). Since more than 80–90% of the leukemias thus induced originate grossly from the thymus, a detailed chronological examination has been made on the thymic histology at intervals of 7 days after the exposure to leukemogens. For comparison, a similar histological analysis was carried out on both spontaneous AKR leukemias and X-ray induced C57BL leukemias.

1. Histogenesis of thymic leukemias in chemical leukemogen-treated Swiss mice

As seen in Fig. 1, a slightly retarded growth of the thymus is noticed before and at the 14th day, and a remarkable thymic atrophy is prominent in the 3rd and 4th week after neonatal exposure to DMBA. The thymic histology at these stages shows that small lymphocytes are virtually absent from the cortex of both lobes causing a great reduction in cortex volume, and that the medulla is not clearly distinguished from the cortex (Photo 1). Figure 1 suggests also that atrophic thymuses are repopulated by the 5–6th week. The cortex is narrow and shows an irregularity in its width because of admixture of persistent subcapsular immature cells and repopulating maturing and mature lymphocytes. It is worth noting that careful histological observation revealed the presence of small nests of atypical, probably neoplastic, cells in the depleted thymus cortex (Photo 2).

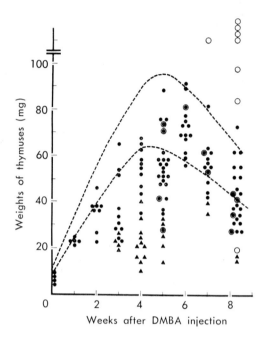

Fig. 1. Thymus weights and neoplastic changes at preleukemic stages in neonatally DMBA-treated Swiss mice
    Dotted lines indicate the average weights in female (upper) and male (lower) control Swiss mice. ▲ complete lymphocyte depletion; ● no leukemia; ◉ microscopic leukemia; ○ macroscopic leukemia.

In not a single case was proliferation of atypical cells confined to a focal cortical area adjacent to the medulla without any involvement of the subcapsular zone. In such a thymus the cortex was not replaced in its entire thickness. The nests later increase in number and size, fuse together, and invade other portions of the cortex and medulla, and the opposite lobe and surrounding tissues. Thus the overt thymic lymphoblastic leukemia develops, with or without spread dissemination (Photo 3).

The exact manner of neoplastic transformation within the thymus is as yet uncertain. It seems likely that thymic leukemic cells originate *in situ* in the thymus, but the possibility that these cells come from the bone marrow after neoplastic transformation cannot be ruled out (2).

A schema of age changes in the histology of carcinogen-exposed thymuses and the size distribution of thymic cells, estimated by the camera lucida method, are given in Fig. 2, which illustrates the initial depletion of small lymphocytes (B) and subsequent repopulation by small and median-sized cells (C) during the preleukemic stages. Larger cells form prominent cellular compartments in the leukemic stages (E). Microscopic leukemias are not infrequently found in small atrophic thymuses at the 6–9th week (Fig. 1). Therefore, there is no direct correlation between the size of thymuses and presence or absence of leukemic foci.

Figure 2 illustrates diagrammatically the histological sequences of development of thymic neoplasms in Swiss mice given DMBA as neonates (*13*). These

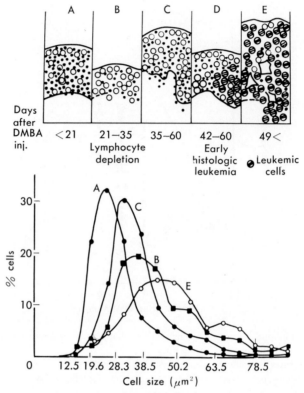

Fig. 2. Schematic illustration of histological changes in thymus and cell size distribution of thymus cells at preleukemic stages in neonatally DMBA-treated Swiss mice

sequences were essentially the same as those in adult mice given BNU (5) or methylnitrosourea (6). In the case of BNU leukemogenesis, in spite of the rapid decrease of thymic weight, no remarkable changes in thymocyte susceptibility to antiserum to the thymus-specific alloantigen θ was found until the 30th day, and a marked reduction and variation in susceptibility were noticed on the 45th day when nests of atypical cells were first found in the atrophic cortex. Similar changes with slightly different time courses have also been observed both in spontaneous viral leukemogenesis in AKR mice (1) and X-ray leukemogenesis in C57BL mice (17).

On the basis of the chronological observations on thymic histology in DMBA-treated Swiss mice, the time course of chemical leukemogenesis could be estimated as follows: the period to clinical leukemia or death from leukemia is 15–30 days from the stage of grossly detectable leukemia by autopsy, 30–45 days from leukemia detectable by histological examination, and 40–70 days from severe lymphocyte depletion in the thymus cortex.

Our previous karyologic study (8) on the hematopoietic tissues demonstrated that chromosome aberrations evoked 24 hr after a single injection of DMBA and urethan were much more abundant in the bone marrow than in the thymus and spleen. Corresponding to this, the most striking cellular damage observed as early as 24 hr after DMBA injection occurs in the bone marrow, not in the thymus. A marked cell depletion in the marrow accompanied by depression of cell maturation is found on the 3rd day. This persists until the 2nd week, at which time active myelopoiesis begins to return. Beginning with the 3rd–4th week there is no longer any appreciable difference in cellularity in the bone marrow between treated and untreated mice. In this system, foci definitely indicating the initial neoplastic change are seen in the bone marrow in only a few cases by the 7–9th week. When the cellular pathway from the bone marrow to the thymus is taken into consideration, the severe reduction of cellularity in the bone marrow prior to thymic aplasia seems to be of significance. This may mean that an insufficient supply of stem cells from the bone marrow is a major cause of the initial lymphocyte depletion in the thymus cortex preceding the occurrence of thymic neoplasms.

2. Leukemias developing outside the thymus in chemical leukemogen-treated Swiss mice

Of interest is the fact that in DMBA-treated Swiss mice, prior to the histological appearance of the initial leukemic nests in the thymic cortex, small foci composed of atypical cells were noted in hepatic sinusoids (Photo 4). These cell aggregates increased in number until the 5th week. Later, they gradually decreased in number and finally disappeared before the occurrence of overt thymic leukemias (Fig. 3). At the 6–7th week some foci were intermingled with phagocytes and neutrophiles. No positive evidence for malignancy of these cell clumps was obtained, because cell transplantation assay with the liver into neonatal and suckling mice was negative at the 5–6th week.

As seen in Table I, non-thymic leukemias can be elicited in young adult Swiss mice given intravenous injections of 6 pulse doses of DMBA, 1.0 mg each, at intervals of 7 days. These leukemias show a slight enlargement of the spleen and lymph nodes, and in a few instances the liver. Histologically, the bone marrow was completely occupied by diffuse proliferation of large, polygonal

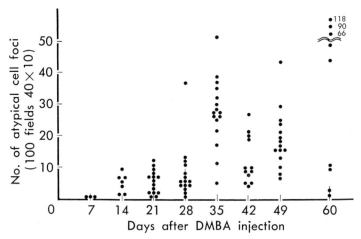

FIG. 3. Variation with age in number of atypical cell foci in hepatic sinusoids after neonatal injection of DMBA in Swiss mice

TABLE I. Leukemia Induction by DMBA in Swiss Mice

Treatments	Incidence of leukemia		Number of mice with		
	Leukemia/ total (%)	Latency (days)	Thymic leukemia	Non-thymic leukemia	Stem cell leukemia
s.c. single injection of DMBA (60 μg) at 3 days of age[a]	29/35 (82.9)	107	28	1	0
s.c. single injection of DMBA (1 mg) at 70 days of age[a]	23/28 (82.1)	102	6	17	0
s.c. single injection of DMBA (1 mg) at 3 days after delivery at 70 days of age in average[a]	21/24 (87.5)	134	15	6	0
i.v. 6 injections of DMBA (1 mg each) at intervals of 7 days from 35 days of age	10/17 (58.8)	89	1	0	9

s.c.: subcutaneous; i.v.: intravenous. [a] Data from Ref. 9.

TABLE II. Incidence and Type of Leukemias Induced by BNU in C57BL/6J Mice

Treatments	Incidence of leukemia		Number of mice with		
	Leukemia/ total (%)	Latency (days)	Thymic leukemia	Non-thymic leukemia	Stem cell leukemia
BNU[a]	30/33 (90.9)	129	26	3	1
Thymectomy[b]+BNU	29/45 (64.4)	172	0	29	0
Splenectomy[b]+BNU	11/13 (84.6)	124	9	1	1
Thymectomy+thymus grafting[c]+BNU	19/22 (86.3)	121	17[e]	2	0
Thymectomy+thymus cell injections[d]+BNU	14/28 (50.0)	197	0	14	0

[a] BNU was given from 37 days of age and continued for 60 days, to a total amount of about 45–60 mg. [b] Thymectomy and splenectomy were done at 32 days of age. [c] Subcutaneous grafting of one pair of whole lobes of 1-day-old isologous thymus was performed at 35 days of age. [d] Intraperitoneal injections of thymus cell suspensions, prepared from 1 to 3-day-old isologous thymus, were given, 7×10^5 cells each, at 35 and 42 days of age. [e] Including leukemias with enlargement of thymus grafts in subcutaneous tissues.

leukemic cells (Photo 5). The thymus was atrophic. Leukemic infiltrations in spleens and lymph nodes were less prominent. Leukemic foci in livers were rather focal and often confined to the neighborhood of blood vessels (Photo 6). The leukemias thus induced can be termed "stem cell leukemia" in the sense that they may originate from stem cells existing in the bone marrow.

The critical role of the thymus in viral and X-ray leukemogenesis is well established (cf. Ref. 9). In AKR mice, thymectomy at preleukemic stages prevents almost completely the development of leukemia. In contrast, thymectomized mice are susceptible to DMBA and develop leukemia (9, 10). This is also seen in BNU leukemogenesis (Table II). About two-thirds of the operated animals developed non-thymic leukemias. Splenectomy had no effect in this system. Histological patterns of the non-thymic type have been previously described (17). In brief, marked enlargement of the spleen and lymph nodes, most frequently the mesenteric nodes, is a conspicuous feature, and neoplastic infiltration into the bone marrow is rather localized and in patches. The leukemic cells are larger, compared with those of the thymic type, and classified as poorly differentiated lymphoblasts. Leukemic infiltration is most prominent in spleens and lymph nodes (Photo 7). In livers and kidneys, leukemic cells tend to aggregate and infiltrate in nodular fashion (Photo 8). The same leukemias could be found not infrequently in non-thymectomized mice, especially in adult mice. The frequency of this type decreased when DMBA was given shortly after the delivery (Table I).

Cellular Origin of Chemically Induced Leukemias

As described above, chemical leukemogens can induce three different types of leukemia; thymic lymphoblastic, non-thymic poorly differentiated lymphoblastic, and bone marrow stem cell types. Studies involving detection of cell markers indicating cellular origin are necessary to determine the precise target cells in chemical leukemogenesis. The techniques for recognition of cell surface markers of lymphocytes and of a chromosome marker for neoplastic cells have been applied for this purpose.

1. Cell surface markers of leukemic cells induced by BNU

It seems difficult to distinguish thymus-derived lymphocytes (T cells) from bone marrow-derived lymphocytes (B cells) by their morphology. However, they have different functional capacities in terms of immune reactions. Recently described cell markers can be used for the segregation of these two cell populations in the mouse. θ-Alloantigen has been shown to be closely associated with the differentiation of T cells (12). Bone marrow stem cells coming into the thymus acquire the θ-antigen and T cells bear it even after peripheralization. On the other hand, B cells can be identified by the presence of easily detectable surface immunoglobulin. Most B cells bear a receptor for antigen-antibody-complement complexes (EAC) not requiring Mg^{2+} (7). It has been suggested that these surface markers could be used for dividing carcinogen-induced mouse leukemias into two categories: T-cell and B-cell leukemias (4, 15, 16).

More than 120 leukemias induced by BNU in Swiss, C57BL/6J, (C3Hf/Bi

TABLE III. T-cell and B-cell Markers on Leukemic Cells Induced by BNU in Mice

Types of leukemia	Incidence of leukemias with markers (positive cases/total cases tested)	
	θ-Antigen[a]	EAC receptor[b]
Thymic leukemia	24/24[c]	0/35[c]
Non-thymic leukemia	0/11[d]	0/39[d]
Stem cell leukemia	0/4	0/9

[a] The method and a part of the data from Ref. 5. [b] EAC complex was prepared by the method of Lay and Nussenzweig (7). In brief, sheep red blood cells (SRBC) were sensitized by IgM-rich mouse anti-SRBC serum and mouse complement, and were suspended in Veronal-buffered saline containing EDTA at a final concentration of 0.01 M (pH 7.5). Positivity of a leukemia for EAC receptor was defined when more than 20% of the leukemic cells bound EAC complex. [c] Including thymectomized mice with thymus graft involvement and splenectomized mice. [d] Including thymectomized mice without thymus graft involvement.

$\times$CBA/H-T6T6)F$_1$, and (C57BL/6J $\times$CBA/H-T6T6)F$_1$ mice were checked for the presence or absence of θ-antigen and EAC receptor on their leukemic cell surface. As summarized in Table III, all the leukemias with thymus involvement bear the θ-antigen. It is of significance that leukemias developing in thymectomized mice with thymus grafts also had the θ-antigen only when involvement of the grafts by leukemic cells was apparent. However, when the grafts were free of leukemia, neoplastic cells did not carry the θ-antigen. All the non-thymic leukemias including 9 cases of stem cell leukemia developing in intact and thymectomized mice bore neither θ-antigen nor EAC receptor. Therefore, it still remains to be clarified whether neoplastic cells of non-thymic leukemia are members of a B-cell subpopulation which lacks the EAC receptor or are derived from immature B cell or T cell precursors before the development of the surface markers. It is likely that the stem cell leukemias are from more primitive cells residing in the bone marrow.

Table II shows also that injections of dissociated thymocytes prepared from 1 to 3-day-old thymuses into thymectomized mice do not restore the capacity for leukemia development. This is in sharp contrast to the effect of thymus grafting which constantly results in an apparent restoration of leukemogenesis. None of 6 leukemias developing in the thymectomized mice that received cell injections bore the θ-antigen.

2. Chromosome analysis for cellular origin of BNU-induced leukemias

Karyological analysis using the T6 chromosome as a cytological marker has been applied for the determination of cellular origin. Although the technique for revealing the T6 marker does not permit the exact identification of leukemic cells, it is likely that the majority of the metaphase plates come from leukemic cells, when the plates examined are prepared from mice not given an injection of colchicine before sacrifice.

Leukemic thymectomized (C3Hf/Bi $\times$CBA/H-T6T6)F$_1$ hybrid mice that received subcutaneous thymus grafts from the parental C3Hf/Bi mice were used. In this system, the cells of the hosts carry the T6 chromosome marker but not the cells of the donors. Thymectomy was done at 32 days of age, thymus grafting

TABLE IV.   Donor and Host Origin of Neoplastic Cells in Hematopoietic Tissues of BNU-induced Leukemias Developing in (C3Hf/Bi$\times$CBA-T6T6)F$_1$ Mice after Grafting with C3Hf/Bi Thymus

Group No.	Type of leukemia	No. of mice	Leukemic tissues			θ-Antigen[a]	
			Thymus	Spleen	Bone marrow	Thymus	Spleen
I	Thymic	6	Donor[b]	Donor	Donor	+	+
II	Thymic	3	Donor	Host	Host	+	NT[c]
III	Thymic	6	Host[b]	Host	Host	+	+
IV	Non-thymic	5	Host (lymph node)	Host	Host	NT	−

[a] The method for the θ-antigen was described in the previous publication (5).   [b] Leukemic cells of donor origin have no T6 chromosome, and those of host origin have T6 chromosome.
[c] NT: not tested.

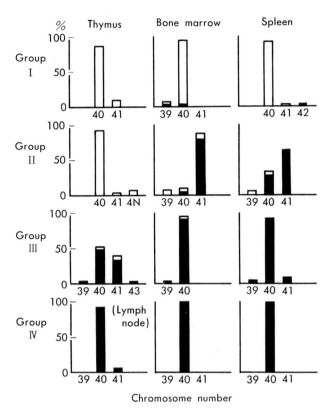

FIG. 4. Percentage distribution and chromosome number of leukemic cells in thymectomized (C3Hf/Bi × CBA/H-T6T6)F₁ mice grafted with neonatal C3Hf/Bi thymuses, followed by oral administration of BNU for 60 days

☐ cells of donor origin; ■ cells of host origin.

at 35 days, and BNU administration was started at 37 days and continued for 60 days. Chromosome analysis was routinely made on the grafted thymus, spleen, and bone marrow. More than 30 metaphase plates were examined in each organ.

Among 20 mice examined, 15 developed leukemias composed of θ-antigen-positive cells together with markedly enlarged thymic grafts (Table IV). Figure 4 shows the cellular origin and chromosome numbers in representative cases. It is clear that 6 of 20 thymic leukemias have neoplastic cells of donor origin in all the three organs tested (Group I), and the 6 others have cells of host origin (Group III). The former cells originate from the thymocytes existing in the grafted thymus when it was placed in the new host. The latter cells probably came from the bone marrow of the hosts and probably multiplied in the grafts. There exists apparently a tendency for leukemias with cells of donor origin to develop earlier and for those with cells of host origin to occur after longer latent periods. Three mice (Group II) had leukemic cells of donor origin in the thymus and cells of host origin in the spleen and bone marrow. This means that leukemic transformation may occur independently in different organs. Five mice (Group IV) developed non-thymic leukemias with neither θ-antigen-positive cells nor enlarged thymic grafts, the leukemic cells being of host origin.

3. Multiple origin of leukemic cells in BNU leukemogenesis

Since multiple cell origin from different organs was strongly suggested by the findings on the leukemias in Group II, a supplemental study on chromosome analysis was carried out on the thymus, lymph nodes, spleen, and bone marrow in a search for the presence of different neoplastic stem lines in these organs. Among 54 leukemic Swiss mice and other inbred mice that were given BNU as young adults, 13 cases showed clear evidence of multiple origin of leukemic cell lines. Some examples of such cases are listed in Table V, in which at least two stem lines with different modal numbers of chromosome are obvious in various leukemic tissues.

TABLE V. Percentage Distribution of Chromosome Numbers in Various Leukemic Tissues in Swiss Mice

Mouse No.[a]	Tissues examined	No. of metaphases analysed	Percentage of cells with chromosome number of							Total No. of hyperdiploids (%)
			39	40	41	42	43	44–45	4n	
136	Bone marrow	26		88	12					12
	Spleen	29		90	7	3				10
	Thymus	27		18	82					82
23	Bone marrow	69		14	23	17	7	18	17	80
	Spleen	79	1	10	14	39	23	9	2	88
	Thymus	41	12	88						0
35	Bone marrow	50	2	18	80					80
	Spleen	38		79	21					21
	Thymus	39		77	20	3				23
58	Bone marrow	23	13	83					4	4
	Spleen	74	27	32	8			1	32	41
	Lymph node	34	3	88	9					9
40	Bone marrow	26		96					4	4
	Spleen	24		96					4	4
	Lymph node	32		28	72					72

[a] Nos. 136, 23, and 35: thymic leukemia. Nos. 58 and 40: non-thymic leukemia.

COMMENTS

It is apparent that three different types of leukemias, thymic lymphoblastic, non-thymic poorly differentiated lymphoblastic, and stem cell leukemias, can be induced in the mouse by chemical leukemogens. The frequency of each type may be correlated in different degrees with host factors such as history of delivery (19) (Table I) and age of the animals when given the carcinogen (19), and with the presence or absence of the thymus (9, 18), and further may be modified by different methods and routes of carcinogen administration. It appears that the marked depletion of lymphocytes from the thymic cortex seems to be a pathognomonic and prerequisite change in preleukemic stages in all the leukemia-inducing systems with chemicals, X rays, and viral agents for the development of thymic leukemia.

There is no doubt that the most prevalent type is thymic leukemia bearing the θ antigen. Studies with chromosome markers suggest that the *in situ* occurrence of neoplastic cells in the depleted thymic cortex is a regular mechanism in the development of thymic leukemia. As described previously (*9*), it appears that the presence of the thymic framework is necessary for the occurrence of the θ-positive leukemia. There was no evidence that T cells circulating in the blood and lodging in the peripheral lymphoid tissues could be transformed into malignant cells. In addition, no definite proof for the presence of B-cell leukemias was obtained, in spite of the rather frequent appearance of non-thymic lymphoblastic leukemias in both thymectomized and intact adult mice. As for the cellular origin of this leukemia, a hypothesis that immature lymphocytes probably committed to T cells residing in the bone marrow and homing into the thymic framework are sensitive target cells and form the non-thymic leukemia unless the suitable thymus is present in the host animal (*cf*. Ref. *9*) must be investigated. Stem cell leukemia, which most probably originates in the bone marrow, appears frequently when the chemical is given in higher doses. The mutiple origin of neoplastic cells in different hematopoietic tissues is clearly demonstrated by the chromosome analysis.

REFERENCES

1. Arnesen, K. Preleukemic and early leukemic changes in the thymus of mice. *Acta Pathol. Microbiol. Scand.*, **43**, 350–364 (1958).
2. Ball, J. K. Role of bone marrow in induction of thymic lymphomas by neonatal injection of 7,12-dimethylbenz[a]anthracene. *J. Natl. Cancer Inst.*, **41**, 553–558 (1968).
3. Dunn, T. B. Normal and pathologic anatomy of the reticular tissue in laboratory mice, with a classification and discussion of neoplasms. *J. Natl. Cancer Inst.*, **14**, 1281–1433 (1954).
4. Haran-Ghera, H. and Peled, A. Thymus and bone marrow derived lymphatic leukaemia in mice. *Nature*, **241**, 396–398 (1973).
5. Hiai, H., Shisa, H., Matsudaira, Y., and Nishizuka, Y. Theta antigen in N-nitrosobutylurea leukemogenesis of the mouse. *Gann*, **64**, 197–201 (1973).
6. Joshi, V. V. and Frei, J. V. Gross and microscopic changes in the lymphoreticular system during genesis of malignant lymphoma induced by a single injection of methylnitrosourea in adult mice. *J. Natl. Cancer Inst.*, **44**, 379–394 (1970).
7. Lay, W. H. and Nussenzweig, V. Receptors for complements on leucocytes. *J. Exp. Med.*, **128**, 991–1009 (1968).
8. Kurita, Y., Shisa, H., Matsuyama, M., Nishizuka, Y., Tsuruta, R., and Yosida, T. H. Carcinogen-induced chromosome aberrations in hematopoietic cells of mice. *Gann*, **60**, 91–95 (1969).
9. Nishizuka, Y. and Shisa, H. Mechanism of leukemogenesis by 7,12-dimethylbenz-[a]anthracene, with special reference to host factors influencing its pathogenesis. *GANN Monograph on Cancer Research*, **12**, 297–307 (1972).
10. Nishizuka, Y. and Shisa, H. Leukemogenesis in thymectomized mice induced by N-butyl-N-nitrosourea. *In* "Topics in Chemical Carcinogenesis," ed. by W. Nakahara, S. Takayama, T. Sugimura, and S. Odashima, University of Tokyo Press, Tokyo, pp. 493–500 (1972).

11. Odashima, S. Leukemogenesis of N-nitrosobutylurea in the rat. I. Effect of various concentrations in the drinking water to female Donryu rats. *Gann*, **61**, 245–253 (1970).

12. Reif, A. E. and Allen, J. M. V. The AKR thymic antigen and its distribution in leukemias and nervous tissues. *J. Exp. Med.*, **120**, 413–433 (1964).

13. Rappaport, H. and Baronic, C. A study of the pathogenesis of malignant lymphoma induced in the Swiss mouse by 7,12-dimethylbenz[a]anthracene injected at birth. *Cancer Res.*, **22**, 1067–1074 (1962).

14. Pietra, G., Spencer, K., and Shubik, P. Response of newly born mice to a chemical carcinogen. *Nature*, **183**, 1689 (1959).

15. Shevach, E. M., Herberman, R., Lieberman, R., Frank, M. M., and Green, I. Receptors for immunoglobulin and complement on mouse leukemias and lymphomas. *J. Immunol.*, **108**, 325–328 (1972).

16. Shevach, E. M., Stobo, J. D., and Green, I. Immunoglobulin and θ-bearing murine leukemias and lymphomas. *J. Immunol.*, **108**, 1146–1151 (1972).

17. Siegler, W., Harrell, W., and Rich, M. R. Pathogenesis of radiation-induced thymic lymphomas in mice. *J. Natl. Cancer Inst.*, **37**, 105–121 (1966).

18. Shisa, H. Studies on the mechanism of 7,12-dimethylbenz[a]anthracene leukemogenesis in mice. II. The role of thymus in DMBA leukemogenesis. *Mie Med. J.*, **19**, 101–109 (1969).

19. Shisa, H. and Nishizuka, Y. Determining role of age and thymus in pathology of 7,12-dimethylbenz[a]anthracene-induced leukemia in mice. *Gann*, **62**, 407–412 (1971).

20. Sugiyama, T., Kurita, Y., and Nishizuka, Y. Biologic studies on 7,12-dimethylbenz[a]anthracene-induced rat leukemia with special reference to the specific chromosomal abnormalities. *Cancer Res.*, **29**, 1117–1124 (1969).

21. Yokoro, K., Imamura, S., Takizawa, S., Nishihara, H., and Nishihara, E. Leukemogenic and mammary tumorigenic effects of N-nitrosobutylurea in mice and rats. *Gann*, **61**, 287–289 (1970).

EXPLANATION OF PHOTOS

PHOTO 1. Thymus of a 35-day-old Swiss mouse given a single injection of DMBA at brith. Note narrow and irregular thymic cortex due to marked depletion of small lymphocytes. Hematoxylin-Eosin stain (H-E). ×156.

PHOTO 2. Localized nest of atypical immature lymphocytes in the thymic cortex of a 49-day-old Swiss mouse given a single injection of DMBA at birth. H-E. ×410.

PHOTO 3. Leukemic thymic lobe (lower) and not neoplastic lobe repopulated by lymphocytes (upper) of a 61-day-old Swiss mouse given a single injection of DMBA at birth. H-E. ×68.

PHOTO 4. Cell aggregates in the hepatic sinusoids found in a 35-day-old Swiss mouse given a single injection of DMBA at birth. H-E. ×530.

PHOTO 5. Stem cell leukemia; diffuse leukemic infiltration in the bone marrow of a Swiss mouse given i.v. injections of 6 pulse doses of DMBA at adult age. H-E. ×156.

PHOTO 6. Stem cell leukemia; leukemic infiltration in the liver of a Swiss mouse given i.v. injections of 6 pulse doses of DMBA at adult age. H-E. ×110.

PHOTO 7. Non-thymic leukemia; massive infiltration in the spleen of a thymectomized C57BL/6J mouse treated with BNU for 60 days at adult age. H-E. ×156.

PHOTO 8. Non-thymic leukemia; localized leukemic infiltration in the liver of a Swiss mouse given a single injectin of DMBA at adult age. H-E. ×110.

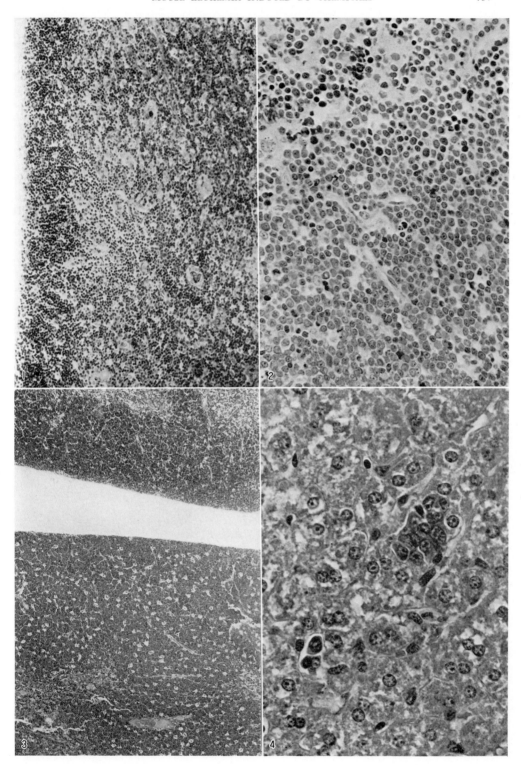

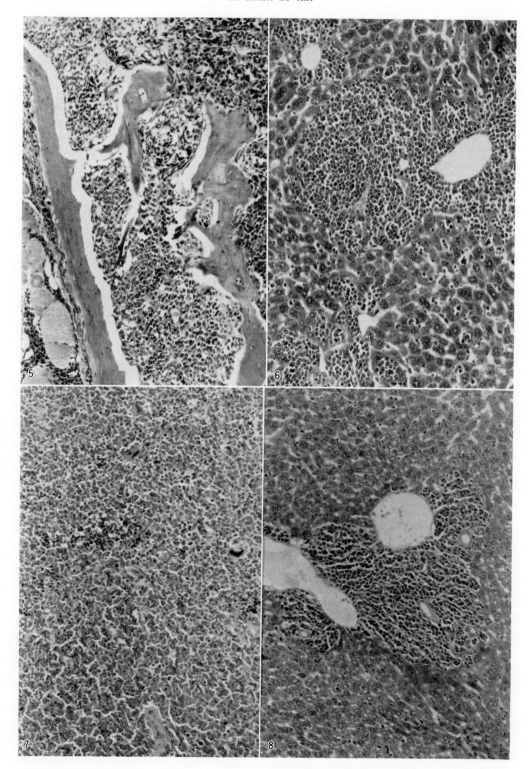

GANN Monograph on Cancer Research 17, 439–448 (1975)

THE EFFECT OF VARIOUS DOSES AND SCHEDULES OF ADMINISTRATION OF N-METHYL-N-NITROSO-UREA, WITH AND WITHOUT CROTON OIL PROMOTION, ON SKIN PAPILLOMA PRODUCTION IN BALB/c MICE

H. B. WAYNFORTH and P. N. MAGEE

*Courtauld Institute of Biochemistry, Middlesex Hospital Medical School**

Various doses of N-methyl-N-nitrosourea (MNU) were applied to the dorsal skin of male and a few female BALB/c mice using 4 administration schedules; (a) a single application, (b) single weekly applications for up to 18 weeks, (c) daily application for up to 5 days, (d) three times weekly application for up to 6 weeks. Some groups were also further treated twice weekly with croton oil. A single dose of MNU alone, even at toxic levels, produced papillomas in only a very few, questionably significant number of mice. A good tumouri-genic response was shown after repeated administration of MNU at a total dose of about 2 mg or more. MNU had a tumour-initiating effect when given as one or three doses of 400 μg but was a complete carcinogen when 5 or more applications were made. A good papil-logenic response was found for mice given a single application of 400 μg every 2 weeks for 18 weeks but this response was reduced when the interval between doses was extended to 4 weeks. Evidence from the present study related to possible repair of DNA damage by MNU is discussed.

N-Methyl-N-nitrosourea (MNU) is a potent carcinogen by various routes of administration and for several organs of a number of different animal species (*10*). Graffi *et al.* (*4, 5*) have shown it to be a potent complete carcinogen for the skin of mice, rats, and hamsters on repeated application. The present work was undertaken to study both the dose-related effect of MNU on the production of skin papillomas and its ability to act as an initiator of skin carcinogenesis, re-quiring subsequent promotion by croton oil for tumourigenesis.

Materials and Methods

Male BALB/c mice bred in this Institute were used, except for a few selected groups utilising female mice. There were generally 20 mice in each dosage group, ranging in age between 6 and 11 weeks. Animals were allocated five to a cage by pooling mice of all ages and then distributing them without conscious selec-

* London W1P 5PR, U.K.

tion. The backs of all mice were shaved prior to the start of treatment and every 1 to 2 weeks subsequently.

Because of the large number of mice required, animals were placed in the experiment in 2 batches approximately 5 months apart. A group of control male mice was associated with each batch and a separate group of female controls was also set up.

MNU was dissolved in acetone at room temperature and used immediately. The required dose was contained in 0.1 ml which was applied to the shaved dorsal surface with a Repette syringe (Jencons Ltd., Hemel Hempstead, Herts., U.K.). Croton oil was similarly prepared as a 0.5% solution and applied twice weekly in 0.1 ml using acetone from the same source as that used to dissolve the MNU. Croton oil treatment was always started in the week following the last MNU application.

The MNU treatment was divided into four administration schedules, with and without subsequent croton oil treatment, as follows.

Control groups: twice weekly applications of croton oil alone, as a 0.5% solution in acetone, for the 36-week duration of the experiment.

Group A: a single application of between 100 μg and 6 mg MNU per mouse.

Group B: single weekly applications of between 40 and 400 μg MNU for 6, 12, and/or 18 weeks. In two cases a single dose of 400 μg was given every 2 and 4 weeks, respectively, for a period of 18 weeks.

Group C: a quantity of 400 μg was given once daily for 3 to 5 days.

Group D: a quantity of 400 μg was applied 3 times weekly on alternate days for between 1 and 6 weeks.

Animals were generally examined weekly for the appearance of papillomas. Those dying during the experiment or killed at its termination were autopsied and the relevant histology obtained. However, because of cannibalism and/or tissue decomposition, the histopathological record of animals dying during the experiment was incomplete.

Statistical analysis

In some groups, animals died without producing papillomas, either from intercurrent disease, toxicity of MNU, or from some other indeterminate cause. In order to take this into account and to effect a more accurate interpretation of the results, the statistical methods described by Peto (*12*) for "non-incidental" tumours were applied, using sub-periods of 1 week. Significance between groups was determined by the χ^2 test. The probability of animals surviving the entire experimental period without producing a papilloma was calculated in a manner similar to that described by Pike and Roe (*13*). Unless otherwise stated, comparisons at the one-tail level of significance were made either between the MNU-treated and the control, croton oil-acetone treated groups or between each MNU-treated and MNU plus croton oil treated group. For significance, the probability level was taken as 0.05 or below.

Results

1. Group A and control groups—Table I

A single dose of 6 mg MNU proved to be toxic and killed about half the mice. A single dose between 400 μg in females or 2 mg in males and 6 mg induced papillomas in a few mice but the numbers were statistically not significant or only just significant. Croton oil alone did not induce papillomas but it significantly increased the number of papilloma-bearing male mice after treatment with 1 mg of MNU and above. It also markedly reduced the time to the first appearance of a papilloma. Doses of 400 μg and 1.0 mg of MNU in male mice had no tumourigenic effect when given alone but did have some activity when combined with subsequent croton oil treatment.

2. Group B—Table II

The non-tumourigenic dose of 400 μg of MNU (Table I) showed a cumulative effect and papillomas were induced after 6 weekly doses. The least probability of mice surviving tumour-free was seen with the longest treatment and animals receiving 4.8 and 7.2 mg total dose also showed an increased incidence of papillomas per mouse. In the highest dosage group, it was impossible to count papillomas accurately towards the end of the experiment because of severe encrustation of the skin. In contrast, no mouse given 100 or 40 μg MNU weekly for 18 weeks showed any papilloma formation but mice receiving 400 μg every 2 or 4 weeks still showed a positive cumulative response.

3. Group C—Table III

Three consecutive daily doses of 400 μg MNU had no tumourigenic effect when given alone but showed good activity when combined with croton oil treatment. There was little increase in tumour activity with 4 doses but 5 daily doses alone produced a marked tumourigenic response.

4. Group D—Table IV

The effect of three 400 μg doses seen in Group C mice was confirmed in this group, with an alternate-day schedule. Weekly application for between 2 and 5 weeks of MNU given three times per week, produced in three of these dosage groups a similar probability of the mice getting a papilloma (i.e., no dose-related increase in response at these dose levels). A marked increase in response was found for male mice treated for 6 weeks. The negligible response of the mice receiving 4 weeks of treatment is puzzling and no explanation could be found. Female mice showed a greater sensitivity to MNU treatment than did male mice and 85 and 100% of the animals were "at risk" (see Ref. 13) for the 5 and 6 weeks of treatment periods, respectively, compared to 35 and 78% for the male mice.

5. Histology

Although malignant skin tumours were found in some mice in all 4 treatment groups, they were rare in Group A where one mouse had a fibrosarcoma at the

TABLE I. Effect of Single Doses of MNU, with and without Subsequent Croton

Group No.	MNU treatment	Total dose (mg)	Croton oil (CO) treatment	No. of mice	Sex	Total No. of mice with papillomas
A 1	6 mg	6		35	M	2
A 2	6	6	CO	35	M	10
A 3	4	4		20	M	2
A 4	4	4	CO	20	M	9
A 5	2	2		20	M	3
A 6	2	2	CO	20	M	9
A 7	1	1		20	M	0
A 8	1	1	CO	20	M	5
A 9	1	1		40	F	2
A10	1	1	CO	40	F	4
A11	400 μg	0.4		30	M	0
A12	400	0.4	CO	30	M	5
A13	400	0.4		40	F	1
A14	400	0.4	CO	40	F	1
A15	100	0.1		20	M	0
A16	100	0.1	CO	20	M	0
A17	Croton oil (1)[c]			20	M	0
A18	Croton oil (2)			20	M	0
A19	Croton oil			20	F	0

NS: not significant.　[a] vs. control.　[b] vs. corresponding MNU group.　[c] Croton oil (1), (2):

TABLE II. Effect of MNU Application Once Weekly,

Group No.	MNU treatment (μg × No. of applications)	Total dose (mg)	No. of mice	Sex	Total No. of mice with papillomas
B1	400 μg × 1/wk/6 wk	2.4	20	M	7
B2	400 × 1/wk/12	4.8	20	M	18
B3	400 × 1/wk/18	7.2	20	M	16
B4	100 × 1/wk/18	1.8	20	M	0
B5	40 × 1/wk/18	0.4	20	M	0
B6	400 × 1/2 wk/18	3.6	20	M	5
B7	400 × 1/4 wk/18	2.0	20	M	3

[a] vs. control.　[b] vs. D5, Table IV.　[c] vs. C5, Table III.

Oil Treatment, and of Croton Oil Alone, on Skin Papilloma Production

No. of papillomas per papilloma-bearing mouse	Earliest appearance of a papilloma (weeks)	No. of mice dying without a papilloma	Probability of mice surviving 36 weeks without producing a papilloma (%)	χ^2	$P<$
1.3	22	17	89.4		NS[a]
2.3	6	22	39.2	11.99	0.001
1.5	13	5	88.7		NS[a]
1.2	6	2	54.5	6.94	0.01
1.0	16	3	84.2	3.16	0.05
1.1	6	0	56.9	5.24	0.05
—	—	0	100		
1.2	8	0	75.0	5.29	0.05
1.0	33	1	94.9		NS[a]
1.5	12	2	86.7	1.72	NS[b]
—	—	3	100		
1.0	15	1	83.0	4.96	0.05[b]
1.0	21	2	97.0		
1.0	6	1	97.2		NS[b]
		0	100		
		0	100		
		2	100		
		1	100		
		0	100		

two separate groups. See Materials and Methods (p. 439).

or Every 2 or 4 Weeks, on Skin Papilloma Production

No. of papillomas per papilloma-bearing mouse	Earliest appearance of a papilloma (weeks)	No. of mice dying without a papilloma	Probability of mice surviving 36 weeks without producing a papilloma (%)	χ^2	$P<$
1.0	23	0	65.0		
4.2	15	0	10.0	14.53	0.0001
4.6	18	4	6.2	2.98	0.05
—	—	3	100		
—	—	6	100		
1.6	23	8	58.3	1) 6.40[a] 2) 0.09[b]	0.01 NS
1.0	23	5	80.0	1) 2.55[a] 2) 7.21[c]	NS 0.005

TABLE III. Effect of Daily MNU Application, with and

Group No.	MNU treatment (μg$\times$No. of applications)	Total dose (mg)	Croton oil (CO) treatment	No. of mice	Sex	Total No. of mice with papillomas
C1	400 μg$\times$3	1.2		20	M	0
C2	400$\times$3	1.2	CO	20	M	6
C3	400$\times$4	1.6		20	M	1
C4	400$\times$4	1.6	CO	20	M	12
C5	400$\times$5	2.0		20	M	10
C6	400$\times$5	2.0	CO	20	M	16

TABLE IV. Effect of MNU Administered Three Times Weekly, with

Group No.	MNU treatment (μg$\times$No. of applications)	Total dose (mg)	Croton oil (CO) treatment	No. of mice	Sex	Total No. of mice with papillomas
D 1	400 μg$\times$3	1.2		20	M	0
D 2	400$\times$3	1.2	CO	20	M	10
D 3	400$\times$3/wk/2 wk	2.4		20	M	7
D 4	400$\times$3/wk/2	2.4	CO	20	M	11
D 5	400$\times$3/wk/3	3.6		20	M	8
D 6	400$\times$3/wk/3	3.6	CO	20	M	15
D 7	400$\times$3/wk/4	4.8		20	M	2
D 8	400$\times$3/wk/5	6.0		20	M	7
D 9	400$\times$3/wk/5	6.0		40	F	28
D10	400$\times$3/wk/6	7.2		20	M	14
D11	400$\times$3/wk/6	7.2		40	F	37

[a] vs. D8.　[b] vs. D8.　[c] vs. D9.　[d] vs. D10.

application site (6 mg MNU+croton oil treatment). An unusual finding was of 2 mice with squamous cell carcinoma of the stomach after treatment with 6 mg MNU alone. This could have arisen by self-licking of the deposits of MNU that occurred on the skin with this dose. In Group B, fibrosarcomas were found in mice treated for 6 to 18 weeks with 400 μg MNU. In addition squamous skin carcinoma formation was seen in the animals treated for 18 weeks, where a large number of the mice showed malignancy. In Group C, only mice treated with croton oil in addition to MNU produced a moderate number of sarcomas and carcinomas while the yield was relatively poor in Group D male mice. Many of the female mice of Group D however showed malignant changes in the dorsal skin.

without Croton Oil Treatment, on Skin Papilloma Production

No. of papillomas per papilloma-bearing mouse	Earliest appearance of a papilloma (weeks)	No. of mice dying without a papilloma	Probability of mice surviving 36 weeks without producing a papilloma (%)	χ^2	$P<$
—	—	1	100		
1.3	6	6	61.0	9.33	0.01
1.0	30	1	95.0		
1.6	6	1	40.9	15.81	0.0001
1.0	6	5	38.0		
2.2	6	0	20.0	4.42	0.05

and without Croton Oil Treatment, on Skin Papilloma Production

No. of papillomas per papilloma-bearing mouse	Earliest appearance of a papilloma (weeks)	No. of mice dying without a papilloma	Probability of mice surviving 36 weeks without producing a papilloma (%)	χ^2	$P<$
—	—	0	100		
1.5	6	2	46.3	14.21	0.001
1.4	6	3	64.2		
1.5	6	1	45.0	2.34	NS
1.5	6	0	60.0		
2.0	6	1	22.0	4.35	0.05
1.5	7	0	90.2		
1.7	7	1	65.0		
2.0	6	7	14.7	12.48[a]	0.0005
2.5	7	3	22.3	6.78[b]	0.01
2.8	6	3	0	1) 13.08[c]	0.0005
				2) 7.01[d]	0.005

DISCUSSION

The potency of MNU as a complete carcinogen for the mouse skin, on repeated application, has been described by Graffi and Hoffman (4) as being at least as great as that of the strongest carcinogenic polycyclic hydrocarbons. This conclusion is endorsed by the results of the present study with BALB/c mice using smaller doses of MNU given over a shorter period (Table IV). When given alone, however, as a single topical application, MNU was an extremely inefficient carcinogen. Even at toxic levels a non-significant number of the surviving mice showed papilloma formation. This is in marked contrast with the action of the polycyclic hydrocarbons where a single, relatively low dose can induce both benign and malignant tumours of the skin in a large percentage of the treated mice (6, 15). This disparity may be related to the different stabilities of these two types of chemical carcinogens. Whereas 9,10-dimethyl-1,2-benzanthracene, for example, remains in the skin for several days (3), MNU is relatively unstable with a half-life at neutral pH of 1.2 hr (2). However, MNU and several other N-nitroso compounds are powerfully carcinogenic in several organs of the rat (10) including the skin (8), after single doses when given orally or parenterally.

Although ineffective as a complete skin carcinogen, a single or a few doses of MNU readily induced changes in the skin which led to the appearance of papillomas after treatment with croton oil. Thus MNU can behave as a typical initiator of skin carcinogenesis.

The dose level below which no skin papillomas were produced was 1–1.2 mg given either as a single dose or as 3 divided doses. It is possible, however, that tumours might have appeared if the animals had been observed longer since Turusov et al. (16) have shown that papillomas arise in mice given very small doses of dimethylbenzanthracene when the observation period is sufficiently prolonged. Nevertheless, application of MNU by the different administration schedules in the present study provides an insight into the ability of skin to recover from changes induced by this carcinogen. A single dose of 400 μg MNU given to male mice did not induce papillomas and had a low degree of initiating activity within the 36-week experimental period. Such a short-lived dose, however, must have had some immediate effect on the epidermal cells since repeated daily applications for 5 days was sufficient to show good tumourigenesis indicating that there was an accumulation of this effect for each 400 μg dose. A good response was also obtained with an alternate-day schedule of administration for 2 or more weeks, suggesting that if any recovery from cellular insult had occurred within the 48 hr between doses, it was slight. Moreover, application of 400 μg once every 2 weeks for 18 weeks (Table II, B3) resulted in the same probability of mice getting papillomas as administration of the same total dose given as 3 weekly 400 μg doses for 3 weeks (Table IV, D5). It seems therefore that any recovery between each 2-week period was probably small and of little significance for the overall tumour yield. A 4-week interval between doses resulted in only a few mice showing papillomas and, when compared with the response to the same total dose given over 5 days (Table III, C5), suggests that considerable recovery had occurred after this interval.

The possibility that carcinogenesis results from interaction of the active form of a carcinogen (ultimate carcinogen) with a cellular receptor has been widely discussed (11). If cancer is a form of somatic mutation, DNA is the likely cellular target and MNU and other N-nitroso compounds have been shown to alkylate this macromolecule in vivo (7, 9, 14). Recently evidence has been reported that liver DNA in rats treated with several nitroso carcinogens undergoes single-strand breaks followed by the repair of these lesions which may take longer than 2 weeks (1). If skin tumours are induced by MNU as a result of an initial interaction with DNA, the evidence for recovery from certain doses of this carcinogen reported here may be a reflection of the capacity for repair of the DNA lesion.

Acknowledgments

It is a pleasure to acknowledge the assistance given by Mr. R. Parkin with the statistics, by Miss P. A. Smith with the preparation of the histological sections, and by Professor A. C. Thackray who undertook most of the histopathology. This work was supported with a grant from the Cancer Research Campaign of Great Britain.

REFERENCES

1. Damjanov, I., Cox, R., Sarma, D. S. R., and Farber, E. Patterns of damage and repair of liver DNA induced by carcinogenic methylating agents *in vivo. Cancer Res.*, **33**, 2122–2128 (1973).

2. Druckrey, H., Preussmann, R., Ivankovic, S., and Schmähl, D. Organotrope carcinogene Wirkungen bei 65 verschiedenen N-Nitroso-Verbindungen an BD-Ratten. *Z. Krebsforsch.*, **69**, 103–201 (1967).

3. Engelbreth-Holm, J. and Iversen, S. On the mechanism of experimental carcinogenesis. II. The effect of different concentrations of 9,10-dimethyl-1,2-benzanthracene on skin carcinogenesis in mice. *Acta Pathol. Microbiol. Scand.*, **29**, 77–83 (1951).

4. Graffi, A. and Hoffman, F. Starke kanzerogene Wirkung von Methylnitrosoharnstoff auf die Mäusehaut im Tropfungsversuch. *Acta Biol. Med. Germ.*, **16**, K1–3 (1966).

5. Graffi, A., Hoffman, F., and Schutt, M. N-Methyl-N-nitrosourea as a strong topical carcinogen when painted on skin of rodents. *Nature*, **214**, 611 (1967).

6. Iversen, O. H. and Iversen, U. A study of epidermal tumourigenesis in the hairless mouse with single and with repeated applications of 3-methylcholanthrene at different dosages. *Acta. Pathol. Microbiol. Scand.*, **62**, 305–314 (1964).

7. Lawley, P. D. The action of alkylating mutagens and carcinogens on nucleic acids: N-Methyl-N-nitroso compounds as methylating agents. *In* "Topics in Chemical Carcinogenesis," ed. by W. Nakahara, S. Takayama, T. Sugimura, and S. Odashima, University of Tokyo Press, Tokyo, pp. 237–256 (1972).

8. Leaver, D. D., Swann, P. F., and Magee, P. N. The induction of tumours in the rat by a single oral dose of N-Nitrosomethylurea. *Brit. J. Cancer*, **23**, 177–187 (1969).

9. Magee, P. N. and Farber, E. Toxic liver injury and carcinogenesis: Methylation of rat liver nucleic acids by dimethylnitrosamine *in vivo. Biochem. J.*, **83**, 114–124 (1962).

10. Magee, P. N. and Barnes, J. M. Carcinogenic nitroso compounds. *Adv. Cancer Res.*, **10**, 163–246 (1967).

11. Miller, J. A. Carcinogenesis by chemicals: An overview—G. H. A. Clowes Memorial Lecture. *Cancer Res.*, **30**, 559–576 (1970).

12. Peto, R. Guidelines on the analysis of tumour rates and death rates in experimental animals. *Brit. J. Cancer*, **29**, 101–105 (1974).

13. Pike, M. C. and Roe, F. J. C. An actuarial method of analysis of an experiment in two-stage carcinogenesis. *Brit. J. Cancer*, **17**, 605–610 (1963).

14. Swann, P. F. and Magee, P. N. Nitrosamine-induced carcinogenesis. The alkylation of N-7 of guanine of nucleic acids of the rat by diethylnitrosamine, N-ethyl-N-nitrosourea and ethyl methanesulphonate. *Biochem. J.*, **125**, 841–847 (1971).

15. Terracini, B., Shubik, P., and Della Porta, G. A study of skin carcinogenesis in the mouse with single applications of 9,10-dimethyl-1,2-benzanthracene at different dosages. *Cancer Res.*, **20**, 1538–1542 (1960).

16. Turusov, V., Day, N., Andrianov, L., and Jain, D. Influence of dose on skin tumors induced in mice by single application of 7,12-dimethylbenz[a]anthracene. *J. Natl. Cancer Inst.*, **47**, 105–111 (1971).

NAME INDEX

SUBJECT INDEX